Food and Lifestyle in Health and Disease

Food and Lifestyle in Health and Disease

Chuong PHAM-HUY, PhD
Bruno PHAM HUY

CRC Press
Taylor & Francis Group
Boca Raton London

CRC Press is an imprint of the
Taylor & Francis Group, an **informa** business

First edition published 2022
by CRC Press
6000 Broken Sound Parkway NW, Suite 300, Boca Raton, FL 33487–2742

and by CRC Press
4 Park Square, Milton Park, Abingdon, Oxon, OX14 4RN

CRC Press is an imprint of Taylor & Francis Group, LLC

Library of Congress Cataloging-in-Publication Data
Names: Pham-Huy, Chuong, author. | Pham Huy, Bruno, author.
Title: Food and lifestyle in health and disease / Chuong Pham-Huy, PhD, Bruno Pham Huy.
Description: First edition. | Boca Raton : CRC Press, 2022. | Includes bibliographical references. | Summary: "This
    book gathers information on various foods and provides an explanation of their nutrient composition,
    sources, and roles and mechanisms in health and diseases. As lifestyle plays important roles in health and
    longevity, this book describes healthy and unhealthy lifestyles regarding choice of diet, physical
    activity, and hobbies"— Provided by publisher.
Identifiers: LCCN 2021049798 (print) | LCCN 2021049799 (ebook) |
    ISBN 9781032112220 (hardback) | ISBN 9781032116303 (paperback) |
    ISBN 9781003220817 (ebook)
Subjects: LCSH: Nutrition—Popular works. | Diet—Popular works. |
    Diseases—Nutritional aspects.
Classification: LCC RA784 .P496 2022 (print) | LCC RA784 (ebook) |
    DDC 613—dc23/eng/20211123
    LC record available at https://lccn.loc.gov/2021049798
    LC ebook record available at https://lccn.loc.gov/2021049799

ISBN: 978-1-032-11222-0 (hbk)
ISBN: 978-1-032-11630-3 (pbk)
ISBN: 978-1-003-22081-7 (ebk)

DOI: 10.1201/9781003220817

Typeset in Times LT Std
by Apex CoVantage, LLC

Table of Contents

Biography

Dr. Chuong Pham-Huy, PhD of Pharmacy, University of Paris René Descartes, France, is an emeritus Associate Professor at the Laboratory of Toxicology, Faculty of Pharmacy, University René Descartes or Paris 5, France. He also worked as Pharmacist Consultant in Bichat Hospital and Necker Hospital, Paris, France.

He is a longtime member of several scientific societies including National Council of Public Health, France; National Information Committee of Drugs of Abuse, France; French Toxicology Society; and American Association for the Advancement of Science, USA.

Dr. Chuong Pham-Huy is Editor of the *Journal of Food, Agriculture and Environment* (section: Food) since 2004, and *International Journal of Biomedical Science* since 2005.

He was a referee for *Basic and Clinical Pharmacology and Toxicology, Journal of Chromatography, International Journal of Biomedical Science*, among others.

He was Director of many PhD theses of Pharmacy, University of Paris, and has published about 100 scientific publications.

Dr. Chuong Pham-Huy has obtained many scientific awards, including:

- Scientific Awards of National Academy of Pharmacy, Paris, France, 1991,
- Scientific Awards of University of Paris René Descartes, France, 1974 and 1980.

Mr. Bruno Pham Huy is an American Engineer currently working in Silicon Valley, California, United States.

He copyedited this work.

Preface

Francois de La Rochefoucauld (1613–1680), a French writer of moralistic maxims, said: 'To eat is a necessity, but to eat intelligently is an art'. The purpose of this maxim is to emphasize that eating for good health is not easy due to the complexity of food and lifestyle choices. Since the ancient times, food and lifestyle always played an important role in health and disease. Nowadays, thanks to the development of different attractive processed foods, the abundant choice of foods present in the market becomes more and more difficult. It is the same for the choice of different lifestyles due to the progress of new technologies.

The aim of the book *Food and Lifestyle in Health and Disease* is to describe different food types, the explanation of their nutrient composition, their sources, their roles and their mechanisms in health and diseases. As lifestyle plays important roles in health, disease, and longevity, this book explains different healthy and unhealthy lifestyles concerning the choice of diet, physical activity, hobbies. Some other factors such as the influence of environmental pollution, the synergistic effects of different foods, as well as the synergy of foods with physical activity or medicines, are also developed. Recently, the discovery of new proteins named sirtuins in the human body, as well as in all animal and vegetal tissues, is also reported because sirtuins and their activators or inhibitors may have important applications in the therapy of various dreadful diseases in the near future. To obtain good health and prevent disease, it is necessary to acquire more scientific knowledge linking the relationships between food, lifestyle, and health.

The book *Food and Lifestyle in Health and Disease* includes nine chapters.

Chapter 1, entitled 'Macronutrients', describes different macronutrients present in the human body as well as in animal and plant foods such as carbohydrates (starch, sugar, fibers), proteins (peptides, enzymes, antibodies), amino acids, lipids (fatty acids, triglycerides, sterols, phospholipids, etc.), and their roles in the human body.

Chapter 2, entitled 'Micronutrients', reports on different macro and microminerals, vitamins, antioxidants, coenzymes, cofactors in foods and their roles in the human body.

Chapter 3, named 'Free radicals and antioxidants in health and disease', explains different free radicals and antioxidants and their roles in health protection and disease development in humans.

Chapter 4, 'Food Types, Beverages, Dietary Supplements and Roles', reports on different food types such as wild foods, natural foods, organic foods, processed foods, genetically modified foods, different beverage types (soft drinks, energy drinks, fruit juices, alcohol, coffee, tea, soy milk, alkaline water), alkaline diet, functional foods, nutraceuticals and dietary supplements, nano-foods, and food cooking types, and develops their roles in health and disease.

Chapter 5, 'Plant source foods', describes plant classification, plant biology (cell wall, chlorophyll, pigments, flavors, primary and secondary metabolites), plant source foods (stable foods, vegetables, fruits, spices), algae, plant-based food products (vegetable oils, cocoa, chocolate), and some medicinal plants, and explains their roles in health and disease. This chapter also describes some medicines extracted from plants and their therapeutic uses in modern or traditional medicine.

Chapter 6, 'Animal source foods', studies animal biology, animal source foods from wild and farm animals, benefits and risks of animal source foods (red meat, white meat, processed meats), and of different animal byproducts (milk and dairy products, eggs, honey, fish oils, krill oils, etc.). This chapter also describes some medicines obtained from different animal organs and their uses in modern or traditional medicine.

Chapter 7, 'Fungi and water', reports on different fungal types such as mushrooms, yeasts and molds and also different types of water like tap water, bottled water, alkaline water, and water used in traditional medicine. Mushrooms are macro fungi, while yeasts and molds are micro fungi. Different species of edible mushrooms and poisonous mushrooms and their roles in health and disease are also developed. Yeasts are unicellular fungi and are used in food preparation and drug production. Molds are multicellular fungi in form of filament and are the cause of many diseases such as allergic asthma and mycoses. Molds are also the source of numerous interesting drugs such as penicillins, cephalosporins, cyclosporins, statins, griseofulvin, and so on. Molds are currently used in food processing and fermentation.

Chapter 8, 'Lifestyle and diets', describes a healthy lifestyle, an unhealthy lifestyle and different famous diets around the world. A healthy lifestyle is the choice of different healthy foods, healthy physical activities and healthy hobbies. Unhealthy lifestyles entail harmful effects such as those of cigarette smoking, drug addiction, alcohol abuse, the different unhealthy foods, the overuse of dietary supplements and over-the-counter medications, the misuse of different household products, and the influence of environmental pollution. This chapter also describes some famous diets like the Mediterranean diet, the Okinawan diet, and the Dietary Approaches to Stop Hypertension (DASH) diet. It cites some factors influencing life expectancy and compares the lifespan of certain populations around the world.

Chapter 9, 'Food interactions, Sirtuins, Genes, Homeostasis, and General Discussion', reports different modes of food interactions, including preliminary studies of some nutrients and physical activity on Covid-19 infection, and the effects of probiotics and prebiotics in gut health. This chapter also relates the functions of different sirtuins, a new class of enzymes recently discovered, in human health, and further develops the roles of genes, p53, homeostasis in the human body. It discusses some main features of this book and gives a brief conclusion for the roles of food and lifestyle in health and disease.

This book, with many recent publications on food and lifestyle, is an interesting document for everybody, in particular, healthcare professionals, students, teachers and researchers. It is also a source for research topics related to health and disease.

Disclaimer

The book *Food and Lifestyle in Health and Disease* is not intended as nutritional or medical advice for any individual problems. It is written solely for informational and educational purposes. Please consult a healthcare professional for any question concerning your health. The authors and publisher of this book are not responsible for any adverse effects or consequences resulting from the use of any of the suggestions cited in this book. The authors do not advocate the use of any particular diet, lifestyle or health program, but report information available in the scientific literature. Any information cited in this book cannot be used in place of a consultation with a competent physician, pharmacist, or nutritionist.

Abbreviation List

A: AA (amino acid); AA (arachidonic acid); ACTH (adrenocorticotropic hormone); ACE (angiotensin-converting enzyme); ACP (Acid phosphatase); AD (Alzheimer's disease); AD (anno Domini); ADH (alcohol dehydrogenase); ADME (absorption, distribution, metabolism, excretion); ADP (adenosine diphosphate); AF (aflatoxin); AGP (arabinogalactanprotein); AHA (American Heart Association); AI (average intake); AIDS (Acquired Immuno-Deficiency Syndrome); ALA (alpha-linolenic acid); ALD (Aldolase); ALDH2 (aldehyde dehydrogenase 2); ALP (alkaline phosphatase); ALT (alanine transaminase); AMD (age-related macular degeneration); AMP (adenosine monophosphate); AMPK (AMP-activated protein kinase); AP-1 (activator protein-1); ASL (argininosuccinate lyase); ASS (argininosuccinate synthase); AST (aspartate aminotransferase); AST (astaxanthin); ATP (adenosine triphosphate).

B: BCR (B-cell receptor); BNP (brain natriuretic peptide); BP (bioactive peptides); BPA (bisphenol-A); BW (body weight).

C: Ca (calcium); CAT (catalase); CHD (coronary heart disease); CK (creatine kinase); CPK (creatine phosphokinase); Cl$^-$ (chloride); Cl (chlorine); CO (carbon monoxide); CO_2 (carbon dioxide); CoA (coenzyme A); COPD (chronic obstructive pulmonary disease); Covid-19 (coronavirus disease 2019); COX (cyclooxygenase); Cr (chromium); CoQ (coenzyme Q); CoQ10 (coenzyme Q10); CsA (cyclosporin A); CTP (Cytidine-5′-Triphosphate); Cu (copper); CVD (cardiovascular disease); cytP450 (cytochrome P450).

D: DASH (Dietary Approaches to Stop Hypertension); DEHP (di-2-ethylhexyl-phthalate); DF (dietary fiber); DHA (docosahexaenoic acid); DHEA (Dehydroepiandrosterone); DHGLA (dihomo-gamma-linolenic); DNA (deoxyribonucleic acid); DMSO (dimethyl-sulfoxide); DRI (Dietary Reference Intake); DXM (dextromethorphan).

E: EA (ellagic acid); EC (epicatechin); ECG (epicatechin gallate); EGC (epigallocatechin); EGCG (epigallocatechin gallate); eNOS (endothelial nitric oxide synthase); EO (essential oil); EPA (eicosapentaenoic acid); ET (ellagitannin).

F: F (fluorine); F- (fluoride); Fab (antigen-binding fragment); FA (fatty acid); Fc (crystallizable fragment); FAD (Flavin Adenine Dinucleotide); FAO (Food and Agriculture Organization); FDA (Food and Drug Administration); Fe (iron); FMN (flavin mononucleotide).

G: GA (Gum Arabic); GABA (gamma aminobutyric acid); GI (gastrointestinal); GI (glycemic index); GLDH (Glutamate dehydrogenase); GLA (gamma-linolenic acid); GM (genetic modification); GMO (genetically modified organism); GPL (glycerophospholipid); GPx or GSHPx (glutathione peroxidase); GRx or GSHRx (glutathione reductase); GSH (glutathione); GSH (glutathione); GSL (glucosinolate); GTP (guanosine triphosphate).

H: HBV (Hepatitis B virus); HCl (hydrochloric acid); HCA (heterocyclic amine); HCN (hydrogen cyanide); HCO_3^- (bicarbonate or carbonate acid); HCV (Hepatitis C virus); HDL (High-Density Lipoprotein); HIV (human immunodeficiency viruses); H_2O_2 (hydrogen peroxide).

I: I (iodine); I- (iodide); IARC (International Agency for Research on Cancer); IDL (intermediate-density lipoprotein); IFN (Interferon); Ig (Immunoglobulin); IL (interleukin); IQ (intelligence quotient); IU (international unit).

K: K (potassium or kalium).

L: L-arg (L-arginine); LA (linoleic acid); LD (lethal dose); LDH (lactase dehydrogenase); LDL (Low-Density Lipoprotein); LOX (lipoxygenase); LSD (lysergic acid diethylamide).

M: MAOI (monoamine oxidase inhibitors); MDA (malondialdehyde); Mg (magnesium); Mn (manganese); MHC (major histocompatibility complex); Mo (molybdenum); MSM (methylsulfonylmethane); mtDNA (mitochondrial DNA).

N: Na (sodium or natrium); NaCl (salt or sodium chloride); NAD (nicotinamide adenine dinucleotide); NADP (nicotinamide adenine dinucleotide phosphate); NADPH (reduced form of Nicotinamide adenine dinucleotide phosphate); NF-kB (nuclear factor-kappa B); NH_3 (ammonia); NK (natural killer); NMN (nicotinamide mononucleotide); NO (nitric oxide); NO_2 (nitrogen dioxide); NOS (nitric oxide synthase); NREM (non-rapid eye movement); NSAID (non-steroidal anti-inflammatory drug); NSP (non-starch polysaccharide); NT-pro-BNP (N-terminal fragment pro- brain natriuretic peptide).

O: O_2 (oxygen); O_3 (ozone); oleic acid (OA); OAT (ornithine aminotransferase); OSA (obstructive sleep apnea); OTC (ornithine transcarbamylase); OTC (over-the-counter).

P: P (phosphor); P5C (pyrroline-5-carboxylate); p53 (protein having 53 kilodalton); PAH (polycyclic aromatic hydrocarbon); PCB (polychlorinated biphenyl); PCDD (polychlorinated dibenzo-p-dioxin); PCDF (polychlorinated dibenzofuran); PD (Parkinson's disease); PDCB (paradichlorobenzene); PG (prostaglandin); PHA (phytohaemagglutinin); PKC (protein kinase C); PL (phospholipid); PLP (pyridoxal phosphate); PMP (pyridoxamine phosphate); PO_4^{-3} (phosphate); PPAR (peroxisome proliferator-activated receptor); PS (Phytosterol); PSA (prostate specific antigen); PSK (polysaccharide Krestin); PSP (polysaccharopeptide); PTH (parathyroid hormone); PUFA (polyunsaturated fatty acid).

R: RAE (Retinol Activity Equivalent); RAR (retinoic acid receptor); RAS (renin – angiotensin system); RDA (Recommended Dietary Allowance); RDI (recommended daily intake); REM (rapid eye movement); RNA (ribonucleic acid); RNS (reactive nitrogen species); ROS (reactive oxygen species); RXR (retinoid X receptor); RYR (red yeast rice).

S: S (sulfur); SAA (sulfur amino acid); SARS-CoV-2 (Severe Acute Respiratory Syndrome Coronavirus-2); Se (selenium); SFA (saturated fatty acid); SGOT (serum glutamate-oxaloacetate aminotransferase); SGPT (serum glutamate-pyruvate aminotransferase); SIR2 (silent information regulator two); Sirt or SIRT (sirtuin); SO_2 (sulfur dioxide); SO_4^{2-} (sulfate); SOD (superoxide dismutase); SPM (specialized pro-resolving mediator); SSRI (serotonin selective reuptake inhibitor).

T: TAG (triacylglycerol); TCM (traditional Chinese medicine); T2D (type 2 diabetes); T2DM (type 2 diabetes mellitus); TFA (trans-fatty acid); *TCDD* (*2,3,7,8*-tetrachlorodibenzo-p-dioxin); TGF-β (transforming growth factor β); THC (tetrahydrocannabinol); THF (tetrahydrofolate); TG (triglyceride); TNFα (tumor necrosis factor α); TP53 (tumor protein 53); TPP (thiamine pyrophosphate); TXA (thromboxane A).

U: UA (uric acid); UA (urolithin A); UDP (uridine diphosphate); UHT (ultra-high temperature); UL (tolerable upper intake level); UNICEF (United Nations International Children's Emergency Fund); UTP (uridine-5´-triphosphate); USDA (United States Department of Agriculture); USP (United States Pharmacopoeia); UV (ultra-violet).

V: Vitamins: A (retinol); B1 (thiamine), B2 (riboflavin), B3 or PP (niacin), B5 (pantothenic acid), B6 (pyridoxine), B7 (biotin), B9 (folic acid), B12 (cobalamin); C (L-ascorbic acid); D2 (ergocalciferol); D3 (cholecalciferol); E (alpha-tocopherol); K1 (phylloquinone); K2 (menaquinone); VLDL (very low-density lipoprotein).

W: WHO (World Health Organization).

Z: Zn (zinc).

1 Macronutrients

1 INTRODUCTION

All foods contain nutrients with different composition and concentration. Nutrients are organic or mineral compounds required by the body to survive and grow. Nutrients must be obtained from diet, since the human body does not synthesize them (1–6). Nutrients are used to produce energy, to move, to respire, to grow, to reproduce, to excrete wastes, and so on. In other words, without the supply of nutrients from foods, the human body does not function normally, and this can lead to disease and even death.

2 CLASSIFICATION OF NUTRIENTS

There are six classes of nutrients required for the body to function and maintain overall health. These are carbohydrates (sugars), lipids (fats), proteins, water, vitamins, and minerals (1–6). They are called essential nutrients because the human body cannot create them and must consume them through foods. Their absence in the diet causes illness and even death to humans.

Nutrients are also divided into two main groups: macronutrients and micronutrients (1–6). Those that are needed in large amounts are called macronutrients. The others in little quantity are named micronutrients. Macronutrients are carbohydrates, proteins, lipids, and are used to produce energy for cellular activity (1–6). Water is also a macronutrient because the body requires a large amount of it, but unlike the other macronutrients it does not yield energy – calories. When necessary, or as a result of disease, proteins can be broken down to generate energy, but carbohydrates and fats are used preferentially for energy (1–6).

Micronutrients are nutrients required by the body in lesser amounts but are still essential for performing bodily functions. Micronutrients include all the essential micro-minerals and vitamins. There are 16 essential minerals and 13 vitamins required to build and maintain all body cells and tissues (1–6). Although classified among the micronutrients, minerals are also divided into two groups: macro-minerals and micro-minerals, depending on the quantity required by the body. A mineral needed in large amounts (i.e., greater than 200 mg per day) is called a macro-mineral, whereas a micro-mineral is required in a quantity lesser than 200 mg per day (2). In contrast to macronutrients, micronutrients are not directly used for making energy, but they help the enzymes in their activities and assist in the process as being part of enzymes. They are called coenzymes (1). These essential macro and micronutrients undergo different complex processes in the body, such as digestion and metabolism, then work together or separately in the body in order to release energy for cell and tissue rebuilding and to maintain the overall health of the individual. Besides, there are non-essential nutrients and semi-essential nutrients. Non-essential nutrients are nutrients that are formed by the human body itself. Their absence in the diet cannot cause problems for the human health, contrary to essential nutrients (1–6). Other nutrients are considered partially essential or semi-essential. Indeed, these nutrients can be furnished by the body, but in certain situation such as age and illness, their production in the body become insufficient; therefore, the supply of these nutrients from food or dietary supplement is necessary for the good functioning of the body. Vitamin D and coenzyme Q10 are some examples of semi-essential nutrients. Another example is amino acids, which are divided into 3 groups: essential, non-essential and conditionally essential or semi-essential nutrients.

Foods also contain other beneficial compounds such as antioxidants, phytochemicals, coenzymes, cofactors, and nucleotides. They are called bioactive compounds or non-nutrients. These

DOI: 10.1201/9781003220817-1

non-nutrients or bioactive compounds are not essential for life in ways that macro- or micronutrients are, but nonetheless have putative health benefits, whether acting directly or indirectly. Diets rich in these compounds significantly reduce our risk of chronic disease, including cancer and cardiovascular disease (2). A lack of non-nutrients or bioactive compounds cited above, or an excess of these, can cause disease.

Malnutrition can be caused by overnutrition (excess nutrient intake) or undernutrition (deficient nutrient intake) (5). It is a major tragedy that millions of people currently live with hunger, and fear starvation (6). In 2010, there were about 925 million undernourished people in the world due to poverty or lack of foods in the market (2). In addition, about 3.5–5 billion people are iron deficient, 2.2 billion iodine deficient, and 140–250 million vitamin A deficient (6). In contrast, overnutrition is observed in developed countries such as the USA (5). Overeating causes excess energy that can lead to overweight, obesity and other diseases.

Antinutrients are natural or synthetic compounds that interfere with the absorption of nutrients (2). For example, oxalates which are present in many plants, particularly star fruit and certain spinach, bind calcium, thereby inhibiting its absorption. Phytic acid in the hull of nuts, seeds, grains, has strong binding affinity for calcium, magnesium, iron, copper, and zinc, thereby reducing their digestive absorption (2).

3   MACRONUTRIENTS

Macronutrients are nutrients that the body needs in large amounts for the production of energy for body activity. There are three classes of macronutrients: carbohydrates (sugars), proteins and lipids (fats). They can be metabolically processed into cellular energy. Water is also an essential nutrient required in a large amount, but unlike the other macronutrients, it does not yield energy. The energy from macronutrients comes from their chemical bonds (1). This chemical energy is converted into cellular energy that is then utilized to perform work, allowing our bodies to conduct their basic functions such as movement, respiration, excretion, growth and reproduction (1). A unit of measurement of food energy is the calorie. Both carbohydrates and proteins provide 4 kcal/gram, and lipids provide 9 kcal/gram for humans (3).

Foods are also divided into two kinds: those rich in calories and those poor in calories. The energetic value of a food depends on the amounts of essential macronutrients (i.e., carbohydrates, proteins and fat) present in this food. For example, vegetables like lettuce, celery, and tomato provide few calories because they are poor in macronutrients, but rich in micronutrients like vitamins, antioxidants, minerals; in contrast, sugar, milk, butter, ice cream, tonic drinks, and so on, provide many calories, and are called energetic foods.

3.1   CARBOHYDRATES

Among the three main macronutrients rich in calories, carbohydrates are the most consumed in the world and also the most abundant in nature, in particular in plants. A carbohydrate is an organic molecule composed of carbon (C), hydrogen (H) and oxygen (O) to form the empirical formula: $C_n(H_2O)_n$, which means hydrate of carbon (1–10).

Carbohydrates are produced during the process of photosynthesis in plants. For example, glucose, a carbohydrate, is formed between carbon dioxide (CO_2) and water (H_2O), under the action of sunlight, inside the chloroplast, to produce glucose ($C_6H_{12}O_6$) and, oxygen (O_2) (7–10).

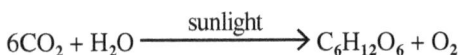

$$6CO_2 + H_2O \xrightarrow{\text{sunlight}} C_6H_{12}O_6 + O_2$$

Glucose (sugar) obtained from photosynthesis can be used immediately to provide energy for plant metabolism or growth, or converted to starch as stock for use later.

$$
\begin{array}{c}
\overset{\displaystyle H}{\diagdown}\overset{\displaystyle O}{\diagup} \\
\underset{|}{C} \\
H\text{-}C\text{-}OH \\
| \\
HO\text{-}C\text{-}H \\
| \\
H\text{-}C\text{-}OH \\
| \\
H\text{-}C\text{-}OH \\
| \\
CH_2OH
\end{array}
$$

D-Glucose

$$
\begin{array}{c}
\overset{\displaystyle H}{\diagdown}\overset{\displaystyle O}{\diagup} \\
\underset{|}{C} \\
H\text{-}C\text{-}OH \\
| \\
HO\text{-}C\text{-}H \\
| \\
HO\text{-}C\text{-}H \\
| \\
H\text{-}C\text{-}OH \\
| \\
CH_2OH
\end{array}
$$

D-Galactose

$$
\begin{array}{c}
CH_2OH \\
| \\
H\text{-}C\text{=}O \\
| \\
HO\text{-}C\text{-}H \\
| \\
H\text{-}C\text{-}OH \\
| \\
H\text{-}C\text{-}OH \\
| \\
CH_2OH
\end{array}
$$

D-Fructose

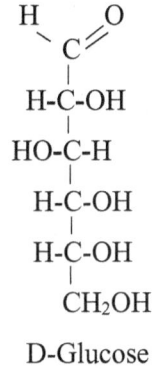

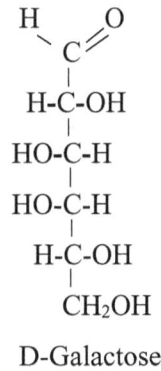

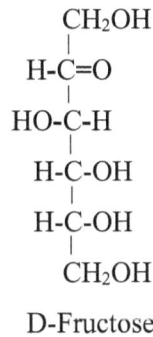

FIGURE 1.1 Chemical structures of 3 monosaccharides: D-Glucose, D-Galactose, and D-Fructose.

Carbohydrates are widely distributed both in animal and plant tissues, where they furnish energy to their host and also exert other functions depending on the type of carbohydrates. After metabolism by the digestive tract, carbohydrates are transformed into glucose, a basic compound for cell activity in our body and provide the major source of energy for people all over the world (5).

Carbohydrates are classified into four main groups: monosaccharides, disaccharides, oligosaccharides, and polysaccharides. The monosaccharides frequently present in food are glucose, fructose and galactose (Fig. 1). The principal disaccharides are sucrose, lactose and maltose (7–10). Both mono- and disaccharides are water-soluble and popularly called sugars. They are rapidly assimilated in the digestive tract and easily broken down with immediate release of energy. Oligosaccharides include α-glucans or malto-oligosaccharides, principally occurring from the hydrolysis of starch and non-α-glucan such as raffinose and stachyose, fructo- and galacto-oligosaccharides and other oligosaccharides (6–10). Polysaccharides may be divided into starch and non-starch polysaccharides (NSPs). NSPs are the major components of the plant cell wall such as cellulose, hemicellulose and pectin, but also include plant gum, mucilage and hydrocolloids (6–12). Dietary fibers consist of intrinsic plant cell wall polysaccharides. They are classified into two groups according to their water-solubility: insoluble dietary fibers like cellulose, hemicellulose, non-starch polysaccharide, and lignin; and soluble dietary fibers such as beta-glucan, pentosan, pectin, gum and mucilage. Some carbohydrates, like inulin, do not fit neatly into this scheme because they exist in nature in multiple molecular forms. Inulin from plants may have from 2 to 200 fructose units; as such, crossing the boundary between oligosaccharides and polysaccharides (8).

In nature, carbohydrate sources include cereal grains, tubers, cane and beet sugars, fruits, vegetables, milk, honey, and so on. From a nutrition point of view, carbohydrates in foods may be divided into three main groups: starch, sugars and dietary fibers.

3.1.1   Starch

Starch, the principal carbohydrate in most diets, consists only of a water insoluble polymer of glucose joined by α-glucosidic bonds and is designated α-glucosan or α-glucan (7, 9). In other words, digestible starch is made up of long chains of glucose and comprises two polymers of glucose: amylose and amylopectin (7–9). Most cereal starches contain about 15 to 30% amylose and 70 to 85% amylopectin by weight (9). Some starches, from maize, rice, and sorghum to barley, contain largely amylopectin and are known as 'waxy' (7). Starch occurs in the form of granules deposited in plant organs. It is relatively dense, insoluble in cold water, and ranges from 1 to 100 μm in size depending on the plant species (7, 9). Starch furnishes energy to the body after digestion into glucose. In the digestive tract, insoluble starch is broken down into soluble glucose by different enzymes (amylases, dextrinase, glucoamylase, maltase, etc.) present in the mouth saliva, small intestine and pancreas secretion. To facilitate this digestion, starch must be cooked before eating. Recent studies suggest that slowly digested starch and enzyme resistant starch have significant implications for human health (7, 9). Starch plays a major part in supplying the metabolic energy that enables the body to perform different functions. It is the basic source of energy for the majority of the world's population.

Among a number of natural foods containing starch, cereal grains like wheat, rice, corn, oats, barley, millet, and rye are the most consumed in the world, and some of them are used as staple food for population of certain areas in this planet. Wheat flour is used to prepare bread and other foods in Western and Middle Eastern countries, while rice is a staple food for more than half of the world's population, especially in Asia. Corn is consumed by people in South American and some African countries. Tubers rich in starch like potato, sweet potato, cassava and yam are also staple food for people in South America, Oceania and tropical areas. Some fruits and vegetables high in starch are banana, plantain, acorn squash, butternut squash, winter squash, water chestnuts and pumpkins. Besides some main starchy foods cited above, dry beans and peas are also vegetable grains rich in resistant starch as well as in fibers and proteins. However, beans and peas are still not considered staple food for people in this planet. The relatively low bean intakes of North Americans and Northern Europeans can be attributed to a negative culinary image as well as to intestinal discomfort attributable to the oligosaccharide content of beans (13).

The chemical composition of cereal grains is characterized by the high content of carbohydrates mainly in the form of starch deposited in the endosperm, amounting to 56–74%, and fiber, mainly located in the bran, to 2–13% (12). The second important group of cereal constituents is the proteins which fall within an average range of about 8–11%. With the exception of oats (~7%), cereal lipids belong to the minor constituents (2–4%) along with minerals (1–3%) (12). Vitamins of group

B are the most abundant, mainly in the bran. Some cereal grains like wheat, rice, corn, oats and some tubers like potato, sweet potato, cassava and yam and their biological effects are described in Chapter 5 of this book.

3.1.2 Sugars

Sugars are the popular name of two important water-soluble carbohydrates: mono- and disaccharides. Sugars are high in calories and present in certain vegetable and animal tissues. The three main monosaccharides are glucose, fructose, and galactose (7–10). Free glucose and fructose occur in small quantities in honey and dried fruit, and in larger amounts in fruits and berries where they are the main energy source (8). Glucose can be used directly by the cells to produce energy, while fructose must first be metabolized in the liver into glucose before absorption by the cells. Fructose needs time to furnish energy; therefore, it cannot replace glucose as a solution for intravenous administration in emergency medicine. Fructose is the sweetest of all the food carbohydrates (8).

Humans and animals can store glucose in excess obtained from the metabolism of starches or other mono- or disaccharides in the form of a very large molecule, glycogen (1, 6). Glycogen, a polymer of glucose, is used in animals and humans as an energy stock furnisher, similar to starch in plants. It is stocked in hepatic and muscular cells, ready to liberate glucose as the body needs energy for its functioning.

TABLE 1.1

Glycemic Index (GI) of Some Carbohydrates in Pure Form and in Natural or Prepared Foods

Food	Glycemic Index (GI)
Glucose	100
Fructose	15 ± 4
Sucrose	65 ± 4
Honey	61 ± 3
White sugar	65 ± 3
Whole wheat	74 ± 2
White wheat bread	75 ± 2
White rice, boiled	73 ± 4
Potato, boiled	78 ± 4
Sweet potato, boiled	63 ± 6
Sweet corn	52 ± 5
Potato, French fries	63 ± 5
Apple, raw	36 ± 2
Banana, raw	51 ± 3
Mango, raw	51 ± 5
Orange, raw	43 ± 3
Orange juice	50 ± 2
Peaches, canned	43 ± 5
Milk, skim	37 ± 4
Milk, full fat	39 ± 3
Soy milk	34 ± 4

Based on Reference 14: Atkinson F.S., Foster-Powell K., Brand-Miller J.C. International tables of glycemic index and glycemic load values: 2008. Diabetes Care, 2008; **31**(12): 2281–2283.

The glycemic index is a value attributed to food that measures the food's effect on the variation of blood glucose level. Values range from 1 (the slowest increase) to 100 (the fastest increase, equivalent to pure glucose) (1, 6, 14).

The food glycemic index allows a diabetic to choose a food corresponding to his/her disease state. As fructose has the lowest glycemic index among carbohydrates, and also the sweetest savor among sugars, it has been proposed to replace sugars by fructose for diabetics. Foods that have a low GI do not increase blood glucose levels quickly as foods that have a higher GI. A diet of low-GI foods has been shown in epidemiological and clinical trial studies to increase weight loss and reduce the risk of obesity, type 2 diabetes, and cardiovascular disease (1, 9).

Sugars are used as a sweetener to improve the palatability of many foods and beverages, and are also used for food preservation and in jams and jellies. Sugars confer functional characteristics to foods, like viscosity, texture, body and browning capacity. They increase dough yield in baked goods, influence starch and protein breakdown, and control moisture thus preventing drying out (8).

The polyols, such as sorbitol, are alcohols of glucose and other sugars. They are found naturally in some fruits and are made commercially by using aldose reductase to convert the aldehyde group of the glucose molecule into the alcohol. Sorbitol is used to replace sucrose in the diet of people with diabetes (8).

The principal disaccharides are sucrose, lactose and maltose. Sucrose is composed of one molecule each of glucose and fructose, while lactose is a combination of glucose and galactose. Sucrose is found widely in fruits, berries and vegetables, and can be extracted from sugar cane or beet sugar for human consumption. Lactose is the main sugar in milk. Maltose is the less abundant of disaccharides; formed by two glucose units, and derived from starch, it occurs in sprouted wheat and barley. Trehalose or mycose, a disaccharide also formed by two glucose units, is found in yeast, mushrooms, bread and honey (8).

Three main chemical physical properties of sugars are: polarity, chirality and reducing power. As sugars have many asymmetric carbon atoms in their chemical structure, they are called chiral compounds and can rotate plane-polarized light through a polarimeter. They may be classified as levorotary (l-isomer) or dextrorotary (d-isomer) depending on whether they rotate this light in a left (-) or right (+) -handed manner, respectively (1, 8, 15). For example, glucose also called dextrose is a dextrorotary, while fructose also named levulose is a levorotary. However, it is remembered that in chiral chemistry, almost all natural carbohydrates in plants and animals have the D-configuration, while all natural amino acids exist in L-form (15). It should be noted that the configurational descriptors D and L do not indicate the direction of rotation of the plane polarized light by soluble carbohydrates (8, 15). For example, D-glucose rotates the polarized light clockwise, it is expressed as D(+)-glucose, while D-fructose turns polarized light counter clockwise, it is designated as D(-)-fructose (4, 8, 15, 16). In plants and animals, all carbohydrates have only D-configuration, while all amino acids have L-configuration. All carbohydrates, proteins, enzymes, amino acids, nucleosides and a number of alkaloids and hormones are chiral compounds (15). The basic law of chemistry says that only the chiral subject may distinguish a chiral object. The human organism is chiral, thus it is not surprising that it can distinguish enantiomers (16). That may explain why many synthetic dietary supplements do not have the same beneficial effects as their corresponding natural compounds because they do not have the same chiral structure as the natural compound. Most synthetic dietary supplements are an equimolar mixture of two enantiomers called racemate, while their natural compounds contain only one enantiomer. The separation of two enantiomers in a racemate is difficult and its manufacturing cost is excessive. It should be noted that D and L configurations are only reserved for carbohydrates and amino acids, respectively. Other chiral compounds such as hormones, enzymes, vitamins, antioxidants, drugs, bio-chemicals, and so on, are designated as S- and R- enantiomers where S means sinister or left and R rectus or right. A racemate is an equimolar mixture of these two enantiomers and designated as R,S (4, 15).

All monosaccharides (glucose, fructose and galactose) are polyhydroxy aldehydes or ketones that confer them the reductive property; they are called reducing sugars. Disaccharides are classified as either reducing or non-reducing sugars, due to the presence or absence of free aldehyde or ketone group in their chemical structure (8). For example, sucrose and trehalose are non-reducing agents, while lactose and maltose are reducing sugars. Reducing sugars, reacting with amino acids present in food by the Maillard reaction during cooking foods at high temperature, can give acrylamide, a flavored and harmful compound (1, 8).

Some main natural sources of soluble carbohydrates are: sugar cane, sugar beet, honey, and milk. Some fruits and vegetables are also rich in glucose, fructose and sucrose. Different sources of carbohydrates are described in Chapters 5 and 6 of this book.

3.1.3 Dietary Fibers

Fibers or dietary fibers consist of intrinsic plant cell wall polysaccharides that are highly branched and cross-linked (7, 17–22). Traditionally, dietary fiber was defined as the edible parts of plant foods that are resistant to digestion and absorption in the human small intestine with complete or partial fermentation in the colon (17–22). The five basic attributes of a dietary fiber are: components of edible plant cell; carbohydrates; resistance to hydrolysis by human alimentary enzymes; resistance to absorption in the small intestine; and hydrolysis and fermentation (partial or total) by the bacteria in the large bowel (17). Dietary fiber consists primarily of carbohydrate polymers (non-starch polysaccharides) that are components of plant cell walls. Dietary fiber may be classified according to its water-solubility into two categories: insoluble fibers and soluble fibers (17–22). The first ones are partially fermented in the large intestine, while the water-soluble fibers are totally fermented in the human large bowel (19). In the market, fibers include both 'dietary fiber', the fiber naturally occurring in foods, and 'functional fibers', which are extracted from plants, then added to foods for human health benefits (17–19).

Dietary fiber is naturally present in cereals, vegetables, fruits, and nuts. The composition and amounts of fibers differ from food to food (7, 18, 19). Oats, fruit, vegetables, and pulses are rich sources of soluble fiber. Gums or hydrocolloids are also a rich source of soluble dietary fiber (17–21). Insoluble dietary fibers include cellulose, hemicellulose and lignin, while other polysaccharides of plant or algal origin, such as hydrocolloids, β-glucans, fucoidan, gum, mucilage, pectin and oligosaccharides (inulin, resistant starches), are soluble dietary fibers (17–21). Simplistically, fibers have been classified as soluble, such as viscous or fermentable fibers like pectin that are fermented in the colon, and insoluble fibers, such as wheat bran, that have bulking action but may only be fermented to a limited extent in the colon.

Dietary fibers are extensively studied in recent years because of their beneficial physiological effects such as lowering of blood cholesterol, improvements in large bowel function, attenuation of post-prandial blood glucose and insulin levels, and cancer prevention – especially colon cancer (17–23). Fiber intake has shown to exhibit chemoprotective effects on cancer proliferation and metastasis that may seem to be very promising (23). This activity of dietary fiber is known as prebiotic activity. Fiber supplementation in obese individuals significantly enhances weight loss. Increased fiber intake benefits a number of gastrointestinal disorders including the following: gastroesophageal reflux disease, duodenal ulcer, diverticulitis, constipation, and hemorrhoids. Prebiotic fibers appear to enhance immune function (20). Date fruit, prune, and pure fruit juice are often used to prevent and fight constipation (18). The recommended dietary fiber intakes for children and adults are 14 g/1000 kcal (20). Prebiotic and probiotic compounds are explained in Chapter 9 of this book.

3.1.3.1 Insoluble fibers

Cellulose, hemicellulose and lignin are insoluble fibers and mainly present in leaves, stems and leafstalks of plants (17). Resistant starch is also included in dietary fibers. All insoluble fibers are fibrous polysaccharides which are non-digestible because humans lack the digestive enzymes necessary to break them down to simple carbohydrates such as sugars like glucose. They form the non-starch polysaccharides (NSPs) (7, 17).

3.1.3.1.1   Cellulose   Cellulose is a non-digestible polysaccharide. Cellulose forms the fibrous component of plant cell walls and is present in fruits, vegetables and cereals (17–23). It is a linear and unbranched polysaccharide consisting of up to 10,000 glucose monomer units per molecule with β-1,4 glucosidic linkages (17, 19). The linear molecules are packed closely together as long fiber and are very insoluble and not digested by the human gastrointestinal enzymes (17, 19). Cellulose forms about one fourth of the dietary fiber in grains and fruit and one third in vegetables and nuts. Wheat bran is a rich source of cellulose or insoluble fiber (17). Being insoluble in water, it has an ability to bind water which helps in increasing fecal volume and thus promoting regular bowel movements. Although humans are not able to digest cellulose, its partial digestion occurs in the colon by beneficial microflora. About 50% of cellulose is degraded by natural fermentation in the colon, producing significant amount of short-chain fatty acids which feed our intestinal cells (17).Cellulose is present in fruits, vegetables, and cereals, and can be found in the cell walls of green algae and membranes of fungi (7, 11). The algal polysaccharides, which include agar, carrageenan, and alginate, are all non-starch polysaccharides (NSPs) extracted from seaweeds or algae (7). They have gel-forming properties. Carrageenan and agar are highly sulphated. Carrageenan is made available to react in combination with milk protein. It is used for making dairy products and chocolate (7). Cellulose is also obtained from agricultural byproducts such as rye, barley, wheat, oat straw, corn stalks, and sugarcane. It is also the major component of cotton bolls (100%), flax (80%), jute (60 to 70%), and wood (40 to 50%) (11).

3.1.3.1.2   Hemicellulose   Hemicellulose differs from cellulose in that it is smaller in size, and contains a mixture of hexose and pentose sugars, often in highly branched chains (7, 19). Hemicellulose contains mostly xylose and glucose, as well as some other sugars such as galactose, mannose, and arabinose. In contrast, cellulose is only constituted of glucose (7, 19). Hemicellulose is an insoluble dietary fiber as cellulose.

For humans, being insoluble in water, cellulose, and hemicellulose are able to bind water which helps to increase fecal volume and thus promote regular bowel movements and help food move faster in the digestive tract. Therefore, both cellulose and hemicellulose may prevent constipation and reduce the risk of diverticular disease development (17). Moreover, cellulose and hemicellulose fibers can bind toxins and cholesterol present in foods to lower the risks of colon cancer development and hypercholesterolemia, respectively (17–23). Some dietary sources of cellulose include green vegetable leaves, whole-grain foods, flax, avocados, prune, and cauliflower.

3.1.3.1.3   Lignin   Lignin, another form of water-insoluble fiber, contains many different chemical species, including ferulic acid, coumaric acid, vanillic acid, vanillin, syringaldehyde and furfural (23). Lignin is mainly present in plant cell walls of wood and bark, and rarely in vegetables and fruits. It has no nutritive value because it is not digestible in the digestive tract (19). Lignin may have beneficial properties to human health, such as their role as antioxidants and in cancer prevention (23). Cell walls containing lignin or suberin adsorb hydrophobic carcinogens particularly well; furthermore, the presence of lignin, and probably suberin, in the walls makes them resistant to degradation in the colon (23).

3.1.3.2   Soluble Fibers

Soluble fibers absorb water and are more easily accessible to bacterial enzymes in the large intestine, so they can be broken down to a greater extent than insoluble fibers. Main soluble dietary fibers are pectin, beta-glucan, fucoidan, inulin, gum and mucilage (20–23). Some examples of soluble fibers are found in peas, beans, oats, barley, rye, fruits, vegetables, mushrooms, algae, and so on. (20–23). Soluble and insoluble fibers are fermented by the luminal bacteria of the colon. In the long term, high-fiber diets reduce incidence of cancer, but the mechanisms involved are not well understood (23). Generally, prebiotic substance such as guar gum, gum acacia, tragacanth gum, fructo-oligosaccharides (FOS) and galacto-oligosaccharides (GOSs) act as food for the intestinal bacteria and thus help in their growth and activity, thereby supporting human health and colon cancer prevention (17, 23).

3.1.3.2.1 Pectins

Pectins are a complex group of polysaccharides composed mainly of chains of galacturonic acid interspersed with units of rhamnose and branched with chains of pentose and hexose units (17, 19). They are structural components of most plant cell walls as well as in the outer skin and rind of fruits and vegetables (17, 19). They also act as intercellular cementing substances and are almost completely metabolized by bacteria in colon. Pectins, highly water-soluble, form gels, and are hence used as gelling and thickening agents in various food products. Increasing pectin intake lowers serum cholesterol levels and blood pressure. Pectin lowers cholesterol by binding the cholesterol and bile acids in the gut and promoting their excretion (17, 19). High intake of pectin improves blood sugar levels and insulin sensitivity in non-diabetic and diabetic individuals (17–20). Due to their gelling behavior, these soluble polysaccharide fibers may decrease the rate of gastric emptying and influence small intestinal transit time (19). This explains their hypoglycemic properties. Pectins are mainly found in fruits and vegetables. For example, the rind of an orange contains 30% pectin, an apple peel 15%, and onion skin 12% (17). Commercial pectins are prepared mostly from some byproducts of the food industry, such as apple pulp, citrus peels, and sugar beet pulp.

3.1.3.2.2 Beta-Glucans

Beta-glucans are polysaccharides of D-glucose monomers linked through beta-glycosidic bonds. Beta-glucan is a viscous, fermentable, soluble dietary fiber (DF), and abundantly found in the cell walls of three main natural sources: cereals (mainly oat and barley), yeast and mushrooms (17, 24–26). They are also present in bacteria, algae, and to a lesser extent, in rye and wheat. Depending on these three main sources, the chemical structure, molecular weight and biological effect of beta-glucans also vary. Beta-glucans from different sources have different molecular weights and chemical structures, therefore, they have different biological activities (24). Beta-glucan from mushrooms and yeasts consists of β-(1, 3) and β-(1, 6) linkages, while β-glucans derived from cereals are polysaccharides of glucose residues with β-(1, 3) and β-(1, 4) linkages. The extraction of β-glucan from oat and barley is more difficult and expensive than that obtained from baker's yeast *Saccharomyces cerevisiae* and mushroom, therefore most beta-glucans sold in the market as dietary supplements are originated from yeast (24–26). Other details concerning β-glucan obtained from yeasts and mushrooms are described in Chapter 7 of this book. Beta-glucan from cereals helps to lower cholesterol and blood glucose (24–25), while β-glucan from fungi has shown effectiveness as an immune system booster and an anti-tumor substance (26). Briefly, anti-hypercholesterolemia of beta-glucans is stronger in oat and barley than in yeasts and mushrooms, while their immunomodulation is stronger in yeasts and mushrooms than in cereals. Moreover, beta-glucans exhibit a broad spectrum of biological activities including anti-tumor, anti-aging, and anti-inflammatory properties, as well as prevention of cardiovascular diseases (24–26). On the basis of its effects on cholesterol and its nontoxicity, the Food and Drug Administration recommended a daily dose of at least 3g of β-glucan from natural oats to prevent hypercholesterolemia and other CVDs (20). The skin health promotion effects of natural β-glucan derived from cereals and micro-organisms has been also reported in the literature (24).

3.1.3.2.3 Fucoidans and Fucans

Fucoidans and fucans are polysaccharides, mainly constituted of sulfated L-fucose (27–28). Fucoidans are a type of homo-polysaccharide, mainly constituted of linked L-fucose with sulfate ester groups, while fucans are complex hetero-polysaccharides containing a majority of sulfated L-fucose, and a minority of other monosaccharides like sugar. Fucoidans are mainly found in the cell wall of brown algae, while fucans occur in echinoderms such as in the egg jelly coat of sea urchins and in the body wall of sea cucumber (27). Main pharmacological properties of fucoidans and fucans include: immune modulator, anti-inflammatory, anticoagulant and antithrombotic, anti-parasites (plasmodium, toxoplasma), anti-viral (influenza, cytomegalovirus, herpes), anti-cancer, liver and kidney protector (27–28). There is growing support for the role of fucoidan as an adjunct dietary therapy in cancer and inflammatory diseases (28). The detail roles of fucoidan are described in Chapter 5 of this book.

3.1.3.2.4   Inulin and Oligofructose   Inulin is a heterogeneous blend of natural fructose polymers as plant storage carbohydrates (29). Oligofructose is a subgroup of inulin, consisting of polymers with a degree of polymerization (DP) inferior or equal to ten. Inulin and oligofructose are dietary fibers and not digested in the upper gastrointestinal tract; therefore, they have a reduced caloric value. They stimulate the growth of intestinal bifido-bacteria (29). The colon is known to be a complex ecosystem with 400 different types of bacteria. Some strains have pathogenic effects such as the production of toxins and carcinogens, whereas others are considered to provide a healthy effect in the large intestine. Among those beneficial bacteria are *Lactobacilli* and *Bifidobacteria* (29). Inulin is, however, digestible by certain microorganisms living in the colon that have inulinase activity including lactobacilli (30). This means inulin can pass though the human digestive system relatively intact, until it reaches the large intestine, where it is digested by bifido-bacteria (30). This encourages growth of a healthy intestinal micro flora that in turn produces important metabolic byproducts including butyric and propionic acid, which suppress colon cancer development (31). Put briefly, inulin, oligofructose and corresponding fermentation products may prevent colon cancer. Thus, this specific type of dietary fiber exerts both blocking agent and suppressing agent types of chemo-preventive activities (30–31). Additionally, inulin has interesting immuno-modulatory properties (30–31). Inulin does not lead to a rise in serum glucose or stimulate insulin secretion. Inulin also induces production of a glucagon-like peptide (GLP)-1 hormone – an important endogenous stimulator of insulin secretion and an appetite suppressant (30). Inulin has relatively low food energy for humans and can be used as a low-calorie bulking agent in food, replacing sugar, flour and fat (30). This makes inulin a valuable probiotic dietary fiber. Moreover, inulin has a significant number of diverse pharmaceutical and food applications. In the food industry it is used as a fat or sugar replacement and soluble dietary fiber, but it also has important pharmaceutical applications, as an excipient or stabilizer, and as an injectable for clinical measurement of kidney function (30). Inulin may also have utility as a slow-release drug delivery medium and as a stabilizer for protein and peptide-based drugs and vaccines (30). Inulin and fructose oligosaccharides are present in more 36,000 plant species (29). Their main natural sources are chicory, Jerusalem artichoke, burdock, dandelion root, wheat, onion, banana, garlic, leek, and asparagus (17, 29, 31).

3.1.3.2.5   Gum   The term 'gum' is used to describe a group of naturally occurring polysaccharides that have numerous interesting applications in different industries (food, pharmacy, textile, cosmetics, etc.) due to their ability either to form the gel or make the viscous solution or stabilize the emulsion systems (32). Water-soluble gums, also known as 'hydrocolloid' are used for various applications as dietary fiber, texture modifiers, gelling agents, thickeners, stabilizers, emulsifiers, coating agents and drug delivery agents (32). Various parts of plants (e.g., plant cell walls, tree exudates, seeds, tuber, roots, seaweeds) have surface cells containing gums, mucilage, and fiber and protein compounds. Plant gum exudates result from the protection mechanisms against mechanical or microbial injury (32). Two well-known plant gums are guar gum and gum Arabic that are dietary fibers and have a large application in industry – mostly in pharmaceutical fabrication (32).

Guar gum is derived from the seeds of the drought tolerant plant Cyamopsis tetragonolobus, a member of Leguminosae family (32–33). This plant is cultivated mostly in Pakistan and India where the plant has been grown for centuries as food for both human and animals (33). Guar gum is a gel-forming galactomannan obtained by grinding the endosperm of cluster bean. It is largely used in the form of guar gum powder as an additive in the food, pharmaceuticals, paper, textile, explosive, and cosmetics industries. Thus, guar gum is chiefly used as thickener and stabilizer. It is also beneficial in the control of many health problems like diabetes, bowel movements, heart disease and colon cancer (33).

Gum Arabic (GA) or *Acacia* gum is an edible biopolymer obtained as exudates of mature trees of *Acacia senegal* and *Acacia seyal* which grow principally in the region of Sahel in Sudan.

The exudate is a non-viscous liquid, rich in soluble fibers, and its emanation from the stems and branches usually occurs under stress conditions such as drought, poor soil fertility, and injury (34). Chemically, GA is a complex mixture of polysaccharides and glycoproteins of different size and composition (34). Gum Arabic is widely used in a wide range of industrial sectors such as food, pharmaceuticals, cosmetics, textiles, ceramics, lithography, glue, and so on. In the food industry, it is used as a stabilizer, a thickener and/or an emulsifier agent for soft drink syrup, gummy candies like chewing gum and creams (34). Gum Arabic slows the rate of absorption of some drugs from the gut. It is water-soluble and considered a physiologically harmless substance. Recent studies have highlighted its antioxidant properties, its role in the metabolism of lipids, its positive results in the treatments of kidney failure and gastrointestinal diseases and its antimicrobial activity in the prevention of dental caries and periodontal disease in tooth decay (34).

3.1.3.2.6 Mucilage Similar to plant gum, mucilage is a gelatinous substance that contains sugars and comprises a wide range of mixed viscous polysaccharides and glycoproteins (19, 35). The difference between them is their mode of formation. Mucilage is generally a normal product of metabolism, formed within the cell (35). Gums are considered to be pathological products, formed by giving injury to the plant or due to unfavorable conditions, such as drought and breakdown of cell walls (35). Gums readily dissolve in water, whereas mucilage form slimy masses. Both gum and mucilage are plant hydrocolloids yielding mixtures of sugars and uronic acids on hydrolysis (35). These hydrocolloids are used in small amounts as gelling, thickening, stabilizing and emulsifying agents in certain food products (17). Mucilage is secreted into the endosperm of plant seeds where they act to prevent excessive dehydration. Mucilage plays a role in the storage of water. Foods rich in mucilage are: aloe vera (leaves of *Aloe barbadensis*), pods of okra (*Abelmoschus esculentus*), fenugreek seeds (*Trigonella foenum-graceum*), hibiscus leaves (*Hibiscus rosa-sinensis*), agar agar (algae), phoenix fruits (*Phoenix dactylifera*), cassia seeds (*Cassia tora*), *Cocculus* mucilage from leaves of *Cocculus hirsute*, mimosa seeds from seeds of *Mimosa pudica*, leaves of broom creeper (*Cocculus hirsute*), seeds of American basil (*Ocimum americanum*), and more (35).

Based on its sustaining capacities, binding properties, and gelling, mucilage could be further exploited in the future as a novel natural polymer for development of different drug delivery systems in the pharmaceutical industry (35). Mixed with water, mucilage has been used to prepare glue.

In summary, carbohydrates are the most abundant and diverse class of nutrients found in nature and play an important role in the maintenance of human health. Starch and sugar are essential nutrients to energy production for cell activity. Dietary fibers are necessary for the prevention of chronic diseases in humans such as constipation, colon cancer, hypercholesterolemia, cardiovascular diseases, diabetes, obesity, and so on.

3.2 Proteins, Peptides and Amino Acids

Proteins and amino acids are essential macronutrients for the human body. Amino acids are commonly called protein's building blocks (1). Proteins from the diet are broken down by different enzymes during human digestion firstly to smaller peptide chains, then finally to different amino acids. The human body reuses these liberated amino acids to construct its proper proteins for its cell or tissue type (3, 5, 36–39). Proteins and their subsidiaries (peptides, amino acids) are organic products mainly constituted of carbon, oxygen, hydrogen, and nitrogen elements in their chemical structure. Like the two other macronutrients, carbohydrates and lipids, proteins are found in a wide variety of foods, plus the human body is able to synthesize them (3). Proteins differ from the carbohydrates and lipids by the permanent presence of amino nitrogen compounds – amino acids in their constitution.

There are 20 different amino acids in proteins (3, 5, 36–39). In each protein, the precise types and amounts of each amino acid are covalently linked in the linear sequence under the instructions of our genetic materials like DNA and RNA (deoxyribonucleic acid and ribonucleic acid) (3, 5). These amino acids are combined by several ways to form many tens of thousands of different proteins in the human body (5, 36–39). Proteins are present in all living organisms from bacteria and yeasts to fungi, plants, and animals. Owing to their presence in every single cell, proteins make up approximately 20% of the human body and are one of the building materials of body tissue (1).

3.2.1   Amino Acids

Amino acids (AA) are organic nitrogenous compounds containing both an acidic carboxyl (-COOH) and a basic amino (-NH2) group attached to a central α-carbon. They are called α-amino acids and are classified as proteins (37–39). The first carbon is part of the carboxyl group. The second carbon, to which is attached the amino group, is called the α-carbon. The α-carbon of most amino acids is joined by covalent bonds to four different groups. Thus, the α-carbon in all the amino acids is asymmetric, except in glycine where the α-carbon is symmetric. In some amino acids, the amine group is attached to the β or γ-carbon, and these are therefore referred to as beta or gamma amino acids (38–39).

Among more than 300 amino acids in nature, only 20 of them serve as building blocks of protein in plants, animals, and humans (38–39). The names of 20 α-amino acids present in proteins are: alanine, arginine, asparagine, aspartic acid, cysteine, glutamic acid, glutamine, glycine, histidine, isoleucine, leucine, lysine, methionine, phenylalanine, proline, serine, threonine, tryptophan, tyrosine, and valine (37–39). Their general chemical structure is the following.

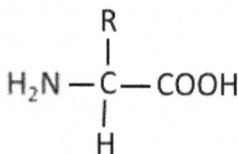

$$H_2N-\overset{\overset{\displaystyle R}{|}}{\underset{\underset{\displaystyle H}{|}}{C}}-COOH$$

FIGURE 1.2   Chemical structure of an L α-amino acid where R represents a side chain specific to each amino acid.

As shown in Figure 1.2, the amino and carboxyl groups are bound to the same atom carbon. It is through the R group that molecules of the 20 amino acids differ from each other. In the simplest molecules of amino acids, glycine, R is a hydrogen atom. Other amino acids have more complex R groups, consisting of atoms of carbon, hydrogen, and in some cases, oxygen, nitrogen, or sulfur (37–39).

In nature, there are some 300 additional amino acids which are never found as constituents of proteins but which either play metabolic roles or occur as natural products (38). Among the important nonprotein amino acids which play metabolic roles are L-ornithine, L-citrulline, β-alanine, creatine, and γ-aminobutyrate. L-ornithine and L-citrulline occur in free state in the animal tissues (38). Arginine, citrulline, and ornithine are metabolic intermediates of the urea cycle and form the urea cycle (36, 38). However, non-protein α-amino acids (e.g., ornithine, citrulline, and homocysteine) and non- α-amino acids (e.g., taurine and β-alanine) also play important roles in cell metabolism (39).

Except for glycine, all AA have an asymmetric carbon, therefore they are chiral compounds – molecules that differ only in the spatial arrangement of their atoms (15, 38). In nature, all 20 α-amino acid constituents of proteins exist in L-stereoisomers according to the configuration by Fischer (15, 36–38). However, certain bacterial species have outer layers composed of polymers made of D-amino acids. Human immune system cells, whose task is to attack and destroy foreign cells, cannot destroy these bacteria containing D-amino acids owing to the difference in stereoisoforms (36–39). Most asymmetric molecules found in living organisms occur in only one stereoisomeric form, either D or L. For example, with a few exceptions, all amino acids found in animal or vegetable proteins only exist as L-stereoisomeric form. It is the same for all carbohydrates, they only exist as D-stereoisomer such as D-glucose, D-fructose, D-galactose (15).

3.2.1.1 Classification of Essential, Nonessential and Conditionally Essential Amino Acids

Amino acids (AA) are further classified based on nutritional aspects (1). The 20 AA constituents of proteins in humans are divided into two main groups: essential and nonessential amino acids (36–39).

There are nine essential amino acids: histidine, isoleucine, leucine, lysine, methionine, phenylalanine, threonine, tryptophan, and valine. These AA are called essential AA because the human body cannot synthesize them. They must be obtained from the diet (1, 3, 9, 36–39).

The 11 AA remaining (alanine, arginine, asparagine, aspartic acid, cysteine, glutamic acid, glutamine, glycine, proline, serine, and tyrosine) are named nonessential AA owing to the auto-synthesis in the human body (36–39). However, in some situations (infancy, growth, diseased states or the elderly), the body cannot synthesize enough of some of the nonessential amino acids and more of them are required in the diet. These types of amino acids are called conditionally essential amino acids or semi-essential amino acids. They mainly include arginine, glutamine, and cysteine (39). Despite the fact that arginine may not be required in the diet to maintain nitrogen balance in the adults of most species, dietary deficiency of arginine can result in metabolic stress, neurological or reproductive dysfunction (39). In addition, arginine becomes an essential amino acid for young mammals. Thus, on the basis of functional needs, arginine is considered an essential amino acid for vascular homeostasis, neurological functioning, spermatogenesis, and fetal growth (39). Glutamine also is a conditionally essential AA in neonates and under stress conditions (39). Cysteine may become essential during metabolic stress (36). Two aromatic amino acids (tyrosine and tryptophan) are important in hormone synthesis. Tyrosine forms thyroxine and the catecholamines, adrenaline and noradrenaline; and tryptophan form serotonin (36, 39).

Growing evidence shows that besides their role as building blocks of proteins and polypeptides, some AA are important regulators of key metabolic pathways that are necessary for growth, reproduction, and immunity in organisms, therefore maximizing efficiency of food utilization, enhancing protein accretion, reducing adiposity, and improving health (36, 39). Called functional AA, they include arginine, cysteine, glutamine, leucine, proline, and tryptophan. Concentrations of AA in plasma are maintained relatively constant in the post-absorptive state of healthy adults.

Additionally, amino acids are classified according to their hydrophobic or hydrophilic property. This characteristic is due to the nature of R group.

Hydrophobic or nonpolar amino acids are:

Glycine (R: H), Alanine (R: CH_3-), Valine (R: $(CH_3)_2$-CH-), Leucine (R: $(CH_3)_2$-CH-CH_2-), Isoleucine (R: CH_3-CH_2-$C(CH_3)H$-), Phenylalanine (R: Phenyl-CH_2-), Tryptophan (R: Indole-CH_2-), Proline (R: (HN)-CH_2-CH_2-CH_2-), Methionine (R: CH_3-S-CH_2-CH_2-) (36, 38–39).

Hydrophilic or polar amino acids include:

Serine (R: OH-CH_2-), Threonine (R: CH_3-$CH(OH)$-), Tyrosine (R: Phenol-CH_2-), Cysteine (R: HS-CH_2-), Asparagine (R: NH_2-CO-CH_2-), Glutamine (R: NH_2-CO-CH_2-CH-), Glutamate (R: COO-CH_2-CH_2-), Lysine (R: NH_2-$(CH_2)_4$-), Arginine (R: $NH=C(NH_2^+)$-NH-$(CH_2)_3$-), Histidine (R: Imidazole-CH_2-), Aspartate (R: COO-CH_2-) (36, 38–39).

Amino acids are also classified according to their pH, and there are three categories: acidic amino acids (glutamic acid, aspartic acid), basic amino acids (arginine, histidine and lysine), and neutral amino acids (the other amino acids) (36). The neutral amino acids may be divided into neutral polar amino acids like serine, threonine, tyrosine, asparagine, glutamine and neutral nonpolar amino acids such as glycine, alanine, valine, leucine, isoleucine, phenylalanine, tryptophan, methionine, cysteine, and proline (36, 39).

The amino acids where R contains S (sulfur) are methionine and cysteine. Amino acids where R is an aliphatic chain are glycine, alanine, valine, leucine, isoleucine, and proline. Amino acids where R is an aromatic ring are phenylalanine (benzene) and tyrosine (phenol) (36, 39).

3.2.1.2 Metabolism of Amino Acids

In general, each AA has its own unique catabolic pathway under the action of different specific enzymes. However, the catabolism of many AA exhibits some common reactions such as transamination, decarboxylation, hydroxylation, reduction, hydrolysis, dehydration, oxidation, and dehydrogenation, via different corresponding enzymes like transaminase, glutamate dehydrogenase, ornithine decarboxylase, NO synthase, arginase, and so on. (36, 39). The metabolism of AA takes place mainly in the small intestine, liver, kidneys, muscle, and immune cells. The main metabolic products of amino acids include urea, creatinine, uric acid, nitric oxide (NO), and other nitrogenous products (36, 39). They are excreted in the urine and also lost in feces, sweat, and other body secretions and in sloughed skin, hair, and nails. A continuous supply of dietary amino acids through foods is required to replace these losses, even after growth has ceased (39). Amino acids consumed in excess of the amounts needed for the synthesis of nitrogenous tissue constituents are not stored but are degraded; the nitrogen is excreted as urea, and the keto acids left after removal of the amino groups are either utilized directly as sources of energy or are converted to carbohydrate or fat (1, 36, 39).

Amino acids and proteins are not a good source of energy production for cell activity, contrary to carbohydrates and fats. Some other metabolites of AA include ammonia, carbon dioxide (CO_2), long-chain and short-chain fatty acids, glucose, hydrogen sulfur (H_2S), ketone, and polyamines. Complete oxidation of AA carbons occurs only if their carbons are ultimately converted to acetyl-CoA, which is oxidized to CO_2 and water (H_2O) via the Krebs cycle and mitochondrial electron transport system. On a molecular basis, oxidation of AA is less efficient for adenosine triphosphate (ATP) production, compared to fat and glucose (39). Thus, the efficiency of energy transfer from L-AA to ATP ranges from 29% for methionine to 59% for isoleucine. However, glutamine is a preferred major fuel for rapidly dividing cells, including lymphocytes, macrophages, enterocytes, and tumors (36, 38–39).

3.2.1.3 Roles of Amino Acids

Amino acids are required for the synthesis of body protein and other nitrogen-containing compounds, such as creatine, peptide hormones, and some neurotransmitters. They also play an important role in regulation of hormone secretion, gene expression, and cell signaling (36–39). The biological roles of some AA and their main metabolites are as follows.

Alanine is directly used in gluconeogenesis, transamination, glucose-alanine cycle, and inhibition of pyruvate kinase and hepatic autophagy.

Arginine takes part in antioxidant activity, regulation of hormone secretion, ammonia detoxification, regulation of gene expression, immune function, methylation of proteins, and citrulline formation for proteins. Its main metabolite, nitric oxide (NO), acts as a regulator of neurotransmission, nutrient metabolism, vascular tone, hemodynamics, angiogenesis, spermatogenesis, embryogenesis, fertility, immune function, hormone secretion, wound healing, tumor growth, mitochondrial biogenesis, and signaling molecule (40).

Aspartate or aspartic acid is the precursor to several amino acids such as isoleucine, lysine, methionine, and threonine. It participates in gluconeogenesis and in the urea cycle. It is a neurotransmitter, but its activity is weaker than that of L-glutamate.

Asparagine is a regulator of cell metabolism, gene expression, and immune function; it plays a role in the ammonia detoxification and the function of the nervous system.

Cysteine is used in disulfide linkage in protein and transport of sulfur. Cysteine is the precursor to taurine, which is not an amino acid. Taurine is an antioxidant and essential for regulation of cellular redox, muscle development, cardiovascular function, the retina, and the central nervous system.

Glutamate (glutamic acid) takes part in glutamine, citrulline, and arginine synthesis, and the urea cycle with the Krebs cycle, transamination, and ammonia assimilation. Its metabolite GABA (gamma amino-butyric acid) is an excitatory neurotransmitter and an inhibitor of T-cell response and inflammation.

Glycine has various functions: precursor to proteins and heme; calcium influx through a glycine-gated channel in the cell membrane; purine, serine and porphyrin synthesis; inhibitory neurotransmitter in central nervous system.

Glutamine plays several roles in the function of the body. Some of the important functions of glutamine include: source of cellular energy; syntheses of protein, purine, pyrimidine, ornithine, citrulline, arginine, proline, asparagine; and production of ammonium to help maintaining the kidney's acid-base balance.

Histidine is the catalytic sites of certain enzymes. Histidine participates in the hemoglobin structure and assists in stabilizing oxyhemoglobin and destabilizing CO-bound hemoglobin. It is a coordinating ligand in metalloproteins and is a precursor for histamine, an amine produced in the body necessary for inflammation and vasodilation.

Isoleucine is necessary for energy production of muscle as well as hemoglobin formation.

Leucine is used in the muscle tissue, adipose tissue, and liver. Leucine directly stimulates the synthesis of muscle proteins. Adipose and muscle tissue use leucine in the formation of sterols.

Lysine has different roles: regulation of NO synthesis, antiviral activity (treatment of Herpes simplex), protein methylation, acetylation, ubiquitination, and O-linked glycosylation.

Methionine is important in angiogenesis, the growth of new blood vessels, and is used to treat and prevent liver disorders and damage in acetaminophen poisoning. It may be used for increasing the acidity of urine, improving wound healing, treating alcoholism, depression, Parkinson's disease, allergies, and asthma.

Phenylalanine directly activates the synthesis of tyrosine as well as neurological development and function.

Proline plays a role in collagen structure and neurological function.

Serine has different roles: syntheses of cysteine, purine, pyrimidine, ceramide and phosphatidylserine; gluconeogenesis (particularly in ruminants); and protein phosphorylation.

Threonine is used in the synthesis of glycine and the mucin protein required for maintaining intestinal integrity and function, and participates in protein phosphorylation as well as immune function.

Tryptophan is a precursor to the neurotransmitter serotonin and the antioxidant melatonin, and inhibits the production of inflammatory cytokines and superoxide.

Tyrosine is directly used in regulation of immune response and protein phosphorylation, nitrosation, and sulfation. It is the precursor of dopamine, a neurotransmitter, and melanin, a pigment and antioxidant. It is also the precursor of thyroid hormones: triiodothyronine (T_3) and thyroxine (T_4), in the thyroid.

Valine directly participates in the synthesis of glutamine and alanine (36–39).

Thus, an optimal balance among amino acids (AA) in the diet and circulation is crucial for whole body homeostasis (39). There is growing recognition that besides their role as building blocks of proteins and polypeptides, some AA regulate key metabolic pathways that are necessary for health maintenance, growth, reproduction, and immunity. They are called functional AA, which include arginine, cysteine, glutamine, leucine, proline, and tryptophan (40). Dietary supplementation with one or a mixture of these AA may be beneficial for ameliorating health problems at various stages of the life cycle like fetal growth restriction, neonatal morbidity and mortality, weaning-associated intestinal dysfunction, as well as wasting syndrome, obesity, diabetes, cardiovascular disease, the metabolic syndrome, and infertility. It is also used for optimizing efficiency of metabolic transformations to enhance muscle growth, milk production, egg and meat quality, and athletic performance, while preventing excess fat deposition and reducing adiposity (39). Thus, amino acids have important functions in both nutrition and health.

Citrulline is a non-essential amino acid under physiological conditions but considered a conditionally essential amino acid in situations where intestinal function is compromised (40). Citrulline functions as an intermediate in the urea cycle and as a precursor of arginine. Citrulline is a non-protein amino acid for which the main source is de novo synthesis in the small intestine (40). Most circulating citrulline derives from glutamine conversion in the enterocyte cells. Glutamine is first converted to glutamate via the enzyme glutaminase. Subsequently, pyrroline-5-carboxylate (P5C) synthase, which is located almost exclusively in the intestinal mucosa, converts glutamate to P5C, which is converted into ornithine via ornithine aminotransferase (OAT) (40). Ornithine is then converted to citrulline via the enzyme ornithine transcarbamylase (OTC), which is expressed only in the liver and intestine. Arginine and proline can also act as intestinal citrulline precursors. All of the enzymes involved in citrulline synthesis are located in the mitochondria of enterocytes. The activities of the two enzymes that catabolize citrulline, argininosuccinate synthase (ASS) and argininosuccinate lyase (ASL), are very low in the intestine (40). Therefore, citrulline cannot be catabolized in enterocytes and is released into the circulation. The majority of citrulline released by the intestine (~70%) is metabolized within the kidney, where it is converted into arginine by the enzymes ASS and ASL present in the proximal convoluted tubule of the nephron. Therefore, endogenous arginine synthesis involves an inter-organ pathway known as the intestinal-renal axis, with de novo arginine synthesis from citrulline representing 5–15% of arginine production. Circulating arginine can be catabolized by liver arginase I to be utilized to fuel the urea cycle via ornithine production (40).

Arginine is another dispensable amino acid with important properties for promoting immune system function. Arginine is the precursor for nitric oxide (NO) synthesis, and it has been proposed as a nutrient for altering immune (37). Although supplementation of specific amino acids or cofactors may produce beneficial responses, on some occasions, supplementation may produce undesirable effects on the disease state. Supplementing glutamine in the diets of patients with cancer may be counterproductive because the glutamine may promote accelerated tumor growth (37). Similarly, arginine supplementation may stimulate nitric oxide synthesis because of the increased availability of the precursor for its formation. However, nitric oxide (NO) production has both helpful and detrimental effects. NO is both antioxidant and free radical (see Chapter 3 of this book). Definition of amino acid and protein requirements in various diseases is difficult to assess and requires a multifactorial approach (37). Consult a doctor before taking an amino acid supplement.

3.2.2 Peptides

In cells, a peptide is formed when two adjacent amino acids are linked together through the carboxyl (COOH) group of one amino acid with the amino (NH_2) group of another to form an amide bond (-CONH-), also called peptide bond. The chain, thus formed, by linking together of many amino acid units is called a peptide chain (36, 38, 41). The two amino acids at the ends of the chain are called N-terminal and C-terminal where the groups NH_2 and COOH are not linked – free or intact. Depending on the number of amino acid molecules composing a chain, the peptides may be termed as a dipeptide (containing 2 amino acid units), a tripeptide (containing 3 amino acid units) and so on. If a peptide is made up of no more than ten amino acids, it is called an oligopeptide; beyond that, it is a polypeptide. Peptide chain may possess from 50 to millions of amino acid units. When they are made up of over 100 amino acids, polypepties are sometimes called macro-peptides. Strictly speaking, proteins are polypeptides with more than 100 amino acids (38). However, this classification is arbitrary, and the number of amino acids can vary according to each author.

Some main polypeptides and peptides in the human body include glutathione, glucagon, insulin, calcitonin, amylin, parathyroid hormone, angiotensin, oxytocin, and brain natriuretic peptide, also known as B-type natriuretic peptide (BNP) (36, 38, 41–46). Peptides can be used in the treatment of various diseases, including endocrine dysfunctions (diabetes, thyroid disorders, osteoporosis, etc.), infectious diseases, cancer, central nervous system disorders, and gastroenterologic diseases, generally by injection (42). Already more than 100 peptide-based drugs have reached the market, and hundreds of peptidergic compounds are in clinical or preclinical studies (42).

The roles of some peptides are as follows.

Glutathione is a tripeptide comprised of three amino acids: cysteine, glutamic acid, and glycine. It is present in all mammalian cells and acts an important antioxidant, a free radical scavenger thanks to the presence of a thiol (SH) group in the cysteine amino acid (36, 38, 42).

Glucagon is a peptide hormone produced by alpha cells of the pancreas and works to raise the level of glucose and fatty acids in blood. Its effect is opposite to that of insulin. Together with insulin, it is a regulator of glucose in blood. Moreover, it hydrolyzes triglycerides into fatty acids and glycerol (38, 42).

Insulin is a peptide hormone produced by beta cells of the pancreas. It regulates the metabolism of sugars, fats, or protein. Injection of insulin is used to lower blood sugar in patients with diabetes of type 1 (36, 38).

Calcitonin is a 32-amino acid linear polypeptide hormone of the thyroid destined to lower blood calcium. Subcutaneous injection of calcitonin is reserved for the treatment of osteoporosis in postmenopausal women. Calcitonin extracted from the ultimobranchial glands of salmon is the most common in therapeutic uses (36–38, 42).

Parathyroid hormone is a polypeptide secreted by the parathyroid glands and used to elevate serum calcium level through its effects on bone, intestine and kidney (36, 38, 42).

Angiotensin is an oligopeptide hormone that causes vasoconstriction leading to increase blood pressure. Blood pressure is regulated by a process known as the renin-angiotensin system and has been the focus of most research on bioactive peptides and functional foods (43). Angiotensin is derived from angiotensinogen, a globulin produced in the liver, and comprises four hormones called angiotensin I, II, III and IV (43–44). The enzyme renin converts the angiotensinogen to angiotensin I, which is then hydrolyzed by the angiotensin-converting enzyme (ACE), releasing the octapeptide angiotensin II (a potent vasoconstrictor). Thus, inhibition of renin or ACE activity plays a significant role in lowering blood pressure during hypertension (43–44). Angiotensin II also signals the release of the hormone aldosterone from the adrenal glands. Aldosterone signals the kidneys to retain sodium and chloride. Because water travels with these two minerals, this results in water retention, which increases blood pressure and decreases urine output (3, 43–44). The renin-angiotensin system (RAS) has important physiological functions such as regulation of blood pressure, maintenance of water and electrolyte balance, and cardiovascular homeostasis. High angiotensin levels cause heart failure. Low angiotensin levels cause hypotension, loss of sodium, retention of potassium and more urine excretion. Drugs containing ACE inhibitors are used for treatment of hypertension and cardiovascular diseases. Recent evidence suggests that inhibition of RAS system may be beneficial in attenuating cognitive deficits observed in aging, Alzheimer's and Parkinson's diseases, and other cognitive impairment diseases (44).

Amylin, a 37-amino-acid-peptide, is a pancreatic β-cell hormone that produces effects in several different organ systems (45). Amylin's major role is as a glucoregulatory hormone, and it is an important regulator of energy metabolism in health and disease. Other amylin actions have also been reported, such as on the cardiovascular system or on bone. Amylin acts principally in the circumventricular organs of the central nervous system and functionally interacts with other metabolically active hormones such as cholecystokinin, leptin, and estradiol. The amylin-based peptide, pramlintide, is used clinically to treat Type 1 and

Type 2 diabetes. Clinical studies in obesity have shown that amylin agonists could also be useful for weight loss, especially in combination with other agents (45).

Oxytocin is a peptide hormone produced by the hypothalamus and released by the posterior pituitary; it causes uterus contraction to facilitate childbirth and also stimulates lactation (36–38).

B-type natriuretic peptide or **Brain natriuretic peptide** (**BNP**) is synthesized as a prohormone named pro-BNP comprising 108 amino acids. Upon release into circulation, it is cleaved in equal proportions into the biologically active 32 amino acid BNP, which represents the C-terminal fragment, and the biologically inactive 76 amino acid N-terminal fragment (NT-pro-BNP) (46). BNP is secreted by the ventricles of the heart in response to excessive stretching of heart muscle cells. Both BNP and NT-pro-BNP are used as biomarkers to establish the diagnosis of heart failure and coronary artery disease (46).

Peptides in natural sources (animal and plant foods), called bioactive peptides (BP), play a significant role in human health by affecting the digestive, endocrine, cardiovascular, immune, and nervous systems. Bioactive peptides are considered the new generation of biologically active regulators; they can prevent oxidation and microbial degradation in foods as well as improve the treatment of various diseases and disorders, thus increasing quality of life. Milk and dairy products (yogurt, cheese) are the main sources of BP. The growing interest in BP has incentivized the scientific community and the food industry to explore the development of new food additives and functional products based on these peptides (41).

3.2.3 Proteins

Proteins are polymers of different amino acids linked together by peptide bonds in the form of long filaments (polypeptide chains). They wrap themselves in a virtually infinite number of spherical or helical forms, which explains the wide variety of functions performed by proteins (36–38, 47). Proteins differ widely in amino acid content. Some amino acids which are in abundance in one protein may be in meagre amounts in others, and may even be lacking in the rest. Tryptophan, for instance, lacks in certain proteins. However, most of the proteins in animal and plant foods contain all the 20 amino acids (36, 38, 47). The proportion of these amino acids varies as a characteristic of a given protein, but all food proteins contain some of each. Collagen, a fibrillar protein that acts like glue between cells, consists of more than one thousand amino acids. Titin or connectin is a giant protein, greater than one μm in length, the largest known protein. It accounts for the passive elasticity of muscles, and consists of more than 25,000 amino acids (1). Titin is known as the largest sarcomeric protein that resides within the heart muscle. Mutations in the titin gene can cause cardiomyopathies, in particular, dilated cardiomyopathy (48). This cardiac disease is characterized by systolic dysfunction and dilation of the left ventricle (48).

3.2.3.1 Protein Intake and Disease

The Recommended Dietary Allowance (RDA) of protein for a healthy adult with minimal physical activity is about 0.8 g protein per kg body weight (BW) per day (3, 36, 49–50). To meet the functional needs such as promoting skeletal-muscle protein accretion and physical strength, dietary intake of 1.0, 1.3, and 1.6 g protein/kg BW/day is recommended for individuals with minimal, moderate, and intense physical activity, respectively. Long-term intake of protein at 2 g/kg BW/day is safe for healthy adults, and the tolerable upper limit is 3.5 g/kg BW/day for well-adapted subjects (49). Chronic high protein intake (>2 g per kg BW per day for adults) may result in digestive, renal, and vascular abnormalities and should be avoided (49). High protein diets appear to only increase the progression of kidney disease and liver malfunction in people who already have kidney or liver malfunction, and not to cause these problems. However, the prevalence of kidney disorders is relatively high and underdiagnosed (1). Concerning colon cancer, an evaluation of more than ten studies performed around the world published in 2011 purports that a high intake of red meat and processed meat is associated with a significant increase in colon cancer risk (1). In contrast, when a person consumes too little protein and energy, the result is protein-energy malnutrition (3). Although severe protein deficiency is rare in the developed world, it is a leading cause of death in children in many poor, underdeveloped countries. There are two main syndromes associated with protein deficiencies, named Kwashiorkor and Marasmus (1, 3). Kwashiorkor disease, caused by a severe deficiency of protein, affects millions of children worldwide. When it was first described in 1935, more than 90% of children with Kwashiorkor died. Although the associated mortality is slightly lower now, most children still die after the initiation of treatment (1). Marasmus caused by the simultaneous deficiency of protein and energy due to severe malnutrition, afflicts very young children who lack both protein and energy foods as well as vitamins and minerals (5). The infant with marasmus appears emaciated but does not have edema. However, residents of developed countries are also at risk, especially homeless, the elderly, people who abuse alcohol or other drugs, and people with AIDS, cancer, and other wasting diseases (3). Genetic disorders involving abnormal proteins include phenylketonuria, sickle cell anemia, and cystic fibrosis (3).

The quantity and quality of protein are the determinants of its nutritional values. Therefore, adequate consumption of high-quality proteins from animal products is essential for optimal growth, development, and health of humans. The protein content of the adult body diminishes with age (50). More specifically, non-muscle mass is little affected by age, whereas muscle diminishes extensively and is compensated for by an increase in body fat. These changes in muscle mass are related to whole-body protein turnover and changes in the rate of protein synthesis. Daily albumin synthesis and serum albumin levels also decrease in elderly people who consume diets with adequate protein (50). Muscle strength is correlated with muscle mass and rapidly declines after the age of 50. For this reason, it is wise to adopt an appropriate diet to prevent or delay the onset of sarcopenia (loss of muscle mass). Protein is known to be more satiating than other macronutrients, and it is unclear whether diets high in plant proteins affect the appetite of older adults, as they should be recommended for individuals at risk of malnutrition (50).

In the body, proteins and other nitrogenous compounds are degraded and resynthesized continuously; indicating that reutilization of amino acids is a major feature of the economy of protein metabolism. This process of recapture is not completely efficient, and some amino acids are lost by oxidative catabolism. Only about 10% of dietary proteins are catabolized each day to make cellular energy (1). If a person's diet does not contain enough carbohydrates and fats their body will use more amino acids to make energy, which compromises the synthesis of new proteins and destroys muscle proteins (1). Alternatively, if a person's diet contains more protein than the body needs, the extra amino acids will be broken down and transformed into fat (1).

3.2.3.2 Classification of Proteins

Because of their diversity, proteins are often classified into two major groups based on their shape and their composition (36, 47).

3.2.3.2.1 Based on the Shape of Proteins

Protein shapes are also divided into two other groups: fibrous proteins and globular proteins (36, 47).

Fibrous or fibrillar proteins are filiform, long and physically tough. They are mainly of animal origin and are insoluble in all common solvents such as water, acid, alkali solution and organic solvents. Fibrous proteins have structural and protective functions. The fibrous proteins are extremely strong and possess the elastomer characteristics. It is a heterogeneous group and includes the keratins and the proteins of connective tissues found in bones, skin, hair, nails, horns, hoofs, wool, and silk (36, 47). The important examples are: collagens, elastins, keratins, and fibroins. Collagens and their analogs elastins are the proteins of connective tissues, skin, cornea of the eyes, tendons, cartilages, and ligaments. They are also called 'cellular glue' as they help give tissues their shape and keep them strong, and are the major proteins of white connective tissues (tendons, cartilage) and of bone. Due to its abundance, strength and its directly proportional relation with skin aging, collagen has gained great interest in the cosmetic industry (51). Elastin has the additional property of being elastic as a rubber band (47). Keratins are rich in cystine, a sulfur amino acid, and are the major components of skin, hair, feathers, hoofs, nails, and horns (47). Fibroins are mainly composed of amino acids; glycine, alanine, and serine and are found in the fibers of silk (47). Fibrin is the protein formed when blood clots.

Globular or corpuscular proteins possess a relatively spherical or ovoid shape and are usually water-soluble (36, 47). Globular proteins are generally more sensitive to temperature and pH change than their fibrous counterparts. Typically, globular proteins play an essential role in metabolism and have several other dynamic functions. Globular proteins include enzymes, cytochrome C, nutrient proteins, reserve proteins, myosin in muscle, and blood proteins such as serum albumin, glycoproteins, hemoglobin, immunoglobulins (antibodies), and hormones (36, 47). Hemoglobin is used to transport oxygen, and albumin is a carrier of fatty acids in blood.

3.2.3.2.2 *Based on Chemical Composition*　Proteins are classified as simple or conjugated (36, 47).

Simple proteins or Holoproteins include proteins containing only amino acids (36, 47). This group include albumins (ovalbumin in egg, lactalbumin in milk, serum albumin in plasma), globulins (in blood plasma, egg white, plant seeds like hemp, soybean, pea, potato), protamines (in herring and salmon sperms), histones (in globin of hemoglobin or in nucleohistones of nuclei), glutelins (gluten from wheat, oryzenin from rice), prolamines (gliadin from wheat, zein from corn, hordein from oat), and scleroproteins (keratin, elastin, collagen, fibroin). Glutelins, prolamines, and scleroproteins are water insoluble (47).

Conjugated proteins or Heteroproteins consist of a simple protein combined with a nonprotein component. The nonprotein component is called a prosthetic group (36, 47). A protein without its prosthetic group is called an apoprotein. A protein molecule combined with its prosthetic group forms a heteroprotein. Prosthetic groups play an important role in the function of proteins. Conjugated proteins are classified according to the nature of their prosthetic groups. They include glycoproteins, lipoproteins, metalloproteins, hemoproteins, phosphoproteins, and so on. Glycoproteins contain a carbohydrate component. Lipoproteins are proteins containing lipid molecules such as cholesterol which are divided into High-Density Lipoprotein (HDL) or 'good' cholesterol and Low-Density Lipoprotein (LDL) or 'bad' cholesterol. Metalloproteins contain metal ions (iron, calcium, copper, zinc, and molybdenum). Phosphoproteins contain phosphate groups, while hemoproteins or chromoproteins possess heme groups such as hemoglobin. Hemoglobin is the metalloprotein containing iron for the transport of oxygen in the red blood cells of all mammals (36, 47).

Moreover, there are soluble proteins and insoluble proteins. Soluble proteins are divided into two groups: proteins soluble in water (such as albumin) and proteins soluble in salt solutions at different pH levels (neutral, acidic or alkaline) (such as globulins). Insoluble proteins are called scleroproteins which are insoluble in any aqueous medium (water, acid, or base) and any organic solvents (such as keratin) (36, 47).

3.2.3.3 *Roles of Proteins*

Proteins are critical to life and have the most diverse functions. Some of their roles include: building and repair of body tissues; defense of the organism; regulation of metabolism and digestion; energy production; transport functions; genetic carriers; detoxification; and catalysts; as well as components of antibodies and some hormones (5, 36–39).

The primary role of proteins is to build and repair body tissues. This is made possible by the provision of the correct type and number of amino acids in the diet. Also, as cells are broken down during metabolism (catabolism) of foods, some amino acids released into the blood are recycled to build new and repair other tissue (anabolism). The body uses the recycled amino acids as efficiently as those obtained from the diet (5). In addition, the fibrous proteins serve as components of the tissues holding the skeletal elements together. Collagen is a structural unit of connective tissues (38).

Proteins are important components of hormones and enzymes that are essential for the regulation of metabolism and digestion of foods, drugs, macronutrients, and micronutrients. For example, cytochromes P450, a diverse group of enzymes present in animals and plants, are typically used to convert xenobiotics (medicines, foods, poisons, chemical contaminants) into less toxic derivatives (36–39).

Proteins help maintain fluid and electrolyte balances in the body and thus prevent edema (abnormal retention of body fluids). Proteins are also essential for the development of antibodies to defend the body against germs, viruses and, therefore, for a healthy immune system (5, 36–39).

Proteins can provide energy if and when the supply of carbohydrates and fats in the diet is insufficient. Each gram of protein provides four calories (5).

Proteins also perform transport functions. Many proteins function as carriers of molecules or ions across membranes or between cells. Examples of membrane proteins include the Na-K-ATPase and the glucose transporter. Other transport proteins include hemoglobin, which carries O2 to the tissues from the lungs, and the lipoproteins LDL and HDL, which transport lipids from the liver and intestines to other organs. Transferrin and ceruloplasmin are serum proteins that transport iron and copper, respectively (36). The mechanism of active transport involves proteins either as catalysts or as adsorbents or as both (38).

The nucleoproteins serve as carriers of genetic characters and hence govern inheritance of traits (38).

3.2.3.4   Types of Proteins

It is estimated that about 20,043 proteins have been detected in the human body, and 1,278 have been measured in a quantitative manner (52). The building of a protein from different amino acids is encoded by a corresponding gene in the cell, i.e., proteins are made according to instructions provided by our genetic materials (3).

Some main types of human proteins include albumins, globulins, enzymes, hormones, antibodies, interferons, collagens, keratins, lipoproteins, glycoproteins, nucleoproteins, p53 protein, and sirtuins. We examine here some important proteins such as enzymes, antibodies, interferons. Sirtuins and p53 protein are explained in Chapter 9 of this book.

3.2.3.4.1   Enzyme   Enzymes are globular proteins which are able to catalyze biochemical reactions. Enzymes accelerate the conversion of substrates into useful products in a buried pocket within the active site of the enzyme (53). In cells and organisms, most reactions are catalyzed by enzymes, which are regenerated during the course of a reaction, although not all reactions in nature require catalysis (53–55). These biological catalysts are physiologically important because they speed up the rates of reactions that would otherwise be too slow to support life (54). Enzymes accelerate the rates of such reactions by well over a million-fold, so reactions that would take years in the absence of catalysis can occur in fractions of seconds if catalyzed by the appropriate enzyme (55). Each enzyme has a specific active site where only one substrate or certain kind of substrate can bind to it for the conversion of the substrate into useful products. This phenomenon may be refered to as 'the lock and key model'. For example, starch is the only substrate of the enzyme amylase which converts starch into soluble glucose, an essential macronutrient and energizing product. Each cell contains thousands of different enzymes that facilitate specific cellular reactions (3, 55). Like proteins, enzymes contain chains of amino acids linked together. The characteristic of each enzyme is determined by the different sequence of amino acid arrangement. When the bonds between the amino acid are weak, they may be broken by high temperatures or high levels of acids, and become inactive.

Although some enzymes consist only of protein, many are complex proteins and require a coenzyme which functions as group transfer reagents (54–55). In this case, the enzymes consist of two parts: the protein part and the non-protein part called the activator. The activator is called a coenzyme, cofactor or prosthetic group. Without a coenzyme or cofactor linked to an enzyme, this enzyme becomes inactive and is called apoenzyme. An enzyme can be bound to one or more activators to become active and useful. Different coenzymes, cofactors and prosthetic groups are described in Chapter 2 of this book.

The name of an enzyme has two parts. The first part is the name of the substrate, and the second part is terminated with a suffix -ase (54). For example, protease is an enzyme of the substrate protein. For the international nomenclature, the name of an enzyme is preceded by the two letters EC (Enzyme Commission) followed by four numbers. For example, E.C.2.7.1.1. The first number denotes one of the six main classes: oxidoreductases, transferases, hydrolases, lyases, isomerases, and ligases. The second number denotes the subclass and the third number denotes the sub-subclass. The last number denotes the serial number of the enzyme in its sub-subclass (53–54). Enzymes are classified based on the reactions they catalyze into six classes cited above. Oxidoreductases such as glutathione reductase, lactate dehydrogenase, and glucose-6-phosphate dehydrogenase are the enzymes that catalyze oxidation-reduction reactions of their substrates. Transferases transfer a functional group between two substrates such as a methyl or phosphate group. Hydrolases catalyze the hydrolysis reactions of carbohydrates, proteins, and esters. Lyases cleave various chemical bonds by other means than hydrolysis and oxidation for the formation of double bonds. Isomerases are involved in isomerization of substrate where interconversion of cis-trans isomers is implicated. Ligases such as alanyl-t-RNA synthetase, glutamine synthetase, and DNA ligases join together two substrates with associated hydrolysis of a nucleoside triphosphate (53–54).

An important function of enzymes is in the digestion of foods. The metabolism of protein foods involves a decomposition into single amino acids by different digestive enzymes (amylase, protease, pepsin, trypsin, and chymotrypsin) from the stomach to the small intestine. Before the absorption in the small intestine, most proteins must be reduced to single amino acid or peptides by specific protein enzymes. Most peptides longer than four amino acids are not absorbed and must be broken into single amino acids. Enzyme production and activity can be decreased with age and illness. Enzymes are present in all foods. However, heat used in cooking, drying, or processing can destroy them. Therefore, fresh foods like fruits and some vegetables are rich in enzymes and help digestion. Some people like to eat raw meat such as raw beefsteak and raw fresh fish; this habit might be helpful for digestion. Enzymes extracted from fruits like papaya, pineapple, kiwifruit, and fig are used as medicines, food-processing agents and dietary supplements. Fruits like papaya, kiwifruit, pineapple and figs are rich in proteases such as papain, actinidin, bromelain, and ficin, respectively, which aid the breakdown of proteins.

Some enzymes are used as markers for the diagnosis of disease. Some enzymes are found only in specific tissues or in a limited number of such tissues (54). For example, lactase dehydrogenase (LDH) is only found in heart and skeletal muscle. An increase of any form of LDH in the blood indicates some kind of tissue damage. A heart attack can usually be diagnosed with certainty if there is an increase of LDH from heart. Also, Creatine Kinase (CK), also called creatine phosphokinase (CPK), is an enzyme that occurs in the brain, heart, and skeletal muscle. An elevated level of creatinine kinase can indicate a stroke, a brain tumor, or a heart attack. After a heart attack, CPK shows up more rapidly in the blood than LDH. Monitoring the presence of both enzymes extends the possibility of diagnosis, which is useful, since a very mild heart attack might be difficult to diagnose (54). LDH is also a valuable prognostic marker in lymphoma, leukemia, and colon cancer (56). Another useful enzyme assayed is acetyl cholinesterase, which is important in controlling certain nerve impulses. Many pesticides affect this enzyme, so farm workers are often tested to be sure that they have not received inappropriate exposure to these important agricultural toxins (54). There are several enzymes that are typically used in the clinical laboratory to diagnose diseases. Commonly assayed enzymes frequently used in diagnosis of heart, liver or brain are the amino transferases including alanine transaminase (ALT), also named serum glutamate-pyruvate aminotransferase (SGPT), and aspartate aminotransferase (AST) or serum glutamate-oxaloacetate aminotransferase (SGOT). SGPT can be found in the liver, skeletal muscle and heart, and its high level in serum is a specific indicator of liver damage. SGOT is a marker of heart attack, while SGPT is an indicator of hepatic diseases (54, 56). In humans, high level of alkaline phosphatase (ALP) indicates an increased osteoblastic activity, as in some bone diseases such as rheumatoid arthritis, rickets, osteomalacia, hyperthyroidism, hyperparathyroidism, and also in hepatobiliary pathology (54, 56). The acid phosphatase (ACP) level found in male prostate gland is 100 times more than in erythrocytes and other body tissue (56). ACP is used in diagnosis of prostate carcinoma (54, 56). ACP assay is supplemented by the prostate specific antigen (PSA) test (56). Glutamate dehydrogenase (GLDH), present in the liver, is used to detect hepatic parenchymal disease. Aldolase (ALD), found in skeletal muscle and the heart, is involved in muscle disease (54). In humans, creatine kinase (CK) is associated with myocardial infarction and muscle diseases (54, 56). Other enzymes are assayed under a variety of different clinical situations. Since these enzymes are relatively easy to determine with precision using automated techniques, they are part of the standard blood test for the rapid diagnosis and treatment of many diseases.

3.2.3.4.2 Immunoglobulin or Antibody Immunoglobulins (Ig) or antibodies, are glycoproteins found in all higher vertebrates and are the major secretory products of the adaptive immune system for the defense against antigens such as bacteria, viruses, parasites, fungi, and so on, to which the host has been exposed (57–59). In the body, immunoglobulins are produced by a class of B cells (white blood cells) called lymphocytes B. The immunogen or antigen reacts with a B-cell receptor (BCR) on the cell surface of B lymphocytes, and a signal is produced that directs the activation of transcription factors to stimulate the synthesis of antibodies, which are highly specific for the immunogen that stimulated the B cell. Furthermore, one clone of B cell makes an immunoglobulin (specificity). Immunoglobulins (antibodies) constitute about 20% of the protein in plasma (59).

The shape of an antibody looks like the letter Y. The two 'arms' of the Y are called Fab or antigen-binding fragment. The tail of the Y is named Fc or crystallizable fragment. Antibodies are heterodimeric proteins composed of two heavy (H) and two light (L) chains (57–59). Each arm is constituted of a light L chain in the outside and a prolonged H chain in the inside.

Since antibodies are glycoproteins, they contain diverse oligosaccharides in the glycosylation site. The immunoglobulins display considerable diversity in the location and number of the conserved N-linked glycosylation sites that are situated both on the Fc (crystallizable fragment) and Fab (antigen-binding fragment) (57). The Fc region mediates biological functions (e.g., the binding capacity to cellular receptors), while the Fab region presides over the antigen-binding sites.

In humans, the immunoglobulins or antibodies are divided into five distinct classes (IgG, IgM, IgA, IgE, and IgD), that share similar structures composed of immunoglobulin domains, but are different in the amino acid sequences in the heavy chains (57–59). In IgG, IgA, and IgD, the Fc and Fab are linked by a flexible hinge region that has no defined secondary structure. In IgM and IgE, this flexible linker is replaced by a more rigid Ig domain. The hinge region can contain N- and O-linked glycans (57).

IgG is the predominant isotype found in the body. It has the longest serum half-life of all immunoglobulin isotypes (58). IgG is synthesized mostly in the secondary immune response to pathogens. IgG is divided in four subclasses including IgG1, IgG2, IgG3, and IgG4. IgG1 is around 65% of the total IgG. IgG2 forms an important host defense against bacteria (58–59). IgG is the only immunoglobulin that crosses the placentae as its Fc portion binds to the receptors present on the surface of the placenta, protecting the neonate from infectious diseases. IgG is thus the most abundant antibody present in newborns (59). However, antibodies in cow milk or other animal milks cannot be used directly because they are destroyed by the digestive tract of the baby. Therefore, breast feeding plays an important role in the baby health. IgG levels increase in all types of infections, liver diseases (viral hepatitis, cirrhosis), rheumatoid arthritis, granulomatous infections, and so on, and decrease in lymphoid aplasia, chronic lymphoblastic leukemia.

IgA serum levels tend to be lower than IgG. Conversely, IgA levels are much higher than IgG at mucosal surfaces and in secretions (saliva, breast milk) (58). IgA protects the epithelial surfaces of the respiratory, digestive, and genitourinary system (58–59). There are two subclasses of IgA, IgA1 and IgA2. IgA2 predominates in the many mucosal secretions, such as the genital tract, whereas more than 90% of serum IgA is in the form of IgA1 (58).

IgM is the first immunoglobulin expressed during B cell development. It is mainly produced in the primary immune response to infectious agents or antigens. It is frequently used to diagnose acute exposure to an immunogen or pathogen (58–59).

IgD is found at very low levels in the serum with a short serum half-life. The function of circulating IgD is unclear. IgD has an unknown function against pathogens (58–59).

IgE is a very potent antibody. It is present at the lowest serum concentration with the shortest half-life. It is associated with hypersensitivity and allergic reactions as well as the response to parasitic worm infections. It also binds to receptors on mast cells and basophils causing allergic reactions (58–59).

Milk contains immunoglobulins, immunomodulatory cytokines such as interleukin-10 (IL-10), and transforming growth factor β (TGF-β), a group of proteins (60). In addition, breastfeeding has been shown to provide protection against gastrointestinal and respiratory tract infections of the newborn (60). Many epidemiological studies have shown a positive association between the consumption of unprocessed cow's milk and a reduced risk for developing allergy like allergic asthma. This association was not found for the intake of heated farm milk and commercial UHT milk (60).

Briefly, adequate protein intake is necessary to support the increased production of antibodies for fighting infection. Insufficient protein intake decreases the resistance of body to microbes, parasites, and chronic diseases. In contrast, eating more protein than we need does not improve immune function (3).

3.2.3.4.3 Interferons Interferons (IFN) are cytokines, a group of glycoproteins, produced mainly by host cells (monocytes and macrophages of the immune system) in response to pathogens, especially viruses. These cytokines are named interferons because they are able to 'interfere' with viral replication by protecting cells from virus infections (61–64). Interferons are a family of autocrine and paracrine cytokines secreted by host cells in response to pathogens, especially viruses. Generally, interferons are comprised of 130–170 amino acids with a molecular weight of 20–100 kD and are easily degraded by proteases, diethyl either, chloroform, and ketones (61). About ten mammalian interferon species have been discovered, but only seven are found in humans (62).

Clinical trials for interferons have focused on cancers and viral diseases. Interferons (IFN) are anti-viral cytokines that have been widely used clinically, especially against Hepatitis B virus (HBV) and Hepatitis C virus (HCV) (61–64). IFN-α-s and IFN-β exhibit a wide breadth of biological activities: antiviral and antiproliferative stimulation of cytotoxic activity of a variety of cells of the immune system (T-cells, natural killer cells, monocytes, macrophages, dendritic cells); increasing the expression of tumor-associated surface antigens and other surface molecules such as major histocompatibility complex (MHC) class I antigens; induction and/or activation of proapoptotic genes and proteins (62). Clinical uses of interferons for treatment of malignancies were greatly stimulated by promising results of limited clinical trials such as renal cancers, malignant melanomas, lymphomas, and leukemia (63). Clinical studies employing interferons were used for the prevention of common colds and the treatment of multiple sclerosis and several herpes virus infections, such as herpes keratoconjunctivitis, the varicella-zoster infections, shingles, and chickenpox (63). In the end of 2020 and the beginning of 2021, some clinical assays employed IFN-β 1b for the treatment of the dreadful Covid-19 infection (64). This research shows encouraging data on IFN-β 1b effectiveness against the corona virus (64). However, the use of this interferon for the treatment of Covid-19 is still not approved by different international healthcare organizations. To date, IFN-αs are approved for the treatment of hairy cell leukemia, follicular lymphoma, malignant melanoma, condylomata acuminata (genital warts), AIDS-related Kaposi sarcoma, and chronic hepatitis B and C; IFN-βs for multiple sclerosis; and IFN-γ for chronic granulomatous disease and malignant osteopetrosis (62). In addition, off-label use of IFN-α is prevalent in many cancers, especially in bladder and renal cancers, often as an adjuvant in conjunction with other therapeutics (62). As immunomodulators, interferons can enhance the function of B and T lymphocytes, the activity of natural killer (NK) cells, and increase the activity of macrophages. They also activate humeral immunity such as interferons and tumor necrosis factor, and regulate the expression of several hundred different genes (61).

A common adverse reaction to the interferons (IFN-α, IFN-β, IFN-γ) is lymphopenia, neuropsychiatric symptoms, anorexia, nausea, diarrhea, mild alanine transaminase elevations, common flu-like symptoms (headache, malaise, fever, chills, fatigue, myalgia, back and joint pain) (61–63). These acute side effects are generally temporary, but other grave side effects are also signaled such as autoimmune hemolytic anemia, collagen vascular disease, and thyroid function decline, as well as immune-related nephritis (61).

Since interferons are mainly produced by many immune cells (macrophages, monocytes), eating some foods rich in immunostimulants such as beta-glucans in yeasts and mushrooms, or probiotics in yogurt, kefir, milk, and cheese, might enhance the production of interferons in normal subjects.

3.2.3.5 Sources of Proteins and Amino Acids

Proteins can be found in a wide range of food (animals, plants, microalgae, mushrooms and their byproducts). However, the quantity of proteins and the distribution of amino acids in proteins can vary greatly in different species. Complete proteins are found in meats, fish, poultry, eggs, milk, and cheese, while proteins present in plant foods are incomplete proteins and are of a lower biologic quality than those found in animal foods (5). Even so, some plant foods are important sources of protein such as soybeans, navy beans, pinto beans, split peas, chickpeas, peanuts corn, grains, nuts, sunflower seeds, and sesame seeds (5). The soybean is notable not only for its total protein content but the quality of soy protein which is higher than that of other plant proteins and similar to animal protein; therefore, soy is often consumed by vegans and vegetarians (47, 65). Soy foods such as tofu, natto (a fermented soybean), and soy milk, have long been recognized as sources of high-quality protein and healthful fat, but over the past 25 years these foods have been rigorously investigated for their role in chronic disease prevention and treatment (65).

There are two kinds of meat: red meat and white meat. Red meats are obtained from mammals such as beef, pork, goat, and rabbit. White meats include poultry and sea foods. Keep in mind that most animal proteins resemble human proteins in their amino acid constitution, especially essential amino acids. Although red meats are high in proteins, they usually are accompanied by bad fats such as saturated fatty acids and low-density lipoprotein (LDL), or bad cholesterol. Therefore, high intake of red meat and processed meats (ham, sausage, bacon, etc.) might increase risks of heart disease, stroke, and cancer (see Chapters 6 and 8 of this book).

Eggs and milk are the best sources of proteins and non-carcinogens. However, egg yolk is rich in cholesterol. Therefore, limiting egg consumption to about seven eggs a week may be helpful for the health of normal adults.

On a worldwide basis, plant protein foods contribute over 60% of the per capita supply of protein, on average (1). Plant sources of proteins include legumes (lucernes, peas, beans, lentils, lupines, soybeans, peanuts, tamarinds, etc.), nuts, seeds, and fruits. These vegetarian foods are high in protein with protein concentrations greater than 7% (1). Other seeds and nuts rich in proteins and amino acids are: kidney beans, white beans, chickpeas, cowpeas, lima beans, pigeon peas, lupines, wing beans, almonds, Brazil nuts, cashews, pecans, walnuts, pumpkin seeds, hemp seeds, sesame seeds, chia seeds, and sunflower seeds. Fruits rich in proteins and amino acids include avocado, jackfruit, banana, cherries, kiwi, orange, pomegranate, raspberries, peaches, nectarines, currants, and grapefruits. Plant foods have advantages over animal foods regarding the prevention of harmful chronic diseases such as cardiovascular diseases, cancer, and obesity thanks to their low saturated fats and cholesterol. Indeed, vegans can obtain all essential amino acids by eating a variety of plant proteins.

For normal consumers, a diet composed of different animal and plant foods with a predominance of vegetables and fruits is the best way to obtain all different amino acids necessary for protein construction in the body and also to avoid some chronic diseases.

3.3 Lipids

Lipids, comprising fats and oils, are essential and nonessential macronutrients for the human body. Lipids are organic compounds mainly constituted of carbon, hydrogen, and oxygen. Lipids perform three primary biological functions within the body: they serve as structural components of cell membranes, function as energy stores within cells, and function as important signaling molecules (66–69). Lipids yield much more energy than carbohydrates and proteins. In fact, one gram of lipid supplies nine kcal, while one gram of carbohydrate or protein gives only four kcal (5, 67–69).

From a chemical point of view, lipids are esters of fatty acids with organic alcohols such as glycerol, cholesterol, and sphingosine. Because lipids are mostly water insoluble, they circulate in the blood stream in the form of lipoproteins, which are composed of cholesteryl esters, triacyl-glycerols, and phospholipids (70). Non-esterified fatty acids are bound to plasma albumin. Fatty acids in the form of phospholipids (mainly phosphatidylcholine, phosphatidylethanolamine, and sphingomyelin) form the backbone of all cell membranes and are essential for their fluidity and functionality (70).

Classification of lipid structures is based on their physical properties, their polarity, their essentiality for humans and their structure (68). For example, at room temperature, oils are liquid and obtained from plants, while fats are solid and often present in animals. Based on polarity, neutral lipids include fatty acids, triglycerides, and sterols, whereas polar lipids include glycerophospholipids and glyceroglycolipids. The separation into polarity classes is rather arbitrary, as some short-chain fatty acids are very polar. Based on their structure, there are simple lipids and complex lipids (68). According to Fahy et al., lipids are divided into different categories such as fatty acyls, glycerolipids, glycerophospholipids, sphingolipids, sterol lipids, prenol lipids, saccharolipids, and polyketides (66). Each category contains distinct classes and subclasses of molecules.

Based on their essentiality for humans, most unsaturated fatty acids are essential, while saturated fatty acids and cholesterol are nonessential.

In general, lipids may be divided into four main categories: fatty acids, triglycerides or triacylglycerols, glycerophospholipids and sterols.

3.3.1 Fatty Acids

Fatty acids are carboxylic acids with a typical RCOOH structure, containing a methyl (-CH$_3$) nonpolar, hydrophobic end that is insoluble in water, a hydrocarbon chain (R), and a carboxylic (-COOH) polar, hydrophilic terminus that is soluble in water (69–72). Fatty acids are the building blocks for simple and complex lipids and constitute the obvious starting point in lipid structures (66–68). Fatty acids have different chain lengths and different compositions. Foods have fatty acids with chain lengths between 4 and 24 carbons (67). When the carbon chain length is shorter, the melting point of the fatty acid becomes lower, and the fatty acid becomes more liquid. Fatty acids are vital for the normal functioning of all body systems such as the circulatory system, respiratory system, immune system, brain, and so on (67).

3.3.1.1 Classification of Fatty Acids

Fatty acids are either saturated or unsaturated carboxylic acids with carbon chains varying between 2 and 36 carbon atoms (70–72). From C2 to C6, fatty acids such as acetic acid (C2), propionic acid (C3), butyric acid (C4), pentanoic acid or valeric acid (C5), and hexanoic acid or caproic acid (C6), are water-soluble or slightly water-soluble. Those more than C6 are water insoluble, but soluble in organic solvents such as alcohols and ethyl ether. The fatty acid components of lipids are classified as short-chain (less than 6 carbons), medium-chain (6 to 10 carbons), or long-chain (12 or more carbons). More than 90% of the fatty acids have an even number of carbon atoms. Fatty acids are also classified as saturated (lacking double bonds), monounsaturated (containing a single double bond), or polyunsaturated (containing more than one double bond) (67, 70). The polyunsaturated fatty acids

(PUFA) are subdivided into those whose first double bond occurs either three carbon atoms from the methyl carbon (n-3 also called omega-3 or ω-3) or six carbon atoms from the methyl carbon (n-6 or omega-6 or ω-6). The major saturated fatty acids in foods include lauric acid (C12), myristic acid (C14), palmitic acid (C16), stearic acid (C18), and arachidic acid (C20). The major monounsaturated omega-7 and omega-9 fatty acids are palmitoleic acid (C16, 1=) and oleic acid (C18, 1=), respectively. The major omega-6 PUFAs in plant foods are linoleic acid (C18, 2=), gamma-linolenic acid (GLA, C18, and 3=), and arachidonic acid (AA, C20, 4 =). The major omega-3 PUFAs are linolenic acid or alpha-linolenic acid (ALA, C18 and 3=), eicosapentaenoic acid (EPA, C20 and 5=), and docosahexaenoic acid (DHA, C22 and 6=) (68, 70–73). EPA and DHA are mainly found in seafood, microalgae, and plankton. Fish cannot produce omega-3 fatty acids by itself, but accumulate them by consuming microalgae or plankton.

Fatty acids are also divided into two groups: essential fatty acids and nonessential fatty acids. Nonessential fatty acids are fatty acids that are made in the human body in sufficient amounts, while essential fatty acids are compounds that cannot be synthetized by our cells and organs and must be imported from the diet. Most saturated fatty acids are nonessential, while a majority of unsaturated fatty acids are essential macronutrients (67). In animal and plant tissues, the most abundant fatty acids are those with 16 and 18 carbon atoms – palmitic, stearic, oleic and linoleic – and half of them are unsaturated and contain 1–6 double bonds in cis configuration (70–72). However, fatty acids with chain lengths shorter than 14 and longer than 22 carbon atoms are present only in minor concentrations (70). Here are the chemical structures of some fatty acids:

- Stearic acid ($C_{18}H_{36}O_2$) is a saturated fatty acid with 18 C and more abundant in animal fats than vegetal fats: CH_3-CH_2-CH_2-CH_2-CH_2-CH_2-CH_2-CH_2-CH_2-CH_2-CH_2-CH_2-CH_2-CH_2-CH_2-CH_2-CH_2-COOH
- Palmitoleic acid ($C_{16}H_{30}O_2$) or $CH_3(CH_2)_5CH=CH(CH_2)_7COOH$, is a C16 omega-7 monounsaturated fatty acid with 1 double bond between C7 and C8 and found in oil of macadamia nut and sea buckthorn.
- Oleic acid ($C_{18}H_{34}O_2$) or $CH_3(CH_2)_7CH=CH(CH_2)_7COOH$, is a C18 omega-9 monounsaturated fatty acid with 1 double bond between C9 and C10. It is present in vegetable oils, especially in olive oil.
- Linoleic acid (LA) ($C_{18}H_{32}O_2$) is a C18 omega-6 polyunsaturated fatty acid (PUFA) with two double bonds at C6 and C9. It is an essential fatty acid and abundant in plant oils, seeds, and nuts:
  - CH_3-CH_2-CH_2-CH_2-CH_2-CH=CH-CH_2-CH=CH-CH_2-CH_2-CH_2-CH_2-CH_2-CH_2-CH_2-COOH
- Gamma-linolenic acid (GLA) ($C_{18}H_{30}O_2$) is a C18 omega-6 PUFA with 3 double bonds at C6, C9 and C12, or all-*cis*-6, 9, 12-octadecatrienoic acid. The human body produces GLA from linoleic acid by an enzyme called desaturase:
  - CH_3-CH_2-CH_2-CH_2-CH_2-CH=CH-CH_2-CH=CH-CH_2-CH=CH-CH_2-CH_2-CH_2-CH_2-COOH
- Arachidonic acid (AA) ($C_{20}H_{32}O_2$) is a C20 omega-6 PUFA with 4 double bonds at C6, C9, C12, and C15. It is a conditionally essential fatty acid:
  - CH_3-CH_2-CH_2-CH_2-CH_2-CH=CH-CH_2-CH=CH-CH_2-CH=CH-CH_2-CH=CH-CH_2-CH_2- CH_2-COOH
- Alpha-linolenic acid (ALA) ($C_{18}H_{30}O_2$) is an essential C18 omega-3 polyunsaturated fatty acid with 3 double bonds at C3, C6, and C9. It is abundant in seed oils (chia, flaxseed, soybean, etc.):
  - CH_3-CH_2-CH=CH-CH_2-CH=CH-CH_2-CH=CH-CH_2-CH_2-CH_2-CH_2-CH_2-CH_2-CH_2-COOH

$$-\overset{\overset{\displaystyle H}{|}}{C}=\overset{\underset{\displaystyle H}{|}}{C}-$$

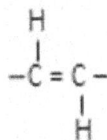

FIGURE 1.3A Trans-isomer.

$$-\overset{\overset{\displaystyle H}{|}}{C}\equiv\overset{\overset{\displaystyle H}{|}}{C}-$$

FIGURE 1.3B Cis-isomer.

Here are the chemical structures of two essential omega-3 fatty acids mainly obtained from seafoods:

- Eicosapentaenoic acid (EPA) ($C_{20}H_{30}O_2$) contains 20 C and 5 double bonds:
  - $CH_3CH_2CH=CHCH_2CH=CHCH_2CH=CHCH_2CH=CHCH_2CH=CH(CH_2)_3COOH$
- Docosahexaenoic acid (DHA) ($C_{22}H_{32}O_2$) contains 22 C and 6 double bonds:
  - $CH_3CH_2CH=CHCH_2CH=CHCH_2CH=CHCH_2CH=CHCH_2CH=CHCH_2CH=CH(CH_2)_2$ COOH

In nature, all double bonds of unsaturated fatty acids are in cis configuration (Figure 1.3A). This means that the two H atoms at the double bond of an unsaturated fatty acid are oriented in the same direction (67–69).

In trans isomers, the 2 H atoms are oriented in the opposite direction of the double bond (Figure 1.3B). They are produced during industrial processing (hydrogenation) of unsaturated oils and in the gastrointestinal tract of ruminants (67–69).

3.3.1.2 Roles of Fatty Acids

Fatty acids (FA) play multiple roles in human and other organisms like plants, animals, bacteria, and so on. Most importantly, FA are a substantial part of lipids, one of the three major components of macronutrients (along with proteins and carbohydrates). Fatty acids are also important energy substrates comprising around 30% of total energy intake for humans (70–75). They can be stored in excess amounts in adipose tissue, especially when increased dietary intake of fat results in obesity (70).

In humans, fatty acids have a number of physiological roles as: energy substrates, structural and functional components of cell membranes, precursors for lipid mediators, and components affecting signal transduction pathways and gene transcription (70–75). Some fatty acids are not only essential dietary nutrients but also contribute to various physiological processes (74). Certain saturated fatty acids are involved in numerous cellular signaling and stabilization processes in the body. For example, myristic acid, a 14-carbon saturated fatty acid, is a source of myristoyl groups utilized within the body to stabilize many different proteins, including proteins in the immune system, and to fight tumors (74). Myristoleic acid, a metabolite of myristic acid, is known to be cytotoxic to tumor cells such as prostate cancer cells (74). Palmitic acid, a 16-carbon saturated fatty acid, is involved in palmitoylation of protein. This palmitoylated protein formed plays important roles in numerous cellular processes, including signaling, apoptosis, and neuronal transmission, and is used to fight degenerative Huntington's disease, T-cell mediated immune disorder, and cancer (74). However, excess consumption of palmitic acid, myristic acid, and other saturated fatty acids, increases the risk of developing hypercholesterolemia, cardiovascular disease and cancer.

Short chain saturated fatty acids, including acetic, propionic, and butyric acids, are formed during fiber fermentation in the proximal colon. They are quickly absorbed by portal circulation and transported to the liver where they are transformed into glucose. Importantly, butyric and partially also propionic acids are used in metabolism, proliferation and restoration of colon cells (70). Other functions of short chain saturated fatty acids in the colon also include stimulation of water, sodium, chloride and bicarbonate absorption and blood flow through mucous membrane of the colon. Other roles are proliferation of colon cells, mucus production, limited reproduction of saprophytic bacteria and putrefaction due to decreased acidity (70). As previously cited, long chain saturated fatty acids such as lauric, myristic, palmitic and stearic acids have significant atherogenic and thrombogenic potentials and increase levels of cholesterol, especially low-density lipoprotein (LDL) cholesterol or 'bad' cholesterol (70). These saturated fatty acids are mainly abundant in butter, lard, beef tallow, poultry skin, coconut oil, cocoa butter, palm kernel oil, chocolate, and so on.

The main unsaturated fatty acids include omega-3, omega-6, omega-7, and omega-9 fatty acids. Only omega-3 and omega-6 are polyunsaturated fatty acids (PUFAs) and are essential nutrients. In contrast, omega-7 and omega-9 FAs are monounsaturated and are nonessential. As the human body cannot make omega-3 and omega-6 fatty acids, it must get them through foods. Otherwise, the body cannot function normally and many diseases may develop. The roles of omega-3 and omega-6 PUFAs are described below.

3.3.1.3 Omega-3 Fatty Acid Family

3.3.1.3.1 Chemical Structure   Omega-3 (ω-3) fatty acids, also called n-3 fatty acids, are polyunsaturated fatty acids (PUFA) having a first double bond (C=C) at the third carbon atom counting the terminal -CH_3 carbon as carbon number one (76–80). As with most natural fatty acids, all double bonds are in the cis-configuration, in other words, the two hydrogen atoms are on the same side of the double bond (73). Other PUFA found in nature are omega-6, omega-7, and omega-9 fatty acids. The two last PUFA are not essential and rarely consumed. Only omega-3 and omega-6 fatty acids are considered essential long-chain PUFA because the human and mammal body cannot synthesize them due to the lack of delta-12 and delta-15 (omega-3) desaturases (80). They are only obtained from food and have an important role in human physiology and health maintenance (76–92).

3.3.1.3.2 Classification   There are three major dietary types of omega-3 fatty acids: alpha-linoleic acid (ALA), eicosapentaenoic acid (EPA), and docosahexaenoic acid (DHA) (76–88). Among these three PUFA, ALA [18:3(n-3)], is the shortest with 18 carbon atoms and three double bonds, then EPA, [20:5(n-3)], with 20 carbon atoms and 5 double bonds, and DHA, [22:6(n-3)], the longest, with 22 carbon atoms and 6 double bonds (76–78). EPA and DHA are long chain PUFA and abundant in seafood (fish, fish oils, crustaceans) and are directly used by the body; while ALA is mostly found in plant foods (nuts, seeds, oils), and needs to be converted into the EPA or DHA to become useful for the human body (73, 75–85). The conversion of ALA to EPA and DHA is regulated by two enzymes, D5 and D6 desaturase in the human liver. However, humans are able to convert only a small portion of fatty acids to more than 20-carbon PUFAs; the conversion rates of 18-carbon fatty acids to EPA and from ALA to DHA were reported to be 5–10% and less than 1%, respectively (73, 78–80). Moreover, this conversion process may be almost non-existent in elderly people. When ALA is not completely converted to EPA or DHA, it remains inactive and is simply stored or used as energy, like other fats. However, EPA and DHA directly produced by the human body from their precursor ALA in vegetable food may become more potent than those prefabricated in seafood or fish oil. Therefore, vegetable food rich in ALA such as flaxseed oils may be reserved for young people, while seafood such as fish, crustacean, seaweeds, and fish oil can be used for everybody and mostly for elderly people. Thus, the health effects of omega-3 fatty acids are due mostly to the active forms of EPA and DHA rather than to their precursor ALA.

In nature, omega-3 fatty acids are mainly esterified either in glycerophospholipids (GPLs) or tri-glycerides (TGs); the carboxylic -COOH group of omega-3 fatty acid is combined with the alcohol -OH of glycerol because free omega-3 fatty acids are highly unstable. TGs are highly hydropho-bic, whereas GPLs are hydrophilic due to the polar head group of phosphate (79, 80). Hence, the physical-chemical properties of these two lipid groups are different, and only glycerophospholipids (GPLs) are able to form micelles and liposomes. There is some evidence that GPLs might be a more efficient delivery form of EPA and DHA omega-3 fatty acids to the brain than TGs (80). In fish and natural fish oil, EPA and DHA are in triglyceride form (TG), while in humans, they are in glycero-phospholipid form (GPL).

3.3.1.3.3   Sources   The main sources of omega-3 fatty acids rich in EPA and DHA include sea-food such as salmon, mackerel, halibut, sardines, tuna, herring, eel, cod, anchovies, menhaden, shrimp, krill, sturgeon, fish roe, and seaweeds. (76–80). Oils extracted from the flesh or the liver of these fish are also a main source of omega-3 fatty acids and are often used as dietary supplements in capsule form. Cod liver oil is a rich natural source of active omega-3 EPA and DHA, as well as vitamins A and D. Squid oil (calamari oil) and krill oil are also other sources of these PUFA. However, certain big fishes like shark, swordfish, and tilefish, are to be avoided because of their high mercury levels (see Chapter 6 of this book). Be sure to buy fish oil supplements made by natural tri-glyceride form and not artificial ethyl ester form obtained from ethanol. Fish oil supplements must be free of heavy metals (mercury, lead, cadmium) and fat-soluble pollutants like polychlorinated biphenyls (PCBs) and dioxins (see Chapter 6 of this book). In general, the overall amount of EPA and DHA is lower in farmed fish than in wild fish because farmed fish feed primarily with grains made by vegetables and vegetable oils, in contrast to wild fish, which feed on natural marine algae and plankton (78, 80). It is noteworthy that marine algae and seaweeds are the unique plants which can directly make active EPA and DHA omega-3 fatty acids, while land plants only make ALA, a precursor of EPA and DHA. Although fish are a dietary source of these PUFA, fish do not synthe-size them; they obtain them from the algae and plankton in their diets. Chicken and beef meat also contain omega-3 fatty acids, but in small amounts (76). The main sources of short ALA omega-3 fatty acids are found in many plant foods such as chia seeds, flax seeds, canola (rapeseed) oil, soy-beans, pumpkin seeds, hemp seeds, purslane, perilla seed oil, peanut, walnuts, walnut oil, kale, and spinach (75–76, 78–80). Brown and green algae are the main plant foods rich in EPA and DHA (see algae in Chapter 5).

Most fish oil supplements are natural byproducts extracted directly from sea fish. The extract containing triglyceride form will be hydrolyzed into free omega-3 fatty acids for their concentra-tion, then the last ones will be recombined again either with glycerol or ethanol for their final stable forms, glyceryl ester or ethyl ester, respectively. Natural triglycerides are the form that occur natu-rally in fish oil, whereas ethyl esters are the synthesized form. Natural triglycerides have somewhat higher bioavailability than artificial ethyl esters (76). Certain producers of fish oil supplements prefer the ethyl form because the preparation from alcohol is cheaper than that of using glycerol. However, the natural form is more efficacious than the artificial form in therapy due to its good absorption in the digestive tract of humans.

3.3.1.3.4   Roles in Human Health   The dietary intake of EPA and DHA is essential as they are extensively associated with optimal human health and protection against disease. Omega-3 fatty acids have been linked to healthy aging throughout life. Deficiency in omega-3 fatty acids is associated with inflammatory diseases, autoimmune diseases, mental diseases, cardiovascular diseases, diabetes, cancer, osteoporosis, macular degeneration, cataract, aging, reproductive sys-tem dysfunctions, skin disorders, and other ailments (76–91). EPA and DHA have a wide range of physiological roles, which are linked to certain health or clinical benefits, particularly related to CVD, cancer, inflammation and neurocognitive function (77). Recently, fish-derived omega-3 fatty acids EPA and DHA have been associated with fetal development, cardiovascular function, weight management, and cognitive function such as Alzheimer's disease (78). Studies have shown that EPA and DHA are important for proper fetal development, including neuronal, retinal, and immune function, and may affect many aspects of cardiovascular function including peripheral artery disease, coronary events, and anticoagulation (78).

Concerning inflammatory diseases and asthma, animal experiments and clinical studies indicate that omega-3 fatty acids have anti-inflammatory properties and, therefore, might be useful in the treatment of asthma, inflammation, and autoimmune diseases (77–84). Animal and human studies support the hypothesis that omega-3 PUFA suppress cell mediated immune responses or Type IV hypersensitivity which is the cause of chronic inflammation like allergic asthma (78–84). There have been a number of clinical trials assessing the benefits of dietary supplementation with fish oils in several inflammatory and autoimmune diseases in humans, including asthma, rheumatoid arthritis, Crohn's disease, ulcerative colitis, psoriasis, systemic lupus erythematosus, multiple sclerosis, and migraine headaches (78, 81–83). Many of the placebo-controlled trials of fish oil in chronic inflammatory diseases reveal significant benefit, including decreased disease activity and a lowered use of anti-inflammatory drugs (78, 83–84). Several studies have reported that the two main bioactive metabolites (resolvin and protectin) of omega-3 fatty acids (EPA, DHA) played beneficial effects in the treatment of allergic asthma and chronic lung inflammation (81). The balance of omega-3 and omega-6 fatty acid levels plays important roles in the trigger of inflammatory diseases like asthma (82). Patients with autoimmune diseases such as rheumatoid arthritis and inflammatory bowel disease usually respond to fish oil supplementation by decreasing the elevated levels of cytokines (78, 83–84). Pure EPA and DHA can inhibit the production of a range of inflammatory proteins, including cyclooxygenase-2 (COX-2), inducible nitric oxide (NO) synthase, tumor necrosis factor α (TNFα), interleukins (IL): IL-1, IL-6, IL-8, and IL-12 in cultured endothelial cells, monocytes, macrophages, and dendritic cells (77–78, 82).

Concerning mental diseases, several epidemiological studies reported a significant inverse correlation between intake of oily fish and depression or bipolar disorders (77–78, 85–86). However, studies conducted specifically on the association between omega-3 intake and depression reported contrasting results, suggesting that the preventive role of omega-3 fatty acids may depend also on other factors, such as overall diet quality and social environment (78, 85–86). As omega-3 fatty acids can cross cerebral membrane, they are highly concentrated in the brain and appear to be important for cognitive (brain memory and performance) and behavioral function. DHA is a major brain ω-3 fatty acid and is also found in the eyeball (retina). The brain is made up of about 60% fat, of which about 50% is DHA. In fact, infants who do not get enough omega-3 fatty acids from their mothers during pregnancy are at risk for developing vision and nerve problems (78). Indeed, omega-3 fatty acids can be effective both in preventing or treating depression and other mental diseases such as age-related cognitive decline or dementia, including Alzheimer disease and attention deficit/hyperactivity disorder (77–78, 85). Moreover, omega-3 fatty acids in seafood and fish oil could improve the intelligence of children as well as the memory of the elderly.

Regarding the beneficial effects of omega-3 fatty acids in cardiovascular disease (CVD), their role is well established (77, 87–90). Clinical studies suggested that omega-3 fatty acids found in fish oil have reduced risk factors for heart disease, including high cholesterol and high blood pressure (87–90). Fish oil has been shown to lower levels of triglycerides (fats in the blood), and to lower the risk of death, heart attack, stroke, and abnormal heart rhythms in people who have already had a heart attack. Fish oil also appears to help prevent and treat atherosclerosis (hardening of the arteries) by slowing the development of plaque and blood clots, which can clog arteries (87–90). Three prospective epidemiological studies within populations reported that men who ate at least some fish weekly had a lower coronary heart disease (CHD) mortality rate than that of men who ate none (88). Inuit peoples in Arctic regions, who get high amounts of omega-3 fatty acids from eating fatty fish, also tend to have increased HDL (good) cholesterol and decreased triglycerides (fats in the blood), hence, their cardiovascular diseases are the lowest in the world (78, 91). Japanese and Inuit have a high dietary intake of fresh seafood rich in long chain omega-3 fatty acids and a low incidence of myocardial infarction and chronic inflammatory or autoimmune disorders, even when compared to their Westernized ethnic counterparts (91). People who follow a Mediterranean-style diet tend to have higher HDL (good) cholesterol levels, which help promote heart health. Other epidemiological studies reported that fish consumption was associated with a reduced risk in cardiovascular mortality, ischemic heart disease, stroke mortality, and cognitive decline with normal aging across the world (87, 91). Some authors reported a dose-response relationship between the frequency of weekly fish intake and reduced CVD risk factors such as hypertension, obesity, and hyperglycemia in a study of Japanese living in Japan or Brazil (87).

The American Heart Association (AHA) recommends eating fish (particularly fatty fish like mackerel, pollock, lake trout, herring, sardines, albacore tuna, and salmon) at least two times a week for the prevention of CVD (87–88). Eating at least two servings of sea fish per week can reduce the risk of stroke by as much as 50%. Some evidence suggests that people with certain circulatory problems, such as varicose veins, may benefit from the consumption of EPA and DHA, which may stimulate blood circulation and increase the breakdown of fibrin, a protein involved in blood clotting and scar formation (87).

Several clinical studies show that fish oil supplements and diets rich in omega-3 fatty acids reduce triglyceride levels and also modestly lower blood pressure in patients, but do not significantly change the level of LDL (bad) cholesterol or HDL (good) cholesterol in the blood (76–78). It is noteworthy that ALA alone, an omega-3 precursor of EPA and DHA, mainly found in seeds and nuts, does not confer the cardiovascular health benefits of EPA and DHA.

According to some authors, antioxidant properties of n-3 PUFAs, along with their anti-inflammatory effect in both blood vessels and cardiac cells, seem to exert beneficial effects in cardiovascular impairment (76–77). In fact, dietary supplementation with n-3 PUFAs has been demonstrated to reduce oxidative stress-related mitochondrial dysfunction and endothelial cell apoptosis, an effect occurring via an increased activity of endogenous antioxidant enzymes (76). However, the explanation about the antioxidant activity of EPA and DHA needs further confirmations.

Briefly, omega-3 fatty acids in sea food, fish oil, some seeds, and nuts, are strong essential nutrients for our body and play important and beneficial roles, mostly in the prevention and treatment of chronic ailments such as inflammation (asthma), cardiovascular diseases, mental disorders and fetal development. Further research investigations are necessary to understand their action mechanisms in these dreadful ailments. However, high doses of fish oil and omega-3 fatty acid supplements along with more than three grams of omega-3 fatty acids per day might increase the risk of bleeding and hemorrhagic stroke. Consult a physician when combining anticoagulant drugs (warfarin, aspirin, heparin, etc.) with fish oil supplement. Fish oil may lower blood pressure, therefore, people with hypotension must inform their doctor before taking fish oil with blood pressure-lowering medications.

3.3.1.4 Omega-6 Fatty Acid Family

3.3.1.4.1 Chemical Structure   Omega-6 (ω-6) fatty acids, also called n-6 fatty acids, are polyunsaturated fatty acids (PUFA) having a double bond (C=C) at the sixth carbon atom from the end of the carbon chain. Omega-6 fatty acids are essential fatty acids because they are necessary for human health, our body cannot produce them, and we must get them through food (73, 92–95).

The parent of omega-6 fatty acid family is linoleic acid (LA) (18:2, *n*−6), with 2 double bonds (C=C) and 18 carbon atoms. Its main metabolic products are gamma-linolenic (GLA) (18:3, *n*−6) with 3 C=C and 18 C, dihomo-gamma-linolenic (DHGLA) (20:3, *n*−6) with 3 C=C and 20 C, and arachidonic acid (AA) (20:4, *n*−6) with 4 C=C and 20 C. Linoleic acid is converted to gamma-linolenic acid in the body, and can then break down further to arachidonic acid, while GLA is metabolized into DHGLA (73, 92–95).

3.3.1.4.2   Biological Roles   The enzymatic oxidation of some omega-6 fatty acids such as arachidonic acid (AA) liberated from phospholipids has been shown to yield potent pathological agents by two major pathways of lipid peroxidation: the cyclooxygenase (COX) or prostaglandin (PG) pathway and the lipoxygenase pathway (93). The first way engenders prostaglandin E2 (PGE2), thromboxane A2, and prostacyclin, which are potential inflammatory mediators (92–93). The second route yields a new class of arachidonic acid oxygenation products called the leukotrienes, which also appear to be important inflammatory mediators (93–94). In contrast, gamma-linolenic acid (GLA) is recently discovered as an anti-inflammatory agent because much of the GLA taken through food or supplement is converted in the body to a substance called DGLA (Dihomo-Gamma-Linolenic Acid) that fights inflammation (73, 92–93). Magnesium, zinc, and vitamins C, B3, and B6 help promote the conversion of GLA to DGLA to fight inflammatory diseases (92). Along with omega-3s, omega-6 fatty acids play a crucial role in health maintenance such as brain function, bone formation, skin stimulation, hair growth, metabolism regulation, and reproductive system maintenance (92–93). Omega-6s also improve diabetic neuropathy, eczema, psoriasis, osteoporosis, and breast tenderness (mastalgia), and aid in breast and prostate cancer treatment (92).

3.3.1.4.3   Source   The major natural source of omega-6 fatty acids is vegetable oils such palm, rapeseed, soybean, and sunflower oils which are richer in omega-6 linoleic acid (LA) than in omega-3 alpha-linolenic acid (ALA) (73, 92–94). Other sources of omega-6s include soybeans, corn, cereals, poultry, eggs, nuts, whole bread, pumpkin seeds, walnuts, and cashews. Gamma-linolenic acid (GLA) is found in several plant-based oils, including evening primrose oil, borage oil, and black currant seed oil. The average diet provides plenty of omega-6 acids, so supplements are usually not necessary, contrary to EPA and DHA omega-3 acids (73, 92). People with ailments such as eczema, psoriasis, arthritis, diabetes, breast cancer, and mastalgia may have to ask their doctors before taking omega-6 supplements (92).

3.3.1.5   Importance of the Ratio of Omega-6/Omega-3 Essential Fatty Acids in the Body
The omega-6 and omega-3 fatty acids are metabolically distinct and have opposing physiologic functions (92–95). Different intakes of omega-6 and omega-3 polyunsaturated fatty acids (PUFAs) result in different levels of PUFAs in cell membrane phospholipids from where they exert actions on cell functions and cell and tissue responsiveness to signals (95). PUFAs may act as antioxidants by regulating the antioxidant signaling pathway and may modulate inflammatory processes (95). In addition to their antioxidant and anti-inflammatory roles, omega-3 fatty acids are considered to regulate platelet homeostasis and lower risk of thrombosis, which together indicate their potential use in Covid-19 therapy (95). Covid-19 is a severe acute respiratory infectious disease caused by a novel coronavirus strain, SARS-CoV-2 (Severe Acute Respiratory Syndrome Coronavirus-2), in 2019. However, the use of omega-3 fatty acids in Covid-19 therapy is still not recognized by different international healthcare organizations; it was only assayed in some clinical studies.

Omega-6 linoleic acid (LA) is abundant in the diets of most people. Diets too high in omega-6 LA and too low in omega-3 fatty acids may lead to chronic inflammation, hypertension and blood clotting tendency that increases the risk of heart attack and stroke. Increased amount of LA slows down the metabolism of ALA to EPA and DHA by inhibiting $\Delta 6$ desaturase which may also decrease with age (73). The increased omega-6/omega-3 ratio in diets most likely contributes to an increased incidence of inflammatory disorders (muscle pain, rheumatoid arthritis, asthma) and cardiovascular disease. A healthy diet must maintain a balance of omega-6 to omega-3 concentrations in the range of 2:1 to 4:1, or even lower ratio at 1:1 (84, 92–94). An inappropriate balance of these two essential fatty acids contributes to the development of disease while a proper balance helps maintain and even improve health (94). Omega-3 fatty acids help reduce inflammation, and most omega-6 fatty acids, except for gamma-linolenic acid (GLA) and dihomo-gamma-linolenic acid (DGLA), tend to promote inflammation (82, 84, 92). The typical American diet tends to contain 14 to 25 times more omega-6 fatty acids than omega-3 fatty acids, which explains the rising rate of inflammatory disorders and cardiovascular diseases in the USA (75, 83–84, 92). In contrast, the Mediterranean diet has a healthier balance between omega-3 and omega-6 fatty acids, comprising a large amount of seafood and other natural food such as fresh fruits and vegetables, garlic and moderate red wine consumption (78). Therefore, most people in the Mediterranean area as well as in Japan have better health and longer life spans than other people in the world (see Chapter 8 of this book).

Besides their opposition properties cited above, the two essential omega-3 and omega-6 fatty acids play an important role in the composition of all cell membranes where they maintain homeostasis for correct membrane protein function and influence membrane fluidity in cell signaling processes, cellular functions and gene expression (93–97). Furthermore, arachidonic acid, an omega-6 fatty acid, is also as important in brain development and cognitive function as DHA, an omega-3 fatty acid (95). In brief, a balanced omega-6/omega-3 ratio is important for health maintenance and in the prevention of many diseases such as obesity, cancer, cardiovascular disease, neurodegenerative diseases, and so on (95–97).

3.3.1.6   Eicosanoids: Prostaglandins, Thromboxanes, Leukotrienes

Eicosanoids, bioactive signaling lipids, are oxidized derivatives of 20-carbon polyunsaturated fatty acids (PUFAs) formed by the action of different enzymes such as the cyclooxygenase (COX), lipoxygenase (LOX), and cytochrome P450 (cytP450) pathways (98–102). Eicosa- comes from the Greek word for 'twenty'. They are also obtained via non-enzymatic free radical mechanisms (99). Arachidonic acid (AA) and other omega-3 or omega-6 PUFAs are the usual substrates for eicosanoid synthesis (95–102).

The cyclooxygenase pathways (COX 1 and 2) initiate the metabolism of omega-6 fatty acids (arachidonic acid, dihomo-gamma-linoleic acid) and omega-3 fatty acids like eicosapentaenoic acid (EPA) to prostanoids, including different prostaglandins, prostacyclins, and thromboxanes (98–102). The lipoxygenase pathways (5-LOX, 12-LOX, 15-LOXa, 15-LOXb) initiate the oxidation of arachidonic acid (AA) of omega-6 fatty acids as well as eicosapentaenoic acid (EPA) of omega-3 fatty acids to different leukotrienes and lipoxins in leukocytes (98–102). The cytochrome P450 pathways comprise a large number of enzymes that contain a heme iron, and are found in the liver and other tissues where they inactivate and eliminate toxins and metabolites and form various epoxy, hydroxy and dihydroxy derivatives. Near hundreds of distinct eicosanoid species are produced from omega-6 and omega-3 metabolism (98–100). Because they are rapidly catabolized (destroyed), eicosanoids mainly act locally to the site of their production. Many eicosanoids have multiple, sometimes pleiotropic, effects on immunity and inflammation (98). They also have roles in the regulation of the vascular, renal, gastrointestinal and female reproductive systems (98). They are also formed when cells are attacked by microbes, viruses, parasites, and so on. The most widely studied is prostaglandin PGE_2. Although eicosanoids are most frequently associated with inflammation, they also have homeostatic functions (99).

Prostanoid includes prostaglandins (PGs) (PGD, PGE and PGF), thromboxane (TXA), and prostacyclin (PGI). These lipids are synthesized from the polyunsaturated fatty acids (PUFAs) dihomo-gamma-linolenic acid (DGLA, precursor of series 1 prostanoids), arachidonic acid (AA, precursor of series 2 prostanoids), and eicosapentaenoic acid (EPA, precursor of series 3 prostanoids). Among these precursors, AA is the most imperative and dominant in humans (102). Prostaglandins, thromboxane, and prostacyclin are universal lipids in animal tissues and organize several pathological and physiological processes. Prostaglandins (PGs) were discovered in 1935 as a blood-pressure-lowering matter from the prostate gland secretion (102). In 1976, prostacyclin was discovered as a powerful repressor of function of platelets, and as a robust vasodilator.

Thromboxane A2 (TXA2) is metabolite of arachidonic acid through thromboxane A synthase 1 action. Thromboxane B2 (TXB2) outcomes from TXA2 degradation and plays an important role in the acetaminophen hepatotoxicity. TxA2 is released by macrophages, neutrophils, and endothelial cells, and has prothrombotic properties such as the activation of platelets and platelet aggregation (102).

Leukotrienes are a family of eicosanoid inflammatory mediators and are synthesized via numerous types of cells comprising leukocytes (white blood cells), spleen, mast cells, and so on. The production of leukotrienes is usually accompanied by the production of histamine and prostaglandins, which also act as inflammatory mediators (102).

Despite their vital role in physiology, these lipid mediators (eicosanoids) are often associated with disease, including inflammatory diseases and cancer (98–102). Inflammation plays a decisive role in various stages of tumor development including initiation, promotion, invasion, and metastasis (101). Dietary fat may contribute to cancer associated inflammation through abnormal arachidonic acid metabolism (100–101). Arachidonic acid can make up to 40% of the fatty acid composition of cancer cell membranes. Eicosanoid biosynthesis and actions can be directly influenced by nutrients in the diet, as evidenced by the emerging role of omega-3 fatty acids in cancer prevention and treatment. The anti-tumorigenic effects of omega-3 polyunsaturated fatty acids (PUFAs) may be partly mediated by their anti-inflammatory effects. Omega-3 PUFAs inhibit carcinogenesis associated with a reduction in proinflammatory cytokines (100).

Since the human body lacks the enzymes needed to synthesize the polyunsaturated fatty acids (PUFAs), α-linolenic (ALA) and linoleic acids (LA) in the diet are its only source. The rate of conversion of α-linolenic omega-3 fatty acid (ALA) into DHA (docosahexaenoic acid) and eicosapentaenoic acid (EPA) is decelerated because of the decreased activity of the $\Delta6$ desaturase in the human body. That is why only 0.2–2% of the dietary ALA is converted into DHA and EPA, while the rest undergoes β-oxidation (102). Therefore, dietary intake of EPA and DHA from fish and crustaceans is needed. EPA and DHA omega-3 acids are also recognized as precursors for the synthesis of novel specialized pro-resolving mediators (SPMs). SPMs include resolvins, protectins, and maresins. Resolvins are synthesized from both EPA and DHA, while maresins and protectins are synthesized from DHA (95). First, EPA and DHA decrease the production of arachidonic acid-derived eicosanoids; then, SPMs activate the resolution of inflammation (95). Hence, a lack of the omega-3 PUFAs, especially EPA and DHA, may not favor resolution of inflammation and may, in fact, promote the pathogenesis of various diseases in which inflammation is involved. Therefore, increased intake of omega-3 fatty acids may decrease inflammation.

Inhibitors that interfere with the synthesis or action of various eicosanoids are used as drugs in disease treatment, especially for inflammatory diseases such as arthritis, asthma, muscular pain, gout, and so on (98–100). Inhibitor drugs including: aspirin; non-steroidal anti-inflammatory drugs (NSAIDs) such as ibuprofen, indomethacin, and diclofenac; and coxibs have been developed for the treatment of pain caused by certain inflammatory diseases. However, the abuse of NSAIDs and coxibs may lead to different side effects such as stomach and duodenum ulcer, ringing in the ears, delays in blood clotting, blood pressure elevation as well as the development of congestive heart failure and acute myocardial infarction (103) (see details in Chapter 8 of this book).

Combining some foods like sea foods, fish oils, seaweeds, resveratrol in red grapes, turmeric, galangal, and omega-3 dietary supplements may prevent or treat some chronic inflammatory diseases. Therefore, many healthcare organizations recommend eating a variety of seafood twice a week for the prevention of many chronic diseases due to inflammation such as arthritis, arthrosis, asthma, and so on.

3.3.1.7 Omega-7 and Omega-9 Monounsaturated Fatty Acids

Omega-7 and omega-9 monounsaturated fatty acids have one carbon-carbon double bond at the C7 and C9 position respectively. The main omega-7 fatty acid is palmitoleic acid, while the main omega-9 is oleic acid (69–71, 104–105). Palmitoleic acid has the formula: $CH_3(CH_2)_5CH=CH(CH_2)_7COOH$ (16 Carbon atoms), while the chemical structure of oleic acid is: $CH_3(CH_2)_7CH=CH(CH_2)_7COOH$ (18 Carbon atoms). Palmitoleic acid (omega-7 FA) is mainly found in oil of macadamia nut and oil of sea buckthorn plant at about 17% and 32–42%, respectively (69, 104). It is also present in salmon (6%), cod liver oil (7%) and in smaller amounts in olive oil, chocolate, and eggs. It is also synthetized by the human body and mainly found in serum and tissues, particularly adipose tissue and liver (104). In the human body, it exists under cis-isoform, but trans-isomer can be found due to exogenous source such as ruminant fat and dairy products (104). Palmitoleate is considered to be a lipokine, because it is released from adipose tissue and exerts its actions on distant organs. Although its role in obesity development and its contribution to liver or cardiovascular health is not clear, decreased incident diabetes is certainly associated with higher palmitoleate concentrations (104).

The primary sources of oleic acid (omega-9 FA) are olive oil, canola oil, rapeseed oil, peanut oil, sweet almond oil, avocado oil, and pistachio (69, 71, 105). Oleic acid has anti-atherogenic and anti-thrombotic properties; it prevents the formation of abnormal fatty deposit on the walls of arteries and it resists the development of blood clot inside blood vessels, respectively (70, 105–106). Oleic acid also increases the resistance to lipid peroxidation, a phenomenon of free radical formation in membrane cells due to the oxidative degradation of lipids. It has been shown to decrease the levels of total cholesterol, low density lipoprotein (LDL)-cholesterol or 'bad' cholesterol, and triglycerides, and is also known to be cardio-protective (70–71, 106). It also regulates insulin sensitivity. Olive oil has also been tested experimentally for its protective role in carcinogenesis and inflammatory phenomena (70–71, 105). Bioactive omega-9 monounsaturated fatty acids, such as oleic acid (OA) and 2-hydroxy oleic acid, also show therapeutic effects in neurotrauma in animal models (106). The relative safe profile of these neuroactive omega-9 fatty acids holds promise for the future clinical development of these molecules as analgesic agents (106).

Both omega-7 and omega-9 fatty acids are nonessential nutrients because the body can make them, and their biological roles occupy a minor place in the body, contrary to omega-3 and omega-6 fatty acids.

3.3.1.8 *Trans-Fatty Acids*

Trans-Fatty Acids (TFA) are unsaturated FAs with at least one unsaturated, non-conjugated double bond in the trans-configuration; two H atoms are oriented in the opposite direction of the double bond (Figure 1.3A). Most unsaturated fatty acids in nature are in the typical cis-configuration (Figure 1.3B) (68, 70–71). However, very small amounts of trans-fat acids are produced by some anaerobic bacteria, predominantly Gram-negative, or are found in beef and cow milk due to the transformation of cis to trans-configuration in the gastrointestinal tract of ruminants (68, 70). But TFA most often comes from the food processing industry, such as margarine and butter manufacturing, and the 'fast-food' (cookies, crackers, chips) industry to prolong shelf-life (67–71, 107).

During food manufacturing, partial hydrogenation of unsaturated fatty acids such as linoleic acid (LA) and alpha-linolenic acid (ALA) in vegetable oils produces trans-fatty acids, which are solid or semisolid at room temperature. The physicochemical properties of TFA are close to those of saturated fatty acids (SFA), therefore TFA affect cell membrane properties similarly to SFA (70). Their atherogenic effect – the formation of fatty deposit in arterial walls – is greater than that of SFA. Also, trans-fatty acids are twice as active in raising LDL-cholesterol and decreasing HDL cholesterol as SFA (67, 70).

Increasing epidemiological and biochemical evidence suggest that excessive trans-fats in the diet are a significant risk factor for coronary heart diseases. A 2% absolute increase in energy intake from trans-fat has been associated with a 23% increase in cardiovascular risk (107). Thus, the American Heart Association recommends limiting trans-fats to less than 1% of energy, and other international healthcare organizations all recommend limiting dietary trans-fat intake from industrial sources as much as possible. Therefore, it is time to promote an effective international intervention to restrict the use of trans-fatty acids in processed foods for the sake of human health.

3.3.2 Triglycerides

Triglycerides belong to the group of glycerolipids formed by the condensation of one, two, or three fatty acids on glycerol, a trihydroxy alcohol. A triglyceride (also called triacylglycerol) is an ester of a glycerol and three fatty acids. It is formed by combining the 3 alcohol -OH groups of a glycerol with the carboxylic -COOH group of 3 fatty acids to give 3 ester bonds (66–68). The 3 fatty acids

(FA) in triglyceride are generally different and most formed by long saturated or unsaturated carbon chain lengths containing from 4 to 24 carbon atoms.

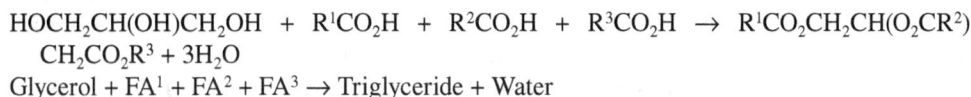

$$HOCH_2CH(OH)CH_2OH + R^1CO_2H + R^2CO_2H + R^3CO_2H \rightarrow R^1CO_2CH_2CH(O_2CR^2)$$
$$CH_2CO_2R^3 + 3H_2O$$

Glycerol + FA^1 + FA^2 + FA^3 → Triglyceride + Water

When the three fatty acids are identical, triglycerides are called homotriglycerides. For example, olein is a triglyceride formed by three oleic acids; stearin, by three stearic acids. Triglycerides are fats and oils in animal and vegetable foods and make up more than 95% of lipids in the diet (67–68). When the esterification of glycerol occurs at one or two alcohol groups, the glyceride formed is called monoglyceride or diglyceride, respectively. However, triglycerides are the most abundant in fat and oil. All glycerides are water insoluble. Vegetable oil is liquid at room temperature because its triglyceride contains a high proportion of unsaturated fatty acids; while fat of animals such as pig, cow, and poultry, is solid because its triglyceride contains a high proportion of saturated fatty acids. However, fat in fish and seafood is liquid because their triglycerides are formed by glycerol with omega-3 fatty acids (EPA, DHA) that are unsaturated fatty acids. Therefore, fish oil supplement and cod liver oil extract are in liquid form.

It is noteworthy that triglycerides come not only from fatty foods, but also from excess of sugar and meat in the diet. Sugar is easily transformed into triglycerides as stock energy in the body when it is in excess.

Lipids, mainly made up of triglycerides, are the strongest source of energy among the macro-nutrients of the diet and provide, on average, 9 kcal/g (67). They provide energy to the body activity, but their main function is to store energy for later use. The excess lipids are mainly stored as triglycerides in adipose tissue. When the body needs calories to function, adipose tissues liberate triglycerides that then are metabolized into energy (67–68). Triglycerides also control the internal body temperature by furnishing energy to the tissues. They also provide a layer of insulation under the skin and protective mattress around the organs. That's why lean people are less resistant to the cold than obese people. Lipids including triglycerides are used to make the myelin sheaths that sur-round nerve cells (67). Myelin sheaths act as insulating agents and help the transmission of nerve impulse and memory storage. More specifically in the brain, fats help brain activity in structure and in function. They help form nerve cell membranes, insulate neurons, and facilitate the signal-ing of electrical impulses throughout the brain (67). It should be remembered that vital organs such as the heart, kidneys, and liver are protected by visceral fat and the brain contains about 60% lipids (67). Triglycerides also help the body produce and regulate hormones. For example, adi-pose tissue secretes the hormone leptin, which regulates appetite. In the reproductive system, fatty acids liberated from triglycerides are required for proper reproductive health; women who lack proper amounts may stop menstruating and become infertile (67). During nutrition, triglycerides (oil, fat) in the diet help the absorption of a numerous fat-soluble micronutrients such as essential vitamins A, D, E, K and antioxidants (carotenes, lycopene, astaxanthin, zeaxanthin, lutein) in the digestive systems, thereby increasing their bioavailability (67–68). Moreover, in cuisine, fat also contributes to the palatability and flavor of food and hence contributes to the enjoyment of eating (68). Although some dietary triglycerides are essential, excess lipids in the diet can be harmful to the body. Current designations of serum triglyceride levels are as follows: less than 150 mg/dL, normal levels; 150–199 mg/dL, borderline high; 200–499 mg/dL, high; and >500 mg/dL, very high (108). When the serum levels of triglycerides become too much, this phenomenon is named hypertriglyceridemia; it can cause cardiovascular diseases (atherosclerosis, stroke, heart attack), obesity, diabetes, cancer, inflammatory diseases, and so on (108–111). Reducing the consumption of animal fat, sugar, and red meat is one of the best ways to reduce these dreadful chronic ailments. Yet, there are two kinds of triglycerides: 'good' triglyceride and 'bad' triglyceride. The first one is predominantly constructed from essential unsaturated fatty acids like oleic acid, linoleic acid, alpha-linoleic acid (ALA), eicosapentaenoic acid (EPA), and docosahexaenoic acid (DHA), and is mainly found in vegetable oil, seed, fish oil, and seafood. The second type is mostly made of saturated fatty acids such as stearic acid and palmitic acid, and is often present in animal fats (lard, butter, cream, milk, etc.). To avoid these chronic diseases due to hypertriglyceridemia, it is recommended to reduce consumption of animal fats and soluble sugars, and to increase the intake of vegetables and seafood. However, it is noteworthy that hypertriglyceridemia has multiple etiology and is not only due to the diet. Some hypertriglyceridemia is originated from genetic disorders, diabetes mellitus, obesity, nephrotic syndrome, hyperuricemia, and systemic lupus erythematosus (108–111). Sedentary lifestyle and certain medicines such as estrogens, certain anti-hypertensives, thiazide diuretics, non-selective beta-blockers, the calcium antagonist (verapamil), and chloroquine may also cause high serum triglyceride levels. Heavy alcohol consumption can elevate triglyceride levels (108–111).

Triglycerides in foods must be metabolized by lipase enzymes in the human digestive system in order to create the proper lipids characteristic of human tissues. Liver cells can synthesize and store triglycerides. As triglycerides are the esters of fatty acids, the sources of triglycerides in the diet are also the same as fatty acids. Triglycerides are commonly found in fried foods, vegetable oil, butter, whole milk, cheese, and some meats (67). Moderate consumption of fats and oils is good for the health.

3.3.3 Lipoproteins

As triglycerides and cholesterol are insoluble in water, they must be transported in combination with proteins to form a complex called lipoprotein (112–113). Lipoproteins are complex particles that have a central hydrophobic core of non-polar lipids, primarily cholesterol esters and triglycerides (112–113). This hydrophobic core is surrounded by a hydrophilic membrane consisting of phospholipids, free cholesterol, and apolipoproteins (112). Apolipoproteins are the proteins on the surface of the lipoproteins. They not only participate in solubilizing core lipids but also play critical roles in the regulation of plasma lipid and lipoprotein transport (109). Apolipoproteins have four major functions including: serving a structural role, acting as ligands for lipoprotein receptors, guiding the formation of lipoproteins, and serving as activators or inhibitors of enzymes involved in the metabolism of lipoproteins (112). These lipoproteins play a key role in the absorption and transport of dietary lipids by the small intestine, in the transport of lipids from the liver to peripheral tissues, and the transport of lipids from peripheral tissues to the liver and intestine (reverse cholesterol transport). A secondary function is to transport toxic foreign hydrophobic and amphipathic compounds, such as bacterial endotoxin, from areas of invasion and infection (112). Plasma lipoproteins are divided into seven classes based on size, lipid composition, apolipoproteins and their density during ultracentrifugation. They include chylomicron, chylomicron remnant, very low-density lipoprotein (VLDL), intermediate-density lipoprotein (IDL), low-density lipoprotein (LDL), high-density lipoprotein (HDL), and lipoprotein (a) (112).

Chylomicrons: These are large triglyceride particles made by the intestine. They transport cholesterol and dietary triglycerides from intestine to peripheral tissues and liver, and are composed of triglyceride, phospholipid, protein, and cholesterol. Their size varies depending on the amount of fat ingested (112).

Chylomicron remnants: The removal of triglyceride from chylomicrons by peripheral tissues results in smaller particles called chylomicron remnants. Compared to chylomicrons, these particles are enriched in cholesterol and are pro-atherogenic (capable of producing atheromatous plaques in artery) (112).

Very low-density lipoproteins (VLDL): These particles are produced by the liver and are triglyceride rich. They are used to transport triglycerides from the liver to the fatty tissue (112).

Intermediate density lipoproteins (IDL): The removal of triglycerides from VLDL by muscle and adipose tissue results in the formation of IDL particles which are enriched in cholesterol. These particles contain apolipoprotein B-100 and E. These IDL particles are pro-atherogenic (112).

Low density lipoproteins (LDL): These particles are derived from VLDL and IDL particles and they are even further enriched in cholesterol. LDL carries the majority of the cholesterol that is in the circulation. An abundance of LDL particles is seen in association with hypertriglyceridemia, low HDL levels, obesity, type 2 diabetes, and infectious and inflammatory states (112). LDL is also known as 'bad' cholesterol because it is associated with progression of atherosclerosis.

High density lipoproteins (HDL): These particles play an important role in reverse cholesterol transport from peripheral tissues to the liver, which is one potential mechanism by which HDL may be anti-atherogenic. In addition, HDL particles have antioxidant, anti-inflammatory, anti-thrombotic, and anti-apoptotic properties, which may also contribute to their ability to inhibit atherosclerosis. HDL particles are enriched in cholesterol and phospholipids (112). HDL is also known as 'good' cholesterol because high concentrations of HDL usually correspond to healthier blood vessels and lower risk of atherosclerosis.

Lipoprotein (a) (Lp (a): Lp (a) is an LDL particle that has apolipoprotein (a) attached to Apo B-100 via a disulfide bond. It is pro-atherogenic; it promotes the formation of fat in the artery (112). Lipoprotein (a) has attracted the interest of researchers and physicians due to its intriguing properties, including an intragenic multiallelic copy number variation in the lipoprotein (a) gene and the strong association with coronary heart disease (CHD) (113). It highlights the role of genetics in establishing lipoprotein (a) as a risk factor for CHD (113). The physiologic function of this lipoprotein is still uncertain (112–113).

In brief, LDL is richer in cholesterol than HDL. HDL is 50% protein and 50% cholesterol and other fats. HDL is smaller, denser, and richer in protein. LDLs carry cholesterol into cells for normal usage, but LDLs can also deposit cholesterol into the walls of blood vessels, which can lead to harmful disease like atherosclerosis (clogging of the arteries). HDLs scavenge excess cholesterol from the cells, tissues, and blood vessels and deliver these back to the liver, where these are either reused or excreted (67). Lipoproteins are vehicles that are used to transport hundreds to thousands of water-insoluble triglyceride and cholesterol molecules in the blood stream and have different composition, size and density depending on the quantity and nature of the transported molecules.

3.3.4 Phospholipids

Phospholipids also known as phosphoglycerides are fat compounds and have a glycerol backbone linked to a hydrophilic phosphate group, and two hydrophobic fatty-acid molecules. The phosphate group can be coupled with a nitrogen-containing compound and is water-soluble (67, 69, 114–115). So, phospholipids are amphipathic molecules, consisting of two hydrophobic fatty acid chains and a phosphate-containing hydrophilic head group, forming the fundamental building blocks of all cell membranes (115–116). By this special structure, phospholipids are amphiphilic compounds; they are both water-soluble and liposoluble. Because their fatty acid tails are insoluble in water, phospholipids spontaneously form stable bilayers in aqueous solutions, with the hydrophobic tails (fatty acids) buried in the interior of the cell membrane and the polar head groups (phosphates exposed to water present in the cell) (115). In blood and body fluids, phospholipids form structures in which fatty acids like omega-3, omega-6 fatty acids, cholesterol, and so on, are enclosed and transported throughout the bloodstream due to their amphiphilic nature (67). In cells, phospholipases hydrolyze phospholipids by releasing the transported fatty acids.

Phospholipids make up only about 2% of dietary lipids and are found in both plants and animals. Phospholipids are crucial for building the protective barrier, or membrane, that makes up the outer layer of all human cells. In fact, phospholipids are synthesized in the body to form cell and organelle membranes (67, 114–116). They play a key role in determining what enters and exits every cell. Phospholipids are important components in central and peripheral nervous systems, in the brain and nerves, all cellular membranes, and animal muscle (115). They are present in three phyla and are synthesized by phytoplanktons.

Phospholipids are divided into two main groups: glycerophospholipids and phosphosphingolipids (69). Glycerophospholipids or phosphoacylglycerols or phosphoglycerides contain a glycerol backbone, while phosphosphingolipids are a subclass of sphingolipid compounds with a sphingo-syl backbone instead of a glycerol (69). These differences in base structure affect their chemical reactivity.

3.3.4.1 Glycerophospholipid

The phospholipids found in most cell membranes are basically glycerophospholipids (GPLs), which consist of fatty acids esterified to a glycerol backbone, a phosphate group and a hydrophilic residue (e.g., choline, ethanolamine, serine, or inositol) (114–115). In GPLs, the alcohol here is glycerol, to which two fatty acids and a phosphoric acid are attached as esters. GPLs are amphiphilic molecules that have a hydrophilic group with a high affinity for water, and lipophilic fatty acid chain with a high affinity for oil, and are therefore are good emulsifiers (69).

3.3.4.2 Sphingolipid

Sphingolipids constitute a class of lipids defined by their 18 carbon-amino-alcohol backbones which are synthesized in the endoplasmic reticulum from non-sphingolipid precursors (66, 117). In sphin-golipids, glycerol is replaced by a group of aliphatic amino alcohol named sphingosine that contains two alcohols with the middle position occupied by an amine. Sphingolipids are complex lipids which yield fatty acids, sphingosine, phosphoric acid, and an alcohol component upon hydrolysis. A sphingosine has three parts, a three carbon chain with two alcohols and amine attached and a long hydrocarbon chain containing 12–22 carbon atoms (69, 115, 117). The main and abundant component of sphingolipids in animals is sphingomyelin that constitutes the membranous myelin sheath surrounding nerve cell axons (114, 117). Sphingomyelin usually consists of a sphingosine linked to a long chain fatty acyl chain called ceramide and attached to a phosphocholine group at the primary alcohol group of a sphingosine (66, 117). Precisely, ceramide is amide of fatty acids with sphingosine. So, sphingomyelin can also be classified as sphingophospholipid (115). Like glyc-erophospholipids and cholesterol, sphingolipids are ubiquitous in the body and found in every cell membrane, particularly nerve cells and brain tissues (114–117).

In brief, brain lipids include glycerophospholipids, sphingolipids, and cholesterol in equimolar proportions.

3.3.4.3 Sources

Sources of phospholipids are commonly found in foods containing lecithin. Lecithin is a mixture of different glycerophospholipids including phosphatidylcholine, phosphatidylinositol, phosphatidic acid, and phosphatidylethanolamine.

Major sources of phospholipids include egg yolks, milk, soybeans and soybean oil, tofu, sun-flower oil, oilseeds, marine sources (fish oil, krill oil, cod liver oil), caviar eggs, krill and fish eggs, liver, brain, lightly cooked meats, wheat germ, and rapeseed (67, 68, 112, 114–115). Leafy vegeta-bles, fruits, and tubers are relatively poor dietary sources of total lipids and phospholipids. Egg yolk contains 10% phospholipid and is used as emulsifying agents for the preparation of mayonnaise and cakes (68). The human body can make phospholipids, but it needs some raw materials such as triglycerides, fatty acids, phosphates, and choline to construct different types of phospholipids.

3.3.5 Sterols: Cholesterol, Phytosterols and Steroids

Sterols are lipid compounds containing a phenanthrene skeleton, and have 27–30 carbon atoms with a hydroxy group (alcohol) at C-3 of the first ring of phenanthrene structure and a side chain of at least seven carbons at C-17. Sterols are quite different from triglycerides and phospholipids made up of fatty acids. Sterols are abundant in nature: animals, plants and fungi (mushrooms) and comprise over 300 compounds (69, 118–119). According to their source, sterols are divided into three groups: zoosterols derived from animals, phytosterols or plant sterols, and mycosterols present in fungi. The most important animal sterol is cholesterol, while phytosterols are abundant in plants. Ergosterol is a common mycosterol found in cell membranes of fungi, yeast and protozoa. Cholesterol in humans and animals is precursor of steroid hormones, vitamin D3 and bile salts. Sterols (cholesterol, phytosterol, mycosterol) play an important role as structural components of cell membranes, and have a broad range of biological activities and physical properties (69, 118–119).

3.3.5.1 Cholesterol

Cholesterol, an important fatty substance, is ubiquitous in human and mammal organisms. Cholesterol is a lipophilic molecule that is essential for human life. It plays many roles that contribute to the normal functioning of cells. It contributes to the structural makeup of the cell membrane as well as modulates its fluidity. Every cell membrane contains cholesterol and phospholipid, another lipid compound for its activity. Cholesterol functions as a precursor molecule in the synthesis of vitamin D, bile acids, adrenocortical hormones (glucocorticoids, mineralocorticoids) and sex hormones (progesterone, testosterone, and estrogens) (118–121). Bile salt is used in digestion to facilitate absorption of fat-soluble vitamins A, D, E, and K. Cholesterol comprises about 0.2% of normal body weight. Most of it (about 33%) is in the brain and myelin of the nervous system, where its function has not been completely explored (119). Thus, it is a crucially important component of our biological activity. It should be noted that every cell in the body can synthesize cholesterol; hence cholesterol is not an essential dietary component. About three quarters of cholesterol are made in the liver. Indeed, the synthesis of cholesterol in the body is very complex and includes 37-step reactions with the intervention of 20 enzymes (118–121). This synthesis begins with the mevalonate pathway and ends with the conversion of its last precursor lanosterol to cholesterol. Furthermore, it can be absorbed directly from animal-based foods. Most ingested cholesterol is esterified, but this esterified form is poorly absorbed from 30 to 70% (118–121). The esterified cholesterol found in muscle may represent a storage compartment and its major function is as an insulator. The percentage of cholesterol ester in muscle increases with age. In the brain, cholesterol is a major constituent of the human brain (with about 35 grams of cholesterol in an adult brain), and the brain is the most cholesterol-rich organ, containing about 20% of the body's total cholesterol (121). Brain lipids consist of cholesterol, glycerophospholipids, and sphingolipids in equimolar proportions. Cholesterol is essential for normal brain development. Cholesterol is required for synapse and dendrite formation and for axonal guidance (121). Within the cell membrane, cholesterol also functions in intracellular transport, cell signaling and nerve conduction. Cholesterol depletion leads to synaptic and dendritic spine degeneration, decreased synaptic plasticity, and failed neurotransmission (121). Defects in cholesterol metabolism lead to central nervous system diseases such as Alzheimer's disease, Parkinson's disease, and Huntington's disease. In addition, cholesterol is involved in learning and memory, but the nature of that involvement appears to be as complex as the synthesis, metabolism, and homeostasis of cholesterol itself (122).

As every rose has its thorn, cholesterol also has its evil effect. It is well known that high blood cholesterol levels called hypercholesterolemia are strongly related to the incidence and risk of atherosclerotic vascular disease, especially coronary heart disease (heart attack) and stroke. Cholesterol forms a large part of the plaque that narrows the arteries in atherosclerosis (118–120, 123). Cholesterols and triglycerides are water insoluble compounds; for their circulation in the bloodstream, they must be linked to a lipoprotein that is an amphipathic compound, as cited earlier (118). Among several types of lipoproteins used to transport cholesterol and triglycerides, low-density lipoproteins (LDL) and high-density lipoproteins (HDL) are the two main carriers of these two fat compounds. Several types of evidence, including clinical dietary and drug trials, show that the cholesterol contained in the plasma's low-density lipoprotein (LDL) fraction is the principal detrimental component, whereas high levels of cholesterol in high-density lipoproteins (HDL) are associated with a reduced risk of coronary heart disease (67). As LDL (size: 18–25 nm) is larger than HDL (size: 5–12 nm) and less water-soluble than HDL, LDL can contain more cholesterol than HDL. Therefore, when the quantity of cholesterol in LDL rises, the risks of the plaque formation in the artery also increase. While HDL is smaller than LDL and more water-soluble than LDL, the complex HDL-cholesterol can easily move in the bloodstream, thereby avoiding the accidents during this transport.

Additionally, LDLs carry cholesterol into cells for normal usage, but when LDL-cholesterol levels are high, LDLs can also deposit cholesterol into the walls of coronary arteries, which can lead to obstruction of blood circulation, thus causing heart attack. HDLs scavenge excess cholesterol from the cells, tissues, and blood vessels and deliver these back to the liver, where these are either reused or excreted (67). Other factors, such as genetic background, cigarette smoking, hypertension, and obesity, also increase the risk of coronary artery disease. The strongest dietary determinant of blood cholesterol level is the saturated fatty acid content. Increased intake of both saturated fatty acids and cholesterol decreases LDL receptor activity in liver cells and increases LDL-cholesterol levels in the blood, thereby causing atherosclerosis. Indeed, all animal-based foods contain cholesterol in varying amounts. Major dietary sources of cholesterol include butter, cheese, egg yolks, pork, beef, poultry, cow milk and breast milk (118–120). Moreover, to avoid this disease, consumption of vegetables and cereals (oat, barley) is another way to reduce 'bad' LDL-cholesterol. Fibers in vegetables clean the intestinal wall and remove at the same time cholesterol liberated from foods. Hypercholesterolemia is mainly treated with a strict diet consisting of low saturated fat, trans-fat-free, low cholesterol foods, more seafoods rich in omega-3 fatty acids, more vegetables and fruits rich in fibers and phytosterols, more natural oats rich in β-glucan, and often followed by one of various hypolipidemic drugs, such as statins or fibrates (118–120). Moreover, regular physical activity may also reduce hypercholesterolemia and obesity. There are several international guidelines on the treatment of hypercholesterolemia and, during the last two decades, also some controversial debates about hypercholesterolemia and its origin as well as the benefits and risks of some anti-cholesterol drugs such as statins (124–126). Thus, only competent doctors can judge the benefits and risks of each anti-cholesterol drug in the treatment of hypercholesterolemia for each patient.

3.3.5.2 *Phytosterols*

Plants manufacture another type of sterols called plant sterols or phytosterols that are bioactive compounds and are the major component contributing to regulation of membrane fluidity in plant cells (127–129). Plant sterols include sterols and stanols, called phytosterols and phytostanols respectively, but combinedly and generally they are called phytosterols (127). Plant sterols resemble mammalian cholesterol in structure but are different in biological activity. Structurally, both phytosterols and cholesterol have sterol rings but the difference resides in the carbon side chains, with or without a double bond (127–128). More than 200 phytosterols have been identified in nature (127, 129). The most abundant plant sterols are: ß-sitosterol (65%), campesterol (32%), and stigmasterol (3%) (127, 129). Brassicasterol is a phytosterol often present in algae such as phytoplankton. In plant tissues, phytosterols (PS) occur in five common forms: free sterols, fatty-acid esters (steryl ester), steryl glycosides, acylated steryl glycosides, and hydroxycinnamic acid steryl esters (127). Stanols do not have double bonds in the sterol ring and are called saturated sterols. Stanols are less abundant in nature than phytosterols. The main stanols are campestanol and sitostanol (127). Plant stanols are also produced by hydrogenating sterols. These phytosterols are normal constituents of the human diet. Cholesterol is often absent or exists in trace levels in plant cells; that's why it is rarely found in plant foods.

Major sources of phytosterols include plant foods and their byproducts such as vegetable oils (rapeseed oil, olive oil, amaranth oil, wheat germ oil, soybean oil, etc.), cereals (oat, barley, rice, wheat germ, wheat bran, rice bran), fruits (avocado, olive, passion fruit, orange), vegetables (broccoli, cauliflower, carrot, soybean, bean, algae, etc.), and grains (peanut, almond, flax seed, chia seed, etc.) (127, 129). Nuts and vegetable oils can contain more than 1% of phytosterols. Phytostanols (saturated sterols) occur in certain cereals (corn, wheat, rye, and rice), fruits, and vegetables, but their concentrations are much lower than those of unsaturated phytosterols (127). Oil and cereal refining processes lead to a loss of phytosterols. Phytosterols (PS) are natural components of human diets.

The average daily intake of PS from natural sources is estimated to be between 150 and 440mg in Western countries (127, 129).

Phytosterols in the human diet can inhibit cholesterol absorption in the intestine, thus contributing to lower serum cholesterol levels (128–130). They compete for the ingestion of dietary cholesterol in the intestines, and also reduce the reabsorption of bile cholesterol in the gut. Clinical studies indicate that the intake of phytosterols (two grams/day) is associated with a significant reduction (8–10%) in levels of low-density lipoprotein cholesterol (LDL-cholesterol or bad cholesterol) with decreased risk of coronary heart diseases (129–130). In addition, plant sterols and stanols may have anti-inflammatory activities, and prevent cancer by induction of apoptosis in cancer cells (130). Thus, several guidelines recommend the intake of two g/day of plant sterols and/or stanols in order to reduce LDL-cholesterol levels (129–130). The United States Food and Drug Administration (FDA) has recognized the roles of phytosterols in the decrease of hypercholesterolemia, thus helping to reduce CVDs (131). However, phytosterols cannot be used as supplements for pregnant women or nursing mothers because they may block absorption not only of cholesterol, but of other important nutrients as well. Moreover, a few adverse effects of phytosterols occur in small group of individuals with phytosterolemia, an inherited lipid disorder, and they may cause decrease in plasma levels of nutrients such as carotenoids (130). In conclusion, phytosterols have several biological activities such as anti-hypercholesterolemia, anti-inflammatory activity, and cancer prevention, so their consumption should be encouraged in the population.

3.3.5.3 Mycosterol: Ergosterol

Like cholesterol and phytosterols, mycosterols are sterols present in fungi (mushrooms) (132–133). Ergosterol (24R-methyl-cholesta-5,7,22(E)-trienol) is the main mycosterol found in cell membranes of fungi, yeasts, and protozoa. Ergosterol is a sterol which was first discovered in 1889, in the plant pathogenic ergot fungus *Claviceps purpurea* (132–133). It is an analog of cholesterol present in mammalian cell membranes. Ergosterol is the major sterol among several sterols present in fungi. Like cholesterol, ergosterol and other mycosterols play similar roles in the permeability and fluidity of fungal cell membranes. They are also needed for fungal growth, a fact that has been exploited in the development of antifungal pesticides widely used in agriculture and antimycotics used to control fungal diseases of humans and animals (132). Ergosterol is converted into vitamin D2 when it is irradiated by sunlight or UV-B. Therefore, cultivated white mushrooms are often exposed to sunlight or UV-B light before marketing to obtain high vitamin D2 levels. Ergosterol also has antioxidant properties (133).

3.3.5.4 Steroids: Hormones, Vitamin D3, Bile

Steroids are biological compounds derived from cholesterol in the human body. The term steroid applies to a wide range of molecules with varying physiological effects. All steroids contain the same fused four ring core structure and have different biological roles as hormones and signaling molecules (66, 69, 134–135). These are subdivided on the basis of the number of carbons in the core skeleton. There are three main groups of steroids: steroid hormones (sex and adrenocortical hormones), secosteroids (various forms of vitamin D), and bile (acids and salts) (66, 69, 134–135).

- **Steroid hormones.** Steroid hormones are subdivided into sex hormones (progesterone, testosterone) and adrenocortical hormones (glucocorticoids, mineralocorticoids) (66, 69, 134–135).

Estrogens are female hormones of which estradiol is the most potent. They maintain the female reproductive tissues in a fully functional condition, promote the estrous state of preparedness for mating, and stimulate development of the mammary glands and of other feminine characteristics. Progesterone is a hormone secreted by the female reproductive system that functions mainly to regulate the condition of the inner lining (endometrium) of the uterus. Progesterone is produced by the ovaries, placenta, and adrenal glands. In the ovaries the site of progesterone production is the corpus luteum. Progesterone prepares the wall of the uterus to accept a fertilized egg that can be implanted and developed into a fetus. Testosterone is an androgen hormone that primarily influences the growth and development of the male reproductive system. It is produced by the male testes (66, 134–135).

Adrenocortical hormones are produced by the adrenal cortex of suprarenal glands and consist of glucocorticoids and mineralocorticoids. Glucocorticoid is a steroid hormone produced by the suprarenal or adrenal gland and known particularly for its anti-inflammatory and immunosuppressive actions. Cortisol is the principal glucocorticoid in many species, including humans. Mineralocorticoids stimulate the retention of sodium in the extracellular body fluids. The most potent mineralocorticoid of all species is aldosterone.

- **Secosteroids: Vitamin D3 or cholecalciferol and vitamin D2 or ergocalciferol.** Vitamin D3 is a secosteroid formed in mammalian skin from one precursor of cholesterol, 7-dehydrocholesterol (66, 134–135). Vitamin D2 is a secosteroid obtained from ergosterol in fungi (mushrooms) under the action of sunlight or UV-B (66, 132–135). In adults, especially in elderly women, the lack of vitamin D3 is one of the causes of some bone diseases such as osteomalacia and osteoporosis. These diseases are different in origin, but they are treated by vitamin D2 or D3 with calcium supplements or by foods rich in these compounds, such as milk. Vitamins D2 and D3 have the same biological activity in humans and a slight difference in chemical structure. Both are widely used in food fortification and dietary supplements. However, vitamin D3 is often preferred because it is better absorbed than vitamin D2 in the human body, thus increasing efficacy in the treatment of vitamin D deficiency (see Chapter 2 of this book).
- **Bile acids and bile salts.** Bile acids are used to facilitate digestion and absorption of lipids in the small intestine as well as regulate cholesterol homeostasis. Bile acids are also involved in the regulation of various metabolic processes such as their own synthesis and enterohepatic circulation, triglyceride, glucose, and energy homeostasis (136). Bile acids promote absorption of fat-soluble vitamins and act as emulsifiers. The synthesis of bile acids occurs exclusively in the liver in a series of enzymatic reactions requiring 17 enzymes that convert hydrophobic cholesterol into more water-soluble compounds (136). Cholic acid and chenodeoxycholic acid are the primary bile acids formed from cholesterol in humans and make up 80% of all bile acids. Before their secretion into the bile canalicular lumen for storage in the gallbladder as mixed micelles with phospholipids and cholesterol, primary bile acids are conjugated with glycine or taurine to form bile salts named glycoconjugates and tauroconjugates, respectively, which become hydrophile (136). These bile salts enter the intestine as sodium salts and assist in the absorption and emulsification of dietary fat. This bile acid secretion is impaired and reduced in some liver diseases and in obstructive jaundice (134). Upon ingestion of a meal, gallbladder contraction releases micellar bile acids into the intestinal lumen to aid digestion. After digestion, a major party of bile acids are reabsorbed in the ileum. Bile acids represent the major route for the elimination of the steroid from the body. Briefly, bile consists of bile acid, cholesterol, conjugated bilirubin, phospholipid, electrolytes and water and aid the absorption of dietary fats and oils and soluble-fat vitamins in the gut. In summary, steroids including steroid hormones, vitamin D and bile acids, are compounds, all derived from cholesterol, and play different roles in the functioning of different organs of sexuality, reproduction, digestion, and the immune and bone systems.

3.3.6 Glycolipids

Glycolipids are glycosyl derivatives of lipids. Glycolipid is any compound containing one or more monosaccharide residues (glucose or galactose) bound by a glycosidic linkage to a hydrophobic moiety such as an acylglycerol, a sphingoid, a ceramide (N-acylsphingoid) or a prenyl phosphate (66, 119, 137–138). Cellular membranes contain several types of glycoproteins, glycolipids, and other lipids, including cholesterol, glycerophospholipids, and sphingomyelin. Glycolipids are essential for biological activities of the cell membrane (137). In addition, the roles of glycolipids are to facilitate cellular recognition, which is crucial to the immune response and the cell connections in tissues.

Glycolipids are divided into glycoglycerolipids and glycosphingolipids. Glycoglycerolipids, also called glyceroglycolipids, are glycolipids containing mono, di or trisaccharides linked glycosidically to the hydroxyl group (OH) of diglycerides. Galactose is the most common carbohydrate molecule in plant glycolipids. Monogalactosyldiacylglycerols and digalactosyldiacylglycerols are the main glycolipid components of the various membranes of chloroplasts, and these are the most abundant lipids in all photosynthetic tissues, including those of higher plants, algae, and bacteria (138). The main functions of glycolipids in the body are to serve as recognition sites for cell contact, as receptor components for proteins and as markers for tumor progression and cell differentiation (138). Glycolipids also act as modulators of signal transduction, cell proliferation, and calcium homeostasis (138). They play important roles in the immune system for the defense against microbes and viruses (137–138).

Glycosphingolipids are lipids containing at least one monosaccharide residue linked to ceramide moiety. They are found in brain and nervous tissue. Ceramides are amides of fatty acids which are long-chain saturated or monounsaturated fatty acids (138).

3.3.7 Waxes

Waxes are esters of long-chain alcohols and long-chain fatty acids and belong to simple lipid group such as sterols and triglycerides. Waxes are long-chain apolar lipidic compounds and often found on the surface of plants and animals (68, 118). Waxes exist in solid or semi-solid form (ointment form) and have melting points from 40° C (104° F) to 120° C (248° F). They are water insoluble, but soluble in organic, nonpolar solvents (118). Waxes are produced by many plants and animals. Beeswax, spermaceti, wool grease, and lanolin are important animal waxes, and used mostly in pharmaceutical and food industries. The vegetable waxes include carnauba wax, candelilla, and sugar cane waxes containing policosanol. The mineral waxes include petroleum waxes, ozokerite, and montan (118).

3.3.7.1 Animal waxes: Beeswax, Lanolin, Human Sweat, Spermaceti

- **Beeswax.** It is a hard amorphous solid, usually light yellow to amber and used in constructing honeycombs. Pure beeswax is the most useful and valuable waxes, and consists of about 80% of long-chain wax esters, 15% of free acids, 10% of hydrocarbon, and small amounts of diols and cholesterol esters. It is used in candle manufacture, and in the food, paper, pharmacy, and rubber industries (118).
- **Lanolin or wool wax or wool grease.** Lanolin is a wax secreted by the sebaceous glands of wool-bearing animals (sheep, lamas, camels, goats, yaks). Lanolin is mostly used in pharmacy and the wool industry (118). Wool wax mainly consists of long chain sterol esters. It is waterproof and aids wool-bearing animals in shedding water from their coats. In humans, lanolin is used to make the skin smooth and shiny. As wool grease is rich in sterols, it is often the raw material for producing cholecalciferol (vitamin D3) by UV irradiation.
- **Sweat or sebum.** Sweat is secreted by sebaceous glands in humans. Sebaceous glands are holocrine glands found over the entire surface of the body except the palms, soles, and dorsum of the feet. They are abundant in the face and scalp where they are the sites of acne. The normal function of sebaceous glands is to produce and secrete sebum, a group of complex oils including triglycerides and fatty acid breakdown products, wax esters, squalene, cholesterol esters, and cholesterol (139).

- **Spermaceti.** It is a white waxy substance found in large amounts in the head cavities of the sperm whale and mainly used in cosmetics and pharmacy for the preparation of ointment and cream (118). It is now not produced because the fishing of whale is banned.

3.3.7.2   Plant Waxes: Sugarcane Wax (Policosanol), Candelilla Wax

Sugarcane wax (Policosanol). Sugarcane wax, an ester of long-chain alcohols and long-chain fatty acids, is a whitish to dark-yellowish powdery deposit on the surface of stalks and leaves of sugarcane, which appears as a cuticle layer (140). Policosanol is a mixture of long chain primary aliphatic alcohols ranging from 2.5–80% extracted from sugar cane waxes. Octacosanol, a major aliphatic alcohol, constitutes 50–80% of the total policosanols. Other major pharmacologically active components of sugarcane wax are long chain aliphatic fatty acids present at lower concentrations. Various phytosterols, steroids, and terpenoids are also found in sugarcane wax (140).

Policosanol is a dietary supplement marketed in the Caribbean, Central and South America, and Canada. Human policosanol consumption is safe and well tolerated and is effective at lowering the blood cholesterol (140–141). Policosanol has been reported to improve blood pressure, lipid profile, and HDL functionality via inhibition of cholesteryl ester transfer protein both in vitro and in vivo in zebrafish and human models (141). However, the anti-hypercholesterolemia effects of policosanol in sugarcane wax are still not officially confirmed by healthcare organizations.

Candelilla wax. It is a vegetable wax produced mainly in Mexico for the manufacturing of chewing gum, cosmetics, and for the production of lubricants, furniture polish, and paper coating (118).

3.3.8   Lipids in Health and Disease

In summary, lipids are the most complex macronutrients because of their different chemical structures and also their multiple roles in human health and disease. There are multitude compounds of lipids present in the human organism such as fatty acids, cholesterol, steroids, bile, vitamins, and so on. Many compounds such as cholesterol, steroids, and bile, are produced in the human body; however, some other compounds, such as omega-3 and omega-6 unsaturated fatty acids, must be provided through foods. Their absence and their excess in the human body causes diseases such as cardiovascular and neurological diseases.

For cardiovascular health, substantial evidence supports the importance of the type of fat consumed, and the elimination of industrially produced trans-fats (119, 142). Much of the evidence suggests that the risk of coronary heart disease is reduced by replacing saturated fat with polyunsaturated fats (119, 142). The lack of omega-3 unsaturated fatty acids is one of the main causes of cardiovascular diseases.

The human brain is composed of 60% different lipidic products such as cholesterol, omega-3 and omega-6 unsaturated fatty acids. The lack of these compounds in the nervous system is the cause of different neurodegenerative diseases such as Parkinson's disease and Alzheimer's disease. Parkinson's disease is characterized by a progressive loss of dopaminergic neurons from the nigrostriatal pathway, formation of Lewy bodies, and microgliosis (143). Recently, some genetic data revealed that lipids were central players in this disease (143). Higher intake of omega-3 fatty acids and alpha-linoleic acid (ALA), but not omega-6 acid or linoleic acid (LA), has been associated with reduced risk of Parkinson's disease (143).

4   DISCUSSION

In summary, all macronutrients, including carbohydrate, protein, amino acid, fat, and fatty acids, are equally essential for life. They are needed in great amounts to produce necessary energy for the functioning of all cells and organs in order to maintain life and health. Fats (lipids) furnish nine calories per gram, while carbohydrates (sugars) and proteins give four calories per gram only. Carbohydrates such as starch in cereals are the most consumed macronutrients in the world because they are transformed into glucose, a basic compound for cell activity. However, excessive consumption of foods rich in sucrose and glucose, such as cake and soft drinks, may cause obesity, diabetes, and so on. Proteins and amino acids are other main macronutrients for the building materials of body tissue and body activity. Antibodies and enzymes are precious proteins for the defense and activity of all organs and tissues. Fatty acids and lipids are the main sources of energy for the body. Essential omega-3 and omega-6 unsaturated fatty acids play an important role in the composition of all cell membranes, and influence membrane fluidity, thus regulating cell signaling processes, cellular functions, and gene expression. Since the discovery of the roles of omega-3 unsaturated fatty acids and the support of their consumption through seafood, fish oil, seeds, soybean and seed oils, a decrease of cardiovascular diseases and inflammatory diseases has been observed. An unbalance of essential omega-3 and omega-6 fatty acids in the diet may be the cause of numerous inflammatory diseases such as asthma and muscular and joint pain, because these fatty acids are the source of different eicosanoids with contradictory biological effects. Indeed, the choice of different macronutrients plays an important role in health maintenance and in disease prevention. A balanced diet and a moderate intake are two necessary conditions to maintain good health. More research is needed on the roles of dietary macronutrients in our health as well as for the discovery of new biological molecules in our body. Briefly, the knowledge of different types of macronutrients allows consumers to choose a good diet for the maintenance of good health and the avoidance of chronic diseases.

5   REFERENCES

1 Zimmerman M., Snow B. (2012). Chapter 1: Nutrition and You, pp. 9–64. In: *An Introduction to Nutrition*, 812 pages. https://2012books.lardbucket.org/pdfs/an-introduction-to-nutrition.pdf.

2. Astley S., Finglas P. (2016). Nutrition and Health. In: *Reference Module in Food Science*. Elsevier Inc. https://doi.org/10.1016/B978-0-08-100596-5.03425-9.

3. Thompson J.L., Manore M.M., Vaughan L.A., Editors. (2011). Chapter 1. The Role of Nutrition in Our Health, pp. 3–38, and Chapter 9. Nutrients Involved in Fluid and Electrolyte Balance, pp. 323–355. In: *The Science of NUTRITION*. 2nd edition. Pearson Benjamin Cummings, San Francisco, 942 pages.

4. Eastwood M., Editor (2003). Part V. Nutrients and Non-Nutrients. In: *Principles of Human Nutrition*. 2nd edition. Blackwell Science Ltd, Oxford, 680 pages.

5. Roth R.A., Editor (2011). *Nutrition & Diet Therapy*. 10th edition. Cengage Learning, Delmar, 608 pages.

6. Gibney M.J., Lanham-New S.A., Cassidy A., Vorster H.H., Editors. (2009). *Introduction to Human Nutrition*. 2nd edition. Wiley-Blackwell, Oxford and Iowa, 386 pages.

7. Cummings J.H., Stephen A.M. (2007). Carbohydrate Terminology and Classification. *Eur. J. Clin. Nutr.*, **61** (Suppl. 1): S5–S18.

8. Izydorczyk M. (2005). Chapter 1. Understanding the Chemistry of Food Carbohydrates. In: *Food Carbohydrates: Chemistry, Physical Properties, and Applications*. Editors: Steve W. Cui. Taylor & Francis Group, CRC Press, 432 pages. https://doi.org/10.1201/9780203485286.

9. Keim N.L., Levin R.J., Havel P.J. (2012). Chapter 2. Carbohydrates, pp. 36–57. In: *Modern Nutrition in Health and Disease*. 11th edition. Editors: A.C. Ross, B. Caballero, R.J. Cousins, K.L. Tucker, T.R. Ziegler. Lippincott Williams & Wilkins, Baltimore, 1646 pages. https://treatment.tbzmed.ac.ir/uploads/User/47/nutrition/1394/modern%20nutrition.pdf.

10. Daniel J.R., Vidovic N. (2018). Carbohydrates, Role in Human Nutrition. In: *Reference Module in Food Science*. Elsevier Inc. https://doi.org/10.1016/B978-0-08-100596-5.02927-9.

11. Izydorczyk M., Cui S.W., Wang Q. (2005). Chapter 6. Polysaccharide Gums: Structures, Functional Properties, and Applications. In: *Food Carbohydrates: Chemistry, Physical Properties, and Applications*. Editor: Steve W. Cui. Taylor & Francis Group, CRC Press, 432 pages. https://doi.org/10.1201/9780203485286.

12. Koehler P., Wieser H. (2013). Chapter 2. Chemistry of Cereal Grains, pp. 11–45. In: *Handbook on Sourdough Biotechnology*. Editors: M. Gobbetti, M. Gänzle. Springer Science & Business Media, New York.

13. Messina V. (2014). Nutritional and Health Benefits of Dried Beans. *Am. J. Clin. Nutr.*, **100** (Suppl.): 437S–442S.

14. Atkinson F.S., Foster-Powell K., Brand-Miller J.C. (2008). International Tables of Glycemic Index and Glycemic Load Values: 2008. *Diabetes Care*, **31**(12): 2281–2283.
15. Nguyen A.L., He H., Pham-Huy C. (2006). Chiral Drugs. An Overview. *Int. J. Biomed. Sci.*, **2**: 85–100.
16. Zawirska-Wojtasiak R. (2006). Chirality and the Nature of Food. Authenticity of Aroma. *Acta Sci. Pol. Technol. Aliment.*, **5**(1): 21–36.
17. Mudgil D., Barak S. (2013). Composition, Properties and Health Benefits of Indigestible Carbohydrate Polymers as Dietary Fiber: A Review. *Int. J. Biol. Macromolec.*, **61**: 1–6.
18. Slavin J.L., Lloyd B. (2012). Health Benefits of Fruits and Vegetables. *Adv. Nutr.*, **3**: 506–516.
19. Dhingra D., Michael M., Rajput H., Patil R.T. (2012). Dietary Fibre in Foods: A Review. *J. Food Sci. Technol.*, **49**(3): 255–266.
20. Anderson J.W., Baird P., Davis Jr R.H., Ferreri S., Knudtson M., Koraym A., Waters V., Williams C.L. (2009). Health Benefits of Dietary Fiber. *Nutr. Rev.*, **67**(4): 188–205.
21. Chawla R., Patil G.R. (2010). Soluble Dietary Fiber. *Compr. Rev. Food Sci. Food Saf.*, **9**: 178–196.
22. Lattimer J.M., Haub M.D. (2010). Effects of Dietary Fiber and Its Components on Metabolic Health. *Nutrients*, **2**: 1266–1289.
23. Papandreou D., Noor Z.T., Rashed M. (2015). The Role of Soluble, Insoluble Fibers and Their Bioactive Compounds in Cancer: A Mini Review. *Food and Nutr. Sci.*, **6**: 1–11.
24. Zhu F., Du B., Xu B. (2016). A Critical Review on Production and Industrial Applications of Beta-Glucans. *Food Hydrocolloids*, **52**: 275–288.
25. Henrion M., Francey C., Lê K.A., Lamothe L. (2019). Cereal B-Glucans: The Impact of Processing and How It Affects Physiological Responses. *Nutrients*, **11**(1729): 1–14.
26. Novak M., Vetvicka V. (2008). B-Glucans, History, and the Present: Immunomodulatory Aspects and Mechanisms of Action. *J. Immunotoxicol.*, **5**: 47–57.
27. Berteau O., Mulloy B. (2003). Sulfated Fucans, Fresh Perspectives: Structures, Functions, and Biological Properties of Sulfated Fucans and an Overview of Enzymes Active Toward This Class of Polysaccharide. *Glycobiology*, **13**(6): 29R–40R.
28. Fitton J.H., Stringer D.N., Karpiniec S.S. (2015). Therapies from Fucoidan: An Update. *Mar. Drugs*, **13**: 5920–5946.
29. Niness K.R. (1999). Inulin and Oligofructose: What Are They? *J. Nutr.*, **129**: 1402S–1406S.
30. Barclay T., Ginic-Markovic M., Cooper P., Petrovsky N. (2010). Inulin – A Versatile Polysaccharide with Multiple Pharmaceutical and Food Chemical Uses. *J. Excipients and Food Chem.*, **1**(3): 27–50.
31. Pool-Zobel B.L. (2005). Inulin-Type Fructans and Reduction in Colon Cancer Risk: Review of Experimental and Human Data. *Br. J. Nutr.*, **93** (Suppl. 1): S73–S90.
32. Mirhosseini H., Amid B.T. (2012). A Review Study on Chemical Composition and Molecular Structure of Newly Plant Gum Exudates and Seed Gums. *Food Res. Int.*, **46**: 387–398.
33. Mudgil D., Barak S., Khatkar B.S. (2014). Guar Gum: Processing, Properties and Food Applications. A Review. *J. Food Sci. Technol.*, **51**(3): 409–418.
34. Montenegro M.A., Boiero M.L., Valle L., Borsarelli C.D. (2012). Gum Arabic: More Than an Edible Emulsifier, Products and Applications of Biopolymers. Chapter 1, pp. 3–27. In: *Products and Applications of Biopolymers*. Editor: Dr. Johan Verbeek. InTech, Rijeka, and Shanghai, 220 pages. http://cdn.intechopen.com/pdfs/31731/intechgum_arabic_more_than_an_edible_emulsifier.pdf.
35. Choudhary P.D., Pawar H.A. (2014). Recently Investigated Natural Gums and Mucilages as Pharmaceutical Excipients: An Overview. *J. Pharm.*, Article ID 204849, 9 pages.
36. McKee T., McKee J.R. (2009). Chapter 5. Amino Acids, Peptides, and Proteins, pp. 108–160. In: *Biochemistry: The Molecular Basis of Life*. 4th edition. Editors: Trudy McKee, James R. McKee. Oxford University Press, Inc., Oxford.
37. Matthews D.E. (2012). Chapter 1. Proteins and Amino Acids, pp. 3–35. In: *Modern Nutrition in Health and Disease*. 11th edition. Editors: A.C. Ross, B. Caballero, R.J. Cousins, K.L. Tucker, T.R. Ziegler. Lippincott Williams & Wilkins, Baltimore, 1646 pages. https://treatment.tbzmed.ac.ir/uploads/User/47/nutrition/1394/modern%20nutrition.pdf.
38. Jain J.L., Jain S., Jain N. (2005). Chapter 9. Proteins-I. General Structure, pp. 132–203. In: *Fundamentals of Biochemistry*. 6th edition. Editors: J.L. Jain, Sunjay Jain, Nitin Jain. S. Chand & Company, New Delhi, 1230 pages.
39. Wu G. (2009). Amino Acids: Metabolism, Function, and Nutrition. *Amino Acids*, **37**: 1–17.
40. El-Hattab A.W., Emrick L.T., Craigen W.J., Scaglia F. (2012). Citrulline and Arginine Utility in Treating Nitric Oxide Deficiency in Mitochondrial Disorders. *Mol. Genet. Metab.*, **107**: 247–252.
41. Sánchez A., Vázquez A. (2017). Bioactive Peptides: A Review. *Food Quality and Safety*, **1**(1): 29–46.

42. Kovalainen M., Mönkäre J., Riikonen J., Pesonen U., Vlasova M., Salonen J., Lehto V-K., Järvinen K., Herzig K-H. (2015). Novel Delivery System for Improving the Clinical Use of Peptides. *Pharmacol. Rev.*, **67**(3): 541–561.

43. Balandran-Quintana R.R., Mendoza-Wilson A.M., Ramos-Clamont Montfort G., Huerta-Ocampo J.A., Mazorra-Manzano M.A. (2021). Chapter 3. Peptides and Proteins. In: *Food Bioactives and Health*. Editor: C.M. Galanakis. Springer Cham, Switzerland. https://doi.org/10.1007/978-3-030-57469-7_5.

44. Jackson L., Eldahshan W., Fagan S.C., Ergul A. (2018). Within the Brain: The Renin Angiotensin System. *Int. J. Mol. Sci.*, **19**(3): 876–898.

45. Hay D.L., Chen S., Lutz T.A., Parkes D.G., Roth J.D. (2015). Amylin: Pharmacology, Physiology, and Clinical Potential. *Pharmacol. Rev.*, **67**(3): 564–600.

46. Weber M., Hamm C. (2006). Role of B-Type Natriuretic Peptide (BNP) and NT-pro-BNP in Clinical Routine. *Heart (British Cardiac Society)*, **92**(6): 843–849.

47. Jain J.L., Jain S., Jain N. (2005). Chapter 10. Protein Classification. In: *Fundamentals of Biochemistry*. 6th edition. Editors: J.L. Jain, Sunjay Jain, Nitin Jain. S. Chand & Company, New Delhi, 1230 pages.

48. Gigli M., Begay R.L., Morea G., Graw S.L., Sinagra G., Taylor M.R.G., Granzier H., Mestroni L. (2016). A Review of the Giant Protein Titin in Clinical Molecular Diagnostics of Cardiomyopathies. *Front. Cardiovasc. Med.*, **3**(21): 9 pages.

49. Wu G. (2016). Dietary Protein Intake and Human Health. *Food Funct.*, **7**(3): 1251–1265.

50. Lonnie M., Hooker E., Brunstrom J.M., Corfe B.M., Green M.A., Watson A.W., Williams E.A., Stevenson E.J., Penson S., Johnstone A.M. (2018). Protein for Life: Review of Optimal Protein Intake, Sustainable Dietary Sources and the Effect on Appetite in Ageing Adults. *Nutrients*, **10**(3): 360–377.

51. Rodriguez M.I.A., Barroso L.G.R., Sanchez M.L. (2018). Collagen: A Review on Its Sources and Potential Cosmetic Applications. *J. Cosmet. Dermatol.*, **17**(1): 20–26.

52. Ponomarenko E.A., Poverennaya E.V., Ilgisonis E.V., Pyatnitskiy M.A., Kopylov A.T., Zgoda V.G., Lisitsa A.V., Archakov A.I. (2016). The Size of the Human Proteome: The Width and Depth. *Int. J. Anal. Chem.*, **2016**, Article ID 7436849, 6 pages.

53. Cuesta S.M., Rahman S.A., Furnham N., Thornton J.M. (2015). The Classification and Evolution of Enzyme Function. *Biophysic. J.*, **109**(6): 1082–1086.

54. Raja M.M.M., Raja A., Imran M.M., Santha A.M.I., Devasena K. (2011). Enzymes Application in Diagnostic Prospects. *Biotechnology*, **10**: 51–59.

55. Cooper G.M. (2000). The Central Role of Enzymes as Biological Catalysts. In: *The Cell: A Molecular Approach*. 2nd edition. Sinauer Associates, Sunderland, MA. www.ncbi.nlm.nih.gov/books/NBK9921/.

56. Hemalatha T., UmaMashewari T., Krithiga G., Sankaranarayanan P., Puvanakhrishnan R. (2013). Enzymes in Clinical Medicine: An Overview. *Indian J. Exp. Biol.*, **51**(10): 777–788.

57. Arnold J.N., Wormald M.R., Sim R.B., Rudd P.M., Dwek R.A. (2007). The Impact of Glycosylation on the Biological Function and Structure of Human Immunoglobulins. *Annu. Rev. Immunol.*, **25**: 21–50.

58. Schroeder Jr. H.W., Cavacini L. (2010). Structure and Function of Immunoglobulins. *J. Allergy Clin. Immunol.*, **125**(2 0 2): S41–S52.

59. Justiz-Vaillant A.A., Jamal Z., Ramphul K. (2021). Immunoglobulin. In: *StatPearls [Internet]*. StatPearls Publishing, Treasure Island, FL, January. www.ncbi.nlm.nih.gov/books/NBK513460/.

60. Ulfman L.H., Leusen J.H.W., Savelkoul H.F.J., Warner J.O., van Neerven R.J.J. (2018). Effects of Bovine Immunoglobulins on Immune Function, Allergy, and Infection. *Front. Nutr.*, **5**(52): 1–20.

61. Wang H., Hu H., Zhang K. (2017). Overview of Interferon: Characteristics, Signaling and Anticancer Effect. *Arch. Biotechnol. Biomed.*, **1**: 001–016.

62. Pestka S. (2007). The Interferons: 50 Years After Their Discovery, There Is Much More to Learn. *J. Biol. Chem.*, **282**: 20047–20051.

63. Friedman R.M., Contente S. (2009). Interferons as Therapy for Viral and Neoplastic Diseases: From Panacea to Pariah to Paragon. *Pharmaceuticals*, **2**: 206–216.

64. Sosa J.P., Ferreira Caceres M.M., Ross Comptis J., Quiros J., Príncipe-Meneses F.S., Riva-Moscoso A., Belizaire M.P., Malanyaon F.Q., Agadi K., Jaffery S.S., Sahajwani J., Arshia A., Senatus A., Verdecia G., Akano L., Razzack A.A., Salam S., Gadamidi V.K., Marian S. (2021). Effects of Interferon Beta in COVID-19 Adult Patients: Systematic Review. *Infect. Chemother.*, **53**(2): 247–260.

65. Messina M. (2016). Soy and Health Update: Evaluation of the Clinical and Epidemiologic Literature. *Nutrients*, **8**(12): 754, 42 pages.

66. Fahy E., Subramaniam S., Brown H.A., Glass C.K., Merrill A.H. Jr., Murphy R.C., Raetz C.R.H., Russell D.W., Seyama Y., Shaw W., Shimizu T., Spener F., van Meer G., VanNieuwenhze M.S., White S.H., Witztum J.L., Dennis E.A. (2005). A Comprehensive Classification System for Lipids. *J. Lipid Res.*, **46**: 839–861.

67. Zimmerman M., Snow B. (2012). Chapter 5, Lipids, pp. 233–281. In: *An Introduction to Nutrition*, 812 pages. https://2012books.lardbucket.org/pdfs/an-introduction-to-nutrition/s09-lipids.pdf.
68. O'Keefe S.F. (2008). 1. Nomenclature and Classification of Lipids, pp. 3–38. In: *Food Lipids: Chemistry, Nutrition, and Biotechnology*. 3rd edition. Editors: C.C. Akoh, D.B. Min. CRC Press, Taylor & Francis Group, Boca Raton, FL, 930 pages.
69. Kalemba D., Dąbrowska M. (2015). 1. Chemistry of Lipids, pp. 1–19. In: *Plant Lipids Science, Technology, Nutritional Value and Benefits to Human Health*. Editors: Grazyna Budryn, Dorota Zyzelewicz. https://studyres.com/doc/15961275/1.-chemistry-of-lipids.
70. Tvrzicka E., Kremmyda L-S., Stankova B., Zak A. (2011). Fatty Acids as Bio-Compounds: Their Role in Human Metabolism, Health and Disease – A Review. Part 1: Classification, Dietary Sources and Biological Functions. *Biomed. Pap. Med. Fac. Univ. Palacky Olomouc Czech Repub.*, **155**(2): 117–130.
71. Castro-Torres I.G., Castro-Torres V.A., Hernández-Lozano M., Ocaña-Sánchez M.F. (2021). Chapter 5. Lipids. In: *Food Bioactives and Health*. Editor: C.M. Galanakis. Springer Cham, Switzerland. https://doi.org/10.1007/978-3-030-57469-7_5.
72. Louda D.W. (2012). Chapter 8. Lipids: Fatty Acids. In: *Biochemistry Review. Overview of Biomolecules*. Florida Atlantic University. http://med.fau.edu/students/md_m1_orientation/Overview.pdf.
73. Kaur N., Chugh V., Gupta A.K. (2014). Essential Fatty Acids as Functional Components of Foods-A Review. *J. Food Sci. Technol.*, **51**(10): 2289–2303.
74. Binienda Z.K., Sarkar S., Silva-Ramirez S., Gonzalez C. (2013). Role of Free Fatty Acids in Physiological Conditions and Mitochondrial Dysfunction. *Food Nutr. Sci.*, **4**: 6–15.
75. Arbex A.K., Bizarro V.R., Santos J.C.S., Araújo L.M.M., de Jesus A.L.C., Fernandes M.S.A., Salles M.M., Rocha D.R.T.W., Marcadenti A. (2015). The Impact of the Essential Fatty Acids (EFA) in Human Health. *Open J. Endocr. Metab. Dis.*, **5**: 98–104.
76. Oppedisano F., Macrì R., Gliozzi M., Musolino V., Carresi C., Maiuolo J., Bosco F., Nucera S., Caterina Zito M., Guarnieri L., Scarano F., Nicita C., Coppoletta A.R., Ruga S., Scicchitano M., Mollace R., Palma E., Mollace V. (2020). The Anti-Inflammatory and Antioxidant Properties of n-3 PUFAs: Their Role in Cardiovascular Protection. *Biomedicines*, **8**(9): 306, 18 pages.
77. Calder P. (2018). Very Long-Chain n-3 Fatty Acids and Human Health: Fact, Fiction and the Future. *Proc. Nutr. Soc.*, **77**(1): 52–72.
78. Swanson D., Block R., Mousa S.A. (2012). Omega-3 Fatty Acids EPA and DHA: Health Benefits Throughout Life. *Adv. Nutr.*, **3**: 1–7.
79. Burri L., Hoem N., Banni S., Berge K. (2012). Marine Omega-3 Phospholipids: Metabolism and Biological Activities. *Int. J. Mol. Sci.*, **13**: 15401–15419.
80. Lee J.M., Lee H., Kang S.B., Park W.J. (2016). Fatty Acid Desaturases, Polyunsaturated Fatty Acid Regulation, and Biotechnological Advances. *Nutrients*, **8**(23): 1–13.
81. Miyata J., Arita M. (2015). Role of Omega-3 Fatty Acids and Their Metabolites in Asthma and Allergic Diseases. *Allergol. Int.*, **64**: 27–34.
82. Wendell S.G., Baffi C., Holguin F. (2014). Fatty Acids, Inflammation, and Asthma. *J. Allergy Clin. Immunol.*, **133**(5): 1255–1264.
83. Simopoulos A.P. (2002). Omega-3 Fatty Acids in Inflammation and Autoimmune Diseases. *J. Am. Coll. Nutr.*, **21**(6): 495–505.
84. Simopoulos A.P. (2002). The Importance of the Ratio of Omega-6/Omega-3 Essential Fatty Acids. *Biomed. Pharmacother.*, **56**: 365–379.
85. Grosso G., Galvano F., Marventano S., Malaguarnera M., Bucolo C., Drago F., Caraci F. (2014). Omega-3 Fatty Acids and Depression: Scientific Evidence and Biological Mechanisms. *Oxid. Med. Cell Longev.*, Article ID 313570, 16 pages.
86. Logan A.C. (2004). Omega-3 Fatty Acids and Major Depression: A Primer for the Mental Health Professional. *Lipids Health Dis.*, **3**(25): 1–8.
87. Kris-Etherton P.M., Harris W.S., Appel L.J. (2002). Fish Consumption, Fish Oil, Omega-3 Fatty Acids and Cardiovascular Disease. *Circulation*, **106**: 2747–2775.
88. Mozaffarian D., Wu J.H.Y. (2011). Omega-3 Fatty Acids and Cardiovascular Disease. Effects on Risk Factors, Molecular Pathways, and Clinical Events. *J. Am. Coll. Cardiol.*, **58**(20): 2047–2067.
89. Torrejon C., Jung U.J., Deckelbaum R.J. (2007). N-3 Fatty Acids and Cardiovascular Disease: Actions and Molecular Mechanisms. *Prostaglandins Leukot. Essent. Fatty Acids*, **77**(5–6): 319–326.
90. Mason R.P. (2019). New Insights into Mechanisms of Action for Omega-3 Fatty Acids in Atherothrombotic Cardiovascular Disease. *Curr. Atheroscler. Rep.*, **21**(2): 11.
91. Stark K.D., Van Elswyk M.E., Higgins M.R., Weatherford C.A., Salem N. Jr. (2016). Global Survey of the Omega-3 Fatty Acids, Docosahexaenoic Acid and Eicosapentaenoic Acid in the Blood Stream of Healthy Adults. *Prog. Lipid Res.*, **63**: 132–152.

92. Maki K.C., Eren F., Cassens M.E., Dicklin M.R., Davidson M.H. (2018). ω-6 Polyunsaturated Fatty Acids and Cardiometabolic Health: Current Evidence, Controversies, and Research Gaps. *Adv. Nutr.*, **9**: 688–700.

93. Patterson E., Wall R., Fitzgerald G.F., Ross R.P., Stanton C. (2012). Health Implications of High Dietary Omega-6 Polyunsaturated Fatty Acids. *J. Nutr. Metab.*, Article ID 539426, 16 pages.

94. Pham-Huy A.L., He H., Pham-Huy C. (2008). Free radicals and Antioxidants in Disease and Health. *Int. J. Biomed. Sci.*, **4**(2): 89–96.

95. Djuricic I., Calder P.C. (2021). Beneficial Outcomes of Omega-6 and Omega-3 Polyunsaturated Fatty Acids on Human Health: An Update for 2021. *Nutrients*, **13**(2421): 1–23.

96. Huerta-Yépez S., Tirado-Rodriguez A.B., Hankinson O. (2016). Role of Diets Rich in Omega-3 and Omega-6 in the Development of Cancer. *Bol. Med. Hosp. Infant Mex.*, **73**(6): 446–456.

97. Abdelhamid A., Hooper L., Sivakaran R., Hayhoe R.P.G., Welch A. (2019). The Relationship Between Omega-3, Omega-6 and Total Polyunsaturated Fat and Musculoskeletal Health and Functional Status in Adults: A Systematic Review and Meta-Analysis of RCTs. *Calcif. Tissue Int.*, **105**: 353–372.

98. Calder P.C. (2020). Eicosanoids. *Essays Biochem.*, **64**(3): 423–441.

99. Dennis E.A., Norris P.C. (2015). Eicosanoid Storm in Infection and Inflammation. *Nat. Rev. Immunol.*, **15**(8): 511–523. Erratum in: *Nat. Rev. Immunol.*, **15**(11): 724.

100. Greene E.R., Huang S., Serhan C.N., Panigrahy D. (2011). Regulation of Inflammation in Cancer by Eicosanoids. *Prostaglandins Other Lipid Mediat.*, **96**(1–4): 27–36.

101. Renata N.G., Felipe C.S., Alison C. (2018). Eicosanoids and Cancer. *Clinics*, **73** (Suppl. 1): e530s, 10 pages.

102. Youness E.R. (2019). Role of Prostaglandins, Thromboxanes and Leukotrienes as Mediators in Inflammations. *Adv. J. Uro. Nephro.*, **1**(1): 1–7.

103. Varga Z., Sabzwari S.R.A., Vargova V. (2017). Cardiovascular Risk of Nonsteroidal Anti-Inflammatory Drugs: An Under-Recognized Public Health Issue. *Cureus*, **9**(4): e1144, 12 pages.

104. Frigolet M.E., Gutiérrez-Aguilar R. (2017). The Role of the Novel Lipokine Palmitoleic Acid in Health and Disease. *Adv. Nutr.*, **8**(1): 173S–181S.

105. Medeiros-de-Moraes I.M., Gonçalves-de-Albuquerque C.F., Kurz A.R.M., de Jesus Oliveira F.M., de Abreu V.H.P., Torres R.C., Carvalho V.F., Estato V., Bozza P.T., Sperandio M., de Castro-Faria-Neto H.C., Silva A.R. (2018). Omega-9 Oleic Acid, the Main Compound of Olive Oil, Mitigates Inflammation during Experimental Sepsis. *Oxid. Med. Cell. Longev.*, **2018**, Article ID 6053492, 13 pages.

106. Galán-Arriero I., Serrano-Muñoz D., Gómez-Soriano J., Goicoechea C., Taylor J., Velasco A., Ávila-Martín G. (2017). The Role of Omega-3 and Omega-9 Fatty Acids for the Treatment of Neuropathic Pain After Neurotrauma. *Biochim. Biophys. Acta*, **1859**: 1629–1635.

107. Remig V., Franklin B., Margolis S., Kostas G., Nece T., Street J.C. (2010). Trans Fats in America: A Review of Their Use, Consumption, Health Implications, and Regulation. *J. Am. Diet. Assoc.*, **110**(4): 585–592.

108. Miller M., Stone N.J., Ballantyne C., Bittner V., Criqui M.H., Ginsberg H.N., Goldberg A.C., Howard W.J., Jacobson M.S., Kris-Etherton P.M., Lennie T.A., Levi M., Mazzone T., Pennathur S. (2011). Triglycerides and Cardiovascular Disease. *Circulation*, **123**: 2292–2333.

109. Laufs U., Parhofer K.G., Ginsberg H.N., Hegele R.A. (2020). Clinical Review on Triglycerides. *Eur. Heart J.*, **41**(1): 99–109.

110. Chapman M.J., Ginsberg H.N., Amarenco P., Andreotti F., Boren J., Catapano A.L., Descamps O.S., Fisher E., Kovanen P.T., Kuivenhoven J.A., Lesnik P., Masana L., Nordestgaard B.G., Ray K.K., Reiner Z., Taskinen M.R., Tokgozoglu L., Tybjaerg-Hansen A., Watts G.F. (2011). Triglyceride-Rich Lipoproteins and High-Density Lipoprotein Cholesterol in Patients at High Risk of Cardiovascular Disease: Evidence and Guidance for Management. *Eur. Heart J.*, **32**: 1345–1361.

111. Seymour C.A., Byrne C.D. (1993). Triglycerides and Disease. *Postgrad. Med. J.*, **69**(815): 679–695.

112. Feingold K.R., Grunfeld C. (2018). Introduction to Lipids and Lipoproteins. In: *Endotext [Internet]*. Editors: K.R. Feingold, B. Anawalt, A. Boyce, et al. South Dartmouth, MA. www.ncbi.nlm.nih.gov/books/NBK305896/.

113. Schmidt K., Noureen A., Kronenberg F., Utermann G. (2016). Structure, Function, and Genetics of Lipoprotein (a). *J. Lipid Res.*, **57**(8): 1339–1359.

114. Küllenberg D., Taylor L.A., Schneider M., Massing U. (2012). Health Effects of Dietary Phospholipids. *Lipids Health Dis.*, **11**(3): 16 pages.

115. Erickson M.C. (2008). 2. Chemistry and Function of Phospholipids, pp. 39–61. In: *Food Lipids: Chemistry, Nutrition, and Biotechnology*. 3rd edition. Editors: C.C. Akoh, D.B. Min. CRC Press, Taylor & Francis Group, Boca Raton, FL, 930 pages.

116. Cooper G.M. (2000). *The Cell: A Molecular Approach*. 2nd edition. Sinauer Associates, Sunderland, MA. Cell Membranes. www.ncbi.nlm.nih.gov/books/NBK9928/.

117. Gault C.R., Obeid L.M., Hannun Y.A. (2010). An Overview of Sphingolipid Metabolism: From Synthesis to Breakdown. *Adv. Exp. Med. Biol.*, **688**: 1–23.

118. Parish E.J., Li S., Bell A.D. (2008). 4- Chemistry of Waxes and Sterols, pp. 99–123. In: *Food Lipids: Chemistry, Nutrition, and Biotechnology.* 3rd edition. Editors: C.C. Akoh, D.B. Min. CRC Press, Taylor & Francis Group, Boca Raton, FL, 930 pages.

119. Kritchevsky D. (2008). 19- Fats and Oils in Human Health, pp. 499–512. In: *Food Lipids: Chemistry, Nutrition, and Biotechnology.* 3rd edition. Editors: C.C. Akoh, D.B. Min. CRC Press, Taylor & Francis Group, Boca Raton, FL.

120. Huff T., Jialal I. (2019). Physiology, Cholesterol. In: *StatPearls.* StatPearls Publishing, Treasure Island, FL. www.ncbi.nlm.nih.gov/books/NBK470561/.

121. Orth M., Bellosta S. (2012). Cholesterol: Its Regulation and Role in Central Nervous System Disorders. *Cholesterol*, Article ID 292598, 19 pages.

122. Schreurs B.G. (2010). The Effects of Cholesterol on Learning and Memory. *Neurosci. Biobehav. Rev.*, **34**(8): 1366–1379.

123. Daniels T.F., Killinger K.M., Michal J.J., Wright Jr. R.W., Jiang Z. (2009). Lipoproteins, Cholesterol Homeostasis and Cardiac Health. *Int. J. Biol. Sci.*, **5**(5): 474–488.

124. DuBroff R., de Lorgeril M. (2015). Cholesterol confusion and statin controversy. *World J. Cardiol.*, **7**(7): 404–409.

125. Gulum A.H., Hume A.L. (2015). Statins: An Update on Clinical Issues and Selected Adverse Effects. *J. Nurse Pract. (JNP)*, **11**(3): 287–294.

126. Stone N.J., Robinson J.G., Lichtenstein A.H., Bairey Merz C.N., Blum C.B., Eckel R.H., Goldberg A.C., Gordon D., Levy D., Lloyd-Jones D.M., McBride P., Schwartz J.S., Shero S.T., Smith S.C., Watson K., Wilson P.W. (2014). 2013 ACC/AHA Guideline on the Treatment of Blood Cholesterol to Reduce Atherosclerotic Cardiovascular Risk in Adults: A Report of the American College of Cardiology/ American Heart Association Task Force on Practice Guidelines. *J. Am. Coll. Cardiol.*, **63**: 2889–2934.

127. Jain T., Bathla S. (2015). Plant Sterols for Human Health- A Review. *J. Appl. Nat. Sci.*, **7**(2): 1081–1087.

128. Cassim A.M., Gouguet P., Gronnier J., Laurent N., Germain V., Grison M., Boutté Y., Gerbeau-Pissot P., Simon-Plas F., Mongrand S. (2019). Plant Lipids: Key Players of Plasma Membrane Organization and Function. *Progress in Lipid Res.*, **73**: 1–27.

129. Cabral C.E., Klein M.R.S.T. (2017). Phytosterols in the Treatment of Hypercholesterolemia and Prevention of Cardiovascular Diseases. *Arq. Bras Cardiol.*, **109**(5): 475–482.

130. Ogbe R.J., Ochalefu D.O., Mafulul S.G., Olaniru O.B. (2015). A Review on Dietary Phytosterols: Their Occurrence, Metabolism and Health Benefits. *Asian J. Plant Sci. Res.*, **5**(4): 10–21.

131. FDA (Food and Drug Administration) (2010). Food Labeling; Health Claim; Phytosterols and Risk of Coronary Heart Disease. *Proposed Rule.*, **75**(235): 76526–76571.

132. Weete J.D., Abril M., Blackwell M. (2010). Phylogenetic Distribution of Fungal Sterols. *PLoS One*, **5**(5): e10899.

133. Dupont S., Fleurat-Lessard P., Cruz R.G., Lafarge C., Grangeteau C., Yahou F., Gerbeau-Pissot P., Abrahão Júnior O., Gervais P., Simon-Plas F., Cayot P., Benet L. (2021). Antioxidant Properties of Ergosterol and Its Role in Yeast Resistance to Oxidation. *Antioxidants*, **10**(1024): 1–21.

134. Shaikh S., Verma H., Yadav N., Jauhari M., Bullangowda J. (2012). Applications of Steroid in Clinical Practice: A Review. *ISRN Anesthesiol. (International Scholarly Research Notices Anesthesiology)*, **2012**, Article ID 985495, 11 pages.

135. Ericson-Neilsen W., Kaye A.D. (2014). Steroids: Pharmacology, Complications, and Practice Delivery Issues. *Ochsner J.*, **14**(2): 203–207.

136. Staels B., Fonseca V.A. (2009). Bile Acids and Metabolic Regulation: Mechanisms and Clinical Responses to Bile Acid Sequestration. *Diabetes Care*, **32** (Suppl. 2), S237–S245.

137. Hanafusa K., Hotta T., Iwabuchi K. (2020). Glycolipids: Linchpins in the Organization and Function of Membrane Microdomains. Front. Cell Dev. Biol., **8**: 589799, 9 pages.

138. Malhotra R. (2012). Membrane Glycolipids: Functional Heterogeneity: A Review. *Biochem. Anal. Biochem.*, **1**: 108, 5 pages.

139. Makrantonaki E., Ganceviciene R., Zouboulis C. (2011). An Update on the Role of the Sebaceous Gland in the Pathogenesis of Acne. *Dermato-Endocrinology*, **3**(1): 41–49.

140. Singh A., Lal U.R., Mukhtar H.M., Singh P.S., Shah G., Dhawan R.K. (2015). Phytochemical Profile of Sugarcane and Its Potential Health Aspects. *Pharmacogn. Rev.*, **9**(17): 45–54.

141. Cho K-H., Kim S-J., Yadav D., Kim J-Y., Kim J-R. (2018). Consumption of Cuban Policosanol Improves Blood Pressure and Lipid Profile via Enhancement of HDL Functionality in Healthy Women Subjects: Randomized, Double-Blinded, and Placebo-Controlled Study. *Oxid. Med. Cell. Longev.*, **2018**, Article ID 4809525, 15 pages.

142. Forouhi N.G., Krauss R.M., Taubes G., Willett W. (2018). Dietary Fat and Cardiometabolic Health: Evidence, Controversies, and Consensus for Guidance. *Br. Med. J. (BMJ)*, **361**: k2139, 1–8.

143. Xicoy H., Wieringa B., Martens G.J.M. (2019). The Role of Lipids in Parkinson's Disease. *Cells*, **8**(27): 1–58.

2 Micronutrients

1 INTRODUCTION

Unlike macronutrients, of which the body needs a few tens to several hundred grams, micronutrients are nutrients required by the body in smaller amounts, from some micrograms (µg) to a few hundred milligrams. Micronutrients include all the vitamins and essential minerals. There are 16 essential minerals and 13 vitamins required to build and maintain all body cells and tissues (1–5). They are essential to life and participate in a wide range of physiological functions, as well as the prevention and treatment of various diseases. Micronutrients play a central part in the metabolism and in the maintenance of tissue function. They are essential components of the human diet and contribute to growth, development, and performance (1–5). Certain minerals or vitamins play a crucial role as co-factors or co-enzymes in the activity of all enzymes to perform their activities in cells and organs. Without them, cell activities will be disturbed or cease to function. Some minerals and vitamins have antioxidant properties which can neutralize the deleterious effects of oxidant species or free radicals. Various minerals are essential for human life.

Micronutrients are organic and inorganic elements that have a physiological function within the body (4). Dietary micronutrients such as vitamin B1, B6, B9, B12, vitamin C, zinc, and copper have certain effects on the structure and certain functions of the brain (5). The functions and effects of micronutrients change throughout the human life cycle and should be ensured by an adequate diet. In particular, the time period of pregnancy and early childhood is critical, and hidden hunger is a worldwide problem, affecting more than two billion people, primarily females and children. The importance of changing micronutrient requirements during the life cycle is usually not considered (2). The lack of essential vitamins and minerals in the diet can cause specific deficiency diseases that can be fatal.

Briefly, micronutrients play important roles in our body such as enzyme activation, hormone production, cell homeostasis, and organ maintenance (immune system, brain, nerve, heart, bone, muscle, fetus, etc.). However, micronutrients yield no energy. Adequate micronutrient intake throughout one's life course is essential for the maintenance of health. Micronutrients are generally not produced by the human body, necessitating an adequate daily intake at levels that have been recommended by various governing bodies. The Institute of Medicine of the USA provides a set of reference values called dietary reference intakes (DRI) that are used to plan and assess nutrient intakes of healthy people, based on age and gender. These values include the recommended dietary allowance (RDA), which is the average daily level of intake that is deemed sufficient to meet the nutrient requirements of nearly all (97%-98%) healthy individuals (2). The adequate or average intake (AI) is a recommended intake value, based on experimentally derived intake levels or approximations of observed mean nutrient intake by a group of healthy people that are assumed to be adequate (2). The tolerable upper intake level (UL) is the highest level of nutrient intake that is likely to pose no risk of adverse health effects for almost all individuals in the general population. As intake increases above the UL, the risk of adverse effects increases (2–3). It should be noted that these values cited previously are recommended to avoid deficiency and toxicity.

The roles and sources of all essential minerals and vitamins will be explained below.

2 MINERALS

Minerals are inorganic elements belonging to either the metal or the metalloid group, and exist in the body either in ionic form (cation or anion), salt, or as component of organic compounds (3–9). They are almost soluble in water. Free mineral ions can be held in water (solubilized) by water dipole-ion interactions. Minerals can also be linked with various substances in the diet such as amino acids, peptides, and volatile fatty acids to form a complex (6). Diet sodium Na$^+$, potassium K$^+$, and chloride Cl$^-$ are absorbed with almost 100% efficiency and enter the blood. Sulfate anion SO_4^{2-} can also be absorbed from the diet, but only with about 60% efficiency. Diet calcium Ca^{2+}, magnesium Mg^{2+}, and phosphate (PO_4^{-3}) are generally absorbed with lower efficiency from the diet than the previous ions (6). Minerals are present in nature from soil, water, microorganisms, parasites, to corals, algae, plants, animals, and humans. Minerals are ubiquitous in the body, but mostly present in blood, cells, and bones. Minerals are used by the body in many ways. Although they yield no energy, they have important roles to play in many activities in the body. They are necessary for the maintenance of certain essential physicochemical processes of cells or organs for the maintenance of life (5–9). Minerals are involved in a number of enzymatic reactions as cofactors for energy production and tissue building. Without the aid of a specific mineral called cofactor, certain enzymes cannot work. They also serve as electrolytes in blood and cells for homeostasis maintenance. Their functions include osmoregulation – maintenance of osmotic pressure between intra-cells and extra-cells – and regulation of acid-base balance. Many minerals are used to build bone tissue, transmit nerve impulses, contract and relax muscles, and synthesize hormones. Certain minerals possess antioxidant activity and are used to protect cells and organs against harmful free radicals. The human body cannot furnish minerals; they must be imported from foods, especially from plant foods. Plant mineral content varies with the mineral levels in soil where they live and also the maturation of the plant. If any of the essential minerals is low or absent in the diet (water, foods), disease will develop in the body. This type of disease is called deficiency disease (1–9).

Although classified among the micronutrients, minerals are also divided in two groups: macrominerals and micro-minerals that depend on the quantity required by the body. A mineral needed in large amounts – around a gram per day or less – is called a macro-mineral, whereas a micromineral is required in a small quantity – microgram to milligram per day. There are 16 essential minerals, 7 of which are macro-minerals including: sodium (Na), potassium (K), calcium (Ca), magnesium (Mg), phosphor (P), chlorine (Cl), and sulfur (S). The rest is micro-minerals such as: iron (Fe), zinc (Zn), iodine (I), selenium (Se), fluorine (F), manganese (Mn), chromium (Cr), copper (Cu), and molybdenum (Mo) (3–9). An excessive intake of minerals through supplements or foods is also harmful to the body as their deficiency. Minerals in vegetal or animal foods are often more assimilated into the body and less toxic than those artificially obtained through supplements. The roles of each essential mineral in the human body will be described as follows.

2.1 MACROMINERALS

2.1.1 Sodium

Sodium (Na) is an alkali metal. In nature and the human body, sodium is in cation form (Na$^+$). Sodium is the principal ion of blood and extracellular fluids. It plays a crucial role in absorption of dietary sugars, amino acids, bile salts, and water (6–9). The recommended daily intake (RDA) for Na$^+$ is 2,300 mg for adult equivalent to 5,800 mg/day of salt (NaCl) for adults (7).

The role of Na$^+$ in human physiology is related to the maintenance of the balance of physiological fluids (blood pressure, kidney function, nerve and muscle functions) through the pump Na$^+$/K$^+$-ATPase enzyme or sodium-potassium adenosine triphosphatase pump (6–9). This enzyme, found in membranes of all animal cells, pumps potassium into cells while pumping sodium out of cells. Because sodium ions are reabsorbed by the kidneys, very little sodium ions (about 200 mg) are required in the diet. The body has very efficient and redundant mechanisms for Na$^+$ absorption (6, 9). A deficiency of Na$^+$ is rare, but it can happen in cases of diarrhea, vomiting, or excessive sweating, and a shortage may lead to nausea, dizziness, poor concentration, muscle weakness, and so on. Excessive presence of sodium cation (Na$^+$) in the body may be due to high intake of sodium salt or kidney alteration, causing high blood pressure and neurological complications. Excessive long-term intake of Na^+ may also cause a secondary loss of calcium (7, 9). In contrast to many minerals, sodium absorption in the small intestine is extremely efficient and in a healthy individual all excess Na^+ is excreted by the kidneys. Kidney reabsorption of Na^+ is hormonally controlled through the mineralocorticoids secreted by the adrenal cortex of suprarenal glands, allowing for a relatively constant Na^+ concentration in the blood. Its metabolism is regulated by aldosterone (8–9). Na^+ excretion occurs mainly through the kidney as sodium chloride or phosphate in the urine. Diuretic drugs are used to help the excretion of Na^+ and water in the urine for the treatment of cardiovascular disease, edema, and hypertension. Na^+ is also excreted in the sweat, and the quantities lost by this route vary rather markedly with environmental humidity and heat (8–9).

Sodium chloride (NaCl), salt, or table salt represents the form of sodium the most present in different foods and dishes consumed by humans. Excessive intake of salt can cause toxicity or diseases to a number of people. The amounts required for toxicity vary and are largely dependent on the availability of water to the body. Normally, the excess of salt is efficiently excreted in healthy individuals, whereas high plasma sodium and chloride levels commonly occur in diabetes insipidus, Cushion's disease, brainstem injury, dehydration through either excessive sweating or deficient water intake, and administration of cortisone, adrenocorticotropic hormone (ACTH), or sex hormones (8). Excessive salt intake may cause hypertension, coronary heart disease, stroke, gastric cancer, osteoporosis, bronchial hyperactivity, and edema. Low level of sodium in the serum is hyponatremia and this occurs in acute Addison's disease, vomiting, diarrhea, nephrosis, severe burns, intestinal obstruction, and diuretic drug intake (8–9). There is scientific evidence supporting that lower-salt diets are preventive against hypertension. Sodium cation is also combined with other anions such as citrate, phosphate, carbonate, fluoride, nitrate, or organic compounds, that are present in the diet or in the body. Briefly, sodium cation is ubiquitous in nature and the human body, and plays important roles in fluid balance in cells, nerve impulsion, and muscle contraction. The main food source for sodium is table salt, but it is also found in sauces (meat sauce, fish sauce, soybean sauce), stock cube, ham, saucisson, sea foods, meat, chips, snacks, dairy products, baking soda, and so on.

2.1.2 Potassium

Potassium (K) is an alkaline metal and exists as a cation (K^+) in the human body. It is the most abundant cation inside cells, and is fully water-soluble. Ninety percent of potassium exists in intracellular fluid, with about 10% in extracellular fluid, and only 1% in blood plasma. As Na^+, K^+ levels in the cells are regulated by the pump Na^+/K^+-ATPase enzyme found in the cell membrane (6–9). More than 90% of dietary K^+ is absorbed in the digestive tract (6). As Na^+, renal K^+ excretion is regulated by aldosterone, which increases Na^+ reabsorption in the kidney in exchange for increased loss of K^+ to the urine. The homoeostasis of K^+ in the body is controlled by renal glomerular filtration and tubular secretion (6, 8–9).

Potassium plays a role in the maintenance of the balance of the physical fluid system and assisting nerve functions through its role in the transmittance of nerve impulses. It is also related to heart activity muscle contraction (7). However, potassium requirements are also dependent on the physiological or pathological environment. Hypokalemia is low level of blood potassium and this occurs in diarrhea, metabolic alkalosis, and familial periodic paralysis (8). It can be caused by a low dietary intake of K^+ or by high salt in the diet, but also by medications like diuretics that increase water excretion. A potassium deficiency may result in fatigue, cramping legs, slow reflexes, muscle weakness, acne, dry skin, mood changes, and irregular heartbeat. Moreover, a reduced level of K^+ produces alkalosis, which makes the kidney less able to retain this mineral (7). Other symptoms of potassium deficiency are cardiac arrythmias, impaired carbohydrate tolerance, and altered electrocardiogram in calves (8). Potassium deficiency affects the collecting tubules of the kidney, resulting in the inability to concentrate urine, and also causes alterations of gastric secretions and intestinal motility (8). Hyperkalemia (increased K^+ level in blood) occurs in Addison's disease, advanced chronic renal failure, shock and dehydration. Excessive potassium intake can be toxic systemically and can cause dilatation of the heart, cardiac arrest, cardiac arrhythmias, and oliguria (7–9).

The recommended intake for potassium is 3500 mg per day for adults (7). An adequate intake of K$^+$ at the normal levels may decrease blood pressure, and maintain a good functioning of the cardiovascular system. However, self-medication of K$^+$ is dangerous. Potassium is only prescribed by health professionals after blood analysis of K$^+$. Sources of potassium include milk, dairy products, vegetables, fruits, and nuts (6–8). Fruits and vegetables that contain high amounts of K$^+$ are spinach, lettuce, broccoli, peas, tomatoes, potatoes, bananas, apples, oranges, and apricots. Whole grains and seeds (cereals, dry beans, chia seeds), certain fish (such as salmon, cod, and flounder), and meats are also high in potassium.

2.1.3   Calcium

Calcium is an alkaline earth metal and exists as a divalent cation (Ca^{++}) in the body. It is often combined with different anions that are present in foods and the human body like phosphate, lactate, chloride, citrate, and carbonate, to form a mineral salt. Calcium is a major component of bones and teeth and the most abundant mineral in the body (3, 4, 6–11). The adult human body contains about 1200 g of calcium, which amounts to about 1–2% of body weight (3). Nearly 99% of total body calcium is located in the bone tissue and teeth. The remaining 1% is found in blood, muscle, extracellular fluid, and soft tissues (3–4).

Calcium cation is needed not only for bone mineralization, but also for tooth health, heart regulation rate and contraction, blood coagulation, parathyroid gland function, muscle contraction, and nerve conduction. In addition, Ca may act as a cofactor in enzyme reactions and is involved in mineral homeostasis and physiological performance in general (3–4, 6–11). In blood coagulation, calcium activates the conversion of prothrombin to thrombin and also takes part in milk clotting. Calcium activates large number of enzymes such as adenosine triphosphatase (ATPase), succinic dehydrogenase, and lipase. It is also required for membrane permeability, and involved in muscle contraction, normal transmission of nerve impulses, and in neuromuscular excitability (8–11). A reduced extracellular blood calcium increases the irritability of nerve tissue, and very low levels may cause spontaneous discharges of nerve impulses leading to tetany and convulsions (8–11). Calcium absorption requires calcium-binding proteins and is regulated by vitamin D, sunlight, parathyroid hormone, and thyrocalcitonin. Parathyroid hormone (PTH) increases the renal tubular reabsorption of calcium, promotes intestinal calcium absorption by stimulating the renal production of 1,25-dihydroxyvitamin D, or calcitriol – the active form of vitamin D – and, if necessary, resorbs bone. In Ca homeostasis, PTH and calcitriol (1,25(OH)2D3) are secreted when plasma Ca is low, whereas thyrocalcitonin is secreted when plasma calcium is high (3–4, 9). Thyrocalcitonin decreases plasma calcium and phosphate levels whereas parathyroid hormone increases them (3, 8–11).

However, the integrity of the system depends critically on vitamin D status; if there is a deficiency of vitamin D, the loss of its calcemic action leads to a decrease in the ionized calcium (Ca^{++}) and secondary hyperparathyroidism and hypophosphatemia. For this reason, vitamin D deficiency results in rickets in children and osteomalacia in adults, while calcium deficiency gives rise to osteoporosis in the elderly (3). Briefly, these two diseases have different origins: osteoporosis is mainly due to lower levels of estrogen in menopausal women or to hormonal change in the elderly for both sexes, whereas osteomalacia or rickets in children is due to the lack of vitamin D that leads to calcium and phosphate deficiency. Osteoporosis is identified by bones becoming porous and weak, while osteomalacia is characterized by softening of the bones that can lead to fractures and severe deformity. Moreover, an increase in Ca intake during pregnancy is recommended to prevent risk of pre-eclampsia. Several studies have shown an association between low calcium intake and increased risks of colon cancer, hypercholesterolemia, and high blood pressure (7, 10). Calcium deficiency also affects the dentition of both children and adult (8–11). In brief, calcium is mainly required for bone and tooth formation, muscle contraction, and nerve transmission. It also plays a role in cellular metabolism, aids blood clotting, and prevents colon cancer in humans (3, 4, 6–11).

Calcium requirements are high during all stages of life. Dietary reference values for individuals over 19 years of age vary from 1000 mg to 1300 mg, depending on the reference guidelines. The

Recommended Daily Allowance (RDA) for Ca is set out in the wide range of 800–1300 mg/day (3, 7–11). The adequate intake (AI) for adults aged 19 to 50 is 1000 mg per day. For adolescents and teens aged 9 to 18, the AI is higher – about 1,300 mg per day – as they are in their growth period. For men and women aged 51 and older, the AI is 1200 mg (3, 7–11). This is why bone health is dependent on the intake of dietary calcium and also why the determination of calcium blood levels does not always reveal the calcium deficiency in the body because the body takes calcium in the bone to compensate for the decrease of calcium in the blood.

About three-quarters of dietary calcium is from dairy products and grains, the rest being accounted for by vegetables, protein-rich foods, fruits, and oil. Other sources of absorbable calcium are: mineral and source waters, nuts, seeds (sesame, chia seed, almond), soybean milk, tofu, broccoli, Chinese cabbage, spinach, kale, and turnip greens (3–4, 7–10). Sardines and other canned fish with bones are additional sources. Among dairy products, hard cheese (parmesan, gouda, cheddar) is the richest source of calcium and can provide one g of Ca per 100 g, whereas milk and yogurt can furnish between 100 mg to 180 mg of Ca per 100 g (9–10). Calcium in milk and dairy foods are more soluble and absorbed in the body than calcium in plant foods because milk contains lactose that helps calcium absorption and transportation. Moreover, phytate, an antioxidant often present in bran of rice and wheat, and oxalate, a mineral often found in some vegetables and fruits like spinach, rhubarb, beet, leek, and star fruit, can partially inhibit the absorption of calcium in the body. The relatively high calcium-phosphate ratio of 2.2 in human milk compared with 0.77 in cow milk may be a factor in the higher absorption of calcium from human milk than cow milk (3). For the growth of children and their rickets prevention, the best way is to consume milk and dairy products daily. Milk and dairy products are also necessary for adults and the elderly since they are not only rich in calcium, but also high in vitamin D, magnesium, fluorine, all phosphorous, which all contribute to the prevention and treatment of a number of diseases (osteoporosis, tooth decay, cramp, etc.). In the United States and in Holland, 72 and 58% of calcium supply comes from dairy products, respectively, whereas in China, only around 7% of total calcium intake comes from dairy products, while most comes from vegetables (30.2%) and legumes (16.7%) (10). The lowest calcium intakes occur in developing countries, particularly in eastern Asia (China, Vietnam, Thailand, Indonesia), and the highest in developed countries, particularly in North America and Europe, because people in eastern Asia do not consume milk and dairy products, contrary to Americans and Europeans (3). The average dietary calcium intake in many countries in Asia is less than 500 mg/day, while that in the United States, Canada and Europe is more than 1500 mg/day (10). Therefore, East Asian people are often small because they do not consume milk and dairy products from infancy to adulthood. In addition, some plant foods such as spinach and star fruit, contain high levels of oxalic acid, an anti-nutrient compound, that interferes with absorption and metabolism of several minerals such as calcium, iron, and magnesium, present in foods or supplements. This oxalic acid can lead to the formation of oxalate stones in urine by impairing kidney function that may cause death. Calcium, magnesium, and iron in foods can also be bound to phytic acid, an antioxidant, often present in the hulls of some nuts, seeds, and grains; the beneficial effects of these minerals become, therefore, diminished or neutralized.

The use of calcium supplements in tablet form is controversial because their efficacy largely depends on their water-solubility. Calcium citrate and lactate are water-soluble, contrary to calcium carbonate and phosphate. The first ones are more absorbed by the intestinal tract than calcium carbonate and phosphate, hence their efficacy is higher than that of carbonate and phosphate. Ca with vitamin D3 supplement is also used to treat some bone diseases. Calcium gluconate is the calcium salt of gluconic acid. It is easily water-soluble and used as an intravenous medication for the treatment of some diseases such as tetany and hypoparathyroidism due to calcium deficiency, and hypocalcemia due to pregnancy or rapid growth of skeleton. The use of Ca supplements also varies between countries. In the United States and Canada, around 40% of the adult population was reported to have taken Ca supplements, and 70% in the older women group (10). In contrast, in Argentina and in Europe, very few people are reported taking Ca supplements, even during pregnancy. This difference is mainly due to the habitude of each population rather than due to the lack of Ca in their diet because both populations have similar diets (10).

The adverse effects of high Ca intakes in humans are primarily from the intake of calcium from nutrient supplements (4). Excessive intake of Ca may cause mineral imbalances because it interferes with the absorption of iron, magnesium, zinc, and so on, and may cause Ca deposits in the bladder and kidneys. Excess Ca depresses cardiac activity and leads to respiratory and cardiac failure; it may cause the heart to stop in systole – although, normally, Ca ions increase the strength and duration of cardiac muscle contraction (8). Excess calcium is excreted by the kidney into the urine. The normal level of calcium in the blood is about 10 mg/dL. When the body cannot maintain this level, a person will experience hypo- or hypercalcemia. Hypercalcemia and its harmful consequences for health are not observed in people who consume natural foods rich in Ca like milk and dairy products. A good illustration of the safety of natural calcium foods is provided by nomadic, pastoralist Masai peoples in East Africa (11). Because their diets consist mostly of the milk of their flocks, they have calcium intakes higher than 5,000 mg/day, roughly 5 to 10 times what people of industrialized nations ingest. Such pastoral peoples are not known to have any unusual incidence of hypercalcemia or kidney stones or other diseases due to overconsumption of calcium (11). However, hypercalcemia, metabolic alkalosis, and possibly renal insufficiency have been observed, especially in postmenopausal and pregnant women when consuming an excessive amount of Ca supplements (typically four g/day), and often in the same time alkaline water, which can raise the pH of the urine and predispose to calcium deposits in the kidneys (11). Therefore, the intake of calcium supplements is not useful when the diet is rich in Ca – rich in dairy products (milk, cheese). Ca supplements are only reserved for people with bone diseases, and not for normal subjects. Consult a doctor before taking calcium supplements. Change your habits by consuming milk and dairy products daily for the sake of your health.

2.1.4 Magnesium

Magnesium (Mg) is an alkaline earth metal and exists as a divalent cation (Mg^{++}) in the body. It is often linked to anions like chloride, phosphate, lactate, and organic complex like chlorophyll in leaves. It is present in vegetables, animals, and the human body. The human body contains about 25 g of magnesium, of which 30–40% is found in the muscle and soft tissues, 1% is present in the extracellular fluid, and the remainder (50–60%) is in the skeleton (3–5, 12). Magnesium has two roles, metabolic and structural. Soft tissue magnesium functions as a cofactor of about 300 enzymes involved in energy metabolism (ionic regulation, oxidation-reduction), protein synthesis, RNA and DNA synthesis, and maintenance of the electrical potential of nervous tissues and cell membranes (3–9, 12). More than half the Mg contained in the nucleus is closely associated with nucleic acids and free nucleotides of DNA. These interactions play a significant role in the stabilization of the secondary and tertiary structure of DNA (12).

Intracellular Mg is indispensable both for the synthesis and action of ATP, and most ATP-dependent enzymatic reactions require Mg, whether for carbohydrate, lipid, nuclear, or protein metabolism (5, 9, 12). Extracellular Mg is vital to normal nerve conduction, muscle function, and bone mineral formation. Adequate blood Mg is also needed to allow normal secretion of parathyroid hormone and its activity (6). In addition, the roles of Mg are to regulate potassium fluxes and to participate in the metabolism of calcium. Mg is essential for normal cellular function, replication, and energy metabolism. Mg homeostasis is maintained by controlling the efficiency of intestinal absorption and Mg losses through the kidneys via the urine (4). Mg with Ca, Na, and K play a role in balance in extracellular fluids for transmission of nerve impulses and muscle contraction (3–9, 12). Mg increases the neuromuscular excitability and has an antispastic and anticonvulsive effect, impairing the contractibility of muscles (12).

The recommended dietary allowance (RDA) of Mg for adult women is 320 mg/day and for adult men is 420 mg/day (4). Normal range of Mg in blood is 0.7–1 mmol/L (1.5–2 mEq/L; 1.7–2.4 mg/dL). Magnesium insufficiency is readily diagnosed by blood Mg concentrations being lower than normal (6). Most of the early pathological consequences of Mg depletion are neurologic or neuromuscular defects. Low intake of Mg below the RDA, but not frank deficiency, is a contributor to the development of chronic maladies such as cardiovascular disease, diabetes mellitus, hypertension, eclampsia and preeclampsia, and osteoporosis. However, the results of studies in this area are ambiguous (4). Malabsorption, alcoholism, chronic or excessive vomiting and diarrhea, as well as kidney disease, may also cause Mg depletion or deficiency (8). Early signs of Mg deficiency are loss of appetite and weakness. Thus, an insufficient Mg level in the body produces anorexia, nausea, muscular weakness, lethargy, staggering, and, if deficiency is prolonged, weight loss. Severe Mg depletion is manifested by muscular spasms (cramps) or spasmophilia, tetany without calcium deficiency, hyperexcitability, hyperirritability, stress, nervousness, and convulsions (3). Cardiac arrhythmia and pulmonary edema frequently have fatal consequences. It has been suggested that an insufficient Mg status may be a factor in the etiology of coronary heart disease and hypertension but additional evidence is needed (3). Visible symptoms of Mg deficiency in healthy people are rare. However, Mg deficiency concerns up to one fifth of the French population: 18% of men and 23% of women have Mg intakes lower than 2/3 of the recommended daily allowance (RDA) (5).

For the toxicity of magnesium, adverse effects in people with normal renal function have been observed upon ingesting foods rich in Mg (4). However, adverse effects of excess Mg intake (e.g., diarrhea, nausea, abdominal cramping, headache, hypotension) have been observed with intakes from nonfood sources such as various Mg salt supplements used for medicinal purposes (4, 7). For this reason, the US Food and Nutrition Board established the maximum usual daily intake level (Tolerable upper intake level) for adults as 350 mg/day of Mg supplements (4). This value for Mg supplements is lower than that of Mg present in natural foods (420 mg/day). Consult a doctor regarding prolonged use of Mg supplements.

For the sources of Mg, milk and dairy products (cheese, yogurt) occupy a privileged position (5). Mineral and source waters are also a good source of soluble magnesium salts. In addition, Mg bioavailability in dairy products and mineral water is excellent (5). Mg is a constituent of chlorophyll, a complex compound in green leaves. Therefore, most green vegetables (lettuce, spinach, broccoli, sorrel, cabbage, green algae, etc.), legume seeds, beans and nuts (haricot beans, soybeans, cocoa beans, walnuts, cashew, peanut, Brazil nut, lentils, etc.), beetroot, and onion, are good source of Mg. Fruits rich in Mg are banana, date, prune, coconut, blackberry, blackcurrant, and kiwi. Seafoods such as whelks, winkles, snails, oysters, mackerel, sardine, and pollock, are also rich in Mg. Tofu, meat, and chili pepper, also contain Mg. Whole wheat, brown rice, potatoes, sweet potatoes, and black chocolate are good sources of magnesium.

2.1.5 Phosphorus

Phosphorus (P), a nonmetallic element, is never found free in nature, but is always combined with other minerals. In the human body, phosphorus is most commonly found in its pentavalent form and often combined with oxygen to form an anion named phosphate (PO_4^{3-}). Phosphorus (as phosphate anion) in pentavalent or trivalent is an essential constituent of almost all plant and animal tissues and carries out all biological roles of P in living beings (4, 6–9). It exists in the form of mineral salts such as calcium or sodium phosphates and also of organic complex compounds like phospholipids, phosphoproteins, adenosine triphosphate (ATP), and nucleic acids like ribonucleic acid (RNA) and deoxyribonucleic acid (DNA) (3, 6–9). Phosphorus is located in every cell of the body and is vitally concerned with many metabolic processes. It functions as a constituent of bones and teeth, and is used as buffering action such as phosphate buffers (8, 9). The major mineral component of bone is calcium phosphate named hydroxyapatite or hydroxylapatite [$Ca_{10}(PO_4)_6(OH)_2$]. The rest (about 4%) is calcium carbonate. In teeth, the hydroxy OH- group of some hydroxyapatite is replaced by ion F- present in tape or mineral water to become fluoroapatite or $Ca_5(PO_4)_3F$ that enhances tooth enamel. In bone formation, vitamin D is probably involved in the control of P absorption and serum levels of P are regulated by kidney reabsorption (8). In addition, P helps digestion and metabolism, improves memory and cognitive activity, regulates hormone balance, increases energy, fights fatigue, stimulates protein synthesis, aids kidney functions, and so on.

Phosphorus makes up about 0.65–1.1% of the adult body (~600 g). In the adult body 85% of phosphorus is in bone and the remaining 15% is distributed in soft tissues (3). Total phosphorus concentration in whole blood is 13 mmol/l, most of which is in the phospholipids of erythrocytes and plasma lipoproteins, with approximately 1 mmol/l present as inorganic phosphate (3). P deficiency is unusual, but symptoms of hypophosphatemia are described as bone pain, irregular breathing, fatigue, anxiety, numbness, changes in body weight and skin sensitivity (7). If Ca supply is also deficient, then the condition may become severe because of increased risks of high blood pressure and bowel cancer (7). Other consequences of P deficiency are rickets in children, osteomalacia in adults, hyperparathyroidism, anorexia, anemia, muscle weakness, De Toni-Fanconi syndrome, general debility, increased susceptibility to infection, paresthesia, ataxia, confusion, and even death (3, 7–8). Ingesting dosages of P exceeding 3–4 g/day may be harmful as it can interfere with Ca absorption (7). Hyperphosphatemia or increased phosphate level in blood is found in chronic nephritis and hypoparathyroidism. It may also lead to bone loss due to hypocalcemia (8). In addition, high phosphorus intakes could decrease calcium absorption by complexing calcium in the chyme, and may be due to high levels of food phosphate additives and cola beverages in the Western diet (3).

The recommended daily allowance (RDA) of P is 700 mg/day for adults, 1250 mg/day for pregnant women and adolescents. The tolerable upper intake level (UL) for P is 4,000 mg/day for adults and 3,000 mg/day for the elderly (4, 7). On a mixed diet, absorption of total P ranges from 55% to 70% in adults. Phosphorus in food is a mixture of inorganic and organic forms. Intestinal phosphatases hydrolyze the organic form contained in food into inorganic form which is then absorbed by the digestive tract (4). Phosphates in foods exist either as natural components of biological molecules or as food additives, such as various phosphate salts added in some fortified foods. About 10% of dietary phosphorus is present as food additives (9). Sources of natural phosphorus include milk and dairy products, sardines, meat, eggs, beans, lentils, whole cereal grains, tofu, nuts, oil seeds, and banana (4, 8). A large percentage (60–80%) of the total P of cereal grains and oil seeds exists as phytic acid. Phytic acid, also called inositol polyphosphate or inositol hexakisphosphate, is found in cereal bran and legume seeds, primarily as the Ca-Mg salt of inositol phosphoric acid named phytin (8). Phytic acid inhibits the absorption of iron, calcium, and zinc, and can cause deficiency in these minerals. However, it is a good antioxidant that might prevent cancer and kidney stones. Sources of artificial P include some junk food, soft drink, and colas. They are added with synthetic phosphoric acid as an acidulant (4).

2.1.6 Sulfur

Sulfur (S) is a nonmetallic and multivalent element. Sulfur, after calcium and phosphorus, is the most abundant mineral found in all living tissues and is essential for life. A large majority of S in the human body is in organic form; the rest is in mineral salt such as sulfate (SO_4^{2-}). The primary sulfur-containing compounds of interest in humans are methionine, cysteine, taurine, methanethiol, S-adenosylmethionine, α-keto-γ-CH3-thiobutyrate (a precursor of methionine), thiamin (vitamin B1), biotin (vitamin B7), alpha-lipoic acid (ALA), coenzyme A, glutathione (GSH), chondroitin sulfate, glucosamine sulfate, fibrinogen, heparin, metallothionein, and inorganic sulfate (6, 8–9, 13–14). Methionine and cysteine are two sulfur amino acids among 20 amino acids present in different proteins of the human body. Methionine is an essential amino acid because it cannot be synthesized by the human body and therefore has to be supplied by the diet. In contrast, cysteine is synthesized from methionine by the human body but the process requires a steady supply of methionine, and therefore, cysteine is a semi-essential amino acid (14). Cystine is an oxidized form of the amino acid cysteine, while homocysteine is a homologue of cysteine with a group -CH_2- in cysteine structure. Methanethiol or methyl mercaptan (CH_3SH) is a putrid gas found in the feces, flatus, bad breath, brain, and blood of animals and humans. It is also the odor of some cheese and fruits. Taurine or 2-aminoethanesulfonic acid (a derivative of sulfur-amino acid) and sulfuric acid are the end products of sulfur metabolism. The taurine is conjugated with cholic acid and excreted in the bile. The sulfuric acid is either neutralized and excreted as inorganic sulfates in the urine or conjugated with phenol, glucuronic acid, or indoxyl. Sulfate from dietary sources and endogenous release from sulfur amino acids is also used to synthesize the chondroitin matrix of cartilage (13). S-adenosylmethionine is mainly used in methyl group transfers, and secondary in trans-sulfuration, and aminopropylation. Proteins contain between 3 and 6% of sulfur amino acids (SAAs). S is present in different proteins, enzymes, and antibodies, mostly in forms of disulfide bonds or disulfide cross-linkages (-S-S-), which are also important in their specific three-dimensional folding (8–9, 13–14).

Methylsulfonylmethane (MSM), a volatile component in the sulfur cycle, is another source of sulfur found in the human diet. Increases in serum sulfate may explain some of the therapeutic effects of MSM, dimethyl-sulfoxide (DMSO), and glucosamine sulfate. Organic sulfur, as SAAs, can be used to increase synthesis of S-adenosylmethionine, glutathione, taurine, and N-acetylcysteine (14). MSM may be effective for the treatment of allergy, pain syndromes, athletic injuries, and bladder disorders. Other sulfur compounds such as S-adenosylmethionine, dimethyl-sulfoxide, taurine, chondroitin sulfate, glucosamine, and reduced glutathione may also have clinical applications in the treatment of a number of ailments such as depression, fibromyalgia, arthritis, interstitial cystitis, athletic injuries, congestive heart failure, diabetes, cancer, and AIDS (13). In addition, sulfur is needed for a number of chemical reactions involved in the metabolism of drugs, steroids, and xenobiotics (13). The other sulfur compounds of biological significance are thiocyanate (SCN) in saliva and other fluids, ergothioneine of the red blood cells, glutathione, present in all cells, and glucosamine and chondroitin sulfate, which serve a structural function in cartilage, bone, tendons, blood vessel walls, and so on (8).

The recommended daily allowance (RDA) committee recommends a combined sulfur amino acids (SAAs) intake of at least 13 mg/kg per day. This is equivalent to 910 mg/day for a 70 kg adult. Other authorities believe this figure to be too low and recommend an intake of 25 mg/kg/day of SAAs for adults (13). Sulfur is the sixth most abundant macro-mineral in breast milk and the third most abundant mineral based on percentage of total body weight. Dietary SAAs analysis and protein supplementation may be indicated for vegan athletes, children, or patients with HIV, because of an increased risk for SAAs deficiency in these groups (13). A sulfur deficiency often leads to various muscle pain and skeletal disorders such as osteoarthritis, rheumatoid and psoriatic arthritis. An adequate sulfur intake through foods rich in sulfur compounds or sulfur supplements such as glucosamine or/and chondroitin, SAAs, may help repair the cartilage or ameliorate bone diseases. Moreover, some sulfur compounds such as glutathione (GSH), alpha lipoic acid (ALA), are strong antioxidants that may prevent many inflammatory diseases such as asthma, arthritis, and rheumatism (9, 13–14). Intake of SAAs (methionine, cysteine), combined with polyunsaturated fatty acids (PUFA) such as omega-3 fatty acids, may be beneficial for people with a variety of joint anomalies associated with inflammation (14). In addition, high levels of GSH inhibit prostaglandin production by a direct interaction with cyclooxygenases or COX enzymes that are responsible for the progression of inflammatory or degenerative states (14).

Dietary sources of sulfur are found in protein-rich animal foods, such as eggs, beef, poultry, seafood, milk, and dairy products. Plant sources of sulfur include garlic, onions, broccoli, turnips, kale, brussel sprouts, cabbage, lettuce, seaweed, nuts, and raspberries (8–9, 13–14). The highest content of sulfur amino acids (SAAs) is found in egg products, the egg white containing around 8% of SAAs (14). Egg yolks are the highest sources of total sulfur organic compounds. The methionine/cysteine ratio is around three to one, in milk and dairy products; it is around four to three in fishes such as canned tuna, and in meats (14). Chicken, fish, and beef proteins contain an average of around 5% of SAA. Dairy products, milk, cheese, and so on, contain lower levels, around 4%, primarily due to the lower content of SAA in casein. The whey protein fraction of milk contains more SAA, and is used therapeutically or as a dietary supplement. Plant proteins are relatively low in SAA, averaging below 4% (14). Fresh garlic contains alliin (a sulfoxide derived from cysteine amino acid), which is responsible for its pungent smell and its strong antioxidant and immunostimulant effect. Fresh garlic is better than dry garlic or odorless garlic because the pungent smell in fresh garlic is rich in sulfoxide antioxidant. Onion is also rich in healthy amino acid sulfoxides. But, when onion is cut or crushed in air, onion produces a lacrimatory gas due to the combined action of air and an enzyme present in onion named alliinase on this sulfoxide found in onion cells. To avoid this disagreeable sensation, cut onion in a basin filled with water. Long exposure to this lacrimatory gas when cutting onion is harmful to the eyes.

2.1.7   Chloride

Chloride is found in the form of anion (Cl^-) in all organisms and combines with cations like sodium ($Na+$) or potassium ($K+$) to form a salt such as sodium chloride ($NaCl$) or potassium chloride (KCl). After sodium, chloride is the most abundant mineral in the body. Chloride is the principal extracellular and intracellular anion (Cl^-) in the body, where it represents 60–70% of the total negative ion content (6, 8, 15–16). Chloride is vital for maintenance of serum electrical neutrality, muscular activity, osmotic pressure, electrolyte balance, acid-base status, renal function, regulation of body fluids (fluid homeostasis), and hydrochloric acid (HCl) production in the gastrointestinal tract (6, 8, 15–16). In addition, it is an essential component for the assessment of many pathological conditions. It maintains the electrical balance in the nervous system and is involved in intracellular and extracellular transport (8, 15–16).

In humans, the main source of chloride is dietary sodium chloride ($NaCl$) or table salt. Recent publication reported that dietary salt intake is the primary Cl^- source with about 6–12 g of $NaCl$ per day, (respectively 100–200 mmol of Cl^- ion per day) (15). The concentration of Cl^- ion is subject to more variation than that of sodium, since other anions, especially bicarbonate (HCO_3^-), can exchange for the chloride (8). Cl^- has an inverse relationship with bicarbonate, which acts as the major acid-base buffer in humans to maintain acid-base balance through reciprocal transport into and out of erythrocytes and renal tubule (15–16).

Chloride is primarily excreted by the kidney. Cl^- undergoes free glomerular filtration with 99% being reabsorbed and about 180 mmol of Cl^- excreted per day (15–16). Most of the reabsorption occurs in the proximal tubule of the kidney, by passive reabsorption, ion conductance or active coupled transport with other ions. Cl^- excretion is an important mechanism in the kidney's adaptation to metabolic acidosis and chronic respiratory acid-base disturbances (15–16). Several preclinical studies showed that Cl^- depletion induced stimulation of renin secretion resulting in increased systemic blood pressure. In addition, Cl^- concentrations may exert direct effects on smooth muscle cells resulting in vasoconstriction (15–16).

Cl^- has two distinct functions in the gastrointestinal (GI) tract. First, it is the chief anion of the gastric juice and is accompanied by hydrogen ions in nearly equal amounts and is secreted in form of HCL (hydrochloric acid) and is required for protein digestion, microorganism homeostasis, and absorption of nutrients (e.g., calcium, zinc, iron, vitamins, folic acid). Second, it is responsible for maintenance of the GI osmotic gradient and fluid secretion (15). The chloride of the gastric secretions is derived from blood chloride and is normally reabsorbed during the latter stages of digestion in the lower intestine (8).

Chloride is an important component of diagnostic tests in different clinical situations. Hypochloremia is usually defined as serum chloride levels below 96–101 mmol/l, while hyperchloremia normally is defined as serum chloride levels higher than 106–111 mmol/l (15). Hypochloremia is often secondary to vomiting, diuretic therapy (furosemide, chlorothiazide), and renal disease. Excessive depletion of chloride ions through losses in the gastric secretions or by deficiencies in the diet may lead to alkalosis due to an excess of bicarbonate, since the inadequate level of chloride is partially compensated for or replaced by bicarbonate (8, 15). Chloride is excreted in the feces, sweat, and urine primarily as sodium or potassium chloride, and secondarily as ammonium chloride when the environment is alkaline (8).

Hyperchloremia in critically ill patients is mainly due to loss of bicarbonate through the gastrointestinal or renal tract, or as a consequence of 'dilution' due to volume loading with fluids with a low bicarbonate concentration (15). Hyperchloremia is also caused by excess infusion of Cl^--rich fluids or by drug intake such as corticosterone, aldosterone, or by consumption of processed foods high in salt like sauce, bacon, ham, sausage, and so on. High intake of dietary salt is often the cause of hypertension (15–16). Essential hypertension is the result of a complex interaction between different regulatory systems which are themselves influenced by a multitude of genetic and environmental factors. Among the environmental factors that affect blood pressure, there is general consensus that increased salt intake increases blood pressure (16). In addition, there is accruing evidence that chloride anion (Cl^-) may have a role in blood pressure regulation which may perhaps be even more important than that of sodium cation (Na^+). Though more than 85% of Na^+ is consumed as sodium chloride, there is evidence that Na^+ and Cl^- concentrations do not go necessarily hand in hand since they may originate from different sources (16). Salt sensitivity is more prevalent in hypertensive individuals (30–50%) compared to normotensives, and the presence of salt sensitivity in normotensives is a risk factor for future development of hypertension (16). Therefore, arterial hypertension is due to the whole molecule NaCl (salt) and not to Na^+ or Cl^- alone. However, sodium iodide (NaI) and sodium bromide (NaBr) can induce hypertension as sodium chloride (NaCl) because iodine (I), bromine (Br) and chlorine (Cl) are in the same family of halogen elements (16). In human body as well as in plants and animals, chlorine only exists as chloride anion (Cl^-) and never as chlorine gas (Cl_2). Chlorine (Cl_2) gas is used as disinfectant for the tap water or like liquid bleach for the household. It is toxic for human health.

The diffusion of Cl^- ion through the cellular membrane is carried by anion channels, also called chloride channels (ClC or CLC). Chloride channels are proteinaceous pores in biological membranes that allow the passive diffusion of negatively charged ions along their electrochemical gradient. CLCs have roles in the control of electrical excitability, extra- and intracellular ion homeostasis, and transepithelial transport (17). The mutations in their genes conduct to diverse pathologies including neurodegeneration, leukodystrophy, mental retardation, deafness, blindness, myotonia, hyperaldosteronism, renal salt loss, proteinuria, kidney stones, male infertility, and osteopetrosis (17).

2.2 MICRO-MINERALS

There are nine micro-minerals: iron (Fe), zinc (Zn), iodine (I), selenium (Se), fluorine (F), manganese (Mn), chromium (Cr), copper (Cu), and molybdenum (Mo).

2.2.1 Iron

Iron (Fe) belongs to the group of transition metals and is found as ferrous ion (Fe^{2+}) and ferric ion (Fe^{3+}). The importance of iron as an element necessary for life derives from its redox reactivity as it exists in two stable, interchangeable forms, ferrous (Fe^{2+}) and ferric (Fe^{3+}) iron. In the human body, iron (Fe^{2+} or Fe^{3+}) mainly exists in complex forms bound to protein. It is a constituent of heme compounds (hemoglobin, myoglobin), various heme enzymes (cytochrome, catalase), non-heme enzymes (NADH hydrogenase, succinic dehydrogenase, flavin-iron enzymes, aconitase), and nonheme compounds (transferrin, ferritin) (3–4, 6, 8–9, 18–19). Iron is required for myelination of spinal cord and white matter of cerebellar folds in brain and is a cofactor for enzymes involved in neurotransmitter synthesis (8). Heme iron (Fe^{2+}) is the essential constituent for oxygen transport in hemoglobin of red blood cells, oxygen storage in myoglobin of diverse muscles, and electron transport for cytochrome function in aerobic respiration of cells (3, 18–19). The second largest pool of iron is found in its storage form ferritin (or also hemosiderin). Ferritin is a large assembly of 24 protein subunits that form a large sphere around a mineralized ferric core of several thousands of iron ions (Fe^{3+}) (9, 19). Newly absorbed iron from food through the digestive tract is bound and transported in the body via transferrin and stored in ferritin molecules in the liver, spleen, or bone marrow. Iron in transferrin and ferritin is ferric ion (Fe^{3+}). Many heme compounds containing ion ferrous Fe^{2+} include hemoglobin, myoglobin, cytochromes, peroxidase, catalase, succinate dehydrogenase, and endothelial nitric oxide synthase (3–4, 8–9, 18–19). Heme is a porphyrin containing an ion ferrous Fe^{2+} in the center of a heterocyclic organic compound such as hemoglobin, myoglobin, while transferrin is a glycoprotein in plasma and contains two ferric ions (Fe^{3+}), and is used for the transport of iron in the blood to the cells. In times of demand, iron is liberated from ferritin or also from hemosiderin to fulfill essential functions in oxygen transport and energy metabolism. Iron is also a component of various tissue enzymes, such as the cytochromes, which are critical for energy production and immune system functioning (4, 8). However, as iron can form free radicals – reactive oxygen species – its concentration in body tissues must be tightly regulated because in excessive amounts, it can lead to tissue damage in the liver, the heart and other metabolically active organs (18). According to Fenton reaction (see Chapter 3 of this book), free iron can change valence easily from Fe^{2+} to Fe^{3+}, depending on the environment, and this phenomenon can generate toxic free radicals including superoxide, thereby causing oxidative stress, a deleterious effect to the body (19). In contrast, iron (Fe^{2+} and Fe^{3+}) bound to proteins or cofactors such as heme or nonheme compounds is safe. Thus, iron is an essential nutrient as well as a powerful toxicant, and it is important to understand how both features are kept in balance (19).

Since iron is required for a number of diverse cellular functions, a constant balance between iron uptake, transport, storage, and utilization is required to maintain iron homeostasis in the body (3, 4, 18–19). The metabolism of iron differs from that of other minerals because the body lacks a defined mechanism for the active excretion of iron through kidneys and urine. Therefore, the maintenance of iron balance is mainly regulated at the point of absorption, namely the digestive tract (4, 18–19). Hepcidin is a circulating peptide hormone secreted by the liver that plays a central role in the regulation of iron homeostasis. It is the master regulator of systemic iron homeostasis, coordinating the use and storage of iron with iron acquisition (18). Thus, when the body needs more iron, absorption is increased, and when the quantity of iron in the body is sufficient, absorption is restricted. This control is not perfect, but is necessary for the prevention of Fe deficiency and excess (4). For maintaining iron balance and preventing iron deficiency and iron overload, the body has three main mechanisms: regulation of iron absorption, storage of iron as ferritin, and reutilization of iron liberated from the destruction of old red blood cells (erythrocytes) (4).

The iron content of an adult man is approximately four to five grams, mainly in complex forms (around 38 mg iron/kg body weight for women and 50 mg iron/kg body for men) (4, 18, 19). Of this content, approximately two-thirds are utilized as functional iron such as hemoglobin (60%), myoglobin (5%), and various heme and nonheme enzymes (5%). The remaining iron is found in body storage as ferritin (20%) and hemosiderin (10%), the two major iron storage proteins. Only very minor quantities of free iron (< 0.1%) are found as a transit chelate with transferrin, the main iron transport protein in the body (4). Humans use 20–25 mg of iron each day for the production of new red blood cells, much of which is recycled from old red blood cells (4, 18–19). About one to two mg of iron is lost every day in feces, urine, sweat, skin, enteric desquamation and some minor accidental blood losses such as epistaxis (scratches) (18–19). Menstruating women suffer an average blood loss of approximately 40 mL/cycle or 0.4 to 0.5 mg/day. Most losses are counterbalanced by the amount of iron provided in the diet.

Iron deficiency is due to the immobilization of iron stores and the absence of iron supply to tissues. It can exist with or without anemia. The primary causes of iron deficiency include low intake of bioavailable iron, increased iron requirements as a result of menstruation, rapid growth in female adolescents, pregnancy, and excessive blood loss caused by pathologic infections, such as hookworm and whipworm causing gastrointestinal blood loss and impaired absorption of iron (9, 18–19). World Health Organization (WHO) estimates that two billion people are anemic worldwide and attribute approximately 50% of all anemia to iron deficiency (18–19). In many developing countries, about 50% of children have anemia, and iron deficiency is present in half of these individuals because their diet is low in meat, which is a good source of heme iron. Iron deficiency during pregnancy is associated with a variety of adverse outcomes for both mother and infant, including increased risk of sepsis, maternal mortality, perinatal mortality, and low birth weight. Iron deficiency anemia results from both a reduction in circulating hemoglobin and a reduction in iron-containing enzymes and myoglobin, and can induce fatigue, restlessness, and impaired work performance (4, 9). Iron deficiency anemia can occur when there are stomach ulcers or other sources of slow, chronic bleeding (colon cancer, uterine cancer, intestinal polyps, hemorrhoids, etc.) (9, 18). It is also associated with aging and causes tiredness, reduced learning ability or increased rates of morbidity (5, 9, 18–19). The brain is quite sensitive to dietary iron depletion because iron is necessary to brain functioning such as protein synthesis, neurotransmitter metabolism, dendritic activity, myelination, and so on. (5, 8, 19).

Excess iron via overuse of iron supplements could pose a possible health risk (4, 19). Ferrous (Fe^{2+}) salts like ferrous sulfate, ferrous fumarate, and ferrous gluconate are often used to prepare oral iron supplements. The mechanism of cellular and tissue injury resulting from excess iron supplement intake is not fully understood (4). Side effects of iron supplements include constipation, dark feces, abdominal pain. Other risks of high iron intake may include increased risks for bacterial infection, neoplasia, arthropathy, cardiomyopathy, and endocrine dysfunctions. However, there is still much debate as to the strength of evidence to support a relationship between dietary iron intake and cancer or cardiovascular disease (4). Gastrointestinal distress does not occur from consuming a diet containing naturally occurring or fortified iron from natural foods. Individuals taking iron supplements at high levels (>45 mg/day) may encounter gastrointestinal side effects (constipation, nausea, vomiting, and diarrhea), especially when taken on an empty stomach. Based largely on the data on gastrointestinal effects following iron supplement intake in healthy adults, the US Food and Nutrition Board established a tolerable upper intake level (UL) of iron of 45 mg/day (4). Iron fortification to prevent nutritional iron deficiency, either through the open market or government-regulated programs, has been successful in developed countries, but it has not proven as effective in less-developed countries where risk for iron deficiency is perhaps more problematic (19). To fight iron deficiency, the best way is to increase food with high iron availability (e.g., meat sources), and to avoid foods that reduce absorption (for example, tea). However, pregnant women, preterm or low birth weight infants, young children, and women in their reproductive years are likely to benefit from iron supplementation. People with kidney failure and inflammatory bowel diseases may also need iron supplements (19). The anemia resulting from hookworm infection and its associated blood loss is also ameliorated by iron supplementation. The use of iron supplements may be contraindicated in anemia of chronic disease, however (19). Iron fortification policies have been criticized because they also may pose problems for people with iron overload or susceptibility for genetic or acquired iron loading such as hemochromatosis and hemosiderosis. Similarly, the benefits of iron supplementation in pregnant women are controversial, given that high iron concentrations can promote oxidative stress and complications such as gestational diabetes, and heart failure (19). As a result, weekly supplementation (as opposed to daily supplementation) and strategies focused on prevention of iron deficiency (rather than treatment of anemia) have been proposed (19). Therefore, the self-medication of iron supplements should be avoided. Consult a healthcare professional for your problem of anemia or iron deficiency. In addition, iron overload is found in two diseases, hemosiderosis and hemochromatosis. Hemosiderosis is an acquired ailment characterized by deposition of excess iron under a complex form called hemosiderin within the body tissues that normally do not contain iron such as lungs, liver, pancreas, heart, and kidneys (8). It is caused by hemolytic anemia (e.g., thalassemia), multiple blood transfusions, or chronic hemodialysis (19). Hemochromatosis is a genetic disorder of iron metabolism characterized by an abnormally high iron absorption owing to a failure of the iron absorption control mechanism at the intestinal level. More than 80% of patients with hereditary hemochromatosis are of Northern European descent, or 1 in 300 in populations of Northern European stock (9, 19). High deposits of iron in the liver and the heart can lead to cirrhosis, hepatocellular cancer, congestive heart failure, and eventual death. Sufferers of this disorder can develop iron overload through consumption of a normal diet but would be at much higher risk if consuming iron-fortified foods or iron supplements. Thus, early detection of the disease via genetic screening followed by regular blood removal has proven to be a successful treatment (4).

The recommended dietary allowances (RDAs) for iron are: 8 mg iron/day for adult men, 18 mg iron/day for adult women (19–50 years), 8 mg iron/day for women 51 years and older, 27 mg iron/day for pregnant women, 7–10 mg iron/day for children (1–8 years), 8–11 mg iron/day for teenage boys (9–18 years) (4, 19).

Many important sources of iron include meat, meat products, eggs, poultry, fish, processed foods from animal blood and organs, cereals, pulses, vegetables and fruits; but, the concentrations of iron in milk, fruits, and vegetables are low (3–5, 9, 18–19). A prime source of iron is black pudding or cooked pork blood sausage (20 mg Fe/100 g), and most foods contain 1–10 mg Fe/100 g (9). There are two types of food iron: nonheme iron, which is present in both plant foods and animal tissues, and heme iron, only coming from the hemoglobin and myoglobin in animal products. Heme iron represents 30–70% of the total iron in lean meat or animal organs (blood, liver, heart) and is always well absorbed. Nonheme iron from meat and vegetable foods depends to a large extent on the iron form (Fe^{2+} or Fe^{3+}) in the food, the presence of enhancing and inhibiting substances in the meal, and on the iron status of the individual (4). Ferrous (Fe^{2+}) ion is better absorbed than ferric ion (Fe^{3+}) in the human gut. Heme iron is highly absorbed (15–35%) and dietary factors have little effect on its bioavailability, whereas nonheme iron absorption is much lower (2–20%) and strongly influenced by the presence of other food components (5, 18). However, nonheme iron generally contributes more to iron nutrition than heme iron. However, major inhibitors of iron absorption are often found in plants and include phytic acid, polyphenols, tannins in tea, calcium, oxalates, and lead. Therefore, lead poisoning is often associated with iron deficiency in children (18–19). In contrast, vitamin C helps the absorption of ferric iron by reducing ferric ion into ferrous ion, a bioavailable form of iron.

In brief, to prevent iron deficiency, the best way is to consume a mixture of foods rich in heme iron and nonheme iron. Iron supplements, mainly made by ferrous sulfate, a nonheme iron, are only reserved for people suffering from significant iron deficiency, and their intake must be supervised by a healthcare professional because iron excess is harmful to the body.

2.2.2 Selenium

Selenium (Se) is an essential micro-mineral (metalloid) for human life. Selenium exists as inorganic salts such as sodium selenite or sodium selenate which are often used for the preparation of Se supplements. Selenate is classified as toxic for the organism. In plants and animals, Se often occurs in organic forms such as selenoproteins, selenoenzymes, or amino acids. In humans, Se forms the active site of several antioxidant enzymes including glutathione peroxidase, thioredoxin reductase, iodothyronine deiodinase, formate dehydrogenase, glycine reductase, and so on. It is also present in many selenoproteins, one of which is selenoprotein P. Se is also a component of the amino acids selenomethionine and selenocysteine, in which Se replaces sulfur (S) of methionine and cysteine respectively. Se is required for immune function and for the synthesis of thyroid hormones. At low doses, the health benefits of Se are as an immunomodulator, antioxidant, and anti-carcinogenic. Se also assists enzymes in protecting cell membranes from damage by oxidative stress. During infection, stress, or tissue injury, selenoenzymes can protect cell membranes against the harmful effects of oxidants like hydrogen peroxide (H_2O_2) or oxygen radicals (3–4, 8, 20–24).

The recommended dietary intake of Se for healthy adults is 60 µg per day for men and 53 µg per day for women (20). According to the World Health Organization (WHO), 19 µg of Se per day is the minimal requirement to prevent the diseases associated with Se deficiency (20). While there are various formulations of supplements available with varying doses and species of Se, the current knowledge advises that people whose serum or plasma Se concentration is 122 µg L^{-1} or higher should not supplement with Se (20). The Tolerable Upper Intake Level (UL) of selenium is 400 µg Se/day (21, 23). Indeed, at low dose – less than 400 µg Se/day – Se is a strong antioxidant, a good immunomodulator, and may be useful for the prevention of some forms of cancers such as prostate cancer and colon cancer (3–4, 20–23). However, at high doses or with prolonged supplementation, Se becomes toxic. Selenium poisoning, called selenosis, is characterized by gastrointestinal disorders, hair and nail loss, cirrhosis, pulmonary edema and death (20–23). Selenium deficiency is observed in patients on total parenteral nutrition (TPN) and in patients with gastrointestinal disorders. Selenium deficiency can occur in people living in areas where soil is poor in selenium, such as in the Keshan region of China, in North America and North Europe, as well as some regions in New Zealand (22–23). Keshan disease is a fatal cardiomyopathy which is cured with Se supplement (3, 22–23). In certain regions where soil is poor in selenium, Se salts are added to chemical fertilizers and feed in order to increase Se contents in animal and vegetable foods. Se levels in soil generally reflect its presence in food and the Se levels in human populations (3, 21). As selenium is found in soil, water and plants are the main sources of Se with different concentrations. Cereals, rice bran, vegetables (garlic, onion, grains, Brazil nuts, soybean), milk, dairy products, sea food, eggs, meat, liver, yeast, and mushrooms (cepes) are the main sources of Se in the human diet (3, 4, 20–23). Some fruits and vegetables with particular odors like durian fruit, jackfruit, garlic, onion, broccoli, and cauliflower, are rich in selenium and sulfur compounds. Se-methylselenocysteine is the major seleno-compound in Se enriched plants such as garlic, onions, broccoli, and leeks (21). Approximately 80% of dietary Se is absorbed depending on the type of food consumed. In general terms, selenium in plant forms is more readily bioavailable than selenium in animal forms (21, 22). Selenium bioavailability is affected by its chemical form. Generally, organic compounds of selenium such as selenocysteine, and selenomethionine are more bioavailable than the inorganic forms like selenide and selenate (21, 22). Plants contain many different selenium compounds, mainly in the form of protein-bound selenomethionine; however, selenocysteine and selenonium have also been reported. Plants also reduce selenate (SeO_4^{2-}) to elemental selenium (Se^0) and selenide (SeO_3^{2-}), and transform them into volatile organic compounds dimethylselenide and dimethyldiselenide, which have the 'garlic' odor characteristic of selenium-plants (22). The role of Se in cancer prevention has been the subject of recent study and debate. Some interesting findings reported an association of Se intake with a reduced prevalence and risk for prostate and colon cancer. However, random trials for other cancer types are inconclusive. Results from clinical and cohort studies about cancer prevention, especially lung, colorectal, and prostate cancers, are mixed (20–23). Some scientists have added selenium salts in soil used for tobacco culture to examine the protective effect of Se against toxic compounds in tobacco smoke tars by in vitro assays on different immunocompetent cells. The results obtained from this experiment were positive and interesting compared to tobacco control without Se supplementation (24).

Briefly, selenium is an essential micro-mineral for human health thanks to its properties as a strong antioxidant and immunostimulant. Se antioxidant activity will be explained in Chapter 3 of this book. It plays a role in the synthesis of thyroid hormones. Its role in cancer prevention needs more investigation. Its deficiency can cause many diseases such as CVDs, infection, and probably cancer. However, auto-supplementation of selenium is to be avoided because selenium is highly toxic when its levels in the body exceed its Tolerable Upper Intake Level (UL). Only health professionals can decide when selenium supplementation is needed after examining symptoms and blood analysis of patient. Selenium supplementation for soil and feed is decided by competent authorities.

2.2.3 Copper

Copper (Cu) is an essential micro-mineral for all living organisms. Copper has the ability to act as an electron donor or acceptor, as it can move between the cuprous (Cu^{1+}) and cupric (Cu^{2+}) oxidation states (6). This makes copper an important component of several enzymes, cofactors, and proteins in the body such as cytochrome c oxidase, ceruloplasmin, monoamine oxidase, diamine oxidase, metallothionein, superoxide dismutase, catalase, peroxidase, tyrosinase, lactase, ascorbic acid oxidase, uricase, and so on. (4–9). Copper is an essential micronutrient necessary for the hematologic and neurologic systems (4–8). It is necessary for the growth and formation of bone and myelin sheaths in the nervous systems, and it helps the incorporation of iron in hemoglobin, as well as assists in the absorption of iron from the gastrointestinal tract, and in the transfer of iron from tissues to the plasma (8). In brain aging and in neurodegenerative disorders, abnormal interactions of iron or copper with metal-binding proteins, such as neuromelanin or amyloid-beta peptide, are important mechanisms leading to oxidative stress. An unbalanced copper metabolism homeostasis (due to dietary deficiency) could be linked to Alzheimer's disease (4–5). Copper and zinc are cofactors participating in the activity of antioxidant enzyme superoxide dismutase (SOD), which is responsible for the elimination of free radical superoxide anion. The combination of Cu/Zn superoxide dismutase protects cells from the deleterious effects of superoxide anion (6). Other antioxidant properties of Cu are cited in Chapter 3 of this book. Ceruloplasmin, a ferroxidase enzyme, is essential for transport of Fe to reticulocytes that produce hemoglobin. It plays a role in iron absorption and facilitates the incorporation of ferric iron into transferrin (4, 6, 8–9). Cupric copper (Cu^{2+}) is more soluble than cuprous (Cu^{1+}), so, its bioavailability is higher than that of cuprous (9).

The recommended dietary allowances (RDAs) for Cu range between 1.0 and 1.6 mg Cu/day for adults. The Tolerable Upper Intake Level (UL) for Cu is 10 mg/day in the US and 5 mg/day in the EU (4, 7, 9).

Rich sources of copper include legumes, whole grains, molasses, nuts, seeds, chocolate, avocado, liver, shellfish (oyster, mollusk), lobster, fishes, and milk (7–9). Deficiencies or excesses of copper are rare in healthy people (4, 9). Therefore, the intake of copper supplements is not necessary for normal subjects because the levels of copper in foods are sufficient for the needs of human body. Briefly, copper participates in the formation of numerous enzymes, proteins, and brain neurotransmitters. It protects the cells from the toxic effects of free radicals and facilitates iron, calcium, and phosphorous fixation.

2.2.4   Zinc

Zinc (Zn) is a trace metal necessary for all living cells, and functions as a cofactor. It serves a catalytic role in enzymes and is present in more than 300 human enzymes, such as lactate dehydrogenase, alkaline phosphatase, alcohol dehydrogenase, glutamic dehydrogenase, carboxypeptidase, carbonic anhydrase, retinene reductase, DNA and RNA polymerase, and so on. (3–8, 25–26). In addition, zinc is a constituent of the cytoplasmic antioxidant enzyme superoxide dismutase (Cu-Zn-SOD), and competes directly with copper and iron, thereby decreasing hydroxyl radical formation to avoid oxidative stress in cells (25–26). Zinc dependent enzymes are also involved in macronutrient metabolism and cell replication (8). Regulations of gene expression and cell signaling pathways are also some of the main biochemical roles of zinc. Zinc participates in nucleic acid and amino acid metabolism as well as in the antioxidant system. The metabolism and bioavailability of Vitamins A and E are dependent on zinc status (8, 25–26). Zinc is abundant in the central nervous system, especially in the sensory receptors and brain regions that perceive and interpret the pleasures of eating. Moreover, zinc plays a role in cognitive development, and participates in the mechanisms for perception of taste and smell; a deficit induces anosmia. Zinc is present in synaptic vesicles for some glutaminergic neurons (5). Moreover, zinc plays a central role in the immune system, affecting several aspects of cellular and humoral immunity (3). Other antioxidant properties of Zn are cited in Chapter 3 of this book.

In humans, the clinical features of severe zinc deficiency are growth retardation, delayed sexual and bone maturation, impotence, eye and skin lesions, diarrhea, alopecia, impaired appetite, depressed immunity and even mental lethargy in grave cases, increased susceptibility to infections mediated via defects in the immune system, and the appearance of behavioral changes (3, 8, 25–26). Many of these symptoms are non-specific and often associated with other health conditions or other micronutrient deficiencies including iron; therefore, a medical examination is necessary to ascertain whether a zinc deficiency is present (4, 26). However, severe zinc deficiency in humans is rare, and more interest has been focused on marginal zinc deficiency. Dietary zinc deficiency has been shown to alter brain zinc homeostasis (5). Zinc deficiency in elderly people leads to reduced appreciation of taste, thereby loss of appetite. Moreover, zinc deficiency impairs the accumulation of polyunsaturated fatty acids throughout the body, which could affect the supply to the brain. A reduction in dietary zinc can induce behavioral changes and some psychiatric problems (5).

The RDA (Recommended Daily Allowance) for zinc is 11 mg/day for adult males and 8 mg/day for adult females (4, 26). The UL (Tolerable Upper Intake Level) is estimated at 40 mg zinc/day for adults (25). Consuming too much zinc can cause zinc poisoning or acute zinc toxicity. Symptoms of zinc poisoning are gastrointestinal irritation, dizziness, vomiting, nausea, abdominal cramps, diarrhea, and headaches in the short term (4, 25–26). Excess of zinc can disrupt absorption of copper and iron, leading to immune system dysfunction in the long term. Zinc supplements are often made with zinc acetate or gluconate (25).

Good sources of zinc include shellfish (oysters, mollusks, whelks), red meat, fish meals, liver, eggs, dairy products, lamb, pork, chicken, toasted wheat germ, spinach, pumpkin seeds, squash seeds, sesame seeds, nuts, dark chocolate, beans, and mushrooms (3–5, 8, 25–26). Phytates, which are present in whole-grain breads, cereals, legumes, and other plant foods, bind zinc and inhibit its absorption (3, 4, 8, 25–26). Thus, the bioavailability of zinc from grains and plant foods is lower than that from animal foods, although many grain- and plant-based foods are still good sources of zinc (26).

2.2.5 Manganese

Manganese (Mn) is a trace metal that plays important roles in the activity of many enzyme-mediated chemical reactions such as pyruvate carboxylase, superoxide dismutase, and arginase. It is a cofactor of many other enzymes, like glycosyl transferases, phosphotransferases, hydrolases, kinases, decarboxylases, and prolinases (4, 8–9). Manganese intervenes in the activity of antioxidant superoxide dismutase within mitochondria and plays important roles in the elimination of harmful free radicals in the body (4, 8). Manganese is a co-factor in phosphohydrolases and phosphotransferases involved in the synthesis of proteoglycans in cartilage (8). Manganese is part of enzymes involved in urea formation, pyruvate metabolism, and the galactotransferase of connective tissue biosynthesis (8). Manganese activates several important enzyme systems for the synthesis of acid mucopolysaccharides, such as chondroitin sulphate, to form the matrices of bones and eggshells (8).

Manganese is stored in liver and bone. Manganese absorption occurs along the entire intestine but overall is only 3–4% (9). The absorption efficiency in the small intestine is low. High concentrations of calcium, phosphorus, fiber, and phytate reduce manganese absorption through interactions. Plasma concentrations of Mn are one to two µg/g, bound to transferrin (9). Manganese deficiency is rare or unknown in humans (4, 8–9). Its toxicity is also uncommon and is most frequently the result of exposure to airborne manganese dust in industry or ore exploitation. Manganese overexposure reportedly may have an adverse effect on central nervous system function and mood (8). Toxicity, disease, or symptoms due to Mn poisoning by inhalation produces psychotic symptoms and Parkinson's syndrome (8). The Tolerable Upper Intake Level (UL) for Mn is 11 mg per day for adults (4). There is currently no RDA set for dietary manganese; instead, there is an AI (average daily intake) value for Mn: 2.3 mg/day for adult men and 1.8 mg/day for adult women (4).

Foods rich in manganese are: cereals (20–30 mg/kg), brown bread (100–150 mg/kg), nuts (10–20 mg/kg), ginger (280 mg/kg), and tea (350–900 mg/kg dry tea) (4). Coffee, dried fruits, fresh fruits, vegetables, seeds, cacao, also contain relatively high levels of Mn. Concentrations of Mn in crops are dependent on soil factors such as pH, whereby increasing soil pH decreases plant uptake of Mn (4). Products of animal origin such as eggs, milk, fish, poultry, and red meat contain low amounts of manganese (4, 8–9).

2.2.6 Fluoride

Fluoride (F⁻) is an essential micro-mineral, along with calcium and phosphate, for the formation of bones and teeth in all vertebrates. Fluoride is the negative ion (anion) of the element fluorine (F), a toxic gas that does not exist in the human body. Nearly 99% of the body's fluoride resides in the bones and teeth (4, 8–9). Fluoride is both a benefic and a toxic mineral for body. It is an essential mineral for bone and tooth health, but an excess can cause diseases for bones, teeth, and other organs. The major mineral component of bone and teeth is calcium phosphate named hydroxyapatite or hydroxyl-apatite $[Ca_{10}(PO_4)_6(OH)_2]$. Fluoride has a high affinity for Ca by forming fluor-hydroxyapatite $[Ca_{10}(PO_4)_6(OH_xF_y)]$ and fluorapatite $[Ca_{10}(PO_4)_6F_2]$, which are harder and more resistant to acidic materials than the hydroxyapatite (4, 8–9). The incorporation of fluoride in bones and teeth is proportional to its total intake. Therefore, fluoride salt like sodium fluoride is often added in tap water or incorporated in toothpaste for the fortification of bone and tooth enamel to prevent osteopathy and treat tooth decay (4, 8–9). The cariostatic action (reduction in the risk of dental caries) of fluoride on erupted teeth of children and adults is owing to its effect in the metabolism of bacteria in dental plaque (i.e., reduced acid production) and on the dynamics of enamel demineralization and remineralization during an acidogenic challenge (4). Fluoride is also used, along with calcium and vitamin D, in the treatment and prevention of osteoporosis in elderly people, especially women after menopause. Fluoride also has the unique ability to stimulate new bone formation (4). When drinking water contains 1 mg/l there is a 50% reduction in tooth decay in children (4, 9).

Fluoride like sodium fluoride (NaF) is often added to water for tap water preparation. This operation is called fluoridation (4, 8–9). The concentrations of fluoride in tap water must be controlled before and after this fluoridation by different analytic techniques because an excess of fluoride in water is also as noxious to health as its deficiency (27–28). Fluoridation of community drinking water to prevent dental caries and osteoporosis is now universal in industrial countries and realized by the public health of each community.

Excessive intake of fluoride gives rise to fluorosis, a disease characterized by excessive bone hardening leading to bones breaking easily. High concentrations of fluoride in drinking water causes corrosion of the enamel of the teeth, a process called mottling (8). Fluorosis is often observed in people living in areas where the soil is too rich in fluoride. Fluorosis has been observed in some region of China such as Tibet in people who have been drinking brick tea for many years. The fluoride concentration of brick tea is 200–300 times higher than ordinary green tea and black tea because brick tea (tea compressed into brick shape) is made from old stems and leaves of the tea tree, but ordinary green tea and black tea are made from tender leaves and buds (29). High intake of fluoride, in excess of one mg/l, results in mottling of the teeth; the enamel is no longer lustrous and becomes rough, an effect particularly marked on the upper incisors. In concentrations well in excess of ten parts per million, fluoride poisoning can occur, causing a loss of appetite and sclerosis of the bones of the spine, pelvis, and limbs (9).

Based on the data on the association of high fluoride intakes with risk of skeletal fluorosis in men, the US Food and Nutrition Board has established a tolerable upper intake level (UL) of fluoride of 10 mg/day for children and adults, as well as pregnant and lactating women (4). The average daily intake (AI) values for fluoride are: infants (7–12 months) 0.5 mg/day, children and adolescents 0.7–2.0 mg/day, male adults 3–4 mg/day, female adolescents and adults 3 mg/day. There is no known RDA requirement for fluoride (9).

Main sources of fluoride include fluorinated drinking water, some natural source or mineral waters such as Vichy water, green tea, toothpaste, dairy products (milk, hard cheese), marine fish consumed with bone (sardine), shrimp, crawfish, and so on (4, 8–9, 29).

2.2.7 Iodine

Iodine (I), a metalloid (nonmetallic) element of the halogen group, is an essential micronutrient for human life. Iodine exists as iodide and complex organic iodine compounds such as thyroxin in the human body.

The main physiological roles known for iodine in the human body are the synthesis of thyroid hormones by the thyroid gland, the nerve development and the thyroid gland growth (2–6, 8–9, 30–31). Thyroid hormones are involved in fetal central nervous system development; therefore, iodine intake during pregnancy plays an important role in the intelligence of infants as they grow. The thyroid gland traps most (about 80%) of the ingested iodine, but salivary glands, gastric mucosa, choroid plexus, and lactating mammary glands also concentrate iodine by a similar active transport mechanism (4). Dietary iodine is converted into the iodide ion before it is absorbed. The iodide ion is 100% bioavailable and absorbed totally from food and water. Iodine enters the circulation as plasma inorganic iodide, which is cleared from circulation by the thyroid and kidney. Iodide is used by the thyroid gland for synthesis of thyroid hormones, and the kidney excretes excess iodine in the form iodide (I^-) with urine (3). In the body, mineral iodine is fixed on tyrosine, an amino acid, to become mono and di-tyrosine, which are the precursors of the hormone L-thyroxine. All biological actions of iodide are attributed to the thyroid hormones (3–6, 31). The thyroid contains two hormones, L-triiodothyronine (T_3) and L-tetraiodothyronine (T_4), or L-thyroxine. Iodine is the critical raw material, because 65% of T_4 and 58% of T_3 weights are iodine (30). The major thyroid hormone secreted by the thyroid gland is T_4. Although T_4 is quantitatively predominant, T_3 is the more active (3–4). The two main physiological roles of thyroid hormones are growth and development and control of metabolic processes in the body (2–6, 8–9, 30–31). Thyroid hormones play a major role in the growth and development of the brain and central nervous system in humans from the 15th week of gestation to 3 years of age. If a deficiency occurs of either iodine or thyroid hormones during this critical period, the consequence is derangement in the development of the brain and central nervous system of the infant. These derangements are irreversible and are the cause of cretinism or mental retardation (2–6, 8–9). In adults, iodine deficiency causes goiter (hypertrophy of thyroid gland) and myxedema (8). Symptoms of myxedema in adults are extreme fatigue, drowsiness, mental depression, goiter development, confusion, and diminution of body temperature (hypothermia). Iodine deficiency perturbs the intellectual and neuro-motor functions even in apparently normal people and affects all populations at all stages of life, from the fetus to the old age (3–6, 9). Consequences of iodine deficiency include goiter, intellectual impairments, growth retardation, neonatal hypothyroidism, and increased pregnancy loss and infant mortality (31).

The other physiological role of thyroid hormones is to control several metabolic processes in the body. These include the metabolism of carbohydrate, fat, protein, vitamin, and mineral. For example, thyroid hormone increases energy production, increases lipolysis, and regulates neoglucogenesis, and glycolysis (3). Moreover, thyroid hormones are used to stimulate enzyme synthesis, oxygen consumption, basal metabolic rate, and a wide variety of other physiological activities such as heart rate and respiratory rate (4). However, under different circumstances, excess iodine intake can cause hyperthyroidism (thyrotoxicosis) and toxic nodular goiter (4, 8). Hyperthyroidism is largely confined to people over 40 years of age. Symptoms of hyperthyroidism include palpitations, trembling, nervousness, weight loss, lack of sleep, tremor, high blood pressure, excessive sweating, and heat intolerance (4). Indeed, too little or too much iodine in the body can cause goiter, an enlargement of the thyroid gland.

Daily iodine intake recommendations by the World Health Organization, United Nations Children's Fund, and International Council for Control of Iodine Deficiency Disorders are: 90 µg/day for infants and children from 0–59 months, 120 µg/day for children from 6–12 years, 150 µg/day for adolescents and adults, 200 µg/day for pregnant women and lactating women (3–4). The UL (Tolerable Upper Intake Level) for adults is set at 600 µg/day (EU) and at 1.1 mg/day (USA) (3–4).

Natural sources of dietary iodine include seafood, such as sea fishes, mussels, oysters, and algae (such as kelp, kombu), cow milk, cheese and eggs. Plants are highly variable in iodine content depending on species and soil type as well as fertilizer and climate (3–6, 8–9). The consumption of vegetables rich in goitrogenic substances such as thioglucosides or cyanoglucosides found in brassica, manioc, kale, cabbage, sprouts, broccoli, turnips, swedes, kohlrabi, rapeseed, mustard, and so on, can decrease the absorption of iodine in the digestive tract (4–5). Iodized salt obtained by adding sodium iodide in table salt is also a good source of iodine for the prevention of iodine deficiency. Moreover, sea air is much richer in iodine gas (I_2) than inland air due to the liberation of I_2 from seaweeds. Many people are regularly exposed to huge amounts of iodine, in the range 10–200mg/day, without apparent adverse effects (3). Japanese people are the highest consumers of iodine in the world. They eat about two to three mg of iodine per day from sea foods – about two to three times the Tolerable Upper Intake Level of iodine without any toxicity (3). This may be explained by the fact that the iodine in seaweeds is not only in iodide (I-) form, but also in I_2 or organic forms (CH_3I, CH_2I_2), which are easily volatilized when cooking, therefore, the iodine levels remaining to consume are not as high as those theoretically calculated. In contrast, the iodine in supplements or other vegetables is in iodide (I-) form, which remains stable when heating. It is of note that populations living far from the sea or near the desert such as in North India, Tibet, West China, Sub Saharan Africa, and Latin America are often subject to iodine deficiency (3). Over one billion people worldwide are estimated to be living in iodine-deficient areas and, therefore, at risk of iodine deficiency disorders such as goiter, cretinism, mental impairment, and intellectual deficiency,. (4). People in iodine-deficient areas can receive iodine as an additive to food or water such as iodinated table salt or iodinated drinking water. Potassium or sodium iodide is often used for the preparation of these fortified foods. Iodine supplementation (150 μg/day) has been recommended in the case of pregnancy (2). Excessive intake of iodine supplements is also harmful to health. Ask a healthcare professional before taking iodine supplements.

Iodine poisoning is also observed in people taking high dose of iodine supplements and medicines containing iodine in their molecules such as amiodarone (3). Amiodarone is used in the treatment of supraventricular and ventricular arrhythmias. Its main side effects include various pulmonary effects such as interstitial lung disease, pulmonary fibrosis, hypothyroidism and hyperthyroidism, and liver disease (31). To prevent these side effects, a therapeutic drug monitoring of amiodarone in serum is necessary (31). Iodine molecules (I_2) in the form of flake or vapor are toxic. Iodine (I_2) diluted in water or alcohol is a good antiseptic, such as in tincture of iodine or povidone-iodine solution, but prolonged use can cause skin burn.

Briefly, iodine is necessary for the production of thyroid hormones that play a major role in the growth and development of the brain and central nervous system and in several metabolic processes in the body. Some main sources of iodine are sea foods (mollusks, oysters, sea fishes, seaweeds), milk, dairy products, and eggs. Iodinated table salt and iodinated drinking water are used by people living in areas with iodine deficiency.

2.2.8 Chromium

Chromium (Cr) is an essential micro-mineral for animals and humans. It is a transition metal that can occur in a number of valence states: 0, +2, +3, and +6. Trivalent chromium (Cr^{3+}) is the most stable form in biological systems, and cannot be oxidized in tissues to hexavalent (Cr^{6+}) form which is toxic (4, 6, 8–9). Some roles of chromium in human nutrition are still uncertain, but chromium may act in an organic complex that influences and extends the action of insulin (9). Trivalent chromium (Cr^{3+}) binds to and activates insulin action, and functions primarily through its role in the regulation of insulin (4, 6, 8–9). Adequate dietary chromium intake may contribute to a normalization of insulin in the body. Chromium (Cr^{3+}) reduces blood glucose levels in subjects with hyperglycemia, increases low blood glucose concentrations in subjects with hypoglycemia, and has no effect on normal subjects (4). It also functions in carbohydrate, lipid, and nucleic acid metabolism (4). It has been found in nucleoproteins isolated from beef liver and also in RNA preparations (8). Chromium is a cross-linking agent for collagen and may have a role in lipoprotein metabolism, in structure of nucleic acids, and in gene expression (9). Chromium deficiencies may exist particularly in children suffering from protein-calorie malnutrition (8). Chromium poisoning in humans is rare and usually limited to accidental ingestion of hexavalent (Cr^{6+}) chromic acid or chromate (CrO_4^{-2}) which is water-soluble and highly toxic (6). Toxicity of hexavalent chrome such as chromate (CrO_4^{-2}) to the liver, kidneys, blood, or nervous system are the major causes of death (8).

There is currently no RDA set for dietary chromium, instead there are AI (average intake) values: adult men 30–35 μg/day and adult women 20–25 μg/day (4). No tolerable UL is set for trivalent chromium (4).

Good sources of chromium include wheat and wheat germ, whole grains, brewer's yeast, nuts, seeds, poultry, eggs, seafood, meat, liver, cheese, beans, peas, lentils, soy products, beer, wine, and dark chocolate (4, 6, 8–9).

2.2.9 Molybdenum

Molybdenum (Mo) is an essential micro-mineral and acts as a cofactor for the activities of several enzymes in the human body including xanthine oxidase, aldehyde oxidase, sulfite oxidase, nitrate reductase, and hydrogenase (4, 6, 8–9). Xanthine oxidase and aldehyde oxidase play a role in iron utilization as well as in cellular metabolism and electron transport. Xanthine oxidase is also used in the uptake and release of iron from ferritin in the intestinal mucosa and in the release of iron from ferritin in the liver, placenta, and erythropoietic tissues to the ferrous form (8). Xanthine oxidase and hydrogenase play a role in the production of uric acid from hypoxanthine and xanthine (4). Aldehyde oxidase oxidizes and detoxifies purines and pyrimidines, while sulfite oxidase containing molybdenum incorporated as part of the molecule, is used for the conversion of sulfite to sulfate (4).

Molybdenum is a cofactor for enzymes necessary for the metabolism of sulfur-containing amino acid and nitrogen-containing compounds present in DNA and RNA, the production of uric acid, and the oxidation and detoxification of various other compounds (8). Both molybdenum deficiency and toxicity are rare (4, 9). Dietary Mo affects copper metabolism in the human body and its high doses inhibit copper absorption (4, 8). This property has been used for the treatment of Wilson's disease, which causes elevated concentrations of copper in the body (4). The amount of Mo in the body is regulated by excretion in the urine and bile. Low Mo intake is a predisposing cause of renal xanthine calculi and gout. Deficiency diseases are secondary to parenteral nutrition (8). However, high intakes of Mo (10–15 mg/day) also cause gout. Mo intake at this level may also be associated with altered metabolism of nucleotides and impaired copper bioavailability (9).

Recommended requirements of Mo are 50–400 µg/day for adults (9). For breast-fed infants a requirement of 0.5–1.5 µg/kg/day has been suggested (9). The tolerable UL for Mo is 2 mg/day for adults (4).

Important dietary sources of molybdenum are wheat flour, wheat germ, whole grains, beans, peas, organ meats, dairy products, and mineral water (4, 8–9). Vegetables grown in neutral and alkaline soils with a high content of organic matter have a higher content of molybdenum (9).

Briefly, the 16 minerals cited previously (sodium, potassium, calcium, magnesium, phosphorus, chloride, sulfur, iron, selenium, zinc, iodine, fluorine, manganese, chromium, copper, molybdenum) are essential micronutrients for the global development of the body or for the activity of specific organs or enzymes. Their deficiency or their excess in the body can cause diverse diseases in humans. Their sources mainly come from plant and animal foods, but also from water.

3 VITAMINS

Vitamins are essential organic compounds that generally cannot be synthetized by the human body and are required in very small daily amounts via food for the functioning of various organs and maintaining good health. The absence of vitamins in food causes diseases. The discovery of vitamins was a major scientific achievement in our understanding of health and disease. In 1912, Casimir Funk (1884–1967, Poland) originally coined the term 'vitamine' instead of 'accessory food factors' because the substance discovered was an amine (thiamine) and vital for life (32). The discovery of most vitamins began in the mid-nineteenth century and ended at the mid-twentieth century. The name of each discovered vitamin was given by an alphabetic letter: A, B, C, D, E, and so on, in the order of its discovery. Nowadays, 13 vitamins are universally recognized as vital for the functioning of the human body because their deficiency can cause diseases. They are divided into two groups: water-soluble vitamins and fat-soluble vitamins. There are in total nine hydro-soluble vitamins that include eight vitamins of group B plus vitamin C (L-ascorbic acid). The eight vitamins of group B are: B1 (thiamine), B2 (riboflavin), B3 (niacin), B5 (pantothenic acid), B6 (pyridoxine), B7 (biotin), B9 (folic acid), and B12 (cyanocobalamin). The four fat-soluble vitamins comprise vitamins A, D, E, and K (33). Water-soluble vitamins like group B and vitamin C are easily eliminated through urine after absorption. In contrast, fat-soluble vitamins (A, D, E, K) are stored for a long time in the body, therefore they become harmful when ingested in large amounts via mostly chemical supplements or artificially fortified foods. A self-supplementation of fat-soluble vitamins without medical prescription is dangerous for the health. The majority of vitamins are not synthesized by the human body, and must be obtained through the diet to avoid diseases and to maintain good health. Almost all vitamins are considered essential. Nevertheless, some vitamins like vitamin D and vitamin B7 (biotin) can be partially synthesized by the body. For example, vitamin D3 or cholecalciferol is obtained from cholesterol by the skin cells under the action of ultraviolet B radiation from sunlight. Biotin is synthesized by the gastrointestinal bacteria in the gut flora. Therefore, these two vitamins, D3 and biotin, can be classified as nonessential or semi-essential. Many animals can synthetize a number of vitamins in their different organs (liver, gut, kidneys) such as vitamin B3, vitamin C, vitamin D, and vitamin K. However, primates, birds, fish, and guinea pigs cannot make vitamin C in their body as humans do because they do not have the enzyme that converts glucose to vitamin C.

The phenomenon caused by vitamin deficiency in the body is called avitaminosis, and is easily cured by vitamin supply through food or supplements. In contrast, an excess of vitamins in human body, called hypervitaminosis, is toxic for the organism and can also cause ailments. It would be interesting to emphasize the difference and the similarity between vitamin and vitamer. Essentially all vitamins exist with multiple nutritionally active chemical species, often called vitamers (34). Vitamer is a member of vitamin. The term vitamin is generally designed for natural compounds found in nature (plants, animals), while different derivatives, artificial synthetic compounds or chemical names of the vitamin are called vitamer. For example, vitamin D has several vitamers which are all fat-soluble, including vitamin D2 or ergocalciferol found in mushrooms, vitamin D3 or cholecalciferol present in the human or animal body, three other vitamers rarely occuring in nature, and four synthetic analogs. Among 13 essential vitamins, there are only three vitamins endowed with antioxidant properties: vitamins A, C, and E. Some vitamins act specifically as coenzymes. The 13 vitamins will be described as follows.

3.1 WATER-SOLUBLE VITAMINS

There are eight water-soluble vitamins of group B (B1, B2, B3, B5, B6, B7, B9, B12) plus vitamin C.

3.1.1 Vitamin B1 (Thiamin)

Vitamin B1, also known as thiamin or aneurin, is one of eight B vitamins called B complex vitamins. Vitamin B1 was the first vitamin B discovered in the beginning of the twentieth century. In 1912, Funk and Cooper isolated a substance from rice bran and called it 'Vitamine' because this substance is an amine necessary for life. This amine was named thiamine and had an anti-beriberi property. It was then crystallized by Jansen and Donath in 1926 (35–36).

Vitamin B1 plays a central role in energy metabolism and especially the metabolism of carbohydrates and sugars (3, 9, 33, 35–36). Therefore, excessive ingestion of sugar automatically increases the need for this vitamin. Thiamin is extremely important for the brain because it facilitates the use of glucose, thus ensuring the production of energy for brain (5). Vitamin B1 functions as the coenzyme thiamine pyrophosphate (TPP) in the metabolism of carbohydrates and branched-chain amino acids and is therefore essential to normal growth and normal function of the heart, nerves, and muscles (3, 9, 33, 35–36). It is used to form adenosine triphosphate (ATP), which every cell of the body uses for energy. In addition, insufficient vitamin B1 decreases not only carbohydrate and amino acid metabolisms, but also the formation of acetylcholine for neural function. Therefore, vitamin B1 is necessary for the brain and nervous system (5). Thiamin diphosphate (also known as thiamin pyrophosphate) is the coenzyme for three oxidative decarboxylation reactions: pyruvate dehydrogenase in carbohydrate metabolism, α-ketoglutarate dehydrogenase in the citric acid cycle, and the branched-chain keto-acid dehydrogenase involved in the metabolism of leucine, isoleucine, and valine (33). Thiamin pyrophosphate is also required for the decarboxylation of α-ketoglutarate in the Krebs citric acid cycle and in the transketolase reaction in the hexose monophosphate shunt

(9). Thiamin triphosphate has a role in nerve conduction (33). Vitamin B1 deficiency causes damage to the brain's thalamus and hypothalamus.

The main disease caused by thiamine deficiency in humans is beriberi, a disease of the peripheral nervous system (3, 9, 33, 35–36). It exists in two forms: dry (paralytic) and wet (edematous) beriberi. Symptoms of wet beriberi are: edema (of the legs, face, trunk, lungs and peritoneal cavity), palpitations, breathlessness, anorexia, dyspepsia, congestive cardiac failure, cardiomegaly, coldness, cyanosis, and sudden death (9). Symptoms of dry beriberi are: paralysis of muscles and legs, great difficulty in walking, weight loss, and Wernicke encephalopathy (9). Another clinical manifestation of vitamin B1 deficiency is neurologic Wernicke-Korsakoff syndrome. This disease is characterized by nerve damage, peripheral neuropathies, uncontrolled eye movements (nystagmus), ataxia (lack of muscle coordination), memory disorder, fatigue, confusion, tremor, tingling, burning sensations in the hands and feet, hypothermia, low blood pressure, trouble breathing, amnesia, disorientation, and coma (3, 9, 33). Beriberi is still endemic in Asia due to the consumption of polished white rice. In industrialized nations, the neurologic manifestations of Wernicke-Korsakoff syndrome are frequently associated with chronic alcoholism and lack of vitamin B1 in the diet (3, 9, 33). Thiamine deficiency has been observed with patients who are on parenteral nutrition, are under diuretic treatment, or long renal dialysis, or have a gastrectomy (3, 9, 33). Vitamin B1 might ameliorate cognitive functions of patients with Alzheimer disease (5, 33). Thiamine is the most efficacious drug to treat and prevent beriberi and other diseases cited above. Alcoholism and hypermetabolism can also cause vitamin B1 deficiency (3, 9, 33, 35–36).

Daily recommendations (RDA) for dietary vitamin B1 are: 1.2 mg/day for men, 1.1 mg/day for women, 0.9 mg/day for children from 9 to 13 years, and 0.5–0.6 mg/day for children from 1 to 8 years (3, 33). Although vitamin B1 is generally safe and nontoxic, self-supplementation of thiamine for the treatment of beriberi or other diseases due to vitamin B1 deficiency is to be avoided because of the potential for side effects and interactions with other medicines (33). Supplementation should only be taken under the supervision of a healthcare professional. Very high doses of vitamin B1 may cause stomach upset. Taking any one of the B vitamins for a long period of time can result in an imbalance of other important B vitamins. For this reason, taking a B-complex vitamin, which includes all the vitamins of group B, is better than taking any vitamin B alone. Eating natural foods rich in thiamine is the best choice to treat and prevent beriberi and other diseases due to vitamin B1 deficiency. Avoid white rice without bran and replace it by brown or normal rice. Vitamin B1 are notably found in whole grains, wheat germs, bran, brown rice, blackstrap molasses, lean pork and other meats, poultry, eggs, fish, liver, potatoes, beans, peas, nuts, and yeast (3, 9, 33–35). Dairy products, fruits, and vegetables contain smaller amounts of vitamin B1. Prolonged cooking of food can cause loss of vitamin B1. Polyphenolic compounds in coffee and tea can inactivate thiamine; high intake of these beverages could compromise thiamine nutrition (35).

3.1.2 Vitamin B2 (Riboflavin)

Vitamin B2 or riboflavin is an essential vitamin of group B. It is a water-soluble, yellow-orange organic compound and is heat stable. Riboflavin is the central component of the coenzymes: flavin adenine dinucleotide (FAD) and flavin mononucleotide (FMN), and acts as a co-factor in numerous enzymatic reactions. It is therefore important for energy production, enzyme function, and normal protein, fatty acid and amino acid synthesis (3, 9, 33, 37–38). It mediates the transfer of electrons in biological oxidation-reduction reactions. It is also involved in the metabolism of folate, vitamin B12, vitamin B6, and other vitamins. It also helps to maintain the integrity of mucous membranes, skin, the eyes and nervous system (38). The role of riboflavin has also been credited in the prevention of a wide array of health diseases like migraine, anemia, cancer, hyperglycemia, hypertension, diabetes mellitus, and oxidative stress, directly or indirectly (38). A deficiency of riboflavin named ariboflavinosis is manifested in swollen tongue, skin eruption, and eye irritation (3, 33, 37–38). Riboflavin deficiency has profound effects on iron absorption, metabolism of tryptophan, mitochondrial dysfunction, the gastrointestinal tract, brain dysfunction, and metabolism of other vitamins

(38). Although riboflavin is involved in all areas of metabolism, and deficiency is widespread on a global scale, deficiency is not fatal (33). Riboflavin deficiency is usually associated with other vitamin B complex deficiencies; isolated riboflavin deficiency is rare (3, 33).

The recommended intakes (RDA) of riboflavin for women and men are 1.1 and 1.3 mg/day, respectively. For infants (0 to 12 months), they vary between 0.3 to 0.4 mg/day, and for children (1 to 9 years), they increase from 0.5 to 1.0 mg/day. For pregnant women and lactating women, they are 1.4 and 1.6 mg/day, respectively (9, 37). This vitamin was initially isolated from milk by English chemist Alexander Wynter Blyth in 1872, but until the early 1930s, it was characterized as riboflavin (37).

The richest natural sources of riboflavin are milk and dairy products (yogurt, cheese), providing 25% or more of total riboflavin intake in most diets (33). Vitamin B2 is also found in foods such as yeast (for instance, brewer's yeast), soybeans, malted barley, whole grains, wheat germ, brown rice, mushrooms, broccoli, Brussels sprouts, spinach, eggs, liver, kidney, and heart. (3, 9, 33, 37–38). As riboflavin is easily destroyed by light, food should be stored away from light to protect its riboflavin content (33). Riboflavin can withstand heat, so there is no problem when cooking foods containing this vitamin.

3.1.3   Vitamin B3 (Niacin)

Vitamin B3 or vitamin PP has two main vitamers: niacin or nicotinic acid and niacinamide or nicotinamide. Nicotinamide is an amide of nicotinic acid. Two secondary vitamers of vitamin B3 are nicotinamide riboside and inositol hexanicotinate. They are all precursors of active coenzymes, nicotinamide adenine dinucleotide (NAD/NADH) and its phosphate analog, the nicotinamide adenine dinucleotide phosphate (NADP/ NADPH), all of which play essential metabolic roles in living cells for energy production. However, vitamin B3 is not strictly an essential vitamin because the organism can synthesize niacin from the essential amino acid tryptophan. Therefore, diseases due to vitamin B3 deficiency can only develop when the diet does not contain both niacin and tryptophan. Chronic dietary deficiency of niacin can cause pellagra (3, 9, 33, 39–42). Therefore, vitamin B3 is also called vitamin PP (pellagra preventive) because it is used to prevent or treat pellagra, which is a chronic wasting disease of the skin, the digestive tract and the nervous system. Pellagra is also called 'the three D disease'. It is characterized by three main symptoms: dermatitis (sun sensitive), dementia, and diarrhea (39–40). Its manifestations include a photosensitive erythematous dermatitis like severe sunburn, a dementia with insomnia and apathy preceding an overt encephalopathy, and a diarrhea resulting from inflammation of the intestinal mucous surfaces. Untreated pellagra can lead to death (3, 9, 33, 39–40). Although this disease has become rare in developed countries, it remains endemic in underdeveloped countries. Pellagra is common in people who mostly eat maize as staple food, because in corn, most nicotinic acid is bound as nicotinoyl esters to a variety of macromolecules such as polysaccharides, polypeptides, and glycopeptides, and the tryptophan content is low (33, 39). Treatment of cereals with alkali (e.g., by soaking overnight in calcium hydroxide solution, as is the traditional method for the preparation of tortillas in Mexico) and baking with alkaline baking powder releases much of the nicotinic acid. This may explain why pellagra has always been rare in Mexico, despite the fact that maize is the dietary staple (33, 40). Pellagra is also observed in malnourished and alcoholic men. Other risk factors leading to vitamin B3 deficiency are nervous anorexia, AIDS, cancer and chemotherapy, as well as Crohn's disease, a chronic inflammation of the digestive tract with abdominal pain, severe diarrhea, weight loss and malabsorptive disorders (40).

In the central nervous system, niacin and nicotinamide play important roles in neuronal development and survival. Nicotinamide, the amide form of vitamin B3 (niacin), has long been associated with neuronal development, survival, and function in the central nervous system (CNS), being implicated in both neuronal death and neuroprotection. Nicotinamide appears to play a role in protecting neurons from traumatic injury, ischemia, and stroke, as well as being implicated in three key neurodegenerative conditions: Alzheimer's, Parkinson's, and Huntington's diseases. A key factor is the bioavailability of nicotinamide, with low concentrations leading to neurological deficits and dementia and high levels potentially causing neurotoxicity (41). In addition, it must be emphasized that niacin bioavailability is also crucial for neuron survival and function, and niacin deficiency has been recognized as a pathogenic factor for neurological deficits and dementia, as well as for neuronal injury and psychiatric disorders (40). It is evident that if tryptophan/niacin deficiency leads to neurological diseases, a cause-effect relationship between niacin and Alzheimer's pathogenesis has not been established (40). More researches are needed to confirm the effects of niacin and nicotinamide in neuropathology cited above.

Niacin (nicotinic acid), but not niacinamide, has been used for decades as a lipid-lowering drug. Niacin is considered a valuable therapeutic agent to boost levels of high-density lipoprotein cholesterol (HDL-C) or good cholesterol. It also lowers levels of low-density lipoprotein cholesterol (LDL-C) or bad cholesterol, as well as decreases hypertriglyceridemia and high lipoprotein A (33, 39, 42). These effects are only observed in high amounts of niacin (two to three g/day). However, the clinical use of niacin to treat hyperlipidemic diseases is limited by its side effects, such as flushing of the skin, liver damage, itching, burning sensation, stomach upset, headache, dizziness, blurred vision, glucose intolerance, paresthesia (tingling), rashes, nausea, mouth pain, and runny nose (33, 39, 42). Moreover, it remains unclear whether niacin, either in the setting of well-controlled LDL-Cholesterol or in combination with other lipid-lowering agents, confers any therapeutic benefit, and if so, by which mechanism (42). The results of recent trials reject the hypothesis that simply raising HDL-Cholesterol is cardioprotective (42). It is of note that nicotinamide does not have the pharmacologic action of the nicotinic acid that is used at high doses to lower blood lipids (3). Therefore, the use of niacin at high doses for the treatment of hypercholesterolemia and hyperlipidemia must be supervised by a cardiologist to calculate the benefits and risks of the treatment.

The recommended dietary allowances (RDAs) range from 2–8 mg/day in infants and children to 14 mg/day in women and 16 mg/day in men (39). The tolerable upper intake levels (ULs) range from 10 to 20 mg/day in children, and up to 35 mg/day in adults (39). The UL values only apply to niacin supplements plus niacin fortification, and they are based on the nicotinic acid – induced skin flush response. High intakes of both nicotinic acid and nicotinamide, in excess of 500 mg/day, also cause liver damage, and prolonged use can result in liver failure (3, 33).

The main food sources of niacin and nicotinamide include nuts, whole cereals, seeds, beets, legumes, brewer's yeast, beef kidney, beef liver, sea foods, fish, meat, poultry, milk, and eggs (3, 9, 33, 39–41).

3.1.4 Vitamin B5 (Pantothenic Acid)

Vitamin B5 or pantothenic acid is an essential micronutrient required for the biosynthesis of coenzyme A. Coenzyme A (CoA) is a key cofactor in the citric acid cycle or the Krebs cycle, as well as in the metabolism of fatty acid. Pantothenic acid is also present at the active site of acyl carrier protein (ACP) (3, 9, 33, 43). About 85% of dietary pantothenic acid is as CoA and phosphopantetheine. All tissues are capable of forming CoA from pantothenic acid (33). Pantothenic acid is required for the synthesis of several essential molecules including sphingolipids, leucine, arginine, methionine, cholesterol, steroid hormones, vitamin A, vitamin D, and heme A. CoA provides the essential acetyl group to the neurotransmitter acetylcholine, to serotonin in its conversion to melatonin, and to the acetylated sugars present in glycoproteins and glycolipids (N-acetylglucosamine, N-acetylgalactosamine, and N-acetylneuramic acid) (33). Pantothenic acid lotion may promote healthy hair. Vitamin B5 has been suggested to aid in wound healing and to prevent acne. Vitamin B5 supplement could also reduce pain in patients with rheumatoid arthritis (33, 43). A deficiency of vitamin B5 is rare, but some benign symptoms may appear such as fatigue, insomnia, acne, dermatitis, irritability, epigastric distress with anorexia and constipation, numbness and tingling of the hands and feet, and stomach pains (3). No toxicity as a result of pantothenic acid excess has been identified at the dosages used (9, 33, 43).

Since a recommended dietary allowance (RDA) could not be set, adequate intake (AI) values for vitamin B5 are as follows: 5 mg/day for adults, 6 mg/day for pregnant women, 7 mg/day for breast-feeding women and 2–4 mg/day for children (1–13 years) (3, 43). No UL (Tolerable Upper Intake Level) is given for vitamin B5 because there is no human data for adverse effects from high doses (43). Excessive doses of vitamin B5 (e.g., 10 g/day) may only give some mild intestinal troubles and diarrhea only. When patients were treated with up to 15 g/day of pantothenic acid, however, symptoms of lupus erythematosus, nausea, and gastrointestinal distress were reported (43).

As vitamin B5 is ubiquitous in all animal and plant tissues, its food sources are large. Some of the richest sources of pantothenic acid include liver, egg yolks, beef, poultry, milk, seafood, royal jelly of honey, brewer's yeast, rice bran, molasses, wheat germ, cereals, cauliflower, kale, broccoli, tomatoes, avocado, lentils, split peas, peanuts, soybeans, potatoes, and sweet potatoes (3, 43).

3.1.5 Vitamin B6 (Pyridoxine, Pyridoxal, Pyridoxamine)

Vitamin B6 comprises six vitamers with vitamin B6 activity: the alcohol pyridoxine, the aldehyde pyridoxal, the amine pyridoxamine, and their three respective 5'-phosphate esters, namely pyridoxine 5' phosphate (PXP), pyridoxal 5' phosphate (PLP) and pyridoxamine 5' phosphate (PMP) (3, 9, 33–44). The two last compounds are the active coenzyme forms of vitamin B6, and perform a wide variety of functions in the body (44). All vitamers of vitamin B6 are multipurpose; involved in more than 100 enzyme reactions, mostly concerned with protein and amino acid metabolisms (44). PLP is also involved in the metabolism of carbohydrates and lipids (3, 9, 33–44). Vitamin B6 also plays a role in cognitive development and brain activity through the biosynthesis of neurotransmitters and in maintaining normal levels of homocysteine, an amino acid in the blood (44). Moreover, vitamin B6 is involved in immune function such as lymphocyte activation and interleukin-2 production, and its deficiency results in an impairment of the immune system (3, 44). It also plays a role in gluconeogenesis and glycogenolysis.

A deficiency of vitamin B6 alone is uncommon because it usually occurs in association with a deficit in other B-complex vitamins, such as vitamin B12 and folic acid (3, 44). Hypovitaminosis B6 may often occur with riboflavin (vitamin B2) deficiency, because riboflavin is needed for the formation of the coenzyme pyridoxal 5'-phosphate (PLP) (3). Infants are especially susceptible to insufficient intakes of vitamin B6, which can lead to epileptiform convulsions (3, 33). Skin changes include dermatitis with cheilosis and glossitis. Vitamin B6 deficiency is associated with normocytic, microcytic, or sideroblastic anemia (3, 44). Other consequences of vitamin B6 deficiency include dermatitis with cheilosis (scaling on the lips and cracks at the corners of the mouth), electroencephalographic abnormalities, and glossitis (swollen tongue), depression and confusion, and weakened immune function (44). Moderate vitamin B6 deficiency results in a number of abnormalities of amino acid metabolism, especially of tryptophan and methionine (33). In infants, vitamin B6 deficiency can cause convulsive seizures and irritability, which may cease rapidly following the administration of vitamin B6 (33–44). Chronic renal insufficiency, homocystinuria, and malabsorption syndromes, such as celiac disease, Crohn's disease, or ulcerative colitis can cause vitamin B6 deficiency. Some medications, such as antiepileptic drugs, can lead to deficiency of vitamin B6 (44). It is the same for isoniazid, an anti-tubercular drug. For that reason, isoniazid is often combined with vitamin B6 in each tablet for the prevention of vitamin B6 deficiency in the treatment of tuberculosis (9).

The Recommended Dietary Allowances (RDA) for men and women are 1.3 mg per day until age 51; then RDAs increase to 1.7 mg per day for men and 1.5 mg per day for women above age 51 (3, 44). For pregnant and lactating women, RDAs are 1.9 mg per day and 2.0 mg per day, respectively. For children for both sexes from 1–8 years, RDAs are 0.5–0.6 mg per day and from 9–18 years, RDAs vary between 1.0–1.2 mg per day (3, 44). The Tolerable Upper Intake Level (UL) for vitamin B6 is 100 mg/day for both sexes (3, 44).

High intakes of vitamin B6 from food sources have not been reported to cause adverse effects (44). However, large doses of vitamin B6 supplement (1–6 g per day for 12–40 months) can cause severe nerve damage and progressive sensory neuropathy characterized by ataxia (loss of control of bodily movements) (44). Other harmful effects of excessive vitamin B6 intake include painful, disfiguring dermatological lesions, photosensitivity, and gastrointestinal symptoms, such as nausea and heartburn (44). The research to date provides little evidence that supplemental amounts of vitamin B6, alone or with folic acid and vitamin B12, can help reduce the risk or severity of cardiovascular disease and stroke or prevent cancer (44). It is the same for the prevention or treatment of cognitive decline in elderly people by vitamin B6 supplement. Therefore, the use of high doses of vitamin B6 must be controlled by a doctor.

The main sources of vitamin B6 are liver, kidney meats, chickpeas, yeast, fishes (salmon, tuna), milk, eggs, bananas, tofu, fruit, cereals, and starchy vegetables like potato and sweet potato (9, 44).

3.1.6 Vitamin B7 (Biotin, Vitamin H)

Vitamin B7, also known as biotin or vitamin H, is a micronutrient that serves as an essential cofactor for several carboxylase enzymes in the metabolism of carbohydrates, fats, and amino acids. Biotin is also recommended for strengthening hair, nails and skin; thus, it is also called vitamin H (H for hair) (3, 9, 33, 45). Like all B vitamins, vitamin B7 is water-soluble, so it is easily eliminated in the urine and cannot be stored for long in the body. It is noteworthy that endogenous bacteria in the human colon can synthesize biotin in large amounts; therefore, biotin is considered nonessential.

Biotin is a growth factor present in small amounts in every cell and plays important roles in numerous carboxylation reactions. The main carboxylase enzymes that need biotin as cofactor include pyruvate carboxylase, acetyl- CoA carboxylase, propionyl-CoA carboxylase, and methylcrotonyl-CoA carboxylase (3, 9, 33). Biotin links covalently to pyruvate carboxylase to form a biotin enzyme complex which then reacts with acetyl coenzyme A in the presence of carbon dioxide ($CO2$) to form intermediates essential to the synthesis of fatty acids (3, 9, 33). Biotin is also important for normal embryonic growth, so, it is an essential nutrient during pregnancy. As biotin is produced by intestinal flora, a natural deficiency of biotin is rare and uncommon (3, 9, 33, 45). Symptoms of biotin deficiency include hair loss, dry scaly skin, cracking in the corners of the mouth (called cheilitis), swollen and painful tongue (glossitis), dry eyes, loss of appetite, fatigue, insomnia, and depression (3, 9, 33, 45). People in parenteral nutrition for a long period, those taking antibiotics, or anti-seizure medication in the long term, and people with Crohn's disease, an inflammatory bowel disease, are subject to be deficient in biotin (3, 9, 33). In addition, people who eat large amounts of uncooked egg for a long period can have biotin deficiency because avidin, a protein in egg white, binds biotin extremely tightly and renders it unavailable for absorption. Avidin is denatured by cooking and then loses its ability to bind biotin (33). Although no major toxicities of excess biotin have been reported, data on the actual benefit of biotin's effect on hair and nail growth is limited (45). So, the interest of biotin supplementation for hair and nail growth in individuals who do not have low levels of biotin is not yet evident. However, biotin supplementation is necessary for some cases of biotin deficiency such as pregnancy, malnutrition, medication effects, and biotinidase deficiency in children (45).

The current Adequate Intakes (AIs) are 30 µg/day for adults and pregnant women and 35 µg/day for breastfeeding women. For infants up to 12 months, the AI is 5–6 µg/day. For children ages 1–18 years, the AI increases with age from 8 to 25 µg/day (3, 45). As there is no human data for toxic effects from high doses for vitamin B7, its Tolerable Upper Intake Levels (ULs) are unknown (3, 45).

The richest sources of vitamin B7 are liver, kidney, pancreas, yeast, milk, brewer's yeast, cooked eggs, especially egg yolk, sardines, nuts (almonds, peanuts, pecans, walnuts), nut butters, soybeans, legumes (beans, blackeye peas), whole grains, cauliflower, bananas, mushrooms and soy flour (3, 9, 33).

3.1.7 Vitamin B9 (Folic Acid, Folate)

Vitamin B9, also called folic acid or folate or vitamin Bc or vitamin M, is a water-soluble vitamin of group B. It was first discovered by Wills and Mehta in 1931 in yeast for the treatment of the macrocytic anemia, then was later isolated from spinach leaves and was given the name folic acid (46). Vitamin B9 was then synthetized in 1935. The term folate is reserved for vitamin B9 obtained from natural foods and biologic organisms such as yeasts, while the name folic acid is given for the synthetic compound (46). The folates found in food consist of a mixture of reduced folate polyglutamates (3, 33). Folates act as enzyme cofactor for the biosynthesis of ribonucleotides and deoxyribonucleotide precursors for DNA synthesis (3, 9, 46). They are also required for amino acid metabolism such as transformation of homocysteine to methionine, and therefore function in the regulation of gene expression by methylation (3, 46). Folates act together with vitamins B6 and B12 and other nutrients to control the levels of amino acid homocysteine in blood because excessive homocysteine levels can cause heart disease and stroke (3). Moreover, vitamin B9 plays important roles in brain function, mental health, and the major growth periods of the body (infancy, adolescence, and pregnancy) (3, 46). It is also necessary for the development of the fetus and for the prevention of spina bifida, a birth defect characterized by a deformation of the spinal column and an incomplete development of the neural tube. Folates and folic acid may also prevent colorectal cancer (46).

Clinically, folate deficiency leads to megaloblastic anemia, the release into the circulation of immature precursors of red blood cells. This anemia develops because of inhibition of DNA synthesis (9, 33). A number of drugs like anticancer (methotrexate), anticonvulsant (phenytoin, phenobarbital, primidone), antibacterial (trimethoprim), and antimalarial (pyrimethamine) agents can cause folate deficiency (3, 9, 33, 46). Celiac disease, inflammatory bowel disease, and alcoholism can cause folic acid deficiency.

The Recommended Dietary Allowances (RDAs) of folic acid are: 400 µg/day for men, women, and teens (14–18 years); 600 µg/day for pregnant women; and 500 µg/day for lactating women. For children ages 1–13 years, the RDA increases with age from 150 to 300 µg/day (3, 46). The Tolerable Upper Intake Level (UL) (the amount that should not cause side effects) of folic acid for adults is 1,000 µg/day (3, 46). At the RDA, side effects from folic acid are rare. Very high doses can cause nausea, loss of appetite, confusion, seizures, and insomnia (46). Consult a doctor before taking high doses of folic acid greater than the RDA.

The main food sources of vitamin B9 are dark green leafy vegetables, avocado, spinach, asparagus, Brussels sprouts, beetroot, grains, fruits and fruit juices, nuts, beans, peas, liver, dairy products, poultry, meat, eggs, and seafood (3, 9, 33, 46). Vitamin B9 (folates) in food is sensitive to high heat and UV light. In the United States and Canada, cereals and flour are fortified with folic acid for the prevention of vitamin B9 deficiency in at-risk populations, such as pregnant women (46).

3.1.8 Vitamin B12 (Cobalamin)

Vitamin B12, or cobalamin, is a water-soluble vitamin of group B that is essential in the synthesis of hemoglobin and the formation of normal red blood cells. Vitamin B12 was discovered in 1926 for the treatment of pernicious anemia, by giving large amounts of liver to patients. It was then identified in the middle of the twentieth century. Vitamin B12 contains a cobalt atom at the center linked to four pyrrole rings (a corrin) and has a high molecular weight of 1350 Da, hence, it is also called cobalamin (3, 9, 33). Vitamin B12 has many vitamers. In mammals, two main vitamers of vitamin B12 are 5-deoxyadenosyl-cobalamin and methyl-cobalamin, while cyanocobalamin and hydroxycobalamin are found in yeast and are used to prepare vitamin B12 supplements. Methyl-cobalamin is found in egg yolk and cheese, and sulfite-cobalamin in some foods. Little or no cyanocobalamin occurs in food, except for cow's milk, which contains three µg/l (3, 9, 33, 47).

Vitamin B12 is found in microorganisms (bacteria, yeast, archaea), seaweeds or algae (spirulina), animals and their products (milk, eggs), but it is absent in plants (vegetables, fruits, tubers, and grains). As vitamin B12 is absent in plant foods, strict vegans are often subject to vitamin B12 deficiency (3, 9, 33, 47). Bacteria, archaea, and yeast can synthesize different forms of vitamin B12. Bacteria in the human colon can produce cobalamin, but this product is not absorbed in the large intestine (9). Vitamin B12 is only absorbed in the duodenum (small intestine). Algae are rich in vitamin B12, but their capacity to synthesize vitamin B12 by different enzymes is still a controversial subject. However, some vegetable fermentation preparations have been reported as being possible sources of vitamin B12, as this fermentation is due to bacteria (3).

Vitamin B12, bound to protein in food, is released by the activity of hydrochloric acid and gastric protease in the stomach. When synthetic vitamin B12 is added to fortified foods and dietary supplements, it is already in free form and, thus, does not require this separation step. Free vitamin B12 then combines with intrinsic factor, a glycoprotein secreted by the stomach's parietal cells, and the resulting complex undergoes absorption within the distal ileum by receptor-mediated endocytosis (47). Therefore, cyanocobalamin and hydroxy-cobalamin are used as supplements to treat anemia due to diseases of the stomach such as pernicious anemia and atrophic gastritis. Pernicious anemia is an autoimmune disease that affects the gastric mucosa and results in gastric atrophy. This leads to the destruction of parietal cells, achlorhydria, and failure to produce intrinsic factor, resulting in vitamin B12 malabsorption. If pernicious anemia is left untreated, it causes vitamin B12 deficiency, leading to megaloblastic anemia and neurological disorders, even in the presence of adequate dietary intake of vitamin B12 (47). Atrophic gastritis with increasing age also leads to progressive failure of vitamin B12 absorption (33). Besides its main role in red blood cell formation, vitamin B12 is required for neurological function and DNA synthesis (47). It participates in the metabolism of folate and helps protect the myelin sheath, the coating that surrounds and protects nerve fibers (3, 47). The neurological symptoms of vitamin B12 deficiency can occur without anemia, so early diagnosis and intervention is important to avoid irreversible damage (47). Neurological changes, such as numbness and tingling in the hands and feet, can also occur. Additional symptoms of vitamin B12 deficiency include difficulty maintaining balance, depression, confusion, dementia, poor memory, and soreness of the mouth or tongue (47). Vitamin B12, folate, and vitamin B6 are involved in homocysteine metabolism. Elevated homocysteine levels have been identified as a risk factor for cardiovascular disease. Insufficiency of vitamin B12 can raise homocysteine levels due to inadequate function of methionine synthase (47). Combinations of vitamin B12 and folic acid supplements with or without vitamin B6 can decrease homocysteine levels in people with vascular disease or diabetes and in young adult women (47). Pernicious anemia is treated with injectable vitamin B12.

The Recommended Dietary Allowances (RDAs) of vitamin B12 are: 2.4 micrograms per day for men, women and children over 14 years, and 0.9–1.8 micrograms per day for children from one to 13 years (3, 47). There are no known toxicity effects of vitamin B12. Intake of 1000μg vitamin B12 per day has never been reported to have any side effects (3).

Vitamin B12 is naturally found in animal products, including fish, meat, poultry, eggs, milk, and milk products. Clams, liver, and beef are the richest foods in vitamin B12. Vitamin B12 is generally not present in plant foods, except algae like spirulina, but fortified breakfast cereals are a readily available source of vitamin B12 with high bioavailability for vegetarians (47). Some nutritional yeast products also contain vitamin B12. Some fermented vegetables can contain vitamin B12 due to the presence of bacteria in these foods. A supplement of vitamin B12 either by tablets or by fortified foods (cereals, soy products) is needed for vegans, especially in pregnancy, infancy, childhood, and adolescence.

3.1.9   Vitamin C (L-Ascorbic Acid)

Vitamin C, also known as L-ascorbic acid or ascorbate, is a water-soluble vitamin, an important essential micronutrient for the human body and a co-factor in at least eight enzymatic reactions in humans. Vitamin C is a six-carbon lactone; a simple sugar with molecular weight of 176 Da. It is synthesized from glucose by many plants and animals. Vitamin C is synthesized in the liver in most mammals and in the kidney in birds and reptiles. However, some vertebrate species: humans, teleost fishes, guinea pigs, bats and some primates such as monkeys, simians and tarsiers are unable to synthesize vitamin C because they lack an enzyme named gulonolactone oxidase used for the conversion of glucose to vitamin C (3, 9, 33, 48–51). Humans lost this capability to synthesize vitamin C endogenously, about 40 million years ago, due to the development of mutations in the gulonolactone oxidase gene leading to stop the vitamin C biosynthetic pathway (49–50). Therefore, the provision of vitamin C via foods is vital for human life. Acute lack of vitamin C leads to scurvy, a disease characterized by blood vessel fragility, connective tissue damage, fatigue, and ultimately, death as result of a general collapse (3, 9, 23, 33, 48–54). As humans cannot obtain this vitamin endogenously, different artificial L-ascorbic acid syntheses have been developed by a combined chemical and microbial method for the production of L-ascorbic acid from D-glucose (55).

In the early 1930s vitamin C was isolated from fruit and vegetables (orange, cabbage, and paprika) and the adrenal gland, and was named 'hexuronic acid'. It was shown to cure scurvy in guinea pigs and was subsequently renamed ascorbic acid to reflect its anti-scorbutic properties. This discovery was performed by Dr. Albert Szent-Gyorgyi (1893–1986, Hungary), who was awarded the Nobel Prize in medicine in 1937. In 1933, its chemical structure and synthesis were realized by the British Sir Norman Haworth, who also obtained the Nobel Prize in chemistry in 1937 (33, 48–49, 52).

Vitamin C is a chiral compound and only the levorotary (L) isomer or L-enantiomer is active and present in humans, animals, and plants. The other dextrorotary (D) isomer or D-enantiomer is not found in nature, but only obtained by artificial synthesis, and has far less vitamin activity than the L-isomer (52). Therefore, most of the enzymatic reactions of vitamin C are stereospecific. In cells, vitamin C can present in two chemically interchangeable forms: ascorbic acid (the reduced form) and dihydro-ascorbic acid (the oxidized form). These forms are both biologically functional and in physiological equilibrium.

L-ascorbic acid is mainly a co-factor for hydroxylases and monooxygenase enzymes involved in the biosynthesis of collagen, L-carnitine, and neurotransmitters (3, 9, 33, 48–49, 53, 54). Collagen represents about one third of the total body protein. Collagen constitutes the principal protein of skin, bones, teeth, cartilage, tendons, blood vessels, heart valves, inter vertebral discs, cornea, and eye lens (48). It is also involved in Hypoxia-Inducible Factor (HIF) degradation, peptide amidation, tyrosine metabolism, and the conversion of dopamine to norepinephrine (50). It is also a key regulator of immune function, cellular growth, and differentiation. Moreover, vitamin C accelerates hydroxylation reactions by maintaining the active center of metal ions (iron, copper) in a reduced state for optimal activity of enzymes: hydroxylase and oxygenase. Vitamin C is essential for the synthesis of muscle L-carnitine by transport and transfer of fatty acids into mitochondria of cell for energy production. Further, ascorbic acid acts as co-factor for the enzyme dopamine-β-hydroxylase, which catalyzes the conversion of neurotransmitter dopamine to norepinephrine. It is also essential for synthesis of neurotransmitters: serotonin and catecholamines (adrenaline, nor-adrenaline, dopamine) (9, 48–49). In addition, L-ascorbic acid catalyzes other enzymatic reactions involving amidation necessary for maximal activity of hormones oxytocin, vasopressin, cholecystokinin, and alpha-melanotripin (3, 33, 48–49). Vitamin C is also necessary for the transformation of cholesterol to bile acids as it modulates the microsomal 7 α-hydroxylation, the rate limiting reaction of cholesterol catabolism in liver. In ascorbic acid deficiency, this reaction becomes slowed down, thus resulting in an accumulation of cholesterol in liver, and an elevation of cholesterol in blood (48). Moreover, other important biological roles of vitamin C reside in its strong antioxidant and reducing properties by donating electrons to various enzymatic and a few non-enzymatic reactions, and by quenching potentially damaging free radicals produced by normal metabolic respiration of the body (23, 48–49). The roles of vitamin C as antioxidant agent are explained in Chapter 3 of this book.

Health benefits of vitamin C are due to its antioxidant, anti-inflammatory, anti-carcinogenic, anti-atherogenic, antiangiogenic, and immunomodulatory properties (3, 9, 23, 33, 48–54). Nobel laureate Pauling and Cameron advocated use of high doses of ascorbic acid (>10 g/day) to cure and prevent common cold, as well as in the treatment of cancer (48). However, its effect in cold treatment remains controversial despite many controlled trials (48–49). Whether vitamin C has anti-cancer properties or not has been debated for decades (50). Daily vitamin C supplementation either as a dietary supplement or in pharmacological doses administered by infusion, can likely reduce the incidence of gastric, esophageal, oral, pharyngeal and cervical cancer, and vitamin C-rich fruits may help prevent colon cancer and lung cancer (48–50). In addition, numerous reports have shown when high doses of vitamin C are combined with conventional chemotherapy drugs, vitamin C enhances the inhibition of cancer cell growth. Interestingly, high doses of vitamin C result in oxidative stress, which preferentially targets cancer cells (50). The positive effect of vitamin C resides in reducing the incidence of stomach cancer, and in preventing lung and colorectal cancer (48–49). In addition, vitamin C intake either from fruits and vegetables or from oral supplements at low doses is also associated with reduced incidence of mortality from cardiovascular diseases (stroke, hypertension, hypercholesterolemia) (48–49, 51–54). However, the role of oral vitamin C in the prevention and treatment of CVDs and cancer remains controversial and is still not evident despite many controlled trials and debates (48–51, 53–54). For other chronic disease prevention, vitamin C may be useful in neuro-degenerative diseases, cataract, diabetes, obesity, and more (48–49, 53). Vitamin C has been shown to stimulate the immune system by enhancing T-cell proliferation in response to infection (48). Ascorbic acid plays a critical role in wound repair and the healing process, as it stimulates collagen synthesis, especially for post-operative patients (48–49, 53). Vitamin C fights fatigue and drowsiness. However, taking vitamin C supplements at night can make sleep difficult. Vitamin C is also known to enhance the availability and absorption of iron from nonheme iron sources possibly by chelation or simply by maintaining the iron in the reduced (ferrous, Fe^{2+}) form; therefore, it may prevent anemia (3). Vitamin C is easily absorbed through the gastro-intestinal tract due to its water-solubility, and is mainly metabolized in the liver and excreted by the kidneys into urine (9, 48–49).

The recommended dietary allowances (RDA) of vitamin C for adults in the United States are: 90 mg/day for men, 75 mg/day for women, 85 mg/day for pregnant women, 120 mg/day for lactating women, 15 mg/day for children 1–3 years, 25 mg/day for children 4–8 years, 45 mg/day for children 9–13 years, 75 mg/day for boys 14–18 years, and 65 mg/day for girls 14–18 years (48, 54). Based on clinical and epidemiological studies, it has been suggested that a dietary intake of 100 mg/day of ascorbic acid is associated with reduced incidence of mortality from heart diseases, stroke, and cancer (48). However, stress, smoking, alcoholism, fever, and viral infections cause a rapid decline in blood levels of ascorbic acid. Intoxication of vitamin C can occur when its daily dose exceeds the Tolerable Upper Intake Level (UL) of 2,000 mg/day, with apparition of different symptoms: insomnia, diarrhea, smarting on urinating, formation of oxalate and uric kidney stones, excessive iron absorption, increase of vitamin B12 deficiency, prickling and irritation of the skin, and more (48–49, 54). In addition, the intake of high doses of vitamin C (2,000mg or more/day) has been the subject of debate, regarding its eventual pro-oxidant or carcinogen property (23, 48, 54). Therefore, the long-term use of ascorbic acid supplementation in high doses may be dangerous. Concerning the bioavailability of synthetic versus natural vitamin C, some studies have reported that overall, a majority of animal studies have shown differences between these two forms of vitamin C, although the results varied depending on the animal model, study design, and body compartments measured (52). In contrast, all steady state comparative bioavailability studies in humans have shown no differences between synthetic and natural vitamin C, regardless of the subject population, study design or intervention used (52). Although synthetic and food-derived vitamin C appear to be equally bioavailable in humans, ingesting natural vitamin C in vegetables is considered preferable because of the concomitant consumption of numerous other macro- and micronutrients and phytochemicals, which will confer additional health benefits. Numerous epidemiological studies have indicated that higher intakes of fruit and vegetables are associated with decreased incidence of stroke, coronary heart disease, and cancers at various sites (52). Concerning coronary heart disease, strong evidence exists for a protective effect of vegetables, moderate evidence for fruit and dietary vitamin C, and insufficient evidence for supplemental vitamin C (52).

The richest fruits in vitamin C, listed in descending order, are acerola cherry, camu camu, kiwifruit, blackberry, strawberry, lemon, blackcurrant, guava, grape, orange, mandarin, grapefruit, cantaloupe, cherry, mango, pineapple, apple, litchi, and banana. Vegetables with high vitamin C concentrations include (arranged in descending order): parsley, red pepper, paprika, Brussel sprout, coriander, broccoli, cauliflower, cabbage, spinach, radish, tomato, and celery (9, 48, 49).

Some animal foods such as lamb liver, pig kidney, lamb heart, lamp tongue also contain significant amounts of vitamin C. Vitamin C is a labile molecule easily lost by heat, light or air oxidation during cooking or long exposure in air, as well as long storage in water such as canned fruit juice (9, 23).

3.2 FAT-SOLUBLE VITAMINS

Fat-soluble vitamins include vitamin A, D, E, and K. As they are lipid soluble, they can be stored for a long time in fat tissues; hence, hypervitaminosis, a toxic form, can occur in long-term intake of these vitamins.

3.2.1 Vitamin A and Carotenoids (Retinoids and Carotenoids)

Vitamin A has two main vitamer forms in foods, which are both fat-soluble: preformed vitamin A or retinoids, and provitamin A or carotenoids. Preformed vitamin A is found only in foods of animal origin, while provitamin A or carotenoids are present in plants, fruits, and vegetables. Preformed vitamin A is a group of fat-soluble unsaturated nutritional compounds called retinoids, including retinol, retinal, retinoic acid and retinyl esters (3, 9, 33, 56). Provitamin A carotenoids are mainly formed by beta-carotene and two other carotenes, alpha-carotene and beta-cryptoxanthin; all are fat-soluble (56). The human body converts these plant pigments, carotenes, into vitamin A. In total, vitamin A includes six to seven vitamers. Both retinoids and provitamin A carotenoids are converted to retinol, which is oxidized to retinal and retinoic acid, the active forms of vitamin A, to support the vitamin's important biological functions (56). Most of the body's vitamin A is stored in the liver in the form of retinyl esters (56). The carotenoid family consists of approximately 100 naturally occurring pigments, which provide the yellow-red color of vegetables and some fruits (9, 57). Only the three carotenoids cited earlier (α-carotene, β-carotene, and β-cryptoxanthin) are converted into retinol, vitamin A; while numerous other carotenoids found in food, such as lycopene, lutein, zeaxanthin, astaxanthin, and so on, cannot be transformed into retinoids (vitamin A) (3, 9, 33, 56, 57). About 90% of ingested preformed vitamin A (retinoids) is absorbed in the small intestine, whereas the absorption efficiency of provitamin A carotenoids varies widely, between 5 and 60%, depending on the type of plant source, the nature of the food, whether it is cooked or raw, and the fat content in the meal, since carotenoids are only absorbed in the presence of fat (3, 33).

Vitamin A is an essential micronutrient for the human body and plays a variety of roles in the visual system, growth and development of the body, regulation of gene expression, immune function, reproduction, and cellular communication (3, 9, 33, 56–61). It is also necessary for brain function, memory, behavior, and learning (60). Vitamin A is critical for vision because it is an essential component of rhodopsin, a receptor protein found in the retinal rod cells. Rhodopsin consists of a membrane-embedded protein, opsin, and a light-sensitive pigment group, retinal. Rhodopsin absorbs light in the retinal receptors and it also supports the normal differentiation and functioning of the conjunctival membranes and cornea (9, 33, 56, 58). Vitamin A deficiency is an important cause of eye malfunction and xerophthalmia (3, 9, 33, 56–59). Clinical signs of xerophthalmia include night blindness or nyctalopia (inability to see in low light or darkness), corneal and conjunctival xerosis (dryness of the eye membranes), keratomalacia (softening of the cornea), Bitot's spots (whitish, opaque deposits on the conjunctiva), and retinopathy (disease of the retina). In developing countries, xerophthalmia due to vitamin A deficiency is the most common cause of childhood blindness, with about three million children having some form of xerophthalmia and another 250 million children having other clinical signs of vitamin A deficiency (3). In addition, supplements containing carotenoids with antioxidant functions, such as beta-carotene, lutein, zeaxanthin and astaxanthin, might be useful for preventing or treating age-related macular degeneration (AMD), another disease of the retina that causes vision loss in older people (56, 58).

Vitamin A also supports cell growth and development of the body. It plays a critical role in the normal formation and maintenance of different organs such as skin, bone, brain, heart, lungs, kidneys, fetus, immune system, and sperm. Retinol and retinoic acid also play a vital part in the development of the human embryo, differentiation of three germ layers, propagation of the signaling process in the formation of the neural tube, organogenesis, and development of limbs during embryogenesis (58). Another role of vitamin A is to promote the body's primary barrier to infection by functioning as a co-factor in enzymatic reactions necessary to the maintenance of healthy functional epithelial tissue (3, 9, 33, 56–58). In infectious diseases, vitamin A supplementation reduced mortality from measles in children younger than two and mortality due to pneumonia in children (56). In addition, retinoid acid, the bioactive metabolite of vitamin A, is a potent signaling molecule in the brains of growing and adult animals, regulates numerous gene products, and modulates neurogenesis, neuronal survival, and synaptic plasticity (60). However, our knowledge of vitamin A effects on behavior and learning, and on neuronal plasticity and cognitive function in adulthood is still emerging (60). Briefly, vitamin A is necessary in vision, bone growth, reproduction, spermatogenesis, fetal development, memory development, immunological response, and more. Other functions of carotenoids, include inhibition of tumor growth, protection against genotoxicity, and modulation of the immune system (9, 33, 56–58). Moreover, vitamin A and carotenoids have antioxidant properties for the prevention of oxidative stress that is the cause of numerous chronic diseases such as cardiovascular disease, cancer, inflammatory diseases. The antioxidant roles of vitamin A and carotenoids are described in Chapter 3 of this book. Because vitamin A has an antioxidant property and plays a role in regulating cell growth and differentiation, several studies have examined the association between vitamin A, or retinoids, and various types of cancer. However, the relationship between serum vitamin A levels or vitamin A supplementation and cancer risk is unclear, and the results of these studies are still contradictory (56, 57). The evidence on the relationship between β-carotene and prostate cancer is also mixed. More research is needed to determine the effects of vitamin A on prostate, lung, and other types of cancer. Vitamin A deficiency is rare in industrial countries, but common in many developing countries, often because people have limited access to foods containing preformed vitamin A from animal-based food sources, and they do not commonly consume available foods containing beta-carotene due to poverty (3, 9, 56). The most common symptom of vitamin A deficiency in young children and pregnant women is xerophthalmia, a form of night blindness (56, 58). Vitamin A deficiency is also due to infectious diseases (diarrhea and measles) mostly in children. It increases the severity and mortality risk of these infections and can lead to anemia due to low iron absorption (3, 56).

The recommended dietary allowances (RDAs) of vitamin A for adults and adolescents over 14 years are: 900 mcg RAE per day for men and 700 mcg RAE per day for women, 770 mcg RAE/day for pregnant women, 1,300 mcg RAE/day for lactating women, 300 mcg RAE/day for children 1–3 years, 400 mcg RAE/day for children 4–8 years and, 600 mcg RAE/day for children 9–13 years of both sexes (56). RAE means Retinol Activity Equivalent and is given as mcg of retinol (56). Because the body converts all dietary sources of vitamin A into retinol, 1 mcg of RAE is equivalent to the following amounts from dietary sources: 1 mcg of retinol, 12 mcg of β-carotene, and 24 mcg of α-carotene or β-cryptoxanthin (56). From dietary supplements, the body converts 2 mcg of β-carotene to 1 mcg of retinol (56). To this day, vitamin A is listed on food and supplement labels in international units (IUs). Conversion rates between mcg RAE and IU are: 1 IU retinol=0.3 mcg RAE, 1 IU β-carotene from supplements=0.15 mcg RAE, 1 IU β-carotene from food=0.05 mcg RAE, 1 IU α-carotene or β-cryptoxanthin=0.025 mcg RAE (3, 56).

Tolerable Upper Intake Levels (ULs) preformed vitamin A are 3,000 mcg RAE/day or 10,000 IU/day for adult men, women, pregnant and lactation women; 2,800 mcg RAE/day or 9,333 IU/day for adolescents of both sexes from 14–18 years; 1,700 mcg RAE/day or 5,667 IU/day for children of both sexes from 9–13 years; 900 mcg RAE or 3,000 IU/day for children of both sexes from 4–8 years; and 600 mcg RAE/day or 2,000 IU/day for baby and children of both sexes from 1 month to 8 years (56).

Retinol and carotenes are yellow or orange pigments. Retinol is stable when exposed to heat and light, but is easily oxidized by air. Vitamin A participates in healing and stimulates the production of melanin, a pigment of skin color. Its bioavailability increases with the presence of vitamin E and other antioxidants.

Since vitamin A is fat-soluble, it can be stored longtime in the body, primarily in the liver. Routine intake of large amounts of vitamin A supplements or polar bear liver over a period of time can result in toxic symptoms, including liver damage, bone fractures, joint pain, increased intracranial pressure, dizziness, alopecia (hair loss), headaches, vomiting, blurry vision, insomnia, fatigue, weight loss, drying of the mucous membranes, skin desquamation, coma, and even death (3, 9, 33, 56–58). Children are more sensitive than adults to a high retinol intake. These toxicities only occur with preformed vitamin A (retinoid), but not with carotenoids such as β-carotene. Hypervitaminosis A is usually a result of consuming too much preformed vitamin A from supplements or therapeutic retinoids (56). High intakes of preformed vitamin A supplement (more than 1,500 μg/day, only slightly higher than the RDA) can reduce bone mineral density, and increase fracture risk (56). In addition, there is also evidence that retinol is teratogenic (causing developmental malformation of the fetus and birth defect). Consequently, it has been suggested that pregnant women or those who are trying to become pregnant should not take vitamin A supplements and should not eat liver or liver products in high amounts (9, 33). Nevertheless, pregnant women are advised not to consume more than 3,000 μg/day (10,000 IU) vitamin A supplement to avoid risk of fetal toxicity (3, 33, 56). Consult a doctor before using vitamin A supplement if you are pregnant.

An excessive intake of food rich in carotenoids such as carrots, tomatoes, can result in a distinct orange-yellow color of the skin, called hypercarotenemia (9, 58). This symptom can be reversed by discontinuing beta-carotene ingestion. Unlike preformed vitamin A, beta-carotene is not known to be teratogenic or lead to reproductive toxicity or birth defect. Carotenes are strong antioxidants. High doses of beta-carotene supplements (20–30 mg/day) or diets with high levels of carotenoid-rich food for long periods are not associated with toxicity (9, 56). However, supplementation with beta-carotene, with or without retinyl palmitate, for five to eight years has been associated with an increased risk of lung cancer and cardiovascular disease in current and former male and female smokers and in male current and former smokers occupationally exposed to asbestos (56). In addition, beta-carotene supplements (20 mg daily) were also associated with increased mortality, mainly due to lung cancer and ischemic heart disease (56). In contrast, natural foods (fruits and vegetables) rich in beta-carotene or carotenoids protect against lung cancer and prevent heart disease (56).

Vitamin A (retinol) is only found in the fatty part of animal foods such as: whole milk, lard, cream, cheese, butter, egg yolk, eels, beef liver, and fatty fish (salmon, tuna) (3, 33, 56, 58). Cod liver oil constitutes one of nature's richest sources of effective vitamins A, E, D, and omega-3 fatty acids. Animal livers contain on average 1.3–40 mg vitamin A/100 g. The liver of the polar bear is the richest in retinol (600 mg/100 g liver) (9). Eating the liver of the polar bear can cause drowsiness, headache, vomiting, and excess peeling of the skin (9). Vegetables contain only provitamin A or carotenoids. Garden vegetables (spinach and similar vegetables), carrots, red capsicum, tomatoes, yellow sweet potatoes, red and yellow fruits (papaya, pumpkins, mango, gac or Momordica cochinchinensis, peach, etc.) are the main sources.

Our ancestors in Egypt, Greece, and China used liver to treat some eye diseases such as night blindness for thousands of years (57). The first discovery of vitamin A was due to the French physiologist François Magendie who conducted a nutritional deprivation experiment with dogs in 1816 that resulted in corneal ulcers and high mortality. In 1880, the Russian Nicolai Lunin, then Carl Socin, showed that there was an unknown substance in milk and egg yolk that was fat-soluble and essential for the survival of mice who could not live on nutrition composed of purified fat, protein, carbohydrate, and salt alone. In 1906, the British biochemist Frederick Hopkins proposed that this substance was necessary for life, then he named this factor 'fat-soluble A' in 1918, and then 'vitamin A' in 1920 (61). In 1929, Sir Hopkins was awarded the Nobel Prize in Physiology or Medicine, with Christiaan Eijkman, for the discovery of this vitamin A (61). Further studies on the chemical structure, the synthesis, and other roles of vitamin A in health and disease continue until today (61).

3.2.2 Vitamin D (Calciferol: Cholecalciferol or Vitamin D3 and Ergocalciferol or Vitamin D2)

Vitamin D, also called calciferol, has several forms (vitamers) that are all fat-soluble. Two main forms of vitamin D present in nature are: vitamin D2 or ergocalciferol, and vitamin D3 or cholecalciferol

7-Cholesterol

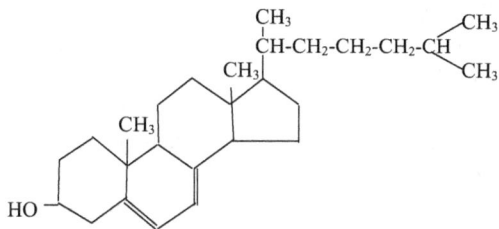

Vitamin D3

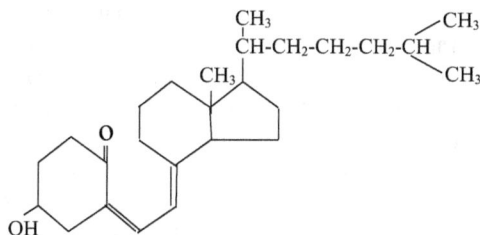

Ergosterol

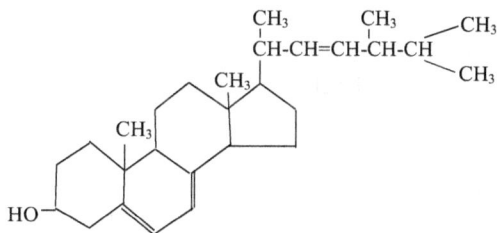

Vitamin D2

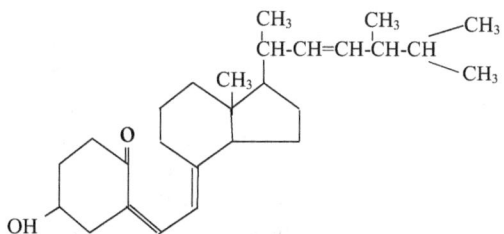

FIGURE 2.1 7-Cholesterol, Vitamin D3, Ergosterol, Vitamin D2.

The precursor of vitamin D2 is ergosterol, mainly found in mushrooms, and that of vitamin D3 is 7-cholesterol, a derivative of cholesterol found in the skin of mammals. The main function of vitamin D (D2 and D3) is to control calcium and phosphate homeostasis; that is, to regulate calcium and phosphate metabolism. Vitamin D is necessary for the health and the growth of the bone and the skeleton. It is used for the prevention and treatment of different ailments such as rickets in children, osteomalacia in adults, and osteoporosis in elderly people (3, 9, 33, 62–66). Apart from vitamin D2 and vitamin D3, vitamin D has three other natural vitamers and four synthetic analogs. Vitamin D analogs are chemically classified as secosteroids, which are steroids with one broken bond (63). The three other natural forms of vitamin D include: vitamin D1 (an equimolar mixture of vitamin D2 and lumisterol and now abandoned), vitamin D4 (22-dihydroergocalciferol), and vitamin D5 (sitocalciferol) (63). The four artificial analogs include: maxacalcitol (22-oxacalcitriol or OCT), falecalcitriol or $1,25-(OH)_2$-26,27-F6-D3, paricalcitol or 19-nor-$1,25(OH)_2$D2, and doxercalciferol or 1-alpha-OH-D2 (63). These analogs are not considered dietary supplements; rather, they are designed for applications in clinical treatment of a specific disease (62). For example, maxacalcitol is only used in Japan for the treatment of psoriasis, while paricalcitol, doxercalciferol, and falecalcitriol are used for the therapy of secondary hyperparathyroidism (63, 66). The two main natural vitamins D2 and D3 are now also obtained by chemical synthesis and used as dietary supplements or fortified foods. The vitamin D2 and vitamin D3 differ only in their side chain structure (62–66). The differences do not affect metabolism (i.e., activation), and both forms function as prohormones. When activated, the D2 and D3 forms exhibit identical roles in the body, and their potency to cure vitamin D deficiency such as rickets is the same (3, 9, 33, 62–66). Vitamin D, in either the D2 or D3 form, is considered biologically inactive until it undergoes two enzymatic hydroxylation reactions. The first takes place in the liver, mediated by the 25-hydroxylase which forms 25-hydroxyvitamin D (25-OH-D) also known as calcidiol. The second reaction takes place in the kidney, mediated by 1α-hydroxylase, which converts 25-OH-D to the biologically active hormone, calcitriol or $1,25$-dihydroxyvitamin D ($1,25-(OH)_2$-D (3, 9, 33, 62). The precursor (25-OH-D) of calcitriol is the major circulating form of vitamin D, and circulates bound to a specific plasma carrier protein, vitamin D binding protein (DBP). DBP also transports inactive D2 or D3 forms and their active metabolite calcitriol. Calcitriol controls the regulation of bone and metabolism of calcium, phosphorus, and other minerals. Low serum phosphorus levels stimulate calcitriol synthesis, whereas high serum phosphorus levels inhibit it (3, 62, 66). Without vitamin D, only 10–15% of dietary calcium and about 60% of phosphorus are absorbed. Vitamin D sufficiency enhances calcium and phosphorus absorption by 30–40% and 80%, respectively (63). Vitamin D promotes calcium absorption in the gut and maintains adequate serum calcium and phosphate concentrations to enable normal mineralization of bone and to prevent hypocalcemic tetany. It is also needed for bone growth and bone remodeling in children. Without sufficient vitamin D, bones can become thin, brittle, or misshapen. Vitamin D sufficiency prevents rickets in children and osteomalacia in adults (64). Together with calcium, phosphorous, and fluorine, it also protects against osteoporosis in the elderly, mostly women after menopause. Other roles of vitamin D in the body include modulation of cell growth, reduction of inflammation, and neuromuscular and immune function (3, 9, 33, 62–65). Many genes encoding proteins that regulate cell proliferation, differentiation, and apoptosis are modulated in part by vitamin D (64).

Vitamin D3 or cholecalciferol is a secosteroid synthesized in the skin cells by sunrays or ultraviolet B light of a precursor cholesterol derivative, 7-dehydrocholesterol, to pre-vitamin D3, which spontaneously isomerizes to vitamin D3. So, to call cholecalciferol a vitamin is inappropriate because it is produced in the human and mammal body with the aid of UV sunlight. Therefore, vitamin D3 may be classified as a steroid compound like some other steroid hormones because they are all made from cholesterol in the body. It is not considered as essential as other vitamins, and may be classified as nonessential or semi-essential. Vitamin D3 is present in human and animal tissues (fish, liver, milk, fish oil, and cod liver oil) (3, 9, 33, 62–66). Vitamin D2 or ergocalciferol is often present in mushrooms found in nature with plenty of sunlight, and in cultivated mushrooms artificially exposed to sunlight or UV-B light. Vitamin D2 is also obtained from the UV irradiation of the yeast sterol, and is naturally present in some invertebrates like oysters. Mushrooms and yeasts are rich in ergosterol (provitamin D2) that is converted to viosterol, a previtamin D2, then to vitamin D2, with the aid of sunlight or UV-B light. Human beings do not make vitamin D2 (3, 33, 62–66).

Vitamin D insufficiency affects almost 50% of the population worldwide. An estimated one billion people worldwide, across all ethnicities and age groups, have a vitamin D deficiency (63). This phenomenon can mainly be attributed to lifestyle and environmental factors that reduce exposure to sunlight, leading to decreased vitamin D production in the skin. Black people absorb more UV-B in the melanin of their skin than do white people and, therefore, require more sun exposure to produce the same amount of vitamin D (63–66). Homebound individuals, women who wear long robes and head coverings for religious reasons, and people with occupations that limit sun exposure are unlikely to obtain adequate vitamin D from sunlight (63). People living in Nordic countries are also subject to vitamin D deficiency due to the lack of sunlight, mostly in winter. Other causes of vitamin D deficiency are low intake of foods rich in vitamin D such as fish, fish oil, milk, and meat, due to poverty, ignorance, or veganism. Vitamin D deficiency is also due to bowel diseases or other diseases of digestive tract (liver disease, cystic fibrosis, celiac disease, and Crohn's disease) that reduce the absorption of vitamin D through foods. Patients on a wide variety of medications, including anticonvulsants and medications to treat AIDS/HIV, are at risk because these drugs enhance the catabolism (degradation) of 25-OH-D and 1,25-(OH)$_2$-D (63). Vitamin D deficiency is also observed in elderly people due to the decrease of hydrolases – enzymes responsible for the metabolism of the inactive vitamin D into its active forms, 25-hydroxyvitamin D (25-OH-D) and calcitriol (1,25-dihydroxyvitamin D). Supplementation of vitamin D either by tablets or fortified foods may reduce this deficiency. A determination of 25-hydroxyvitamin D (25-OH-D), a precursor form of calcitriol, in serum is necessary to evaluate this treatment because the metabolite (25-OH-D) is present in circulating blood, while the active calcitriol is generally fixed in tissues.

Besides the main roles of vitamin D in the prevention and treatment of some bone diseases cited above, vitamin D may have other effects in the prevention of some chronic diseases such as cancer, diabetes, hypertension, and multiple sclerosis (62–66). Regarding cancer prevention of vitamin D, the results in the literature are still contradictory. Strong biological and mechanistic bases indicate that vitamin D plays a role in the prevention of colon, prostate, and breast cancers (64). However, clinical studies did not show a protective effect of vitamin D on cancer. A recent review found an increased risk of pancreatic cancer associated with high levels of serum 25-OH-D ($\geq$100 nmol/L or $\geq$40 ng/mL) (64). Further research is needed to determine whether vitamin D inadequacy in particular increases cancer risk, whether greater exposure to the nutrient is protective, and whether some individuals could be at increased risk of cancer because of vitamin D exposure (62, 64). Indeed, studies to date do not support a role for vitamin D, with or without calcium, in reducing the risk of cancer (62, 64). Recently, vitamin D was proposed by some therapists in the prevention and treatment of Covid-19 which is a viral infection worldwide in 2020 and 2021. However, this proposal was not accepted by healthcare organizations (see Chapter 9 of this book).

Inversely, high intake of vitamin D mostly by supplementation can cause toxicity to the body because vitamin D is fat-soluble and can be stocked long-term in fatty tissues and organs. Vitamin D toxicity can cause non-specific symptoms such as anorexia, weight loss, polyuria, and heart arrhythmias. More seriously, it can also raise blood levels of calcium which leads to vascular and tissue calcification, with subsequent damage to the heart, blood vessels, and kidneys (64). A study observed that the use of supplements of both calcium (1,000 mg/day) and vitamin D (400 IU) by postmenopausal women was associated with a 17% increase in the risk of kidney stones over 7 years (64). A 25-OH-D concentration in serum consistently >500 nmol/L (>200 ng/mL) is considered to be potentially toxic (64). The use of vitamin D supplements for therapeutics must be done by a professional healthcare agent. Intakes of food rich in vitamin D are safer than high intakes of dietary supplements containing vitamin D.

The recommended dietary allowances (RDAs) of vitamin D for adults, adolescents, children from 1 to 70 years are: 600 UI or 15 mcg per day for both sexes and for pregnant and lactating women (64). The RDAs are 800 UI or 20 mcg per day for elderly people of both sexes over 70 years (64). Even though sunlight may be a major source of vitamin D for some, the RDAs of vitamin D are set on the basis of minimal sun exposure (64). The Tolerable Upper Intake Levels (ULs) for vitamin D are 4,000 IU (100 mcg) per day for children from 9 years to adults of both sexes (64). They are 2500–3000 UI (63–75 mcg) per day for children from 1 year to 8 years (64). Long-term intakes above the UL increase the risk of adverse health effects. For the relation between serum 25-hydroxyvitamin D (25-OH-D) concentrations and health, it is established that 25-OH-D concentration in serum >50 nmol/L (>20 ng/mL) is generally considered adequate for bone and overall health (64). It becomes toxic when levels are greater than 125 nmol/L (>50 ng/mL). When 25-OH-D levels decrease <30 nmol/L (<12 ng/mL), rickets are observed in infants and children, and osteomalacia in adults (64). Between 30 to <50 nmol/L (12 to <20 ng/mL), these levels are generally considered inadequate for bone and overall health in healthy individuals (64).

The Food and Nutrition Board (FNB) concluded that serum 25-OH-D levels above approximately 125–150 nmol/L (50–60 ng/mL) should be avoided, because of increases in all-cause mortality, greater risk of cancer at some sites like the pancreas, greater risk of cardiovascular events, and more falls and fractures among the elderly. So, recommended vitamin D intakes do not exceed 5,000 IU/day (64).

Regarding the toxicity of vitamins D2 and D3, some experimental animal data from a number of mammalian species ranging from rodents to primates support the concept that the D2 form is less toxic than D3, but there is no evidence available in humans (62). At this time, firm conclusions about different effects of the two forms of vitamin D cannot be drawn; however, it would appear that at low doses, D2 and D3 are equivalent, but at high doses, D2 is less effective than D3, but probably less toxic than D3 (62). Despite the importance of the sun for vitamin D synthesis, it is prudent to limit exposure of skin to sunlight and UV radiation from tanning beds because UV light is a carcinogen responsible for about 1.5 million skin cancers and 8,000 deaths due to metastatic melanoma that occur annually in the United States (64–66).

Sources of vitamin D in nature are limited. Fatty fishes such as salmon, tuna, mackerel, snapper, herring, roe, sardine, and cod liver oil are among the best sources. Small amounts of vitamin D are found in beef liver, cheese, milk, yogurt, and egg yolks. Vitamin D in these foods is primarily in the form of vitamin D3 and its metabolite 25-OH-D3. Fish have the highest natural vitamin D content because their main food are microalgae (67). Microalgae belonging to the plant kingdom contain cholesterol and some provitamin D3 sterols like sitosterol, desmosterol, fucosterol, and so on (67). In general, fruits and vegetables contain a small amount of vitamin D2 due to the contamination of plants with fungi (62–67). Some mushrooms and yeasts provide vitamin D2 in variable amounts. The vitamin D2 levels in mushrooms can be increased when they are exposed to sunlight or UV-B light, even after harvesting (3, 9, 33, 62–67).

At the beginning of the twentieth century, many scientists such as Sir Edward Mellanby in Great Britain in 1918, Pr. Elmer McCollum in the United States in 1918, and Pr. Adolf Windaus in Germany in 1920, contributed to the discovery and identification of vitamin D. In 1922, Elmer McCollum in the United States found that the factor in cod liver oil which cured rickets in dogs is a new vitamin; he named it vitamin D because it was the fourth vitamin discovered in this period after vitamins A, B, and C (68). The chemical structures of the various forms of vitamin D were determined in the 1920s and 1930s by Windaus and colleagues in Germany. Windaus was awarded the Nobel Prize in Chemistry in 1928 for his research concerning the constitution of different sterols and their connection with the vitamins (68).

In brief, vitamin D3 is made in the skin from 7-dehydrocholesterol, a derivative of cholesterol present in human body, under the action of UV sunlight. Vitamin D2 (ergocalciferol) is derived from the plant sterol named ergosterol, present mostly in mushrooms. Vitamin D is considered a semi-essential steroid hormone because it is made in the body when human biological condition is normal. Long-term intakes of high doses of vitamin D are dangerous for the health and must be managed by a healthcare professional.

3.2.3 Vitamin E (Alpha-Tocopherol)

Vitamin E is the collective name for a group of fat-soluble compounds found in many foods, fats, and vegetable oils. Vitamin E is a chiral compound and naturally exists in eight chemical forms: α-, β-, γ-, δ-tocopherol and α-, β-, γ-, δ- tocotrienol, which are synthesized by plants from homogentisic acid, and stored in leaves and seeds. Only α-tocopherol is the most bioactive form in humans and the most abundant in human blood (3, 9, 33, 69–74). Other forms of vitamin E are active in animals, and their biological properties cannot be extrapolated to humans (69). Tocopherols and tocotrienols have the same basic chemical structure, which is characterized by a long isoprenoid side chain attached at position two of a six-chromanol ring. Their chemical difference consists in the number and position of the methyl groups of the chromanol ring. Tocopherols have a saturated side chain while tocotrienols contain an unsaturated side chain with three double bonds (33, 69–71). Natural vitamin E in plants occurs in dextrogyre (d) stereoisomer only and is called RRR-alpha-tocopherol, commonly labeled as d-alpha-tocopherol. The synthetic vitamin E in supplements is a mixture of d- and l-stereoisomers and contains eight different stereoisomers which are called 'all-rac'-α-tocopherol (commonly labeled as dl-alpha-tocopherol). Therefore, synthetic α-tocopherol does not have the same biological potency as the corresponding natural compound. This is because the side chain of tocopherol has three centers of asymmetry, and when it is synthesized chemically the result is a mixture of d and l-isomers or R and S-stereoisomers. In natural vitamin E, all three asymmetric centers have the R-configuration – the three methyl groups are in the same side of the lateral chain. Hence, natural α-tocopherol is called all-R, or RRR-α tocopherol (33). R means rectus or right and is equivalent to d or dextrogyre of the ancient nomenclature, while S means sinister or left and is equivalent to l or levogyre. 'Rac' or dl or RS means racemate which is an equal mixture of dextrorotary (d) and levorotary (l) compounds or a mixture of R and S stereoisomers (75). The receptors and enzymes in the body are highly stereoselective and interact exclusively with one of the enantiomers of a chiral molecule in a process called chiral recognition. As a result, only one enantiomer has the desired effect on the body, while the others may have either no effect or an adverse effect (75). Vitamin E isoforms are not interconvertible inside the human body. Moreover, natural RRR-α-tocopherol is nearly twice as active as synthetic racemic RS-α-tocopherol supplements (71, 73). Briefly, only one, RRR-α-tocopherol or d-α-tocopherol, satisfies the criteria of being a vitamin, and is the most bioactive form in humans to protect the human body against disease produced by its absence.

Vitamin E has two main functions including enzymatic and antioxidant activities (23, 69–74). As an enzymatic activity regulator, vitamin E inhibits the activity of protein kinase C (PKC), an enzyme involved in cell proliferation and differentiation in smooth muscle cells, platelets, and monocytes (69–74). Vitamin E also increases the expression of two enzymes, namely cytosolic phospholipase A2 and cyclooxygenase-1, that suppress arachidonic acid metabolism, thereby increasing the release of prostacyclin from the endothelium, which, in turn, dilates blood vessels and inhibits platelet aggregation in humans (70–71). A few other studies suggest that tocopherols appear to inhibit platelet aggregation through the inhibition of protein kinase C (PKC) and the increased action of nitric oxide synthase (71). Another main activity of vitamin E is its antioxidant property. Alpha-tocopherol is a strong peroxyl radical scavenger and an inhibitor of oxidative stress, which can cause numerous chronic diseases like cancer, inflammatory diseases, and CVD. Thanks to its antioxidant effect, natural vitamin E in foods may prevent cardiovascular disease (CVD) and cancer. Details of the antioxidant property of vitamin E and its mechanism are developed in Chapter 4 of this book. In addition, natural vitamin E (RRR-α-tocopherol) possesses anti-inflammatory, anti-platelet aggregating, and immunostimulant properties, and is a regulating cell signaling agent as well as a modulating gene transcription compound (69–74).

Frank vitamin E deficiency is rare and overt deficiency symptoms have not been found in healthy people who obtain little vitamin E from their diets (33, 70, 73). Premature babies of very low birth weight (<1,500 grams) may be deficient in vitamin E. Vitamin E supplementation in these infants may reduce the risk of some complications, such as those affecting the retina, but they can also increase the risk of infections. Because the digestive tract requires fat to absorb vitamin E, people with fat-malabsorption disorders are more likely to become deficient than people without such disorders. People with Crohn's disease, cystic fibrosis, biliary secretion insufficiency or chronic diarrhea, for example are also subject to vitamin E deficiency (70). Deficiency symptoms include muscular dystrophy, peripheral neuropathy, ataxia (loss of muscle movement control), skeletal myopathy, retinopathy, and impairment of the immune response (69–74). Ataxia and vitamin E deficiency (AVED) is another rare, inherited disorder in which the liver's alpha-tocopherol transfer protein is defective or absent. People with AVED have such severe vitamin E deficiency that they develop nerve damage and lose the ability to walk unless they take large doses of supplemental vitamin E (69–70).

About the roles of vitamin E supplement in disease cited in the literature, there are four main ailments in which vitamin E may be involved: heart disease, cancer, eye disorders, and cognitive decline (69–71). Concerning coronary heart diseases, many population studies have found that people with higher levels of vitamin E in their bodies have a lower risk of heart ailment. Supplementation with vitamin E is considered to provide health benefits against CVD through its antioxidant activity, the prevention of lipoprotein oxidation, and the inhibition of platelet aggregation (74). Several observational studies have associated lower rates of heart disease with higher vitamin E intakes (70). However, the results from large prospective, randomized, placebo-controlled clinical trials with synthetic alpha-tocopherol supplements have been largely negative and have not shown any benefit (69–74, 76–81). A recent meta-analysis suggests that alpha-tocopherol supplements may actually increase all-cause mortality; however, the mechanism for this increased risk is unknown (33, 69–71, 74). Among healthy people who were at low risk for heart disease, two large trials also found no protection from vitamin E supplementation (70, 74). The Heart Outcomes Prevention Evaluation (HOPE) study, and the HOPE-TOO follow-up study, found no significant protection by vitamin E supplement against heart attacks, strokes, unstable angina, or deaths from cardiovascular disease, and found that it may even increase the risk of heart failure (69, 70, 78–80). Furthermore, regular supplementation of vitamin E was often associated with a higher risk of hemorrhagic stroke (70, 71, 74, 78). In contrast, one large clinical study suggested that foods rich in vitamin E may reduce the risk of death from stroke in postmenopausal women, but did not support a protective role for vitamin E supplement or other antioxidant vitamins (77). Perhaps, this difference may be due to the chiral forms of vitamin E, since synthetic vitamin E is a racemate compound, while natural vitamin E in foods is a pure stereoisomer. In general, routine use of vitamin E supplements does not prevent cardiovascular disease or cannot reduce its morbidity and mortality. But, in healthy women, a study showed that vitamin E did not affect the overall risk of heart failure (81). Long-term vitamin E supplementation can cause hemorrhagic stroke because vitamin E possesses anticoagulant properties and is an antivitamin K (70, 73, 77–78).

Concerning cancer prevention, population studies suggest that eating foods high in vitamin E and other antioxidants may help prevent cancer. Other studies show that people with cancer often have lower levels of vitamin E in the blood. Vitamin E might also block the formation of carcinogenic nitrosamines formed in the stomach from nitrites in foods, and protect against cancer by enhancing immune function. Unfortunately, human trials and surveys that have attempted to associate vitamin E supplement intake with cancer incidence have found that vitamin E is not beneficial in most cases (69–71, 79). Both the Heart Outcomes Prevention Evaluation-The Ongoing Outcomes (HOPE-TOO) trial and the Women's Health Study (WHS) study evaluated whether vitamin E supplements might protect people from cancer and found no significant reduction in the risk of developing cancer in individuals taking daily doses of 400 IU or 600 IU of vitamin E (69–71, 79). Vitamin E supplements also did not protect or reduce breast, prostate, lung, pancreatic, and colorectal cancers. A clinical study of more than 29,000 men reported no association between dietary or supplemental vitamin E intake and prostate cancer risk (69). However, another trial found that vitamin E supplements, taken for about five and a half years, not only did not prevent prostate cancer, but instead substantially increased the risk of developing prostate cancer (69). In contrast, another study found that among current smokers and men who had quit, vitamin E intakes of more than 400 IU/day were associated with a statistically significant 71% reduction in the risk of advanced prostate cancer (70). In general, many experts believe getting antioxidants such as vitamins C and E from foods may be the best way to protect against cancer and to avoid side effects that often occur when taking antioxidant supplements. Moreover, the use of long-term vitamin E supplementation should be approached cautiously because it is fat-soluble and can accumulate for a long time in different tissues.

Concerning eye disorders, prospective cohort studies have found that people with relatively high dietary intakes of vitamin E (e.g., 30 IU/day) have an approximately 20% lower risk of developing age-related macular degeneration (AMD) than people with low intakes (e.g., <15 IU/day) (70). Vitamin E (400 IU) combined with other antioxidants, including zinc (80 mg), beta-carotene (15mg), vitamin C (500 mg), and copper (2 mg), compared to participants taking a placebo over 5 years, seems to protect against developing AMD (69–70). However, two randomized controlled trials in which participants took supplements of vitamin E (500 IU/day D-alpha-tocopherol in one study, and 111 IU/day DL-alpha-tocopheryl acetate combined with 20 mg/day beta-carotene in the other) or a placebo failed to show a protective effect for vitamin E on AMD (69–70). Researchers do not know whether this combination of nutrients helps prevent AMD or helps people with less advanced AMD. Vitamins E and C may also help treat uvea inflammation (uveitis). Several observational studies have revealed a potential relationship between vitamin E supplements and the risk of cataract formation. One prospective cohort study found that lens clarity was superior in participants who took vitamin E supplements and those with higher blood levels of the vitamin (70). In another study, long-term use of vitamin E supplements was associated with slower progression of age-related lens opacification. Overall, the available evidence is inconsistent with respect to whether vitamin E supplements, taken alone or in combination with other antioxidants, can reduce the risk of developing AMD or cataracts (69–70). Briefly, the effects of vitamin E supplement in the prevention of AMD or cataracts are mixed and still not evident.

Concerning cognitive decline, evidence is mixed as to whether vitamin E can help prevent or treat age-related diseases in humans such as Alzheimer's disease (69–70, 76). As vitamin E is an antioxidant, some researchers believe that antioxidants may help prevent Alzheimer's disease. However, most research results do not support the use of vitamin E supplements by healthy or mildly impaired individuals to maintain cognitive performance or slow its decline with normal aging (69). As far as the use of vitamin E in protecting against neurodegenerative disease, based on a Cochrane Dementia and Cognitive Improvement's Specialized Register, it has been concluded that there is no evidence of efficacy of vitamin E in the prevention or treatment of people with Alzheimer's disease or Mild Cognitive Impairment (69). Vitamin E was also ineffective in preventing dementia incidence among asymptomatic men (69). Clinical intervention trials have also demonstrated that supplementation with vitamin E is neutral or even harmful for preventing age-related diseases in humans. Therefore, the role of vitamin E as an 'anti-ager' has been called into question (76). The best way to prevent aging and age-related diseases is to consume natural foods rich not only in vitamin E, but also in other antioxidants. More research is needed to identify the role of vitamin E in the management of cognitive impairment.

In summary, vitamin E supplementation has not been shown to have significant benefit for people who are healthy. Moreover, it appears to be harmful with prolonged use. It does not improve CVDs, diabetes mellitus, or decrease the risk of cancer, and it may cause hemorrhagic stroke. It cannot stimulate spermatozoid production. There is no benefit to mother or child taking vitamin E supplements during pregnancy. In contrast, vitamin E may increase risk of having early rupture of membranes at term. There is also no significant benefit for eye disorders (AMD, cataract) with vitamin E supplementation.

Regarding health risks from excessive vitamin E intake, research has not found any adverse effects from consuming natural vitamin E in food (69–71, 77). However, high doses of alpha-tocopherol supplements can cause hemorrhage and interrupt blood coagulation in animals, and *in vitro* data suggest that high doses inhibit platelet aggregation. Two clinical trials have found an increased risk of hemorrhagic stroke in participants taking alpha-tocopherol supplement (70, 77, 78). Hypervitaminosis E may also counteract vitamin K leading to a vitamin K deficiency (70, 73). In high doses, vitamin E has pro-oxidant properties that are harmful to the body and may cause nausea, diarrhea, or vision troubles. Also, vitamin E supplementation combined with chemotherapy or radiotherapy for cancer therapy is to be avoided.

The U.S. Food and Nutrition Board has set a tolerable upper intake levels (ULs) of vitamin E at 1,000 mg (1,500 IU) per day for adults of both sexes (70). The Recommended Dietary Allowances (RDAs) for vitamin E are 15 mg/day or 22.4 IU for women and men ages 14 and up and 19 mg/day for lactating women (70). For children ages 1–13 years the RDA increases with age from 6 to 11 mg/day (70). To convert from mg to IU: 1 mg of alpha-tocopherol is equivalent to 1.49 IU of the natural form or 2.22 IU of the synthetic form. To convert from IU to mg: 1 IU of the natural form is equivalent to 0.67 mg of alpha-tocopherol. One IU of the synthetic form is equivalent to 0.45 mg of alpha-tocopherol (70). As with all supplements, consult a health care provider before taking vitamin E to avoid toxicity and undesirable effects due to its fat-solubility and its high accumulation in the body.

The main food sources of vitamin E include vegetable oils (wheat germ oil, almond oil, rapeseed oil, sunflower oil, olive oil, soybean oil, and sesame oil), wheat germ, soybean, almond, peanut, spinach, turnip, broccoli, avocado, kiwi, mango, cod liver oil, liver, fish, meat, and butter. Consuming natural vitamin E in food is the best choice to avoid its deficiency in the body and also to prevent some chronic diseases (33, 69–71).

Vitamin E was discovered in 1922 by Evans and Bishop in the United States as a necessary dietary factor for reproduction in rats. Later, several other scientists completed the research on the chemical structures, antioxidant properties, and biological activities of vitamin E (69, 72).

3.2.4   Vitamin K (Phylloquinone and Menaquinones)

Vitamin K is a group of fat-soluble vitamins with a common chemical structure of 2-methyl-1, 4-naphthoquinone, and includes two natural vitamers: vitamin K1 or phylloquinone and vitamin K2 or menaquinones (3, 9, 33, 82–88). In addition, menadiol and menadione, called vitamin K3, are synthetic compounds that can be metabolized to phylloquinone in the body (33, 85). However, they are reported to have adverse effects such as hemolysis and liver toxicity and are not used in therapy (82, 85). Therefore, only vitamin K1 and vitamin K2 are called vitamin K and naturally exist in some foods and are available as dietary supplement.

Vitamin K functions as a coenzyme for the activity of numerous enzymes and proteins in the body, such as the coagulation factors (II, VII, IX, X and protein C and protein S), osteocalcin (a bone-forming protein) and matrix-Gla protein (MGP – an anti-calcification protein) (82, 83). It is best known for its role in helping blood coagulate or clot to prevent and stop bleeding or hemorrhage through prothrombin and vitamin K-dependent carboxylase, an enzyme required for the synthesis of proteins involved in hemostasis (blood clotting) (3, 9, 33, 82–88). Prothrombin is a vitamin K-dependent protein in plasma that is directly involved in the body's blood clotting mechanism – blood coagulation (3, 82). It is often used in the treatment and prevention of hemorrhages and also as an antidote to counteract the excess effects of anticoagulant drugs such as warfarin. Vitamin K also plays an important role in bone health. Osteocalcin is another vitamin K-dependent protein that is present in bone and may be involved in bone mineralization or turnover. Matrix Gla-Protein (MGP), a vitamin K-dependent protein present in vascular smooth muscle, bone, and cartilage, might help reduce abnormal calcification (83, 86). Vitamin K supplements, especially vitamin K2, can decrease inactive MGP levels and slow the progression of Coronary Artery Calcification (CAC) in healthy older adults with pre-existing CAC, as well as improve arterial stiffness (86). Furthermore, vitamin K2 in the form of MK-7 has been shown to be a bioactive compound in regulating osteoporosis, atherosclerosis, cancer, and inflammatory diseases, without risk of negative side effects or overdosing (85). Vitamin K exerts its anabolic effect on the bone turnover in different ways such as promoting osteoblast differentiation, upregulating transcription of specific genes in osteoblasts, and activating the bone-associated vitamin K-dependent proteins which play critical roles in extracellular bone matrix mineralization. Therefore, vitamin K improves bone health and reduces the risk of bone fractures, particularly in postmenopausal women who are at risk for osteoporosis (84).

Vitamin K2 (menaquinone) could be used to treat bone loss and osteoporosis caused by high doses or long-term corticoid treatment. However, currently few guidelines recommend vitamin K therapy for prevention or treatment of osteoporosis (83). Vitamin K is also helpful to lower hyper-cholesterolemia in people on dialysis only. In any case, consult a doctor before taking vitamin K1 or K2, because excessive vitamin K may cause dangerous blood coagulation. Vitamin K is also present in the liver and other body tissues, including the brain, heart, pancreas, blood, and bone (82–88). It intervenes in other diverse physiological functions such as the synthesis of sphingolipids that are now known to play key roles in the central and peripheral nervous systems (87).

People are generally encouraged to get their daily requirement of vitamin K through dietary foods because deficiency in vitamin K is rare. In addition, fat-soluble vitamins A, D, E, and K, are stored long-term in the body's fat tissues, and can cause hypervitaminosis, which is toxic for the body. Vitamin K1 (phylloquinone) is present primarily in green leafy vegetables because it is synthesized in plants through photosynthesis. Vitamin K1 is the main dietary form of vitamin K. Vitamin K2 (menaquinones) have several related chemical subtypes with different unsaturated isoprenyl side chains and are designated as MK-4 through MK-13, based on the length of their side chain. MK-4, MK-7, and MK-9 are the most well studied menaquinones (3, 9, 33, 82–88). Menaquinones, which are predominantly of bacterial origin, are present in modest amounts in various animal-based and fermented foods. Almost all menaquinones, in particular the long-chain menaquinones, are also produced by bacteria in the human gut (82).

Like dietary lipids and other fat-soluble vitamins, ingested vitamin K is incorporated into mixed micelles via the action of bile and pancreatic enzymes, and it is absorbed by enterocytes of the small intestine (82). Vitamin K is rapidly metabolized and excreted. This rapid metabolism accounts for vitamin K's relatively low blood levels and tissue stores compared to those of the other fat-soluble vitamins (82). Vitamin K deficiency is rare because vitamin K is present in dietary foods, mostly in leafy green foods, and the bacteria in human intestines can make vitamin K (3, 9, 33, 82–86). Sometimes taking antibiotics can kill the bacteria and lead to a temporary mild deficiency. Vitamin K deficiency can lead to bleeding and hemorrhage, such as oozing in the nose, gums, and intestines. Other diseases may lead to vitamin K deficiency such as celiac disease, Crohn's disease, liver disease, bleeding disorders, gallbladder or biliary disease, cystic fibrosis, long-term hemodialysis, treatment by warfarin (an anticoagulant drug), and serious burns (33, 82–86). Because vitamin K is required for the carboxylation of osteocalcin in bone, vitamin K deficiency could also reduce bone mineralization and contribute to osteoporosis, and is associated with a higher risk of osteoarthritis (82–84). Allergic reaction to vitamin K supplementation is possible.

According to the U.S. Dietary Reference Intake, the daily adequate intake (AI) of vitamin K is 120 micrograms for men 19 years and older. For women including pregnant and lactating women, the amount is 90 micrograms/day; for infants 6–12 months, it is 2–2.5 micrograms/day; for children (1–13 years), the requirement is 30–60 micrograms/day; and for adolescents (14–18 years), it is 75 micrograms/day (82).

Several food sources rich in vitamin K1 (phylloquinone) include vegetables, especially green leafy vegetables, vegetable oils (olive oil, soybean oil), lucerne (*Medicago sativa*), green tea, turnip greens, broccoli, kale, spinach, cabbage, asparagus, dark green lettuce, and some fruits. Meat, dairy foods, chicken, and eggs yolks contain low levels of phylloquinone but modest amounts of vitamin K2. Natto (a Japanese fermented soybean food) and tofu have high levels of vitamin K2 (3, 9, 33, 82–86). Freezing foods may destroy vitamin K, but heating does not.

Vitamin K was discovered in 1929 by the Danish biochemist Henrik Dam (1895–1976) in studying cholesterol metabolism in chicks. This vitamin K was designed by the letter 'K' because coagulation is written as 'Koagulation' in German (85, 88). Ten years later, Edward Adelbert Doisy and his colleagues in the United States succeeded in isolating the vitamin and determining its structure. Both Dam and Doisy received the Nobel Prize for medicine in 1943 for their discovery (88).

4   ANTIOXIDANTS

Antioxidants are micronutrients present in a variety of food, and can also be made by the body. There are two kinds of antioxidants: endogenous antioxidants and exogenous antioxidants. That means that some antioxidants are produced in our tissues and some others must be obtained through the diet. Antioxidants are also categorized as essential antioxidants, nonessential antioxidants and semi-essential antioxidants. There are about ten antioxidants furnished by our body and called endogenous antioxidants, while some ten hundred other antioxidants found in nature are named exogenous antioxidants. Some of them, like vitamins C, A, and E, as well as some minerals such as iron and selenium have been cited in this chapter. Other types and roles of antioxidants are explained in Chapter 3 of this book.

5   COENZYMES AND COFACTORS

5.1   DEFINITION

In general, an enzyme cannot function alone; it must be activated by one or many small molecules called coenzymes and cofactors. Some enzymes require several coenzymes and cofactors. Coenzymes and cofactors are small organic molecules or metal ions that are used by enzymes to help catalyze reactions (89–93). In other words, coenzymes are typically organic molecules that contain functionalities not found in proteins, while cofactors are catalytically essential molecules or ions that are covalently bound to enzymes (91). The term holoenzyme refers to an active enzyme complex: an enzyme combined with a coenzyme or a cofactor. An apoenzyme is an inactive enzyme: an enzyme without an activator (coenzyme or/and cofactor). The term prosthetic group is used to refer to minerals, activated vitamins, or other nonprotein compounds that are required for full enzyme activity (89–93). The prosthetic group remains bonded for the enzyme during the reaction. In some cases, the prosthetic group is covalently bound for its apoenzyme, while in other cases it is weakly bound to the active center by numerous weak interactions (93).

Coenzymes, also called organic cofactors, are small organic non-protein compounds. They are used to initiate or aid in the function of enzymes. A coenzyme cannot function alone; it requires the presence of an enzyme. It can be reused several times when combined with an enzyme. Coenzyme is not considered part of an enzyme's structure (90–93). Coenzymes participate in numerous biochemical reactions involving energy release or catabolism, as well as accompanying anabolic reactions. Coenzymes are required for the biosynthesis of amino acids and proteins (89). Many (not all) coenzymes are vitamins or are derived from vitamins, such as all water-soluble vitamins (B group and C) and two of the fat-soluble vitamins, A and K (90–93). In addition, vitamin coenzymes are involved in vision functioning, blood coagulation, hormone production, and collagen synthesis (90). Coenzymes may be separated from the enzyme by dialysis. Coenzymes transport chemical groups from one enzyme to another. For example: Nicotinamide Adenine Dinucleotide (NAD), Adenosine Tri-Phosphate (ATP), Flavin Adenine Dinucleotide (FAD), NAD, ATP, and so on can be produced by several distinct cellular processes in the body, while FAD, TPP (thiamine pyrophosphate), and THF (tetrahydrofolate), are usually derived from vitamins (90–93). There are many nucleoside triphosphates which behave as coenzymes. Among them, adenosine triphosphate (ATP) is the most abundant, and an important cofactor for storing and transferring energy in cells (92). Other frequent examples are GTP (guanosine triphosphate), *S*-adenosyl methionine, and nucleotide sugars such as uridine diphosphate glucose (UDP-glucose) (93).

Coenzymes can be classified into two groups depending on their interaction with apoenzymes. The coenzyme of the first type – often called a **co-substrate** – is a substrate in the reactions catalyzed by enzymes. A co-substrate changes during the reaction, and disassociates from the active center (93). So, a co-substrate is a coenzyme that binds temporarily to an enzyme or protein, and can be released, binding again at some point (93). The second type of coenzyme is called the **prosthetic group**. The prosthetic group includes small organic groups like vitamins or mineral elements like metal, and remains bonded for the enzyme during the reaction. In general, the prosthetic group is tightly or even covalently, and permanently bound to its apoenzyme, and is often involved in the active site of the enzyme for its functioning (90–93).

Some coenzymes derived from vitamins which act as a prosthetic group (fixed compounds) include: biotin or vitamin B7, vitamin K, flavin mononucleotide (FMN) and flavin adenine dinucleotide (FAD) from riboflavin (vitamin B2), thiamine pyrophosphate (TPP) from thiamine (vitamin B1), pyridoxal phosphate (PLP) from pyridoxine (vitamin B6), adenosyl-cobalamin and methyl-cobalamin from cobalamine (vitamin B12), and retinal from vitamin A. Lipoamide is a non-vitamin compound and acts as prosthetic group (93). Other coenzymes derived from vitamins which act as co-substrates (labile compounds) are: nicotinamide adenine dinucleotide (NAD) and nicotinamide adenine dinucleotide phosphate (NADP) from niacin (vitamin B3), coenzyme A (CoA) from pantothenate (vitamin B3), and tetrahydrofolate from folic acid (vitamin B9). Co-substrates non-derived from vitamins include: adenosine triphosphate (ATP), uridine diphosphate glucose, S-adenosyl methionine, and ubiquinone (coenzyme Q10) (93).

Cofactors are inorganic molecules such as metal ions or nonprotein compounds that are bound to an enzyme for its functioning. Cofactors tightly bound to the protein form metalloenzymes, while those that are loosely associated with the protein are termed activator ions (90–92). Metalloenzymes are enzyme proteins containing metal cofactors, which are covalently bound to the enzyme. About one-third of all enzymes are metalloenzymes. For example: iron in cytochrome oxidase, copper in catalase, zinc in alcohol dehydrogenase, alkaline phosphatase, and so on (91–93). In humans, the metalloid selenium forms the active site of several antioxidant enzymes including glutathione peroxidase, thioredoxin reductase, iodothyronine deiodinase, formate dehydrogenase, and glycine reductase. Some cofactors are essential at the active site of a reaction, while others help maintain the structural integrity of an enzyme or protein (90). Therefore, when these mineral activators are absent in foods, enzymes become inactive and diseases appear.

5.2 CLASSIFICATION OF COENZYMES

In the body, there are two types of coenzymes: vitamin-derived coenzymes and non-vitamin organic coenzymes, also called metabolite coenzymes or nucleotide coenzymes (89–93).

5.2.1 Vitamin-Derived Coenzymes

All the water-soluble vitamins and two of the fat-soluble vitamins, A and K, function as coenzymes (90). Some vitamins act directly as coenzymes, but some vitamins help the body to produce coenzymes. Therefore, vitamin deficiency in food leads to enzyme inactivity. Enzymes are the key to all activities of cells for the production of energy that is vital for life. Most coenzymes derived from vitamins are obtained by enzymatic transformation in the body. Water-soluble vitamins, which include all B complex vitamins and vitamin C, lead to the production of coenzymes. The coenzymes derived from B complex vitamins are essential for enzymes to form fats, carbohydrates, and proteins. The most important vitamin-derived coenzymes are nicotinamide adenine dinucleotide (NAD) and coenzyme A (90–93).

5.2.1.1 Nicotinamide Coenzymes (NAD and NADP)

They include nicotinamide adenine dinucleotide (NAD) and nicotinamide adenine dinucleotide phosphate (NADP). Both are derived from vitamin B3 or niacin or nicotinic acid and differ only in the presence or absence of a phosphate group on the 2'-C of the adenosyl moiety (90–96). NAD and NADP coenzymes are diffusible co-substrates that take part in oxidation-reduction reactions. NAD^+ and $NADP^+$ are the oxidized forms of the co-substrate, and function as hydrogen acceptors in dehydrogenation reactions in the presence of dehydrogenase enzymes, and are converted into the reduced form NADH and NADPH, respectively. Life cannot exist without NAD; therefore, it is often called coenzyme 1. This coenzyme is not only a co-substrate in electron transfer during oxidation-reduction reactions, but it also plays a key role in cell signaling, regulating several pathways from intracellular calcium transients to the epigenetic status of chromatin (94). Thus, NAD is a molecule that provides an important link between signaling and metabolism, and serves as a key molecule in cellular metabolic sensing pathways. Importantly, it has now been clearly demonstrated that cellular NAD levels decline during chronological aging. This decline appears to play a crucial role in the development of metabolic dysfunction and age-related diseases (94). NAD and NADH assist dehydrogenase enzymes in the catabolism of fat, carbohydrates, and amino acids, and in the enzymes involved in the synthesis of fats and steroids and other vital metabolites (90, 93). If an organism has a NAD^+ deficiency, then mitochondria become less functional and provide less energy for cell activities. Thus, a lack of nicotinamide coenzymes results in widespread fatigue due to energy deficits in cells (90–96). All sirtuin (silent mating-type information regulation) enzymes are dependent on NAD^+ (96). The roles of sirtuin enzymes are described in Chapter 9 of this book. In addition, enhancing NAD^+ biosynthesis by using NAD^+ intermediates, such as nicotinamide mononucleotide (NMN), effectively ameliorates age-associated physiological decline. NMN has been shown to enhance NAD^+ biosynthesis, ameliorate various disease models as well as slow down aging in mice (95). Without any obvious toxicity, NMN was shown to enhance energy metabolism, promote physical activity, improve insulin sensitivity and plasma lipid profile, ameliorate eye function, and prevent other ailments in mice (95). Some natural food sources rich in NMN are: edamame (immature soybeans), avocado, broccoli, cabbage, whole cucumber peel and seed, and tomato (95–96).

5.2.1.2   Coenzyme A

Coenzyme A (abbreviated CoA or CoA-SH), also known as acetyl-CoA, naturally derives from vitamin B5 or pantothenic acid. It has three main components: a 2-mercaptoethylamine unit with free -SH group, pantothenate vitamin (vitamin B3), and ADP part (93). This coenzyme is involved in the reactions of acyl group transfers. Coenzyme A is involved in the biosynthesis of some carbohydrates and fats. Acetyl CoA is an energetically rich compound because of the high energy of the thioester bond (93).

5.2.1.3   Other Coenzymes Derived from Vitamins

Thiamine pyrophosphate (TPP) is a coenzyme derived from thiamine (vitamin B1) and is used for the transfer of acyl group in decarboxylation and transketolase reactions (90–91).

The flavin coenzymes including flavin adenine dinucleotide (FAD) and flavin mononucleotide (FMN) are derivatives of riboflavin (vitamin B2). Like the nicotinamide coenzymes, the flavin coenzymes participate in redox reactions that affect energy nutrients in the citric acid cycle and in the electron transport system.

Pyridoxal phosphate (PLP) and pyridoxamine phosphate (PMP) are the coenzyme forms derived from pyridoxine (vitamin B6), and participate in the metabolism of amino acids, including transamination, racemization, deamination and desulfhydration, and the conversion of tryptophan to nicotinic acid (90).

Biotin (vitamin B7) is a prosthetic group for enzymes which catalyze the reactions of the transfer of the carboxyl group and the reaction of carboxylation dependent on ATP. It is covalently bound to the active center of its host enzyme by amide bond through the amino group of a lysine residue of the enzyme (93).

Adenosyl and methylcobalamin coenzymes are derived from cobalamin or vitamin B12 and assist in the conversion of homocysteine to the amino acid methionine. They also participate in the oxidation of amino acids and odd-chain fatty acids, and the removal of a methyl group from methyl folate, which regenerates tetrahydrofolate (90–91). Tetrahydrofolate serves as a key coenzyme in the biosynthesis of purines and pyrimidines.

Vitamin C (ascorbic acid) is a coenzyme for the hydrolases. Some examples are the hydroxylation of proline and lysine to create cross-links from intramolecular hydrogen bonds during collagen biosynthesis. Hydrolases are also used in the hydroxylation of cholesterol to form bile acids, and the hydroxylation of tyrosine to form the hormone norepinephrine (noradrenaline) (90, 92).

Retinal, the aldehyde form of vitamin A, is a cofactor for opsin, an apoprotein in the eye. Opsins are responsible for dim-light vision in the rods (rhodopsin) and are involved in color and bright-light vision in the cone of the retina (iodopsin). Retinoic acid is the metabolite form of vitamin A that regulates genes. It binds to proteins called retinoic acid receptors (RARs) and retinoid X receptors (RXRs). These proteins are transcription factors belonging to the steroid/thyroid hormone receptor superfamily of proteins and are found throughout the body. The RAR/RXR proteins regulate the transcription of numerous target genes important for cell development (90).

Vitamin K acts as a coenzyme for γ-carboxylases, enzymes that transfer CO_2 groups that are available for calcium binding and for the formation of osteocalcin, a protein important in bone remodeling, and prothrombin, a coagulation factor (II) involved in blood clotting (90).

It is notified that the list of coenzymes cited here is not exhaustive.

5.2.2 Metabolite Coenzymes

Metabolite coenzymes or non-vitamin coenzymes typically aid in chemical transfer for enzymes. These coenzymes can be produced from nucleotides such as adenosine, uracil, guanine, or inosine. There are many nucleoside triphosphates which behave as coenzymes. Among them, adenosine triphosphate (ATP) is the most abundant. Other metabolite coenzymes are Guanosine-5′-Triphosphate (GTP), Uridine-5′-Triphosphate (UTP), Cytidine-5′-Triphosphate (CTP), ubiquinone (coenzyme Q) (91–93). All metabolite coenzymes act as co-substrates.

5.2.2.1 *Adenosine Triphosphate (ATP)*

Adenosine Triphosphate is an example of an essential non-vitamin coenzyme. In fact, Adenosine Triphosphate or Adenosine-5′-Triphosphate (ATP) is a nucleoside triphosphate composed of three compounds: a nitrogenous heterocyclic base (adenine), the sugar β-D-ribose, and three phosphate groups (92–93, 97–98). ATP is considered the single most important molecule in the cell and is often referred to as a molecule of intracellular energy transfer and as a universal coenzyme (type co-substrate) for a large number of enzymes, especially kinases (92, 98). In general, ATP carries both phosphate and energy to different places within a cell for the release of energy in situ by losing one or two of its phosphate groups, becoming adenosine diphosphate (ADP) or adenosine monophosphate (AMP), respectively. Much of the chemical energy used by cells is stored in the two phosphor-anhydride bonds of ATP which are high in energy (92, 97–98).

Adenosine-5′-Diphosphate (ADP) is formed when the phosphor-anhydride bond between the γ and β phosphate is hydrolyzed. Adenosine-5′-Monophosphate (AMP) is formed when both high energy phosphor-anhydride bonds are hydrolyzed. AMP is the lowest energy molecule (92). ATP is universally seen as the energy exchange factor that connects anabolism and catabolism but also fuels processes such as motile contraction, phosphorylation, and active transport. It is also a signaling molecule both inside and outside the living cell, and its universal importance in biology reaches well beyond its most familiar role as an energy metabolite (97–98). ATP transports substances and supplies energy needed for necessary chemical reactions and muscle contraction, as well as for different processes that range from neurotransmission to the chemotaxis of immune cells (98). Briefly, without the coenzyme ATP, normal life functions could not occur.

5.2.2.2 *Guanosine-5′-Triphosphate (GTP)*

Guanosine-5′-Triphosphate is a nucleotide containing the heterocyclic base Guanine. Like ATP, GTP carries energy in phospho-anhydride bonds. In terms of co-substrate/coenzyme activity, GTP is the 'energy source' for the reactions of protein synthesis. GTP also serves an important role in the cellular response to signal molecules, for instance, hormones (92).

5.2.2.3 Uridine-5′-Triphosphate (UTP)

Uridine-5'-Triphosphate is a nucleotide with the heterocyclic base Uracil. UTP is used as a co-substrate and activator/carrier molecule for monosaccharide isomerization (epimerization) reactions and for the biosynthesis of disaccharides and polysaccharides (92).

5.2.2.4 Cytidine-5′-Triphosphate (CTP)

Cytidine-5′-Triphosphate is a nucleotide containing the heterocyclic base Cytosine. CTP is used as a co-substrate and activator/carrier molecule during the biosynthesis of phospholipids and sphingolipids (92).

5.2.2.5 Coenzyme Q

Another example of a non-vitamin coenzyme is the coenzyme Q. Coenzyme Q (CoQ) or ubiquinone is the only fat-soluble antioxidant that is synthetized in mammals by every cell and its biosynthesis is a very complex process which involves the participation of at least nine gene products in all species studied. Its chemical structure comprises a benzoquinone derivative with an isoprenoid side chain. In mammals, CoQ has ten isopren units; hence, it is called coenzyme Q10 (Q: quinone), and it is abundant in the heart and liver (99–100). It is ubiquitous in nature from microorganisms and yeasts to plants, animals, and humans. In microorganisms and yeasts, the side chain contains only three isopren units. In humans, coenzyme Q10 is synthetized in situ and has important functions such as antioxidant activities. The different biological roles of coenzyme Q10 in humans will be explained in Chapter 3.

5.3 CLASSIFICATION OF COFACTORS

Unlike coenzymes, true cofactors are inorganic compounds. Usually, cofactors are metal ions. Thousands of enzymatic reactions require metal ion cofactors in functions ranging from Lewis acid catalysis to redox catalysis and electron transfer (91).

In general, metal cofactors are divided into two groups: metalloenzymes and metal activated enzymes. In the first case, metal ion cofactors are tightly bound to the enzyme via coordination of amino acid side chains, and are not dissociable from the complex (91). Enzymes with more loosely bound metal ion cofactors are commonly called metal activated enzymes (91). Metals must be obtained in the diet as the body cannot naturally synthesize metal ions. Some of the main metals and metalloids used by the body for the syntheses of cofactors are iron, copper, zinc, magnesium, manganese, nickel, and selenium (metalloid).

5.3.1 Iron Cofactor

Iron is ubiquitous in the body. Iron plays important roles in different processes of biological systems, including oxygen transport and utilization, electron transfer, metabolism of nucleic acids, and many other key biological molecules (91). A number of enzymes such as peroxidase, xanthine oxidase, catalase, and cytochrome oxidase require an iron cofactor and utilize both the accessibility of multiple redox states of iron (both Fe^{2+} and Fe^{3+}). Iron is also commonly found bound tightly to hem groups, for example in the ubiquitous cytochrome enzymes such as cytochrome P450 and hemoglobin (91). Metalloenzymes containing iron catalyze an enormous variety of reactions, mostly redox reactions.

5.3.2 Copper Cofactor

Copper, like iron, has two oxidation states (I and II) that are readily available under physiological conditions, and therefore can participate in catalysis of redox reactions of many enzymes, like superoxide dismutase, cytochrome oxidase, tyrosinase, and lysyl oxidase. It is also a cofactor in dopamine β-monooxygenase and peptidylglycine α-amidating enzyme used in monooxygenation (91).

5.3.3 Zinc Cofactor

Zinc is a cofactor of numerous enzymes including alcohol dehydrogenase, carbonic anhydrase, alkaline phosphatase, lactate dehydrogenase (LDH), carboxy peptidase, and some sirtuins (91).

5.3.4 Other Metal Cofactors

Other metals such as magnesium, manganese, and nickel are cofactors of enzymes like hydrolase, isomerase, or oxidase (91).

6 DISCUSSION

In summary, our body regularly needs about 16 minerals and 13 vitamins in small amounts for the good functioning of cell and organs. They come from plant and animal foods; some minerals can be found in natural water such as spring water. Many micronutrients are essential because our body cannot make them. Their absence can cause diseases and even death. In contrast, an excessive intake of micronutrients (mineral or vitamin) is also harmful to our health and can cause diseases and eventually death. Poisoning due to micronutrients is frequently observed in people taking high doses of vitamin or mineral supplements, or taking some micronutrients with accumulative properties for a long period. Therefore, water-soluble vitamins, such as vitamins of B group and vitamin C, are safer than fat-soluble vitamins (A, D, E, K) because the first ones are not stored long-term in the body and are easily eliminated via urine. Moreover, taking a B-complex vitamin supplement, which includes all the B vitamins, is better than taking any vitamin B alone. Always ask a healthcare professional before taking any vitamin or mineral at high doses or for long-term use, especially fat-soluble vitamins A, D, E, and K, or minerals such as selenium and fluorine. Eating natural foods rich in vitamins and minerals is better than taking synthetic vitamin supplements. For example, eating hard cheese is better than taking a tablet of calcium supplement, because calcium in hard cheese is an organic compound which is easily absorbed and transported in the body, while calcium in tablet form is made by inorganic compounds such as calcium citrate, carbonate, or phosphate. Dietary supplements are only necessary in specific cases of vitamin deficiency due to diseases or to the absence of a micronutrient in natural foods such as iodine, vitamin B1, in a specific region. However, some synthetic micronutrients are not chemically identical to their corresponding natural compounds. For example, synthetic vitamin E is a racemate (R,S) compound, while natural vitamin E in foods is a pure stereoisomer (R only). Selenium in plants is a complex organic compound, while selenium in tablet supplement is in simple mineral form (selenite or selenate). The bioavailability between these two organic and mineral forms is also different; therefore, selenium supplement is more dangerous than selenium present in vegetables. For vegans, the consumption of some dietary supplements such as vitamin B12 or iron becomes necessary because vitamin B12 exists in animals only, except in some seaweeds such as spirulina, brown algae, while iron in plants is not easily assimilated. Choosing a good diet for each health situation also requires some scientific knowledge because there are interactions between different nutrients in the diet. Such a phenomenon is called a synergistic effect. Moreover, each food is rich in particular vitamins and/or minerals. It should be noted that some vitamins and antioxidants are destroyed by heat or air, such as vitamin C, therefore cooking and storage can influence the efficacy of these labile compounds.

According to International Agency for Research on Cancer (IARC) of the World Health Organization, the low consumption of fruit and vegetables in many regions of the world, especially in the developing countries, may be the cause of cancer development (101). Moreover, micronutrient-supplementation randomized controlled intervention trials have largely failed to show an effect on chronic disease risk. In contrast, whole foods that are rich in micronutrients, like fruit and vegetables, or some complete dietary patterns such as Mediterranean diet, have been associated with increased survival and reductions in cardiovascular diseases and cancer end points (92, 102). Recently, some scientists revealed the coenzyme nicotinamide adenine dinucleotide (NAD) and its intermediate nicotinamide mononucleotide (NMN) can slow down aging, obesity, diabetes, hypercholesterolemia in mice (95–96). These products NAD and NMN are present in certain vegetables such as edamame, soybeans, broccoli, cucumber, cabbage, and some fruits like avocado and tomato (95). These observations are based on the fact that fresh fruits and vegetables obtained from natural sources are rich in essential micronutrients like vitamins, minerals, coenzymes, and antioxidants. These natural micronutrients in food act synergistically to enhance the effect of each nutrient alone which becomes more efficacious in the prevention of cancer and other chronic ailments such as cardiovascular diseases, diabetes, obesity, aging, neuro-degenerative diseases, and so on. It is good to remember that deficiency as well as excess of micronutrients (vitamins, minerals, and antioxidants) can cause disease and even death. In brief, the best way to maintain a good health is to consume a variety of natural vegetable and animal foods with moderation.

7   REFERENCES

1. Shenkin A. (2006). Micronutrients in Health and Disease. *Postgrad. Med. J.*, **82**(971): 559–567.
2. Biesalski Hans K., Jana T. (2018). Micronutrients in the Life Cycle: Requirements and Sufficient Supply. *NFS J.*, **11**: 1–11.
3. WHO FAO (The World Health Organization and the Food and Agriculture Organization of the United Nations). (1998). Vitamin and Mineral Requirements in Human Nutrition. 2nd edition. Report of a joint FAO/WHO expert consultation, Bangkok, Thailand, 21–30 September 1998, 341 pages. https://apps. who.int/iris/bitstream/handle/10665/42716/9241546123.pdf?sequence=1.
4. Strain J.J., Cashman K.D. (2009). 9- Minerals and Trace Elements. 188–237. In: *Introduction to Human Nutrition*. 2nd edition, Edited on Behalf of the Nutrition Society by Michael J. Gibney, Susan A. Lanham-New, Aedin Cassidy, Hester H. Vorster. Wiley-Blackwell (John Wiley & Sons Ltd), Oxford, United Kingdom, 371 pages.
5. Bourre J.M. (2006). Effects of Nutrients (in Food) on the Structure and Function of the Nervous System: Update on Dietary Requirements for Brain. Part 1: Micronutrients. *J. Nutr. Health Aging*, **10**(5): 377–385.
6. Goff J.P. (2018). Mineral Absorption Mechanisms, Mineral Interactions That Affect Acid – Base and Antioxidant Status, and Diet Considerations to Improve Mineral Status. *J. Dairy Sci.*, **101**: 2763–2813.
7. Martínez-Ballesta M.C., Dominguez-Perles R., Moreno D.A., Muries B., Alcaraz-López C., Bastias E., Garcia-Viguera C., Carjaval M. (2010). Minerals in Plant Food: Effect of Agricultural Practices and Role in Human Health. A Review. *Agron. Sustain. Dev.*, **30**(2) 295–309.
8. Soetan K.O., Olaiya C.O., Oyewole O.E. (2010). The Importance of Mineral Elements for Humans, Domestic Animals and Plants: A Review. *Afr. J. Food Sci.*, **4**(5): 200–222.
9. Eastwood M., Editor (2003). Part V. Nutrients and Non-Nutrients. In: *Principles of Human Nutrition*. 2nd edition. Blackwell Science Ltd, Oxford, United Kingdom, 680 pages.
10. Cormick G., Belizán J.M. (2019). Calcium Intake and Health. *Nutrients*, **11**(7): 1606, 16 pages.
11. Weaver C.M., Heaney R.P. (2012). B. Minerals. Chapter 7. Calcium, pp. 133–149. In: *Modern Nutrition in Health and Disease*. 11th edition. Editors: A.C. Ross, B. Caballero, R.J. Cousins, K.L. Tucker, T.R. Ziegler. Lippincott Williams & Wilkins, Baltimore, 1646 pages. https://treatment.tbzmed.ac.ir/uploads/ User/47/nutrition/1394/modern%20nutrition.pdf.
12. Pasternak K., Kocot J., Horecka A. (2010). Biochemistry of Magnesium. *J. Elementol.*, **15**(3): 601–616.
13. Parcell S. (2002). Sulfur in Human Nutrition and Applications in Medicine. *Altern. Med. Rev.*, **7**(1): 22–44.
14. Nimni M.E., Han B., Cordoba F. (2007). Are We Getting Enough Sulfur in Our Diet? *Nutr. Metab.*, **4**(24): 12 pages.
15. Pfortmueller C.A., Uehlinger D., von Haehling S., Schefold J.C. (2018). Serum chloride levels in critical illness-the hidden story. Intensive Care Med. Exp., **6**(1): 10, 14 pages.
16. McCallum L., Lip S., Padmanabhan S. (2015). The Hidden Hand of Chloride in Hypertension. *Pflugers Arch. – Eur. J. Physiol.*, **467**(3): 595–603. doi:10.1007/s00424-015-1690-8.
17. Jentsch T.J., Pusch M. (2018). CLC Chloride Channels and Transporters: Structure, Function, Physiology, and Disease. *Physiol. Rev.*, **98**: 1493–1590.
18. Abbaspour N., Hurrell R., Kelishadi R. (2014). Review on Iron and Its Importance for Human Health. *J. Res. Med. Sci.*, **19**(2): 164–174.
19. Wessling-Resnick M. (2012). B. Minerals. Chapter 10. Iron, pp. 176–188. In: *Modern Nutrition in Health and Disease*. 11th edition. Editors: A.C. Ross, B. Caballero, R.J. Cousins, K.L. Tucker, T.R. Ziegler. Lippincott Williams & Wilkins, Baltimore, 1646 pages. https://treatment.tbzmed.ac.ir/uploads/ User/47/nutrition/1394/modern%20nutrition.pdf

20. Wrobel J.K., Power R., Toborek M. (2016). Biological Activity of Selenium: Revisited. *IUBMB Life*, **68**(2): 97–105.

21. Navarro-Alarcon M., Cabrera-Vique C. (2008). Selenium in Food and the Human Body: A Review. *Sci. Total Environ.*, **400**: 115–141.

22. Fordyce F. (2013). Selenium Deficiency and Toxicity in the Environment. Chapter 16, pp. 373–415. In: *Essentials of Medical Geology*. Editors: O. Selinus, et al. Springer, London.

23. Pham-Huy A.L., He H., Pham-Huy C. (2008). Free radicals and Antioxidants in Disease and Health. *Int. J. Biomed. Sci.*, **4**(2): 89–96.

24. Pham-Huy C., Nguyen P., Marchand V., Claude J.R., Duc H.T. (2001). Selenium and Tobacco Smoke Tars: In Vitro Effects on Different Immunocompetent Cells. *Toxicology*, **164**: 111–112. Presented in International Congress of Toxicology XI, Brisbane (Australia), July 7–12.

25. King J.C., Cousins R.J. (2012). B. Minerals. Chapter 11. Zinc, pp. 189–205. In: *Modern Nutrition in Health and Disease*. 11th edition. Editors: A.C. Ross, B. Caballero, R.J. Cousins, K.L. Tucker, T.R. Ziegler. Lippincott Williams & Wilkins, Baltimore, 1646 pages.

26. National Institutes of Health (NIH). (2021). Zinc, March 26. https://ods.od.nih.gov/factsheets/Zinc-Health Professional/.

27. Pham-Huy C., Nadji F., Postaire M., Hamon M. (1991). Determination of Fluorides and Fluorophosphates in Drugs, Toothpastes and Mineral Waters by Gas Liquid Chromatography. *Ann. Pharm. Fr.*, **49**(3): 139–150. French.

28. Bouygues-de-Ferran A.M., Pham-Huy C., Postaire M., Hamon M. (1991). Determination of Trace Amounts of Fluoride in Raw Materials for Pharmaceuticals by Gas-Liquid Chromatography. *J. Chromatogr. A*, **585**(2): 289–295.

29. Pham-Huy N.L.A., He H., Pham-Huy C. (2008). Green Tea and Health. An Overview. *J. Food Agric. Environ. (JFAE)*, **6**: 6–13.

30. Rousset B., Dupuy C., Miot F., Dumont J. (2015). Chapter 2. Thyroid Hormone Synthesis and Secretion. In: *Endotext*. Editors: L.J. De Groot, G. Chrousos, K. Dungan, et al. South Dartmouth, MA. www.ncbi.nlm.nih.gov/books/NBK285550/.

31. Pearce E.N., Andersson M., Zimmermann M.B. (2013). Global Iodine Nutrition: Where Do We Stand in 2013? *Thyroid*, **23**(5): 1–6.

32. Semba R.D. (2012). The Discovery of the Vitamins. *Int. J. Vitam. Nutr. Res.*, **82**(5): 310–315.

33. Bender D.A. (2009). 8- The Vitamins, pp. 132–187. In: *Introduction to Human Nutrition*. 2nd edition, Edited on Behalf of the Nutrition Society by Michael J. Gibney, Susan A. Lanham-New, Aedin Cassidy, Hester H Vorster. Wiley-Blackwell (John Wiley & Sons Ltd), Oxford, United Kingdom, 371 pages.

34. Gregory J.F. (2012). Accounting for Differences in the Bioactivity and Bioavailability of Vitamers. *Food Nutr. Res.*, **56**: 5809, 11 pages. doi:10.3402/fnr.v56i0.5809.

35. Lonsdale D. (2006). A Review of the Biochemistry, Metabolism and Clinical Benefits of Thiamin(e) and Its Derivatives. *Evid. Based Complement Alternat. Med.*, **3**(1): 49–59. doi:10.1093/ecam/nek009.

36. Lonsdale D. (2018). Thiamin. *Adv. Food Nutr. Res.*, **83**: 1–56.

37. Northrop-Clewes C.A., Thurnham D.I. (2012). The Discovery and Characterization of Riboflavin. *Ann. Nutr. Metab.*, **61**: 224–230.

38. Thakur K., Tomar S.K., Singh A.K., Mandal S., Arora S. (2017). Riboflavin and Health: A Review of Recent Human Research. *Crit. Rev. Food Sci. Nutr.*, **57**(17): 3650–3660.

39. Kirkland J.B. (2014). Chapter 23. Niacin, pp. 331–340. In: *Modern Nutrition in Health and Disease*. 11th edition. Editors: A.C. Ross, B. Caballero, R.J. Cousins, K.L. Tucker, T.R. Ziegler. Lippincott Williams & Wilkins, Baltimore, 1646 pages.

40. Gasperi V., Sibilano M., Savini I., Catani M.V. (2019). Niacin in the Central Nervous System: An Update of Biological Aspects and Clinical Applications. *Int J Mol Sci.*, **20**(4): 974, 26 pages.

41. Fricker R.A., Green E.L., Jenkins S.I., Griffin S.M. (2018). The Influence of Nicotinamide on Health and Disease in the Central Nervous System. *Int. J. Tryptophan Res.*, **11**: 1–11.

42. Song W-L., FitzGerald G.A. (2013). Niacin, an Old Drug with a New Twist. *J. Lipid Res.*, **54**: 2586–2594.

43. Trumbo P.R. (2012). Chapter 25. Pantothenic Acid, pp. 351–357. In: *Modern Nutrition in Health and Disease*. 11th edition. Editors: A.C. Ross, B. Caballero, R.J. Cousins, K.L. Tucker, T.R. Ziegler. Lippincott Williams & Wilkins, Baltimore, 1646 pages.

44. National Institutes of Health (NIH). (2021). Vitamin B6, March 26. https://ods.od.nih.gov/factsheets/VitaminB6-HealthProfessional/.

45. Patel D.P., Swink S.M., Castelo-Soccio L. (2017). A Review of the Use of Biotin for Hair Loss. *Skin Appendage Disord.*, **3**(3): 166–169.

46. Stover P.J. (2012). Chapter 26. Folic Acid, pp. 358–367. In: *Modern Nutrition in Health and Disease*. 11th edition. Editors: A.C. Ross, B. Caballero, R.J. Cousins, K.L. Tucker, T.R. Ziegler. Lippincott Williams & Wilkins, Baltimore, 1646 pages.

47. National Institutes of Health (NIH). (2021). Vitamin B12, April 6. https://ods.od.nih.gov/factsheets/VitaminB12-HealthProfessional/.

48. Naidu A.K. (2003). Vitamin C in Human Health and Disease Is Still a Mystery? An Overview. *Nutr. J.*, **2**: 1–10.

49. Li Y., Schellhorn H.E. (2007). New Developments and Novel Therapeutic Perspectives for Vitamin C. *Critical Review. J. Nutr.*, **137**: 2171–2184.

50. Wang J., Wu F., Corpe C. (2019). Editorial: Vitamin C in Cancer and Infectious Diseases: Physiological, Biochemical and Therapeutic Interventions. *Front Physiol.*, **10**: 734, 3 pages.

51. Ashor A.W., Brown P., Keenan P.D., Willis, N.D., Siervo M., Mathers J.C. (2019). Limited Evidence for a Beneficial Effect of Vitamin C Supplementation on Biomarkers of Cardiovascular Diseases: An Umbrella Review of Systematic Reviews and Meta-Analyses. *Nutr. Res.*, **61**: 1–12.

52. Carr A.C., Vissers M.C.M. (2013). Synthetic or Food-Derived Vitamin C – Are They Equally Bioavailable? *Nutrients*, **5**: 4284–4304.

53. Grosso G., Bei R., Mistretta A., Marventano S., Calabrese G., Masuelli L., Giganti M.G., Modesti A., Galvano F., Gazzolo D. (2013). Effects of Vitamin C on Health: A Review of Evidence. *Front Biosci.*, **18**: 1017–1029.

54. Yang J., Liu J., Liu J.P. (2009). Chapter VIII. Vitamin C: Daily Requirements, Dietary Sources and Adverse Effects, pp. 237–260. In: *Handbook of Vitamin C Research: Daily Requirements, Dietary Sources, and Adverse Effects*. Editors: Hubert Kucharski and Julek Zajac. Nova Science Publishers, Inc., New York, 415 pages.

55. Pappenberger G., Hohmann H.P. (2014). Industrial Production of L-Ascorbic Acid (Vitamin C) and D-Isoascorbic Acid. *Adv. Biochem. Eng. Biotechnol.*, **143**: 143–188.

56. National Institutes of Health. Office of Dietary Supplements. (2021). Vitamin A, March 26. https://ods.od.nih.gov/factsheets/VitaminA-HealthProfessional/.

57. Bushue N., Wan Y.J. (2010). Retinoid Pathway and Cancer Therapeutics. *Adv. Drug Deliv. Rev.*, **62**(13): 1285–1298.

58. Noh M.F.M., Gunasegavan R.D.N., Mustar S. (2019). Chapter 2. Vitamin A in Health and Disease. In: *Vitamin A*. Editors: Leila Queiroz Zepka, Eduardo Jacob-Lopes and Veridiana Vera de Rosso. IntechOpen. http://dx.doi.org/10.5772/intechopen.84460.

59. Mendu V.V.R., Nair K.P.N., Athe R. (2019). Systematic Review and Meta-Analysis Approach on Vitamin A Fortified Foods and Its Effect on Retinol Concentration in Under 10 Year Children. *Clin. Nutr. ESPN*, **30**: 126–130.

60. Olson C.R., Mello C.V. (2010). Significance of Vitamin A to Brain Function, Behavior and Learning. *Mol. Nutr. Food Res.*, **54**(4): 489–495.

61. Semba R.D. (2012). On the Discovery of Vitamin A. *Ann. Nutr. Metab.*, **61**(3): 192–198.

62. Ross A.C., Taylor C.L., Yaktine A.L., Del Valle H.B., Editors. (2011). 3. Overview of Vitamin D. In: *Dietary Reference Intakes for Calcium and Vitamin D. Institute of Medicine; Food and Nutrition Board*. The National Academies Press, Washington, DC. www.ncbi.nlm.nih.gov/books/NBK56061/.

63. Nair R., Maseeh A. (2012). Vitamin D: The "Sunshine Vitamin". *J. Pharmacol. Pharmacother.*, **3**(2): 118–126.

64. National Institutes of Health (NIH). Office of Dietary Supplements. (2021). Vitamin D, March 26. https://ods.od.nih.gov/factsheets/VitaminD-HealthProfessional/.

65. Bouillon R., Carmeliet G., Verlinden L., van Etten E., Verstuyf A., Luderer H.F., Lieben L., Mathieu C., Demay M. (2008). Vitamin D and Human Health: Lessons from Vitamin D Receptor Null Mice. *Endocr. Rev.*, **29**(6): 726–776.

66. Bikle D.D. (2014). Vitamin D Metabolism, Mechanism of Action, and Clinical Applications. *Chem. Biol.*, **21**: 319–329.

67. Japelt R.B., Jakobsen J. (2013). Vitamin D in Plants: A Review of Occurrence, Analysis, and Biosynthesis. *Front Plant Sci.*, **4**: 136, 1–20.

68. Norval M. (2005). A Short Circular History of Vitamin D from its Discovery to Its Effects. *Res. Medica*, **268**(2): 57–58.

69. Azzi A. (2018). Many Tocopherols, One Vitamin E. *Mol. Aspects Med.*, **61**: 92–103.

70. National Institutes of Health (NIH). Office of Dietary Supplements. (2021). Vitamin E, March 26. https://ods.od.nih.gov/factsheets/VitaminE-HealthProfessional/.

71. Rizvi S., Raza S.T., Ahmed F., Ahmad A., Abbas S., Mahdi F. (2014). The Role of Vitamin E in Human Health and Some Diseases. *Sultan Qaboos Univ. Med. J.*, **14**(2): e157–e165.

72. Traber M.G., Atkinson J. (2007). Vitamin E, Antioxidant and Nothing More. *Free Radic. Biol. Med.*, **43**(1): 4–15.

73. Romero A.C., Olvera Hernández E.G., Cerón T.F., Chávez A.Á. (2013). Chapter 2. The Exogenous Antioxidants, pp. 33–57. In: *Oxidative Stress and Chronic Degenerative Diseases – A Role for Antioxidants*. Editor: José A. Morales-González. InTech Europe, Rijeka, Croatia, 512 pages.

74. Clarke M.W., Burnett J.R., Croft K.D. (2008). Vitamin E in Human Health and Disease. *Crit. Rev. Clin. Lab. Sci.*, **45**(5): 417–450.

75. Nguyen A.L., He H., Pham-Huy C. (2006). Chiral Drugs. An Overview. *Int. J. Biomed. Sci.*, **2**: 85–100.

76. Ochi H., Takeda S. (2015). The Two Sides of Vitamin E Supplementation. *Gerontology*, **61**(4): 319–326.

77. Yochum L.A., Folsom A.R., Kushi L.H. (2000). Intake of Antioxidant Vitamins and Risk of Death from Stroke in Postmenopausal Women. *Am J Clin Nutr.*, **72**: 476–483.

78. Schürks M., Glynn R.J., Rist P.M., Tzourio C., Kurth T. (2010). Effects of Vitamin E on Stroke Subtypes: Meta-Analysis of Randomised Controlled Trials. *BMJ.*, **341**: c5702.

79. Lonn E., Bosch J., Sheridan P., Pogue J., Arnold J.M., Ross C., Arnold A., Sleight P., Probstfield J., Dagenais G.R., HOPE and HOPE-TOO Trial Investigators. (2005). Effects of Long-Term Vitamin E Supplementation on Cardiovascular Events and Cancer: A Randomized Controlled Trial. *JAMA.*, **293**(11): 1338–1347.

80. Marchioli R., Levantesi G., Macchia A., Marfisi R.M., Nicolosi G.L., Tavazzi L., Tognoni G., Valugussa F. on Behalf of the GISSI-Prevenzione Investigators. (2006). Vitamin E Increases the Risk of Developing Heart Failure After Myocardial Infarction: Results from the GISSI-Prevenzione Trial. *J. Cardiovasc. Med.*, **7**(5): 347–350.

81. Chae C.U., Albert C.M., Moorthy M.V., Lee I.M., Buring J.E. (2012). Vitamin E Supplementation and the Risk of Heart Failure in Women. *Circ. Heart Fail.*, **5**(2): 176–182.

82. National Institutes of Health (NIH). Office of Dietary Supplements. (2021). Vitamin K, March 29. https://ods.od.nih.gov/factsheets/VitaminK-HealthProfessional/.

83. DiNicolantonio J.J., Bhutani J., O'Keefe J.H. (2015). The Health Benefits of Vitamin K. *Open Heart*, **2**(1): e000300, 7 pages.

84. Akbari S., Rasouli-Ghahroudi A.A. (2018). Vitamin K and Bone Metabolism: A Review of the Latest Evidence in Preclinical Studies. *Biomed Res Int.*, **2018**: 4629383.8 pages.

85. Halder M., Petsophonsakul P., Akbulut A.C., Pavlic A., Bohan F., Anderson E., Maresz K., Kramann R., Schurgers L. (2019). Vitamin K: Double Bonds Beyond Coagulation Insights into Differences Between Vitamin K1 and K2 in Health and Disease. *Int. J. Mol. Sci.*, **20**(896): 1–15.

86. Sharafi Miab M., Masoumi S.J., Haghighat N., Zare M. (2019). The Effects of Vitamin K Supplementation in Vascular Calcification: A Systematic Review. *Int. J. Nutr. Sci.*, **4**(2): 54–58.

87. Ferland G. (2012). Vitamin K and the Nervous System: An Overview of its Actions. *Adv. Nutr.*, **3**: 204–212,

88. Ferland G. (2012). The Discovery of Vitamin K and Its Clinical Applications. *Ann. Nutr. Metab.*, **61**: 213–218.

89. Kirschning A. (2021). The Coenzyme/Protein Pair and the Molecular Evolution of Life. *Nat. Prod. Rep.*, **38**: 993–1010.

90. Freeland-Graves J.H., Bavik C. (2003). Coenzymes, pp. 1475–1481. In: *Encyclopedia of Food Sciences and Nutrition*. 2nd edition. Editor in Chief: Benjamin Caballero. Academic Press, Maryland, 6000 pages.

91. Broderick J.B. (2001). Coenzymes and Cofactors. In: *Encyclopedia of Life Sciences*. Editors: John Wiley & Sons, Ltd. Nature Publishing Group, Chichester, UK. https://doi.org/10.1038/npg.els.0000631.

92. Thapa M., Dallmann G. (2020). Role of Coenzymes in Cancer Metabolism. *Semin. Cell Dev. Biol.*, **98**: 44–53.

93. Arsic B. (2018). Mechanisms of Actions of Coenzymes. *Chemia Naissensis*, **1**(1): 153–183.

94. Chini C.C.S., Tarragó M.G., Chini E.N. (2017). NAD and the Aging Process: Role in Life, Death and Everything in Between. *Mol. Cell Endocrinol.*, **455**: 62–74.

95. Mills K.F., Yoshida S., Stein L.R., Grozio A., Kubota S., Sasaki Y., Redpath P., Migaud M.E., Apte R.S., Uchida K., Yoshino J., Imai S-I. (2016). Long-Term Administration of Nicotinamide Mononucleotide Mitigates Age-Associated Physiological Decline in Mice. *Cell Metabolism*, **24**: 795–806.

96. Imai S-I., Guarente L. (2014). NAD$^+$ and Sirtuins in Aging and Disease. *Trends Cell Biol.*, **24**(8): 464–471.

97. Bonora M., Patergnani S., Rimessi A., De Marchi E., Suski J.M., Bononi A., Giorgi C., Marchi S., Missiroli S., Poletti F., Wieckowski M.R., Pinton P. (2012). ATP Synthesis and Storage. *Purinergic Signal.*, **8**(3): 343–357.

98. Rajendran M., Dane E., Conley J., Tantama M. (2016). Imaging Adenosine Triphosphate (ATP). *Biol Bull.*, **231**(1): 73–84.

99. Garrido-Maraver J., Cordero M.D., Oropesa-Ávila M., Vega A.F., de la Mata M., Pavón A.D., de Miguel M., Calero C.P., Paz M.V., Cotán D., Sánchez-Alcázar J.A. (2014). Coenzyme Q10 Therapy. *Mol. Syndromol.*, **5**: 187–197.

100. Motohashi N., Gallagher R., Anuradha V., Gollapudi R. (2017). Co-enzyme Q10 (Ubiquinone): It's Implication in Improving the Life Style of the Elderly. *Med. Clin. Rev.*, **3** (Suppl. 1): 10 pages.

101. International Agency for Research on Cancer of World Health Organization (IARC) (2003). *Handbooks of Cancer Prevention. Fruit and Vegetables*, Volume 8. IARC Press, Lyon, France, 384 pages.

102. Woodside J.V., McCall D., McGartland C., Young I.S. (2005). Micronutrients: Dietary Intake v. Supplement Use. *Proc. Nutr. Soc.*, **64**(4): 543–553.

3 Free Radicals and Antioxidants

1 INTRODUCTION

The theory of free radicals has been known for about a century now. The knowledge of organic free radicals was discovered for the first time by Moses Gomberg when he inadvertently synthesized triphenylmethyl, a mysterious, highly reactive, unstable substance. Gomberg published his findings about free radicals in 1900, but the scientific community recognized their existence 30 years later (1). In 1954, the presence of free radicals in biological materials was demonstrated for the first time by Commoner, Townsend and Pake (2). Like many great discoveries, the first antioxidant named superoxide dismutase (SOD) was discovered by accident in the late 1960s when Joe McCord and his mentor, Irwin Fridovich, were studying the function of different enzymes. In the beginning, both researchers did not know this mysterious enzyme and its exact role in the body (3). They named it superoxide dismutase (SOD), then later found its important role as an antioxidant in the body. Thanks to these monumental findings, an explosion of research about antioxidants and free radicals in the animal, vegetable, and mineral kingdoms has been sparked worldwide from academic research to industrial development, mostly during the last two decades.

Oxygen is an element indispensable for life. However, it is ironic that oxygen can, under certain situations, have severely deleterious effects on the human body. When cells use oxygen to generate energy, free radicals are created as a consequence of ATP (adenosine triphosphate) production by the mitochondria (4–6). Most of the potentially harmful effects of oxygen are due to the formation and activity of a number of chemical compounds, known as reactive oxygen species (ROS), which have a tendency to donate oxygen to other substances. Many such reactive species are free radicals and have a surplus of one or more free-floating electrons rather than having matched pairs and are, therefore, unstable and highly reactive (5–7). These byproducts are generally reactive oxygen species (ROS) as well as reactive nitrogen species (RNS) that result from the cellular redox process. These free radicals play a dual role as both harmful and beneficial compounds. The delicate balance between their two antagonistic effects is clearly an important aspect of life (6–9). At low or moderate levels, ROS and RNS exert beneficial effects on cellular responses and immune function. At high concentrations, they generate oxidative stress, a deleterious process that can damage all cell structures (6, 10). Oxidative stress plays a major part in the development of chronic and degenerative diseases such as cancer, cardiovascular and neurodegenerative diseases, arthritis, autoimmune disorders, aging, chronic renal failure, diabetes mellitus, cataract, and so on (11–17). The human body requires both free radical (oxidant included) and antioxidant species for normal metabolism, signal transduction, and regulation of cellular functions. Therefore, each cell maintains a condition of homeostasis *in situ* between free radical and antioxidant species. Nature has endowed the human body with several mechanisms to counteract any harmful effects of free radicals and oxidative stress by producing antioxidants, which are either naturally produced *in situ* (endogenous antioxidants) and/or externally supplied through foods (exogenous antioxidants) (17–21). The main role of antioxidants is to prevent damage to cellular components arising as a consequence of chemical reactions involving free radicals (14). In recent years, a substantial body of evidence has developed supporting a key role for free radicals in many fundamental cellular reactions and suggesting that oxidative stress might be important in the pathophysiology of several common diseases cited above. Endogenous and exogenous antioxidants act as 'free radical scavengers' by preventing and repairing damages caused by free radicals (ROS and RNS), and can therefore enhance immune defense and lower the risk of cancer and degenerative diseases (12–15). Some exogenous antioxidants are essential for life because their absence in foods can cause illness and eventual death. Dietary supplements including artificial antioxidants and vitamins are now marketed in order to prevent their eventual deficiency in the body. However, the excessive use of exogenous antioxidants such as supplements could be harmful to the body because beneficial free radicals are completely destroyed by these supplements; thereby cells and organs, especially the immune system, can become dysregulated by the lack of this material. Also, antioxidant supplements can act as pro-oxidants – as oxidative stress inducers – if they are consumed at levels significantly above the recommended dietary intakes (RDI) (6). Therefore, the knowledge of free radicals and antioxidants allows to distinguish 'good' food and 'bad' foods, as well as to determine appropriate lifestyle choices, as these factors may play an important role in the maintenance of health.

2   FREE RADICALS AND OXIDANTS

2.1   CHARACTERISTICS

In chemistry, a free radical, also called a radical, is an atom, molecule, or ion that has one or more unpaired electrons (14, 16). Electrons normally exist in pairs in specific orbital in atoms or molecules. Free radicals, which contain only a single electron in any orbital, are usually unstable toward losing or picking up an extra electron, so that all electrons in the atom or molecule will be paired (16). Unpaired electrons cause radicals to be highly reactive. Radicals can have positive, negative, or neutral charge. Free radicals are classified into two main species: reactive oxygen species (ROS) and reactive nitrogen species (RNS). Reactive oxygen species (ROS) and reactive nitrogen species (RNS) are the terms collectively describing free radicals and other non-radical reactive derivatives, also called oxidants, which are capable of generating free radicals. Radicals are less stable than non-radical species (oxidants), although their reactivity is generally stronger (6). In general, free radicals are very short lived, with half-lives in milli-, micro- or nanoseconds, contrary to oxidants which are stable (17). The reactive sulfur species (RSS) occupy a minor place of free radicals.

Reactive oxygen species (ROS) include superoxide anion (O_2^-) or superoxide anion radical ($O_2^{\cdot-}$), singlet oxygen ($^1O_2$), hydroxyl radical (HO$^\cdot$), peroxyl radical (ROO$^\cdot$), and lipid peroxyl radical (LOO$^\cdot$). They are very highly reactive and their half-life is also very short from 10^{-9} sec to one sec.

Reactive nitrogen species (RNS) comprise nitric oxide (NO$^\cdot$), peroxynitrite (ONOO$^-$), and nitrogen dioxide (NO$_2^\cdot$). They are highly reactive and their half-life varies from 10^{-3} sec. to one sec.

Some reactive sulfur species (RSS) are thiyl radical (RS$^\cdot$) and peroxysulfenyl radical (RSOO$^\cdot$). Furthermore, some ROS such as hydrogen peroxide (H_2O_2), ozone (O_3), singlet oxygen ($^1O_2$), lipid peroxide (LOOH), and hypochlorous acid (HOCl), are not considered free radicals, and are generally called oxidants because they are more and less stable. It is the same for some RNS like nitrous acid (HNO$_2$), dinitrogen trioxide (N$_2$O$_3$), and some RSS such as sulfite (SO$_3\_$), disulfide (DSSO), and sulfenic acid (RSOH). However, these oxidants can easily lead to free radical reactions in living organisms and can yield reactive species – active free radicals (6, 15, 17–19).

2.2   FORMATION

Reactive oxygen species (ROS) include superoxide anion (O_2^-) or superoxide anion radical ($O_2^{\cdot-}$), singlet oxygen ($^1O_2$), hydroxyl radical (HO$^\cdot$), peroxyl radical (ROO$^\cdot$), and lipid peroxyl radical (LOO$^\cdot$). They are very highly reactive and their half-life is also very short, from 10^{-9} sec. to one sec.

Free radicals are formed from molecules via the breakage of a chemical bond such that each fragment keeps one electron, by cleavage of a radical to give another radical and, also via redox reactions (6). Intracellular generation of free radicals mainly comprises superoxide ($O_2^{\cdot-}$) radicals and nitric oxide (NO$^\cdot$) radicals. Under normal physiologic conditions, nearly 2% of the oxygen consumed by the body is converted into free radicals through mitochondrial respiration, phagocytosis, and more such processes (20). However, free radical levels considerably increase during infections, diseases, fatigue, excessive exercise, stress, aging, exposure to pollutants, UV light, ionizing radiation, some medication, bad alimentation, and so on. Formation of ROS and RNS can occur in the cells by two ways: enzymatic and non-enzymatic reactions.

2.2.1 By Enzymatic Reactions

Enzymatic reactions generating free radicals include those involved in the respiratory chain, the phagocytosis, the prostaglandin synthesis, and the cytochrome P450 systems (4–6). For example, the production of superoxide anion radical ($O_2^{\bullet-}$) occurs mostly within the mitochondria of a cell via several cellular oxidase systems such as NADPH oxidase, xanthine oxidase, and peroxidases. The generation of ROS in cells such as activated phagocytic cells (e.g., neutrophils and monocytes) is realized with rapid uptake of oxygen (O_2), activation of NADPH oxidase, and the production of the superoxide anion radical ($O_2^{\bullet-}$) according to equation one:

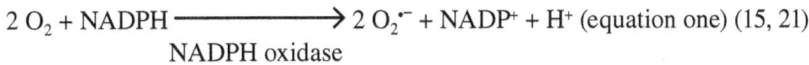

$$2\ O_2 + NADPH \xrightarrow{\hspace{2cm}} 2\ O_2^{\bullet-} + NADP^+ + H^+ \text{ (equation one) (15, 21)}$$
$$\text{NADPH oxidase}$$

The superoxide radical ($O_2^{\bullet-}$) is then rapidly converted to hydrogen peroxide (H_2O_2) by superoxide dismutase (SOD) according to equation two:

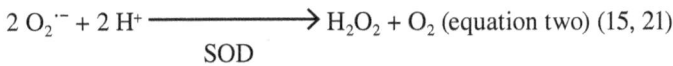

$$2\ O_2^{\bullet-} + 2\ H^+ \xrightarrow{\hspace{2cm}} H_2O_2 + O_2 \text{ (equation two) (15, 21)}$$
$$\text{SOD}$$

Hypochlorous acid (HOCl) is produced by the neutrophil-derived enzyme myeloperoxidase (MPO), which oxidizes chloride ions in the presence of H_2O_2 (equation three):

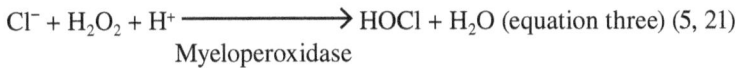

$$Cl^- + H_2O_2 + H^+ \xrightarrow{\hspace{2cm}} HOCl + H_2O \text{ (equation three) (5, 21)}$$
$$\text{Myeloperoxidase}$$

The production of reactive nitrogen species (RNS), such as nitric oxide ($NO^{\bullet}$), is performed by action of the enzyme nitric oxide synthase on the amino acid arginine (equation four):

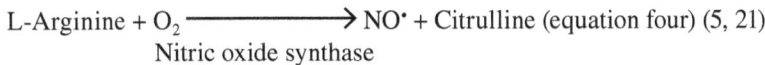

$$L\text{-Arginine} + O_2 \xrightarrow{\hspace{2cm}} NO^{\bullet} + Citrulline \text{ (equation four) (5, 21)}$$
$$\text{Nitric oxide synthase}$$

An inducible nitric oxide synthase (iNOS) is capable of continuously producing large amounts of nitric oxide radical ($NO^{\bullet}$), which act as a superoxide anion radical ($O_2^{\bullet-}$) quencher. The $NO^{\bullet}$ and $O_2^{\bullet-}$ react together to produce peroxynitrite ($ONOO^-$), (equation five), a very strong oxidant, hence, each can modulate the effects of the other. Although neither $NO^{\bullet}$ nor $O_2^{\bullet-}$ is a strong oxidant, peroxynitrite is a potent and versatile oxidant that can attack a wide range of biological targets.

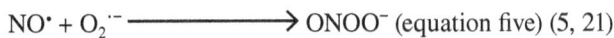

$$NO^{\bullet} + O_2^{\bullet-} \xrightarrow{\hspace{2cm}} ONOO^- \text{ (equation five) (5, 21)}$$

Peroxynitrite reacts with aromatic amino acid residues within enzymes, resulting in nitration of the aromatic amino acids. Such a change in the amino acid residue can result in enzyme inactivation (21).

2.2.2 By Non-Enzymatic Reactions

Two non-enzymatic reactions can form hydroxyl radical ($^{\bullet}OH$), the most reactive free radical *in vivo*, by the reaction of $O_2^{\bullet-}$ with H_2O_2 in the presence of Fe^{2+} or Cu^+ (catalyst) by Fenton reaction (equation six) and/or Haber-Weiss reaction (equation seven):

$H_2O_2 + Fe^{2+} \longrightarrow {}^{\cdot}OH + OH^+ + Fe^{3+}$ (equation six= Fenton reaction) (5, 21)

$O_2{}^{\cdot-} + H_2O_2 \longrightarrow {}^{\cdot}OH + OH^+ + O_2$ (equation seven= Haber-Weiss reaction) (21)

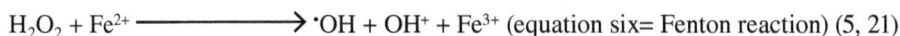

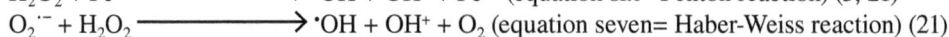

Free radicals ${}^{\cdot}OH$ can also be produced by ionizing radiations (cosmic rays, X-rays, radioactive chemicals) (equation eight):

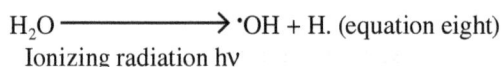

$H_2O \longrightarrow {}^{\cdot}OH + H.$ (equation eight)
      Ionizing radiation hv

The non-enzymatic process may also generate organic radicals from contact biomolecules, or occur during oxidative phosphorylation (i.e., aerobic respiration) in the mitochondria (5, 8).

2.3 SOURCES

The generation of ROS and RNS comes from two types of origins: endogenous sources and exogenous sources (6, 21–22). Biological sources of ROS and RNS are mainly located in mitochondria, endoplasmic reticulum, peroxisomes, cytosol, plasma membrane, and extracellular space of mammalian cells (22). Major sources of ROS include metabolic processes and cellular respiration processes (21–22).

2.3.1 Endogenous Free Radical Sources

The formation of ROS is a natural consequence of aerobic metabolism to maintain tissue oxygen homeostasis. Two types of endogenous free radicals are formed in the body. The first type are generated from normal essential metabolic processes such as immune cell activation (monocytes, neutrophils, and macrophages), cellular differentiation (mitochondria, microsomes), enzymatic reactions, and neuronal activity. The second type of endogenous free radicals come from abnormal states of organs or tissues due to pathology such as inflammation, infection, cancer, stroke, cardiovascular diseases, mental stress, insomnia, excessive exercise, ischemia, and aging. (6, 22).

2.3.2 Exogenous Free Radical Sources

Exogenous sources of ROS and RNS are numerous and various, such as exposure to cigarette smoke, incense smoke, 'bad' foods or cooking (alcohol, fast food, conserve, smoked meat, fat, used oil, preservative, artificial colorant, sweetener, etc.), air and water pollutants (ozone, smog, car exhaust fumes, mercury, lead, pesticides), radiations (X-rays, thermonuclear reaction, UV, microwave radiation, etc.), industrial vapors or chemicals in workplace, chemical deodorants, mothball (naphthalene), and certain drugs (cisplatin, gentamycin, bleomycin, cyclosporine, tacrolimus, etc.). Recently, the development of nanotechnology in industries using different nanoparticles such as carbon nanotubes, carbon nanofibers, metals, superparamagnetic iron oxide (Fe_3O_4) nanoparticles and fullerenes, may be the cause of occupational lung diseases in workers, like asbestos pathology (14, 23–24). It should be noted that numerous nanoparticles are cytotoxic, and this toxicity has been linked to free radicals and oxidative stress (14).

After penetration into the body by different routes, these exogenous toxic compounds are decomposed or metabolized into free radicals (4–8, 14, 22). When these exogenous ROS and RNS become too elevated, oxygen homeostasis is not maintained; this phenomenon becomes harmful to the cellular environment and causes a phenomenon called oxidative stress.

In summary, free radicals are generated in biological systems both as a result of normal cellular aerobic metabolism as well as from abnormal reactions stimulated by some disease processes and xenobiotics (14). Although free radicals can explain the pathology of many toxicities and disease processes, their causal role in specific disorders continues to be difficult to determine. Thus, determining whether free radicals are a cause, effect or both, in toxicity and disease, can be problematic (14).

2.4 ROLES OF FREE RADICALS AND OXIDANTS

In human body, ROS and RNS have two contradictory roles: they are both beneficial and toxic compounds, with varying effects according to circumstance. At low and moderate concentrations, they are indispensable for life; however, at high levels they become harmful for cells and organs, leading to the development of many dreadful ailments such as cancer, diabetes, neurodegenerative diseases, cardiovascular diseases, and immune function decrease (4–15, 22, 25).

2.4.1 Beneficial Effects of Free Radicals and Oxidants

The beneficial effects of ROS and RNS occur at low and moderate concentrations and are involved in several normal physiological function and cellular responses (10, 15, 22, 25). Also, free radicals are necessary for the maturation process of cellular structures and can act as weapons for the host defense system. Indeed, in the immune system, phagocytes (neutrophils, macrophages, monocytes) release free radicals to destroy invading pathogenic microbes as part of the body's defense mechanism against disease (5, 10, 15). ROS have been shown to trigger proliferation of T cells through NF-κB activation. Macrophages and neutrophils generate ROS in order to kill the bacteria that they engulf by phagocytosis. Furthermore, tumor necrosis factor (TNF-α) destroys tumor and virus through ROS generation by induction of apoptosis (process of programmed cell death) (20). The importance of ROS production by the immune system is clearly exemplified by patients with granulomatous disease. These patients have a defective membrane-bound NADPH oxidase system which makes them unable to produce the superoxide anion radical ($O_2^{\cdot-}$), thereby resulting in multiple and persistent infection (4–6). Most cells can produce superoxide radical, hydrogen peroxide and nitric oxide constitutively, while others have inducible ROS/RNS release system (22, 10). For example, defense against infectious agents by phagocytosis, killing of cancer cells by macrophages and cytotoxic lymphocytes, detoxification of xenobiotics by cytochrome P450, generation of ATP in mitochondria (energy production), cell growth, and the induction of mitogenic responses at low concentrations are some key beneficial activities of ROS and RNS. They also play important roles in different cellular signaling at low concentration, such as activation of several cytokines and growth factor signaling, non-receptor tyrosine kinases activation, protein tyrosine phosphatases activation, release of calcium from intracellular stores, and activation of nuclear transcription factors (22). ROS exert vital actions such as gene transcription and regulation of soluble guanylate cyclase activity in cells. In mammalian cells, the biological sources of ROS are as follows: mitochondria, endoplasmic reticulum, peroxisomes, cytosol, plasma membrane, and extracellular space (10). Major sources of ROS include metabolic processes and cellular respiration processes. During metabolic processes the peroxisome catabolizes biomolecules that remove hydrogen in an oxidative reaction creating hydrogen peroxide oxidant (H_2O_2). ROS also act as the stimulating agents for biochemical processes within the cell. ROS exert their effects through the reversible oxidation of active sites in transcription factors such as nuclear factor-kappa B (NF-kB) and activator protein-1 (AP-1) leading to gene expression and cell growth (10, 20). ROS can also cause indirect induction of transcription factors by activating signal transduction pathways. One example of signal transduction molecules activated by ROS is the mitogen activated protein kinases (MAPKs) (20). ROS also participate in the biosynthesis of molecules such as thyroxin and prostaglandins. It is noteworthy that in thyroid cells, regulation of H_2O_2 concentration is critical for thyroxine synthesis, as it is needed to catalyze the binding of iodine atoms to thyroglobulin (20).

Nitric oxide (NO·) radical, an important RNS, a small, unstable and highly lipophilic gas, endogenously formed by action of the enzyme nitric oxide synthase on the amino acid L-arginine, or produced by neurons, has emerged as a fundamental signaling device regulating virtually every critical cellular function, as well as a potent mediator of cellular damage in a wide range of conditions (6, 26–29). Nitric oxide (NO) is a double-edged sword. NO at low concentrations is beneficial, but has harmful effects on body health in high levels (6, 28). Protective effects occur at pico- to nanomolar NO concentrations. At higher levels (micromolar) or in the presence of reactive oxygen species (ROS) such as hydrogen peroxide (H_2O_2), superoxide anion ($O_2^{\cdot-}$), NO, and its derivatives become cytotoxic (27, 28). For example, nitric oxide (NO) at low concentrations is an intercellular messenger for modulating blood flow, thrombosis, and neural activity (6, 26–29). Moreover, NO produced by endothelial cells is essential for vasodilatation, blood pressure regulation, angiogenesis, leukocyte adhesion, thrombosis, and platelet aggregation (26–28). Physiological NO levels act as neuromodulators or neurotransmitters in response to different brain stimuli within the central nervous system (CNS), and it plays an important role in long-term potentiation of the hippocampus and synaptic plasticity by controlling appetite, sleep, neurosecretion, and body temperature (29). So, nitric oxide (NO) is an intercellular messenger for modulating blood flow and neural activity. It is probably important in memory and learning (28). NO generated by activated macrophages is also a key mediator of the immune response and an important cytotoxic effector molecule in nonspecific host defense against tumor cells, various protozoa, fungi, helminths, and mycobacteria (26, 28). Paradoxically, excessive NO production is cytotoxic and destroys mitochondrial function. Mitochondria are primary cellular targets for NO (27). For example, the same molecule NO at high levels can become highly damaging to the same neurons within a few minutes during pathological challenges as occur after cerebral ischemia (26). Elevated production of nitric oxide takes place in numerous pathological conditions, such as neurodegenerative diseases (Parkinson's disease, Alzheimer's disease, Huntington's disease, amyotrophic lateral sclerosis), inflammation, and ischemia, which occur concurrently with elevated nitrosative/oxidative stress (29). High amounts of NO can evoke profound vasodilation, refractory hypotension, acute catecholamine-resistant cardiac pump failure, and failure of multiple end-organs (27). Recent evidence indicates that most of the cytotoxicity attributed to NO is rather due to peroxynitrite ($ONOO^-$), produced from the diffusion-controlled reaction between NO and another free radical, the superoxide anion ($O_2^{\cdot-}$) (26). In addition, nitric oxide (NO) effects on mitochondria have considerable implications for cell physiology and cell death (apoptosis). Other roles and properties of NO and L - arginine (L- arg), also called arginine, is classified as a semi- essential, proteinogenic amino acid, meaning the human body can normally produce a sufficient amount through biosynthesis to meet its demands (26 -27, 88 - 89).

   In summary, free radicals and oxidants play an important role in biological regulation. Their important physiological functions include: regulation of vascular tone, sensing of oxygen tension and regulation of functions that are controlled by oxygen concentration, enhancement of signal transduction from various membrane receptors including the antigen receptor of lymphocytes, and oxidative stress responses that ensure the maintenance of redox homeostasis (4). Briefly, free radicals and oxidants (ROS, RNS) at low or moderate levels are vital to human health.

2.4.2   Deleterious Effects of Free Radicals and Oxidants: Oxidative Stress and Pathogenesis

At high concentrations, ROS and RNS can cause structural damage to cells, proteins, lipids, lipoproteins, deoxyribonucleic acid (DNA), nucleic acid, and so on. All the biological molecules present in our body are at risk of being attacked by free radicals. Such damaged molecules can impair cell functions and even lead to cell death, eventually resulting in diseased states (17, 30). The excessive production of free radicals and oxidants comes from two main sources: endogenous and exogenous origins as cited previously, such as infections, inflammation, aging, stress, cigarettes smoke, radiation, medication, poor diet, 'bad' food, alcohol use, and pollution. The presence of significant quantities of free radicals in cells results in a stressed condition at the cellular level called oxidative stress (20–22, 30–31). Oxidative stress can arise when cells cannot adequately destroy the excess of free radicals formed. In other words, oxidative stress results from a serious imbalance between formation and neutralization of ROS/RNS (6, 8). Lipids, proteins, DNA, RNA, and carbohydrates are all targets for oxidative stress. The body has several mechanisms to counteract the excess of free radicals by using DNA repair enzymes and/or antioxidants in order to maintain a balance between free radicals and antioxidants. This phenomenon is called redox homeostasis (4, 6).

2.4.2.1   *Lipid Peroxidation*

When lipids and lipoproteins in cell membranes are targets of oxidative stress caused by an excess of hydroxyl radical and peroxynitrite, for example, this process is called lipid peroxidation (32). The overall process of lipid peroxidation consists of three stages: initiation, propagation, and termination (32). Once formed, peroxyl radicals (ROO•) can be rearranged via a cyclization reaction to endoperoxides (precursors of malondialdehyde) with the final product of the peroxidation process being malondialdehyde (MDA). Malondialdehyde, $CH_2(CHO)_2$, mainly exists in the enol form (32):

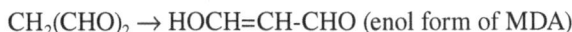

$$CH_2(CHO)_2 \rightarrow HOCH=CH\text{-}CHO \text{ (enol form of MDA)}$$

In general, lipid peroxidation is considered the main molecular mechanism involved in oxidative damage to cell structures and in the toxicity process that leads to cell death (30). Lipid peroxidation occurs by a radical chain reaction; once it has started, it spreads rapidly and damages a great number of lipid molecules, especially polyunsaturated fatty acids (PUFA) (6, 14, 30). This chain reaction is initiated by the hydrogen abstraction or addition of an oxygen radical, resulting in the oxidative damage of PUFA. Since polyunsaturated fatty acids are more sensitive than saturated ones, it is obvious that the reactive oxygen species (ROS) target the carbon-carbon double bond of PUFA (4, 9, 30). Lipid peroxidation leads to the eventual destruction of membrane lipids, with the production of a variety of breakdown products, including alcohols, ketones, alkanes, aldehydes (MDA), and ethers. MDA and other conjugated diene compounds formed are cytotoxic, mutagenic in mammalian cells, and carcinogenic in rats (6, 30).

Proteins may also be damaged by ROS/RNS, called protein oxidation, leading to structural changes and loss of enzyme activity (9, 14). Oxidative damage to DNA, called DNA oxidation, leads to the formation of different oxidative DNA lesions which can cause mutations.

The mechanism of biological damage and the toxicity of these reactive species on biological systems are currently explained by the sequential stages of reversible oxidative stress and irreversible oxidative damage. Oxidative stress is understood as an imbalance situation with increased oxidants or decreased antioxidants (30–31). The concept implies the recognition of the physiological production of oxidants and the existence of operative antioxidant defenses (30). If not regulated properly, oxidative stress can induce a variety of chronic and degenerative diseases as well as the aging process and some acute pathology (trauma, stroke). In humans, oxidative stress is thought to be involved in the pathogenesis of different dreadful ailments such as cancer, neurodegenerative, cardiovascular and pulmonary diseases, arthritis, nephropathy, inflammation, diabetes, aging, cataract, and so on.

Moreover, drug-induced oxidative stress is implicated as a mechanism of toxicity in numerous tissues and organ systems, including the liver, kidney, ear, cardiovascular and nervous systems. Well-characterized drugs associated with adverse events to which oxidative stress may contribute include chemo agents, antiretroviral agents, antipsychotics, and more (33). Metabolism of a drug may generate a reactive intermediate that can reduce molecular oxygen directly to produce ROS/RNS. By long-term therapy, accumulation of free radicals formed by drug metabolism could develop oxidative stress in different tissues and organs.

In pharmaceutical industries, 56% of the drugs currently in use are chiral products, and 88% of the chiral drugs are marketed as racemates consisting of an equimolar mixture of two enantiomers (isomers) such as β-blockers, calcium channel antagonists (verapamil, nicardipine, etc.), non-steroidal anti-inflammatory drugs (ibuprofen, ketoprofen, etc.), bronchodilators (salbutamol, salmeterol, terbutaline), analgesics (methadone), and so on (34). However, the majority of these racemic drugs only have one active isomer; the other isomer is pharmacologically inactive or toxic (34). The prolonged consumption of these racemic drugs may induce toxicity because the unnecessary energy used for the metabolism of the inactive isomer could engender free radicals leading to oxidative stress in the body. Therefore, the elimination of the inactive isomer in a racemic drug may be helpful for the sake of the patient's health.

2.4.2.2   Oxidative Stress and Pathogenesis

Oxidative stress may be the cause of many diseases, as follows.

Lungs:	**Kidneys:**	**Sperms:**
Asthma	Glomerulonephritis	Infertility
COPD	Chronic renal failure	Spermatozoon Motility

Joints:	**Oxidative Stress**	**Eyes:**
Arthritis		Cataract
Rheumatism		Glaucoma

Brain:	**Multi-organs:**	**Heart-Vessels:**
Alzheimer's	Cancer	Arteriosclerosis
Parkinson's	Aging	Hypertension
Memory loss	Diabetes	Ischemia
Depression	Inflammation	Cardiomyopathy
Multiple sclerosis	Infection	Heart failure

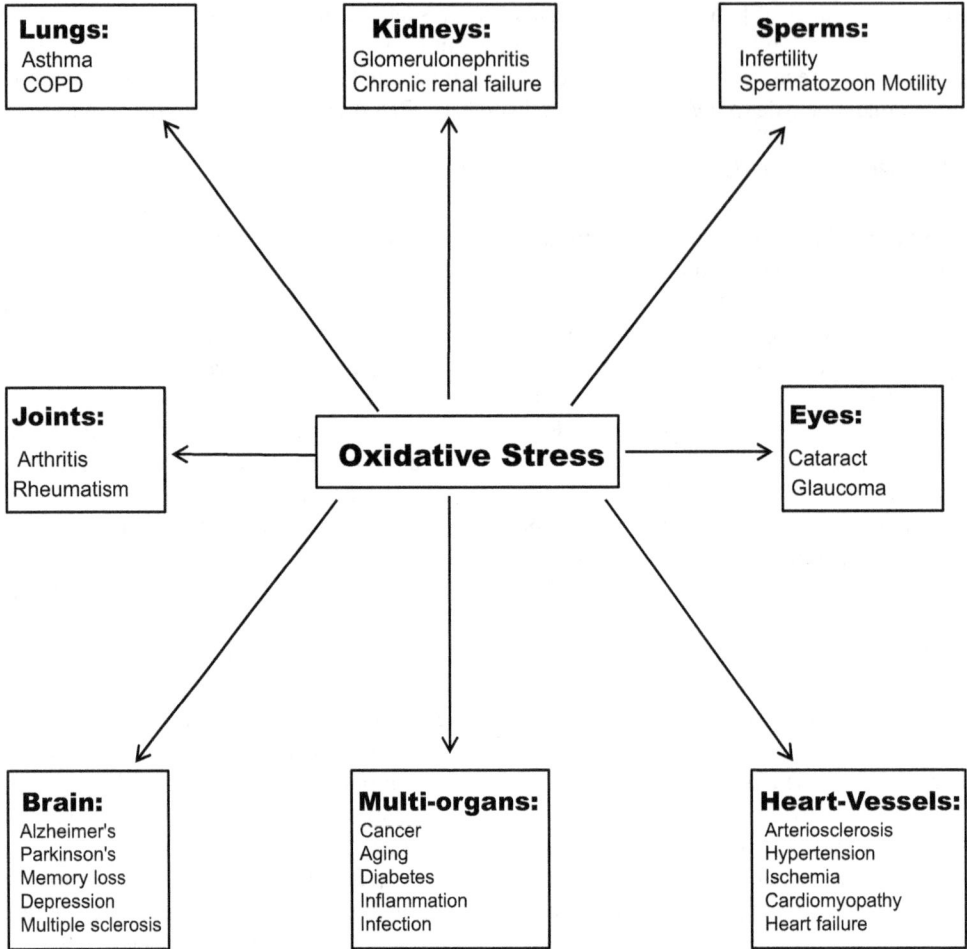

FIGURE 3.1 Oxidative stress-induced diseases in humans (6).

2.4.2.2.1 Cancer The development of cancer in humans is a complex process including cellular and molecular changes mediated by diverse endogenous and exogenous stimuli. It is well established that oxidative DNA damage is responsible for cancer development (5, 6, 14, 31–33, 35–36). ROS are mutagenic to human cells and may function as tumor initiators (14). ROS can alter the activities of kinases, and oxidative DNA modifications may activate oncogenes or inactivate tumor suppresser genes (14, 35). Cancer initiation and promotion are associated with chromosomal defects and oncogene activation induced by free radicals (6). A common form of damage is the formation of hydroxyl bases of DNA, which are considered an important event in chemical carcinogenesis (7, 35–36). This adduct formation interferes with normal cell growth by causing genetic mutations and altering normal gene transcription. Oxidative DNA damage also produces a multiplicity of modifications in the DNA structure including base and sugar lesions, strand breaks, DNA-protein cross-links and base-free sites (6, 31). Free radicals (ROS/RNS) can both inhibit and stimulate cell proliferation, depending upon cell type and condition, but a direct interaction of free radicals with DNA is not required to affect cell proliferation (14). Thus, in addition to genotoxic effects, free radicals can affect the development of cancer through non-genotoxic mechanisms, such as through modulation of signal transduction pathways (14, 37). It is noteworthy that approximately 5–10% of all cancers are considered to be hereditary (38–39). Unlike most cancer, hereditary cancer results from gene defects (mutations) inherited from a parent (38–39). It can also be due in part to other factors, like obesity, that tend to run in families and influence cancer risk. Overall, endogenous and exogenous free radical sources play an important role in the development of most cancer forms.

Exogenous free radical compounds such as cigarette smoke, incense smoke, alcohol, chemical deodorant, mothball (naphthalene, 1,4-dichlorobenzene), and so on, become carcinogenic with prolonged use or exposure. Some processed foods such as smoked meat, ham, saucisson, fat, and canned foods, are also harmful to the body and can cause cancer with long-term consumption because they contain preservative, sweetener, smokes, acrolein, polycyclic aromatic hydrocarbons (PAHs), trans-fats, and so on (40–42). They must be reduced for the sake of health. The highly significant correlation between consumption of fats and death rates from leukemia and breast, ovary, rectum cancers among elderly people may be due to strong lipid peroxidation (6, 22). Exogenous carcinogenic free radicals generated from industry and car fumes, pesticides, herbicides, plastics, chemicals in polluted air, water or food, ionizing radiation from X-rays, nuclear reactors for electricity production, must be eliminated or reduced for the sake of people's health (43). In addition, stress is an important source of free radicals for the trigger and the development of cancer. Endogenous free radicals are mainly due to aging, infections, hormone imbalance, vitamin deficiency, and so on.

Medication is also an exogenous source of oxidative stress, mostly used in the long term. The late Professor René Truhaut of our laboratory of Toxicology (University of Paris 5, France) was among the first scientists who have discovered the potential carcinogenic hazards from numerous drugs in the 1960s (44). Long-term uses of some medicines such as analgesics, tranquilizers, corticoids, and antineoplastic agents (adriamycin, cis-platin, methotrexate, cyclophosphamide, doxorubicin), could develop tumors (45). Recently, among 105 commonly used drugs never screened before by epidemiology, 61 showed possible increased cancer risk regarding hyoscyamine, nortriptyline, sulindac, oxazepam, fluoxetine, paroxetine, nifedipine, and more (46). However, this last statistical study is still not confirmed. The immune system, the main organ of host defense against tumor and infection, is also weakened by drug-induced oxidative stress, thereby developing cancer. In summary, endogenous and exogenous ROS/RNS are potential carcinogens because they facilitate mutagenesis, tumor promotion, and progression.

2.4.2.2.2 Cardiovascular Diseases Cardiovascular disease (CVD) is of multifactorial etiology associated with a variety of risk factors for its development, including drugs, infection, smoking, diabetes, poor diet, stress, hypercholesterolemia, aging, and physical inactivity, among others (5, 6, 47). Recently, research data has raised a passionate debate as to whether oxidative stress is a primary or secondary cause of many cardiovascular diseases (48). Further in vivo and ex vivo studies have provided precious evidence supporting the role of oxidative stress in a number of CVDs such as atherosclerosis, ischemia, hypertension, cardiomyopathy, cardiac hypertrophy, and congestive heart failure (48). The major sources of oxidative stress in the cardiovascular system involve: the enzymes xanthine oxidoreductase (XOR), NAD(P)H oxidase and NOS, as well as mitochondrial cytochromes and hemoglobin (5). Oxidative stress is associated with increased formation of ROS that modifies phospholipids and proteins leading to peroxidation and oxidation of thiol groups (5, 47). The assaults by ROS lead to changes in membrane permeability, membrane lipid bilayer disruption, and functional modification of various cellular proteins. In addition to cellular protein and lipid damage, abnormalities in myocyte function due to increased oxidative stress are considered to be associated with the effects of ROS on subcellular organelles (5).

Atherosclerosis is a multifactorial disease characterized by hardening and thickening of the arterial wall. The vascular areas affected by this disease contain mononuclear cells, proliferating smooth muscle cells, and extracellular matrix components. Atherosclerosis is commonly viewed as a chronic inflammatory disease and is associated with certain risk factors such as hyperlipidemia, diabetes, and hypertension. Excessive ROS production has been implicated in the pathogenesis of atherosclerosis and hypertension. The invasion of the artery wall by monocytes and T lymphocytes is one of the earliest events in the development of atherosclerotic lesions (4). Lipid peroxidation and atherogenesis may be ameliorated by vitamin E (4).

The critical role of intracellular Ca^{2+} overload in the genesis of myocyte dysfunction has been well established (5, 47). In general, Ca^{2+}-overload can be induced by direct effect of ROS on Ca^{2+}-handling proteins or indirectly, by inducing membrane lipid peroxidation. In addition, other mechanisms involving an increase in the concentration of Na^+ and accumulation of long chain fatty acids in cardiac membranes should be considered (5). Deficiency in ATP in the ischemic heart may also induce Ca^{2+}-overload. Intracellular Ca^{2+}-overload seems to be a common denominator for many CVDs such as atherosclerosis, hypertension, myocardial cell damage, and cardiac hypertrophy (5, 47–48). Evidence for the participation of oxidative stress in these types of cardiovascular disease is recognized by many authors (4–8, 34, 47–48).

2.4.2.2.3 Neurodegenerative Diseases Oxidative stress-induced neurodegenerative diseases include Alzheimer's disease, Parkinson's disease, multiple sclerosis, amyotrophic lateral sclerosis (ALS), memory loss, and depression (49). Alzheimer's disease (AD) is a neurodegenerative disorder characterized by a progressive decline in cognitive function and extensive neuronal loss (50). The brains of affected patients show numerous amyloid plaques and neurofibrillary tangles. The production of ROS in the brains of AD patients and its implication in AD pathogenesis are implicated by the significant amount of lipid peroxidation detected in the brain as well as by the increased levels of 4-hydroxynonenal found in postmortem cerebrospinal fluid of AD patients (4–5, 7, 51). In AD, oxidative damage plays a key role in the loss of neurons and the progression to dementia (6). The production of ß-amyloid, a toxic peptide often found present in Alzheimer's patients' brains, is due to oxidative stress and plays an important role in the neurodegenerative processes (4, 51–54). Parkinson's disease (PD) involves a selective loss of neurons in an area of the midbrain called the substantia nigra (5, 54). The cells of the substantia nigra use dopamine (a neurotransmitter-chemical messenger between brain and nerve cells) to communicate with the cells in another region of the brain called the stratium. Thus, a reduction in nigral dopamine levels results in a decrease in stratial dopamine that is believed to cause PD symptoms (52). A majority of studies explored the effect of oxidative stress that contributes to the cascade of events leading to dopamine cell degeneration in PD (5, 53–54). The occurrence of oxidative stress in Parkinson's disease is supported by both postmortem studies and by studies demonstrating the capacity of oxidative stress to induce nigral cell degeneration. However, other factors involving inflammation, excitotoxicity mechanisms, nitric oxide toxicity, and mitochondrial dysfunction play roles in the etiology of Parkinson's disease (5, 54).

Levodopa (L-dopa), a dopamine precursor and the most commonly used medicine to treat Parkinson's disease, may cause oxidative damage and toxicity to brain cells in prolonged periods. If this observation turns out to be true, it would further suggest the addition of antioxidants to standard PD therapy (5). Since oxidative stress appears to represent a portion of a cascade of biochemical changes leading to dopaminergic death, further studies are necessary to understand the complicated pathogenesis of Parkinson's disease (5, 54).

2.4.2.2.4 Pulmonary Diseases It is well known that inflammatory lung diseases such as asthma and chronic obstructive pulmonary disease (COPD) as well as pulmonary cancer initiation and promotion have been linked to a series of systemic and local chronic inflammation and biochemical pathways of oxidative stress (6, 55). The lungs are exposed daily to oxidants generated either endogenously or exogenously such as cigarette smoke and air pollutants. It has been demonstrated that lung cancer increases substantially for tobacco smokers due to the synergistic effects in the generation of free radicals ROS, leading to oxidative stress and inflammation with high DNA damage potential (56).

Free radicals may play a role in enhancing inflammation through the activation of different kinases and redox transcription factors such as the Nuclear Factor-kappa B (NF-kB) and the Activator Protein-1 (AP-1) (6, 52–55). The NF-kB activation has been linked to a wide spectrum of extracellular stimuli and oxidants and subsequent involvement in the carcinogenic process through promotion of angiogenesis and tumor cell invasion and metastasis. The AP-1 contributes to basal gene expression in biological systems. ROS can also activate AP-1 through several mechanisms (56).

The mechanisms by which ROS exacerbate asthma could be due to both effects of free radicals on airway smooth muscle and mucin secretion by decreasing β-adrenergic function in lungs and also by sensitizing airway muscles to acetylcholine induced contraction (57). Hydrogen peroxide (H_2O_2) can also stimulate tracheal smooth muscle to contract. Finally, ROS/RNS have been reported to stimulate mucin secretion. A recent study indicated that development of an oxidant/antioxidant imbalance in asthma leads to activation of the redox-sensitive transcription factor NF-kB (nuclear factor-kappa B) (57).

For chronic obstructive pulmonary disease (COPD), considerable evidence now links this chronic ailment with increased oxidative stress. The most striking relationship is between cigarette smoking and COPD. Nearly 90% of all COPD patients are smokers (58). Yet, for unknown reasons, only about 20% of cigarette smokers develop COPD (58). Maybe, the other smokers have strong immune systems or consume good diets rich in natural antioxidants. The role of iron has become increasingly significant in understanding the development of COPD.

Overall, it is evident that many chronic pulmonary diseases are in relationship with oxidative stress caused by exogenous and/or endogenous free radicals. Knowledge of the mechanisms of ROS regulation may allow for the use of some natural antioxidants as adjuvants in the treatment of some lung inflammation and injury such as chronic asthma, COPD, or tumor.

2.4.2.2.5 Diabetes Mellitus   There are two main types of diabetes mellitus: insulin-dependent diabetes mellitus or juvenile diabetes or type 1 diabetes; and non-insulin-dependent diabetes mellitus or type 2 diabetes mellitus (5). The first type is rare (about 10% of patients) and results from the pancreas' failure to produce enough insulin. However, the majority of diabetes patients are non-insulin-dependent and capable of producing insulin at least initially, but are deficient in their cellular response. This type 2 diabetes mellitus is the most common form of diabetes. Obesity, particularly truncal obesity (abdominal obesity), is closely correlated to the prevalence of type 2 diabetes. Hyperglycemia is a hallmark of both non-insulin-dependent (Type 2) and insulin-dependent (Type 1) diabetes mellitus.

Increased oxidative stress has been proposed to be one of the major causes of the hyperglycemia-induced trigger of diabetic complications (4). Hyperglycemia in the body stimulates ROS formation from a variety of sources. In this case oxidative stress is associated with a pro-oxidative shift of the glutathione redox state in the blood (4–5). Elevated glucose levels are associated with increased production of ROS by several different mechanisms. In addition, superoxide is generated by the process of glucose auto-oxidation that is associated with the formation of glycated proteins in the plasma of diabetic patients (4, 7). The interaction of advanced glycation end-products with corresponding cell surface receptors stimulates ROS production and decreases intracellular glutathione levels (4, 11). The increase in ROS production contributes to the development of diabetic complications such as atherosclerosis, hypertension and other vascular diseases (4–5, 59). In addition, hyperglycemia enhances cell-mediated low-density lipoprotein (LDL) peroxidation in endothelial cells. Treatment with antioxidants such as alpha lipoic acid as dietary supplement in experimental diabetes ameliorates diabetic complications such as nerve and vascular dysfunction (59).

2.4.2.2.6 Rheumatoid Arthritis   Rheumatoid arthritis is a systemic autoimmune disease characterized by chronic joint inflammation with infiltration of macrophages and activated T cells (60). The pathogenesis of this disease is due to the generation of ROS and RNS at the site of inflammation (4–6). Oxidative damage and inflammation in various rheumatic diseases were proved by increased levels of isoprostanes and prostaglandins in serum and synovial fluid compared to controls (5). The migration of monocytes and lymphocytes into the rheumatoid arthritis synovium is mediated by the abnormal expression of several adhesion molecules including ELAM-1, VCAM-1, ICAM-1, and ICAM-2. Oxidative conditions in synovial tissue are also associated with a higher incidence of p53 gene mutations (4). This may be explained by the abnormal induction of redox-sensitive signaling pathways (4–5, 60).

2.4.2.2.7 Nephropathy   Oxidative stress plays a role in a variety of renal diseases such as glomerulonephritis and tubule-interstitial nephritis, chronic renal failure, proteinuria, uremia, and diabetic nephropathy (6, 61). Various metals such as heavy metals (Cadmium, Chrome, Mercury, Lead, Uranium), transition metals in excessive concentrations (Cobalt, Cupper, Iron, Zinc), or metals used in cancer therapy (Platine, Vanadium), accumulate in the mammalian kidney, largely in the proximal tubule cells, and cause functional and structural damage that results in reabsorptive and secretory defects (62). The intracellular mechanisms of their toxicity in the proximal tubule cells are not well-known. Recent studies have indicated an oxidative stress with associated lipid peroxidation, apoptosis, and necrosis as common phenomena in the course of nephrotoxicity of these metals (62).

The nephrotoxicity of certain drugs such as cyclosporine, tacrolimus (FK506), gentamycin, bleomycin, and vinblastine is mainly due to oxidative stress via lipid peroxidation (63–65). Recently, some findings suggest a major role for ROS, oxidative stress, and mitogen-activated protein kinase (MAPK) signaling in promoting Cyclosporine A-induced glomerular dysfunction and subsequent nephrotoxicity (66).

Diabetic nephropathy is a leading cause of end-stage renal failure worldwide. A large body of evidence indicates that oxidative stress is the common denominator link for the major pathways involved in the development and progression of micro- as well as macrovascular complications of diabetes. New generations of antioxidants may be more effective in reducing renovascular complications of diabetes.

2.4.2.2.8 Ocular Diseases   Oxidative stress is one of the multifactorial causes of some ocular diseases mostly developed in elderly people such as cataracts, glaucoma and age-related macular degeneration by altering various cell types in the eye either via photochemical or non-photochemical action (6, 67–70). Free radicals can cross-link and aggregate the crystalline proteins in the lens, leading to the formation of cataracts (6, 67–68). In glaucoma, antioxidant levels decrease in the aqueous humor in patients with primary open-angle glaucoma (POAG), compared to the aqueous humor of patients with cataracts, suggesting that peroxidation may be involved in the development of glaucoma (69–70). The potential role of oxidative stress in relation to age-related macular degeneration (AMD) is also discussed because in the retina, long-term exposure to radiation can inhibit mitosis in the retinal pigment epithelium and damage the photoreceptor outer segments (71). The retina is particularly susceptible to lipid peroxidation because of its high consumption of oxygen, its high proportion of polyunsaturated fatty acids, and its exposure to visible light (72). The association between cigarette smoking and many ocular diseases such as Graves' ophthalmopathy, AMD, and cataract, is due to the enhancement of superoxide radical formation and the decrease of antioxidants in the eyes (73).

2.4.2.2.9 Aging   Aging is a natural and universal biological process causing vulnerability of the organism to internal and external aggression (74–75). Its etiology is multifactorial and linked to genetic programming, as well as the modifications that occur at a cellular-molecular level (76). This process may also relate to the presence and action of the free radicals such as ROS, which is one of the primary determinants of aging (76).

The widely popular free radical theory of aging states that the age-related degenerative process is to a large extent the consequence of free radical damage (4). The 'oxidative stress theory' holds that a progressive and irreversible accumulation of oxidative damage caused by ROS impacts on critical aspects of the aging process and contributes to impaired physiological function, increased incidence of disease, and a reduction in life span (4, 76). Other theories of aging have been proposed, including the free radical and mitochondrial theories of aging (76–78). Both theories speculate that cumulative damage to mitochondria and mitochondrial DNA (mtDNA) caused by reactive oxygen species (ROS) is one of the causes of aging. Oxidative damage affects replication and transcription of mtDNA and results in a decline in mitochondrial function which in turn leads to enhanced ROS production and further damage to mtDNA (76–78).

Indeed, the production of radicals and their role in aging is well understood. Further research may apply this knowledge in the development of a practical method to prevent or repair mtDNA radical damage in order to extend life span. However, according to Yan (79), a moderate level of oxidative stress, induced by a variety of stressors, can yield great beneficial effects on adaptive cellular responses to pathological challenges in aging and aging-associated disease tolerance such as ischemia tolerance.

2.4.2.2.10 Male Infertility Among many causes of male infertility, oxidative stress has been attributed to affect fertility status, and thus it has been studied extensively in recent years (80). Oxidative stress in the male germ line is thought to affect male fertility and impact upon normal embryonic development. Administration of some antioxidants like vitamin C, zinc, L-Carnitine, or N-acetyl-L-cysteine alone or in combination to infertile men has been assessed in numerous clinical studies. Strong evidence supports improved motility, particularly in asthenospermic patients (81). However, these observations are still preliminary. More studies are needed to confirm these promising results. Finally, a résumé of oxidative stress-induced diseases in humans is described in Figure 3.1.

3   ANTIOXIDANTS

3.1   Definition

Antioxidants are molecules that can inhibit and neutralize free radicals (ROS, RNS) by accepting or donating electrons to eliminate the unpaired condition of the radical (82–84). Indeed, an antioxidant could be considered a 'generous' molecule in donating its electron to a 'poor' free radical, for transforming the last one into a stable and inoffensive molecule. Antioxidants are also known as 'free radical scavengers' because they delay or inhibit cellular damage mainly through their free radical scavenging property (82). Briefly, the roles of antioxidants are to neutralize the excess of free radicals, to protect the cells against their toxic effects, and to contribute to disease prevention (5–6, 21, 82–87).

Regarding the chemical structure of an antioxidant, the number of double bonds or conjugated double bonds in the side chain and/or in the heterocyclic ring plays an important role in its antioxidant activity. In general, the higher the number of double bonds, the better the activity. In vegetables, the color, savor or odor of fruits, tubers, and leaves, are also due to the presence of conjugated double bonds in their chemical structures. Indeed, the more pronounced the color, the better the antioxidant activity. For example, blackberry contains more antioxidants than strawberry, black or red grapes are better than green grapes, and so on.

3.2   Mechanisms of Antioxidant Activity

Nature has endowed each cell with adequate protective mechanisms against any harmful effects of free radicals: superoxide dismutase (SOD), glutathione peroxidase, glutathione reductase, thioredoxin, thiols and disulfide bonding are buffering systems in every cell. Vitamin E (α-tocopherol) is an essential nutrient which functions as a chain-breaking antioxidant, preventing the propagation of free radical reactions in all cell membranes in the human body. Ascorbic acid (vitamin C) is also part of the normal protecting mechanism. Other non-enzymatic antioxidants include carotenoids, flavonoids and related polyphenols, α-lipoic acid, glutathione, and so on (17).

When an antioxidant destroys a free radical, this antioxidant itself becomes oxidized – an antioxidant radical. Therefore, the antioxidant resources must be constantly replenished in the body either by regenerating in situ or replacing by external supply such as foods or dietary supplements in order to maintain redox homeostasis (6). In general, the antioxidant radical is relatively unreactive and unable to attack further molecules (16). Two main mechanisms have been proposed for antioxidant activity: chain-breaking and chain-removing (6, 12, 16, 82, 87).

For the chain-breaking mechanism, the primary antioxidant donates an electron to the free radical present in the systems by interrupting the propagation of the autoxidation chain reaction (12, 82). The second mechanism involves removal of free radical initiators (secondary antioxidants) by quenching chain-initiating catalysts (6, 82). Antioxidants may exert their activity on biological systems by other mechanisms including the prevention of ROS formation by preventive enzymatic antioxidants (like superoxide dismutase, catalase, and glutathione peroxidase), inhibition of pro-oxidative enzymes (like NADPH oxidase, xanthine oxidase, and NO synthase), chelation of transition metal radicals (such as copper and iron), gene expression regulation, co-antioxidants, and electron donation (5, 6, 17, 82, 85–87).

However, while in one particular system an antioxidant is effective against free radicals, in other systems the same antioxidant could become ineffective. Also, in certain circumstances such as prolonged intake or overload of dietary supplements, an antioxidant may even act as a pro-oxidant, generating harmful free radicals (6, 16, 85–87).

3.3 CLASSIFICATION

In the human body, the production of antioxidants occurs in two ways: endogenous antioxidants and exogenous antioxidants.

3.3.1 Endogenous Antioxidants

Endogenous antioxidants or in vivo antioxidants are compounds naturally generated in the body or in cells. They exist in two forms: enzymatic antioxidants and non-enzymatic antioxidants (6, 87).

3.3.1.1 Enzymatic Antioxidants

Different antioxidant enzymes directly involved in free radical neutralization include: superoxide dismutase (SOD), catalase (CAT), glutathione peroxidase (GPx), and glutathione reductase (GRx) (5–6, 21, 83, 87). Enzymatic antioxidants work by breaking down and removing free radicals. The antioxidant enzymes convert dangerous oxidative products to hydrogen peroxide (H_2O_2) and then to water, in a multi-step process, in the presence of cofactors such as copper, zinc, manganese, and iron. They also reduce the levels of lipid hydroperoxide and H_2O_2, thus they are crucial in the prevention of lipid peroxidation and the maintenance of cell membrane structure and function (21).

3.3.1.1.1 Superoxide Dismutase   Superoxide dismutase (SOD) is an important endogenous antioxidant enzyme and the first line of defense against free radicals in the body. It is located in the cytosol and mitochondria, and can exist in several common forms (6, 21–22). SOD catalytically converts the superoxide anion radical ($O_2^{\cdot-}$) into hydrogen peroxide (H_2O_2) by reduction in the presence of metal ion cofactors such as copper (Cu), zinc (Zn), or manganese (Mn) (12, 14, 21, 87):

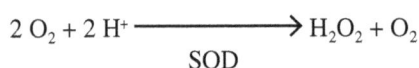

$$2\,O_2 + 2\,H^+ \xrightarrow{\quad\quad} H_2O_2 + O_2$$
$$\text{SOD}$$

The hydrogen peroxide (H_2O_2) must then be removed by catalase or glutathione peroxidase, as described below.

In human tissues, there are three forms of superoxide dismutase, each with a specific subcellular location and different tissue distribution and also depending on the presence of metal cofactor: SOD1 is located in the cytoplasm, SOD2 in the mitochondria, and SOD3 is extracellular (12, 22, 82). They are proteins containing copper and zinc, or manganese, iron, or nickel. SOD1 and SOD3 contain copper and zinc, while SOD2 has manganese in its reactive center (82).

3.3.1.1.2 Catalase (CAT) is a common, highly efficient antioxidant enzyme mainly located within cells in peroxisomes (12, 22). It is a tetramer containing four porphyrin heme groups and a molecule of NADPH, allowing the enzyme to decompose the oxidant hydrogen peroxide (H_2O_2), formed above by SOD, to water and oxygen. The rate constant for this reaction is extremely high (~10^7 M/sec), so that each catalase molecule can decompose millions of hydrogen peroxide molecules to water and oxygen in every second (12, 22, 87).

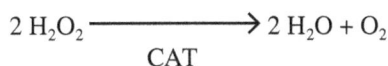

$$2\,H_2O_2 \xrightarrow{CAT} 2\,H_2O + O_2$$

3.3.1.1.3 Glutathione Peroxidases (GSHPx) Glutathione peroxidases (GSHPx) are found both in the cytoplasm and extracellularly in almost every human tissue (22). The biochemical activity of glutathione peroxidase is to reduce free hydrogen peroxide (H_2O_2) to water (H_2O) and to reduce lipid hydroperoxides to their corresponding alcohols. They protect the cell against oxidative injury caused by H_2O_2 and prevent the formation of hydroxyl radical ($^{\bullet}$OH) from H_2O_2 (21). GSHPx convert the oxidant H_2O_2 into water with the aid of its coenzyme glutathione (GSH). The last one is oxidized into glutathione disulfide (GS-SG) (21, 22, 87).

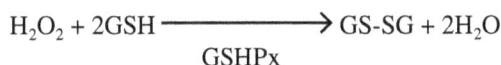

$$H_2O_2 + 2GSH \xrightarrow{GSHPx} GS\text{-}SG + 2H_2O$$

The enzyme GSHPx has strong activity towards both H_2O_2 and fatty acid hydroperoxides. Glutathione peroxidases catalyze the oxidation of glutathione (GSH) at the expense of a hydroperoxide (ROOH), which might be hydrogen peroxide (H_2O_2), or another species such as a lipid hydroperoxide (LOOH) (12):

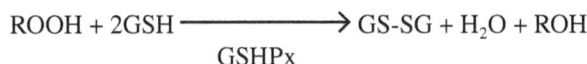

$$ROOH + 2GSH \xrightarrow{GSHPx} GS\text{-}SG + H_2O + ROH$$

Other peroxides, including lipid hydroperoxides, can also act as substrates for these enzymes which might therefore play a role in repairing damage resulting from lipid peroxidation. GSHPx is formed by four protein subunits, each of which contains one atom of selenium (Se) at its active site. So, deficiency of GSHPx might occur in the body when there is severe selenium deficiency in food and environment (12, 21, 87). The plasma form of glutathione peroxidase is believed to be synthesized mainly in the kidney. Within cells, the highest concentrations are found in the liver, although glutathione peroxidase is widely distributed in almost all tissues. The predominant subcellular distribution is in the cytosol and mitochondria, suggesting that GSHPx is the main scavenger of hydrogen peroxide in these subcellular compartments (12). The activity of the enzyme is dependent on the constant availability of reduced glutathione (GSH).

3.3.1.1.4 Glutathione Reductase (GSHRx) GSHRx is a ubiquitous flavoprotein enzyme and can regenerate GSH from GS-SG, with NADPH (reduced form of Nicotinamide Adenine Dinucleotide Phosphate: NADP) as a source of reducing power (12, 22, 87). The oxidized glutathione, glutathione disulphide (GS-SG), is reduced back to GSH by the presence of glutathione reductase (GSHRx), which uses NADPH as an electron donor. The ratio of GSH/GSSG is an important general measure of oxidative stress of an organism, because very high concentrations of GS-SG may damage many enzymes (12, 22).

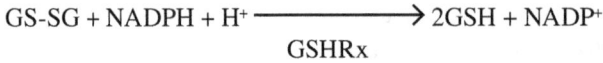

$$GS\text{-}SG + NADPH + H^+ \xrightarrow{\hspace{2.5cm}} 2GSH + NADP^+$$
$$\text{GSHRx}$$

3.3.1.2 Non-Enzymatic Antioxidants

The non-enzymatic antioxidants are divided into endogenous metabolic antioxidants and exogenous nutrient antioxidants (6, 22).

3.3.1.2.1 Endogenous Metabolic Antioxidants Metabolic antioxidants belonging to endogenous antioxidants are produced during normal metabolism in the body, such as glutathione, L-arginine, coenzyme Q10, lipoid acid, uric acid, melatonin, bilirubin, L-carnosine, dehydroepiandrosterone (DHEA), taurine, cysteine, metal-chelating proteins such as transferrin, and so on (9, 22, 84, 87–88). Some main endogenous metabolic antioxidants are described below.

3.3.1.2.1.1   Glutathione   Glutathione (GSH) is an endogenous antioxidant peptide composed of three amino acids: cysteine, glycine, and glutamate; and can be found in every cell (except in epithelial cells) of the human body (82). Its antioxidant properties are due to the thiol group present in its cysteine moiety which is a reducing agent and can be reversibly oxidized and reduced (82). In cells, glutathione is maintained in the reduced form by the enzyme glutathione reductase and in turn reduces other metabolites and enzyme systems as well as reacting directly with oxidants (82). Due to its high concentration and central role in maintaining the cell's redox state, glutathione is one of the most important cellular antioxidants (82). GSH has a central role in biotransformation and elimination of xenobiotics and protects cells against oxidative stress. It is not required in the diet, but it is also present in vegetable and animal foods and can be partially absorbed by the human small intestine (22).

3.3.1.2.1.2   L-arginine   L-arginine (L-arg) is classified as a semi-essential, proteinogenic amino acid, meaning the human body can normally produce a sufficient amount through biosynthesis to meet its demands (26–27, 88–89). However, under certain stressful situations (burns, aging, liver disease, sepsis, trauma, childhood, etc.), the body cannot produce enough of this amino acid antioxidant, and supplementation through food or synthetic arginine becomes necessary for optimal health (26–27, 88). Thus, L-arginine is both an endogenous and exogenous antioxidant. The L- appellation of arginine means levorotary (L) isomer (enantiomer) of a chiral molecule (35).

L-arginine (L-arg), is the main precursor of nitric oxide (NO), an endogenous messenger molecule involved in a variety of endothelium-mediated physiological effects in the nervous, immune, and cardiovascular systems (88–89). L-arginine is metabolized by two major pathways under the action of two specific enzymes: nitric oxide synthase and arginase. The nitric oxide synthase (NOS) pathway converts L-arg to NO and L-citrulline by three distinct isoforms of this enzyme: neuronal NOS (nNOS), inducible NOS (iNOS), and endothelial NOS (eNOS) (26–29, 88–89). The arginase pathway catalyzes the hydrolysis of L-arg to urea and ornithine in the liver through the urea cycle with the genesis of different polyamines (putrescine, spermidine and spermine). Briefly, L-arg plays a central role in the biosynthesis of nitric oxide, creatinine, agmatine, polyamines, proline, glutamate, and so on (26–27, 88–89). Most tissues in the body must be supplied with adequate intracellular levels of L-arg from circulation for their good function. All animal and vegetable proteins from the diet can be catabolized by the body into L-amino acids, of which L-arg. L-arginine is found abundantly in meat, milk, seafood, poultry, egg, soybeans, nuts, seeds, and more (88). In contrast, cereals are comparatively devoid of L-arginine, with only 3–4% of their low protein content being L-arginine (88). About 5 g of L-arginine is ingested each day in a normal Western diet (88).

It is of note that nitric oxide (NO), a main metabolite of L-arginine, is a highly reactive free radical gas which has been shown to possess an extraordinary variety of biological functions. It can be toxic or beneficial, depending on the amount and where in the body it is released (26–29, 88–89). There are three types of NO: brain-derived NO (bNO), endothelial-derived NO (eNO), and macrophage-derived NO (mNO). Brain-derived NO (bNO) is an important neurotransmitter in both the central as well as peripheral nervous systems, affects several types of nerve cells and regulates the release and production of many hormones (26–29, 88–89). Endothelial-derived NO (eNO) diffuses out of endothelial cells lining arteries and veins and into muscle cells of arteries enhancing relaxation, dilatation, and other activities of vascular physiology. It also acts on platelets to inhibit blood clotting. Macrophage-derived NO (mNO) plays a key role in the immune system by helping macrophages and other phagocytes (neutrophils, monocytes) to kill bacteria, viruses, and tumor cells for host defense. Therefore, NO is considered a messenger molecule involved in a variety of physiological organ functions. It can intervene in everything and everywhere in the body, such as digestion, sense of sight and smell, and eventually memory and learning. It may also participate in disease processes such as stroke, hypertension, septic shock, depression, diabetes, and impotence. So, the deficiency of L-arginine, a semi-essential amino acid, due to poor nutrition, aging or diseases (gastro-intestinal or hepatic troubles) may be the origin of some neurotransmitter disorders such as memory loss, trembling hand (26–28). Although the presence of NO is crucial for all physiological functions, its overproduction leads to serious adverse reactions, called oxidative stress (26–29, 88–89). For example, during a massive bacterial infection, excess NO produced by phagocytes can cause a dramatic decrease in blood pressure by excessive vasodilatation, which may lead to possibly fatal septic shock. The overproduction of NO in the brain may be involved in the pathogenesis of stroke and other neurodegenerative diseases such as Alzheimer's disease, Parkinson's disease, Huntington's disease, amyotrophic lateral sclerosis (26–29, 88–89). Recent evidence indicates that most of the cytotoxicity attributed to NO is rather due to powerful oxidant peroxynitrite (ONOO−) (26).

In brief, at low or moderate concentrations (nano molar), nitric oxide (NO), a main metabolite of L-arginine, is vital to human health; in contrast, at high levels (micromolar), it becomes harmful to the body through a biochemical process called oxidative stress. Therefore, adequate production of NO from L-arginine is vital for human health, especially in the elderly (6, 26–29, 88–89). Supplementation of L-arginine through food is the best way for the elderly. Consult a specialist or nutritionist if you use L-arginine supplement.

3.3.1.2.1.3 Coenzyme Q10   Coenzyme Q10 (CoQ10) is a coenzyme – an organic, non-protein molecule. Because of its ubiquitous presence in nature and its quinone structure, CoQ10 is also known as ubiquinone. The name coenzyme Q10 derives from its chemical structure, a benzoquinone ring with a side chain composed of ten isoprene units in humans, and from six to ten isoprene units in various animal species. Coenzyme Q10 is a lipophilic molecule and uses lipoprotein mediated transport for circulation. It exists in three oxidation states: the fully reduced form (ubiquinol or CoQ10H2), the radical semiquinone intermediate or partially reduced state or ubisemiquinone (CoQ10H), and the fully oxidized form (ubiquinone) (90–95). First, CoQ10 is a cofactor for mitochondrial enzyme complexes involved in oxidative phosphorylation in the production of adenosine triphosphate (ATP) (90–91). Hence, it has a fundamental role in cellular bioenergetics, which has led to its clinical application in problems involving tissues with high metabolic requirements, such as heart muscle. Second, beyond its role in generating ATP, CoQ10 serves as an antioxidant or free radical scavenger (90). In its reduced form, ubiquinol, it is itself a potent lipophilic antioxidant, and can recycle and regenerate other antioxidants in the body. Numerous other functions of CoQ10 have been described, such as cell signaling, gene expression, and membrane stabilization (90). Every cell in nature, from microorganisms and yeasts to plants, animals, and humans, has the ability to synthesize CoQ10. It is mainly found in the heart and

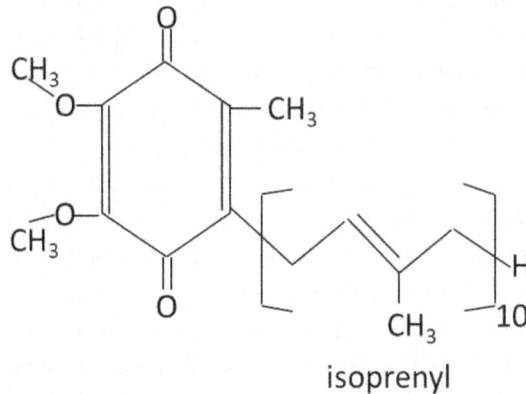

isoprenyl

FIGURE 3.3   cenzyme Q10, Oxidized form of Co10 orUbiquinone,Reduced from of Co10 or Ubiquinol

liver of mammals (cow, pig), the flesh of fish (sardines, mackerel), and the thighs of poultry. It is also abundant in soybean oil, olive oil, grapeseed oil, canola, and in nuts, avocados, and parsley. In humans, CoQ10 is synthesized in all tissues in varying amounts, with the highest concentrations seen in tissues with high energy requirements or metabolic activity, such as the heart, kidney, liver, and muscle. However, endogenous biosynthesis tends to decline with age. So, in humans, CoQ10 has both endogenous and exogenous sources. CoQ10 levels are highest between 20–25 years old, then decline with advancing age, and this decline may contribute in part to some of the manifestations of aging (90–93). Numerous disease processes associated with CoQ10 deficiency can benefit from CoQ10 supplementation, including primary and secondary CoQ10 deficiencies, mitochondrial diseases, cardiovascular diseases (cardiomyopathy, chest pain, heart failure, hypertension), neurodegenerative diseases (Parkinson's disease), aging, cancer, diabetes, male infertility, fibromyalgia, chronic fatigue, and periodontal disease (90–95). CoQ_{10} has also been used to treat muscle pain due to the side effects of statin medications. However, clinical evidence supporting the use of CoQ_{10} supplement in the treatment of statin-induced myopathy is limited and controversial (92). CoQ10 is not considered a dietary essential nutrient because it is synthesized in our body. The best sources of CoQ10 are heart or liver of beef or pork, and some vegetable oils.

Microorganisms that produce CoQ10, including photosynthetic bacteria and yeasts, were selected and used for the fermentation production of CoQ10. In industry, CoQ10 supplement is mainly manufactured by fermentation of yeast (Saccharomyces cerevisiae) and to a smaller extent by bacterial fermentation (95). In Japan, CoQ10 has been regulated as a drug for heart disease therapy.

As CoQ10 is a chiral compound, it occurs in two isomeric forms, namely the 'trans' and the 'cis' forms. The natural endogenous CoQ10 is in the trans form only, whereas the synthetic CoQ10 contains a mixture of both trans- and cis-isomers (94). According to the US Pharmacopoeia (USP), the presence of inactive CoQ10 cis-isomer and other impurities must be less than 1.5% for CoQ10 supplement. Therefore, only CoQ10 supplement products marked 'Conform to USP' on their labels are considered safe to use.

3.3.1.2.1.4 Alpha-Lipoic Acid   A-Lipoic acid (ALA) or thioctic acid is a sulfur-containing endogenous antioxidant, characterized as a 'thiol' or 'biothiol' molecule. ALA is produced naturally by most organisms, including plants, animals, and humans (96–97). ALA is readily absorbed from the diet and is converted rapidly to its reduced form, dihydrolipoic acid (DHLA) (83, 96–97). ALA and DHLA are essential and universal antioxidants for the function of different enzymes that take part in the oxidative metabolism of mitochondria. As ALA and DHLA are both soluble in fat and water, they are capable of quenching free radicals in both these domains. Moreover, they have many other biochemical functions, acting as metal chelators, reducing the oxidized forms of other antioxidant agents such as vitamins C and E and glutathione (GSH), and modulating the signaling transduction of several pathways, like insulin and nuclear factor kappa B (NFkB); also, they do not exhibit any serious side effects (83, 96–97).

The therapeutic action of ALA is based on its antioxidant properties. Studies have shown that ALA has potential therapeutic uses in preventing, reducing or treating many chronic diseases, such as diabetes mellitus type 2, neurodegenerative diseases, CVDs, hypertension, atherosclerosis, osteoporosis, cataracts, glaucoma, anti-aging, autoimmune diseases, cancer and AIDS (83, 96–97).

Due to the presence of asymmetrical carbon atom, ALA and DHLA are chiral compounds and exist only under R-isomer in the body and in foods. Synthetic compounds used as supplements are under racemic form – a mixture of R- and S-isomers – and are less active than natural R-alpha-lipoic acid (96, 97). Recently, some manufacturers can synthetize the active R-isomer alone. Dietary natural R-alpha-lipoic acid (R-ALA) is obtained from both animal and plant sources. R-ALA is found primarily in animal-derived foods, such as red meat and liver, heart, and kidney. The most abundant plant sources of R-ALA are spinach, broccoli, tomatoes, Brussel sprouts, potatoes, garden peas, and rice bran (97). The supplementation of synthetic ALA is not necessary because ALA is produced in humans, animals, and plants. The use of high amounts ALA supplements for the co-treatment of some chronic diseases cited earlier requires the management of a healthcare professional. It has also been suggested that food intake reduces the bioavailability of ALA supplement. Therefore, ALA supplements should be taken 30 minutes before or 2 hours after eating (97).

3.3.1.2.1.5   Uric Acid   Uric acid (UA) is the end of purine metabolism catalyzed by the enzyme xanthine oxidase in the human liver, then excreted in human urine and feces; therefore, uric acid is an endogenous antioxidant (21, 98–99). Purines are found in high amounts in animal food products, such as liver and sardines, and also in moderate quantity in beef, pork, poultry, fish, seafood, and vegetables (asparagus, cauliflower, spinach, mushrooms, green peas, etc.). Due to the presence of double bonds in its chemical structure, uric acid has excellent antioxidant capacity and strong radical scavenging activity (100). Uric acid is the most abundant aqueous antioxidant found in humans and it can be responsible for two thirds of total plasma antioxidant capacity (21, 98–99). Uric acid is a powerful scavenger of carbon-centered radicals and peroxyl (ROO.) radicals in the hydrophilic environment but loses its radical scavenging activity within lipid membranes (21, 98). Moreover, UA is an exceptional scavenger of peroxynitrite (ONOO⁻) in extracellular fluid. However, it is important to note that uric acid cannot scavenge the superoxide anion radical ($O_2^{•-}$) (21). An excess of UA in plasma causes hyperuricemia, which is usually associated with gouty arthritis or nephrolithiasis (formation and deposition of UA crystals in urine and kidneys). The synthesis of fatty acids (triglycerides) in the liver is associated with the de novo synthesis of purine, accelerating UA production. The role played by diet on hyperuricemia has not yet been fully clarified, but high intake of fructose-rich industrialized food and high alcohol intake (particularly beer) seem to influence uricemia. There is still no consensus regarding whether UA is a protective or a risk factor, however, it seems that acute elevation is a protective factor, whereas chronic elevation a risk for disease (99). Some authors suggest that uric acid may function either as an antioxidant (primarily in plasma) or pro-oxidant (primarily within the cell). At high levels of UA, its pro-oxidative effects could engender some diseases such as hypertension, stroke, and obesity (98).

3.3.1.2.1.6   Melatonin   Melatonin (N-acetyl-5-methoxytryptamine) is an indoleamine neuro-hormone, initially found in the pineal gland for the control of circadian rhythms, sleep induction, regulation of seasonal reproduction, and immune enhancement in vertebrates (83, 100–102). Recently, numerous studies have shown the presence of this endogenous antioxidant in other organs, including gut, retina, ovary, testes, bone marrow and lens (100–102). Melatonin has also been identified in bacteria, alga, fungi, and other plants (vegetables, fruit, nuts, cereals), and humans can absorb it via foods (101–102). Nowadays, melatonin has been shown to protect against oxidative stress in various, highly divergent experimental systems (83, 100–102). One major function of melatonin is to scavenge free radicals in oxygen metabolism, thereby potentially protecting against free radical-induced damage to DNA, proteins, and membranes, thus it has the potential to play an important role in the reduction of free radical mediated diseases (83). Signaling effects comprise the upregulation of antioxidant enzymes, such as superoxide dismutases, peroxidases, and enzymes of glutathione supply, down-regulation of pro-oxidant enzymes, such as nitric oxide synthases and lipoxygenases, and presumably also the control of quinone reductase (100). Other mechanisms are based on direct interactions with several reactive oxygen and nitrogen species (101). In humans, melatonin production not only diminishes in the aged but also is significantly lower in many age-related diseases including Alzheimer's disease and cardiovascular disease (102). Melatonin has been and is being used in several clinical trials with different therapeutic approaches such as improvements of sleep, amyotrophic lateral sclerosis, and treatment of neurodegenerative disorders (Alzheimer's disease) (101).

3.3.1.2.1.7 Bilirubin Bilirubin is a major product of heme catabolism in humans and vertebrates. This endogenous process is necessary for the elimination of aged red blood cells (9, 83). Numerous studies have been published showing bilirubin is a strong lipophilic antioxidant that protects cellular membranes from lipid peroxidation (9, 83, 103–104). It is also potent against superoxide and peroxyl radicals for the protection of membrane proteins from oxidation. At physiological plasma concentrations, bilirubin is effective in preventing some chronic diseases such as atherosclerosis, as well as stimulating the immune system and cardiovascular organs including vascular smooth muscle and endothelial cells (9, 83, 103–104). Bilirubin is excreted in bile and urine and its elevated levels are toxic and may indicate certain diseases such as jaundice and hepatitis (9, 83, 103–104).

3.3.1.2.1.8 Carnosine Carnosine or L-carnosine is a dipeptide composed of two amino acids: beta-alanine and L-histidine. It is an endogenous nitrogenous water-soluble compound mainly present in the non-protein fraction of skeletal muscle and other tissues (brain, olfactory epithelium) of humans, mammals, and other vertebrates. Carnosine is an endogenous metabolic antioxidant and a non-enzymatic free radical scavenger in humans. It is also able to inactivate reactive oxygen species and chelate pro-oxidative metals (105–106). Moreover, it is a strong immunomodulator, neuroprotector against free radicals, and may be a good neurotransmitter (106). Recent data report that carnosine is able to rejuvenate senescent cells and can delay eyesight impairment for the prevention and treatment of senile cataract by eye drops (105).

3.3.1.2.1.9 Dehydroepiandrosterone (DHEA) DHEA and its sulfated metabolite, DHEA-S, together represent the most abundant endogenous circulating steroid hormones in the human body. Both DHEA and DHEA-S are produced from cholesterol in the adrenal cortex glands, the gonads (testis, ovary), and the brain (107–110). The body converts them into two other well-known male and female sex hormones, testosterone and estrogen, respectively. The circulating levels of both DHEA and DHEA-S (in plasma and cerebrospinal fluid) peak at about age 25, and then progressively decline with age in both men and women. By age 65 to 75 years, elderly people exhibit 10 to 20% of young adult DHEA levels (107, 109). DHEA is also called juvenile hormone or antiaging agent or 'fountain of youth hormone'.

Some main biological actions of endogenous DHEA and DHEA-S include neuroprotection, neurite (axon, dendrite) growth, and antioxidant effects (107–110). DHEA is a neuro-steroid, and directly affects the brain. It has important effects on neurological and psychological functioning. Its activities are not fully understood, but some researchers believe it helps protect neurons from toxins and after injuries, such as strokes. Despite the considerable increase in DHEA and DHEA-S research in recent years, its role in neuropsychiatric diseases and its place in clinical therapeutics remain uncertain (107).

As an antioxidant, DHEA is able to prevent lipid peroxidation (107). DHEA levels may have implications for Alzheimer's disease, since DHEA was also shown to be neuroprotective against amyloid β protein toxicity *in vitro*; this neuroprotective effect could be due to DHEA's antioxidant effects (107). Recently, some authors suggested that DHEA and DHEA-S may have a role in trauma, sepsis, wound healing and burns (110). However, its physiological significance, its mechanisms of action and its possible roles in human diseases are not well understood (107, 108). In Canada, Australia, and many European countries, DHEA is a prescribed drug; in contrast, it is sold as an over-the-counter supplement in the United States.

3.3.1.2.2. Exogenous Nutrient Antioxidants   The nutrient antioxidants are compounds which cannot be produced or partially produced in the human body and must be provided through natural vegetable and/or animal foods or artificial supplements. The exogenous nutrient antioxidants are divided into two groups: essential nutrient antioxidants and semi-essential nutrient antioxidants. The essential nutrient antioxidants include vitamins, carotenoids, trace metals, and so on. These antioxidants are essential for human life because they are not synthetized in human cells and their absence can cause diseases or even death. Most of them are present in different organs of vegetables, while some others are rich in different organs of animals. The semi-essential group contains substances partially produced in the human body by metabolism or synthesis, but in certain conditions such as aging or illness, they are absent or in very low quantity; therefore a supply of these antioxidants through foods is necessary. They are also called metabolic antioxidants, as cited above, such as L-arginine, coenzyme Q10, and L-carnosine. In nature, there are several hundred antioxidants in plants and animals – only some of them are essential for human life like vitamins, carotenoids, and so on. The others are not considered essential; however, many of them have therapeutic and preventive properties such as polyphenols, flavonoids, and terpenoids. Though the antioxidant groups are different from species to species, the presence of antioxidant defense is universal in all living beings (21, 111–116).

Antioxidants from our diet play an important role not only in helping endogenous antioxidants for the neutralization of oxidative stress, but also in preventing or treating a number of ailments (111–116). The nutrient antioxidant deficiency is one of the causes of numerous chronic and degenerative pathologies such as cancer, cardiovascular diseases, neuro-degenerative diseases, diabetes, arthritis, aging, and ocular diseases. Each nutrient is unique in terms of its structure and antioxidant function (6, 38). Natural antioxidants are very abundant in food (greens, spices, fruits, tubers, animal meat, sea foods, yeasts, algae, mushrooms, honey, etc.) and exist in a multitude of chemical compounds. So, this natural treasure may help us live better. A natural food such as an orange contains not only vitamin C, but also other vitamins, antioxidants, minerals, and coenzymes which exert their action both individually and collectively – synergistically. Some action mechanisms of antioxidants for disease prevention are (115):

- Antioxidant activity through free radical scavenging and reduction of oxidative stress
- Inhibition of cell proliferation and of oncogene expression for cancer prevention
- Anti-angiogenesis for cancer prevention
- Induction of cell differentiation and of apoptosis
- Enhancement of immune functions
- Regulation of steroid hormone and estrogen metabolisms
- Antibacterial and antiviral effects
- Prevention of DNA binding and inhibition of cell adhesion and invasion for cancer prevention (115).

Although there are numerous antioxidants in nature, only the following main dietary antioxidants will be studied: vitamin C, vitamin E, vitamin A, carotenoids (β-carotene, lycopene, lutein, astaxanthin), some flavonoids, terpenoids, and antioxidant minerals (zinc, manganese, iron, and selenium).

3.3.1.2.2.1 Vitamins Vitamins are organic components in food that are needed in very small amounts for growth and for maintaining good health. They are essential for human life. The majority of vitamins are not synthesized by our organism and must be supplied through the diet for maintaining health (111–115). Nowadays, about 13 vitamins are found present in human body including 8 vitamins of group B (B1, B2, B3, B5, B6, B7, B9, B12), vitamin C, vitamin A, vitamin E, vitamin D, and vitamin K. They are divided into two groups: water-soluble vitamins (vitamin C and 8 vitamins of group B) and fat-soluble vitamins (A, D, E, and K). The properties and roles of different vitamins have been described in Chapter 2 of this book. Only three vitamins endowed with antioxidant properties, namely vitamins C, E and A are described below.

3.3.1.2.2.1.1 Vitamin C Vitamin C also known as L-ascorbic acid is a water-soluble vitamin, a strong antioxidant, a good reducing agent, and an important chiral molecule. Only the levorotary (L) isomer of vitamin C is active and present in humans, animals, and plants. The other dextrorotary (D) isomer or D-enantiomer is not found in nature, but only obtained by artificial synthesis and has far less vitamin activity than the L-isomer (6, 115–118). Vitamin C is easily oxidized by air and heat to become inactive. Therefore, foodstuffs containing vitamin C must be consumed in whole original form. For example, vitamin C in orange fruit is more abundant and active than its corresponding processed foods such as orange juice.

Vitamin C is best known for its role as the primary small molecule antioxidant in aqueous environments. Here it assists other enzymatic and nonenzymatic components of the antioxidant defense system in providing protection against free radical-mediated attack, in an effort to minimize oxidative stress (117). As a potent water-soluble antioxidant acting within plasma, vitamin C is a strong free radical scavenger, quenching an array of aqueous reactive oxygen species, namely hydroxyl, alkoxyl, peroxyl, superoxide anion, hydroperoxyl radicals, and reactive nitrogen radicals such as nitrogen dioxide, nitroxide, and peroxynitrite, leaking from activated neutrophils and macrophages, as well as other lipid peroxidation products (117–118). In addition, vitamins C can regenerate other antioxidants such as α-tocopherol, urate, and β-carotene radical cation from their radical species. It also transforms the catalytic metallic ions (iron, copper) of specific biosynthetic enzymes under their reduced forms (117–118). Thus, ascorbic acid is a co-antioxidant for vitamin E (α-tocopherol) and both vitamins C and E play a key role as chain breaking antioxidants during lipid peroxidation, acting in both the aqueous and lipid phase, respectively (117–118).

In brief, due to its highly effective antioxidant properties, vitamin C can protect proteins, enzymes, lipids, carbohydrates, and nucleic acids (DNA and RNA) from damage by free radicals. Apart from its antioxidant roles, other health benefits of vitamin C are anti-inflammatory, anti-angiogenic, anti-atherogenic, anti-carcinogenic, and immunomodulatory (6, 115–118). In addition, vitamin C could reduce the incidence of stomach cancer and might prevent lung, prostate, esophagus, pharynx, and cervical cancer (112, 117). However, vitamin C, under certain conditions such as the intake of high doses of vitamin C supplement and/or in the presence of free transition metals such as copper and iron, may function as a pro-oxidant (117–118). Metal ions are indeed reduced by ascorbate and, in turn, may react with hydrogen peroxide leading to the formation of highly reactive and damaging hydroxyl radicals (118). The pro-oxidant activity of vitamin C leads to the formation of ROS or glycated proteins (118). The intake of high doses of vitamin C supplement has been the subject of debate for its eventual pro-oxidant or carcinogen property (6, 112, 117–118). The use of vitamin C for the treatment of human diseases, as well as for prevention of disease development is a subject of many scientific debates. Some scientists suggest that vitamin C (and other antioxidants) are mischaracterized by describing them solely as antioxidants. They are in fact redox agents, antioxidants in some circumstances (like the physiological quantities found in food), and pro-oxidants (producing billions of harmful free radicals) in other cases (often so in the pharmacologic quantities found in ill-designed supplements) (117). Therefore, the use of high doses of vitamin C supplement as well as other antioxidant vitamins (A, E, carotenes) must be prudent because they become pro-oxidant compounds which are harmful to DNA and other cell constituents. In contrast, some studies on healthy human volunteers found that consuming fruits and vegetables rich in vitamin C decreased levels of oxidative DNA damage and may prevent cancer (112, 117). Recent studies suggest that well-known antioxidants (vitamin E, C, beta carotene) contribute a relatively small portion of all total antioxidants. It should be noted that the protective effect of a certain diet is not equivalent to the protective effect of antioxidants in the diet (117). Positive effects of the protective substances that originate from food are greater because of the synergic activity between individual antioxidant substances (vitamins, minerals, polyphenols, terpenoids, etc.), nutritional fibers, and secondary vegetal and animal substances (sugars, proteins, enzymes, cofactors, fats, etc.). The thesis that the pro-oxidant effect of vitamin C depends on its unbalance with other antioxidants, minerals, and other nutrients, among them many still unknown, opens many questions regarding the best way to minimize oxidative damage through food intake (117). Therefore, the choice of the diet for the maximal obtention of essential macro and micronutrients is the best way to maintain health and prevent disease. Vitamin supplements are only necessary in specific diseases due to vitamin deficiency and must be used in a defined period. Other roles, dosage and dietary source of vitamin C have been described in Chapter 2 of this book.

3.3.1.2.2.1.2   Vitamin E   Vitamin E is a fat-soluble vitamin and consists of four tocopherols and four tocotrienols. The main biological functions of vitamin E in humans are antioxidant and enzymatic activities (119–120). Alpha-Tocopherol (αT) is the predominant form of vitamin E in tissues and its deficiency leads to ataxia in humans. All tocopherols and tocotrienols are potent antioxidants with lipoperoxyl radical scavenging activities. As an antioxidant, vitamin E acts as a peroxyl radical scavenger, inhibiting the production of free radicals in tissues and terminating the lipid peroxidation chain reactions. Due to its fatty solubility, this efficient antioxidant functions as a 'chain breaker' during lipid peroxidation in cell membranes and various lipid particles including low-density lipoprotein (21, 119–120). Vitamin E can be incorporated into cell membranes by protecting them from oxidative damage. Its antioxidant properties are due to its phenolic hydroxyl group, which provides hydrogen to peroxyl radicals, resulting in the formation of stable lipid species (111, 119–120). As an enzymatic activity regulator, α-tocopherol inhibits the activity of protein kinase C (PKC), an enzyme involved in cell proliferation and differentiation in smooth muscle cells, platelets, and monocytes. It has a stimulatory effect on the dephosphorylation enzyme, protein phosphatase 2A, which in turn, cleaves phosphate groups from PKC, leading to its deactivation, bringing the smooth muscle growth to a halt (111, 120). In addition, it is also involved in immune function, cell signaling, regulation of gene expression, and other metabolic processes (119–120).

Due to its high antioxidant activity, vitamin E has been proposed for prevention against colon, prostate and breast cancers, some cardiovascular diseases, ischemia, cataract, arthritis and certain neurological disorders (6, 119–120). However, a recent meta-analysis suggests that alpha-tocopherol supplements may actually increase all-cause mortality; however, the mechanism for this increased risk is unknown (120).

The deficiency of vitamin E is rare and can be due to two causes: not consuming a certain food rich in vitamin E, or poor fat absorption, because this vitamin needs fat to be absorbed in the intestine under micelle particles (120). Moreover, vitamin E levels can fall due to a zinc deficiency (111). Cooking and storage may destroy natural vitamin E in foods (6). Other roles, dietary source, dosage, and side effects of vitamin E such as stroke have been described in Chapter 2 of this book.

3.3.1.2.2.1.3   Vitamin A and Carotenes   Two forms of vitamin A are available in the human diet: preformed vitamin A or retinoids and provitamin A carotenoids (114, 121–122). Preformed vitamin A is a group of fat-soluble unsaturated nutritional compounds called retinoids, including retinol, retinal, retinoic acid, and retinyl esters (111, 121–122). Provitamin A carotenoids are mainly formed by beta-carotene and two other, less important, carotenes, namely alpha-carotene and beta-cryptoxanthin, present mainly in persimmon fruits and leaves (114, 121). The body converts these plant pigments, carotenes, into vitamin A. Both retinoids and provitamin A carotenoids are converted to retinol, which is oxidized to retinal and then to retinoic acid, the active forms of vitamin A, to support the vitamin's important biological functions (114, 121–122). Vitamin A is an essential micronutrient for vision, immune function, reproduction, fetal development, epithelial cell integrity, lipid metabolism, cellular communication, spermatogenesis, cellular proliferation, bone growth, and so on (111, 121–122). Vitamin A is also an important antioxidant, a property shared with vitamins E and C, respectively (121). As a good antioxidant, vitamin A eliminates free radicals and protects the DNA from their mutagenic action, thus continuing to halt cellular aging. Its oxygen sensitivity is due to the large amount of double bonds present in their structure. Its biological activity is attributed to all-trans retinol (111). Antioxidant activity of vitamin A, retinoids, and β-carotene in small doses showed anti-cancer effect. It appears to stem from its ability to scavenge for reactive oxygen species (ROS) and can improve immune function in addition to eliciting an anti-proliferative effect through the retinoic acid receptor (RAR) and retinoid X receptor (RXR). ROS are the most important free radicals in biological systems and the most harmful byproducts generated during normal cellular functions. In this way, they can block certain carcinogenic processes and thus inhibit tumor cell growth (121–122).

Among the functions attributed to β-carotene and carotenoids are: inhibition of tumor growth, protection against genotoxicity, and modulation of the immune system (114). The antioxidant properties of β-carotene and carotenoids are particularly important in protecting lipids and can act in conjunction with vitamin E in preventing lipid peroxidation, being fat-soluble compounds. Carotenoids may also act to protect DNA against the action of free radicals and stimulating repair mechanisms (114).

New biological functions of vitamin A such as lipid metabolism, insulin response, energy balance, and the nervous system, are continuously being discovered. Detailed roles, dosage, side effects, dietary sources of vitamin A and β-carotene are described in Chapter 2 of this book.

3.3.1.2.2.2 Carotenoids   Carotenoids are a family of naturally occurring organic pigmented compounds that are produced by fungi, several bacteria, and plastids of algae and plants (123). More than 600 carotenoids have been identified in nature. However, only about 50 carotenoids are found in a typical human diet. Carotenoids are divided into two main groups, namely carotenes and xanthophylls, according to their chemical constituents (123). The first group includes all unsaturated hydrocarbon compounds containing only carbon and hydrogen atoms, such as α-, β-, δ-, γ- carotenes and lycopene. The second big carotenoid-group is constituted of xanthophylls or oxy-carotenoids, which contain oxygen in their structure, such as lutein, β-cryptoxanthin, astaxanthin, zeaxanthin, fucoxanthin, and more. Due to a long chain adjacent with multiple conjugated double bonds in their chemical structure, carotenoids are known as a strong quencher of singlet oxygen and a potent scavenger of free radicals (123). They can protect the body against oxidative stress that is the cause of numerous chronic ailments such as cancer, CVDs, aging, eye diseases, neurodegenerative diseases, and inflammatory diseases. However, most carotenoids, except β-carotene, are considered nonessential micronutrients. Some main carotenoids are cited as follows.

3.3.1.2.2.2.1 Lycopene   Lycopene is a carotenoid possessing antioxidant and anti-proliferative properties (124–130). Lycopene is an acyclic isomer of beta-carotene, but cannot convert to vitamin A due to the lack of a terminal β-ionone ring; so, it is not a provitamin A (124–129).

Lycopene is a tetraterpene hydrocarbon containing 40 carbon atoms and 56 hydrogen atoms. It is also a highly unsaturated compound due to a straight chain hydrocarbon containing 11 conjugated and two non-conjugated double bonds. Thanks to the presence of numerous conjugated double bonds in its chemical structure, lycopene possesses strong antioxidant activity (124–129). It is a natural red pigment synthesized by plants and microorganisms (126). Lycopene is a non-essential micronutrient, contrary to beta-carotene. As a polyene, lycopene undergoes cis-trans isomerization induced by light, thermal energy, or chemical reactions (125). Lycopene from natural plant sources such as tomato exists predominantly in trans-configuration, the most thermodynamically stable form (125–126). The lycopene isomers found in human blood plasma, liver, testes, prostate tissue, adrenal glands, adipose tissues, breastmilk, and human tissues are mainly of the cis-isomer type (124–127). However, trans-isomer lycopene also exists, but in smaller amounts, in the human body. This observation suggests that tissue isomerases might be involved in *in vivo* isomerization of lycopene from all *trans* to *cis* form. It is hypothesized that prostate cancer patients perhaps lack the ability to isomerize dietary lycopene and therefore do not absorb it efficiently (127). The biological significance of these isomers of lycopene is still unclear. Lycopene, ingested in its natural trans form found in tomatoes, for example, is poorly absorbed. Recent studies have shown that heat processing of tomatoes and tomato products induces isomerization of lycopene to the cis form which in turn increases its bioavailability (124–127).

Due to the presence of numerous conjugated double bonds in its straight chain hydrocarbon, lycopene is known to be the most potent oxygen quenching reagent among carotenoids (124–126, 128–129). Antioxidant activity of lycopene is superior to α-tocopherol and β-carotene. The system of conjugated double bonds allows lycopene molecules to efficiently quench different deleterious forms of oxygen (singlet oxygen) and to scavenge a large spectrum of free radicals, like OH^- or peroxyl radicals (125–126, 128). Lycopene has been reported to deactivate *in vitro* an array of free radicals, such as hydrogen peroxide, nitrogen dioxide, thyl, and sulphonyl (128). It has also been suggested that lycopene might act as an antioxidant in vivo by repairing vitamin E and vitamin C radicals. It can stimulate the production of cellular enzymes such as superoxide dismutase, glutathione S-transferase, and quinone (126). So, lycopene should be able to protect against oxidative stress, a deleterious phenomenon which can cause cancer and other chronic diseases such as CVDs, aging, neurodegenerative diseases, and inflammatory diseases. As lycopene exists in cis- or/and trans-isomer forms, the antioxidant potential of lycopene also depends on its isomer form. It is reported that 5-cis lycopene has been found to be most potent, followed by 9-cis lycopene. The weakest antioxidant properties have been reported for the all-trans isomer (125). Therefore, the antioxidant potential of lycopene depends on its cis-isomer concentrations, and also on the involvement of tissue isomerases in the body to transform all trans isomer into cis form, since lycopene in fresh fruits and vegetables are almost all in trans isomer form (129). In addition, cooking or processing can transform trans into cis form.

Several studies based on in vitro and animal experiments have demonstrated the anti-proliferative properties of lycopene on prostate cancer cells, and other cancer cells like breast or lung cancer. However, its anticancer activity in humans is still not clearly proven and remains controversial (124–130). These experimental findings demonstrate that lycopene not only enhances the antioxidant response of prostate cells, but that it is even able to inhibit proliferation, induce apoptosis, and decrease the metastatic capacity of prostate cancer cells (125). However, there is still no clearly proven clinical evidence supporting the use of lycopene supplement in the prevention or treatment of prostate cancer or other cancer forms. In contrast, dietary intakes of tomatoes and tomato products containing lycopene have been shown to be associated with decreased risk of chronic diseases such as cancer, aging, and cardiovascular diseases in several recent studies (124, 127). Serum and tissue lycopene levels have also been inversely related with the chronic disease risk. Although the antioxidant properties of lycopene are thought to be primarily responsible for its beneficial properties, evidence is accumulating to suggest other mechanisms such as modulation of intercellular gap junction communication – hormonal and immune system and metabolic pathways may also be involved (127). In addition, lycopene can also inhibit cell invasion, angiogenesis, and metastasis. Despite these promising reports, it is difficult at the moment to directly relate available experimental data to human pathophysiology. More well controlled clinical intervention trials are needed to further clarify the exact role of lycopene in the prevention of lung cancer cell growth and other cancer forms (128). The benefits of lycopene supplementation in prostate cancer patients are still not evident (130). Consumption of processed tomato products like tomato juice and ketchup, containing lycopene, is the best way to prevent oxidative stress and carcinogenesis in healthy and Type 2 diabetic patients, as well as prostate cancer patients (129).

As a fat-soluble compound, lycopene is mainly distributed to fatty tissues and stocked in different organs such as the adrenal glands, liver, prostate, and testes. Lycopene absorption is greatly affected by dietary composition. Due to its lipophile property, lycopene is easily absorbed in the digestive tract in the presence of fat compounds. For example, consuming salads with full-fat dressing results in higher blood carotenoid levels than eating salads with reduced fat dressing (124). Lycopene is nontoxic and is commonly found in the diet, but excessive carotenoid intake can cause yellow coloration of the skin temporarily. Some cases of allergic reaction to dietary lycopene are also reported, with symptoms such as diarrhea, nausea, stomach pain or cramps, gas, vomiting, and loss of appetite (124).

Red or pink fruits are generally high in lycopene; some of them ranged in descending order are as follows: gac (*Momordica cochinchinensis*), tomatoes, watermelon, rosehip, cherry, papaya, pink guava, strawberry, pomegranate, pink grapefruit, persimmon, and autumn olive (124–125, 128). Gac fruit, originally from Southeast Asia, mostly in Vietnam, hence its name, is the richest fruit in lycopene. However, tomato is the most lycopene-rich fruit consumed in the world, either as fresh fruit or as processed foods like ketchup sauce or tomato juice. The amount of lycopene present in processed foods is often much higher than that found in fresh foods given that processing often involves concentration via water loss. For example, ketchup contains 9.9–13.44 mg lycopene/100 g, whereas fresh tomatoes contain anywhere from 0.88–7.74 mg lycopene/100 g wet weight (124). Animals cannot synthesize lycopene and this carotenoid is not an essential nutrient, contrary to beta-carotene, a precursor of vitamin A.

Briefly, lycopene is a strong antioxidant and can inhibit prostate or lung cancer cells in in vitro and animal experiments. However, lycopene is still not proven to treat prostate cancer and other cancer forms in humans. Consuming fruits and vegetables rich in lycopene may prevent chronic ailments.

3.3.1.2.2.2.2 Lutein and Zeaxanthin Lutein and its isomer zeaxanthin belong to the xanthophyll family of carotenoids or oxy-carotenoids, which contain oxygen in their structure, contrary to the carotenes, and lycopene, which are strictly hydrocarbons (131–134). They are synthesized only by plants. Animals obtain them from plants and stock them in different organs. Lutein and zeaxanthin are yellow or orange pigments present in various common foods such as kale, spinach, parsley, peas, lettuce, squash, edamame beans, sprouts, pistachio, cantaloupe, corn, carrots, orange pepper, kiwi fruit, grapes, orange juice, zucchini, broccoli, pasta, egg yolk, fish, salmon, and animal fats (131–134). There is 44 mg of lutein per cup of cooked kale, 26 mg/cup of cooked spinach, and 3 mg/cup of broccoli (133). In humans and primates, lutein and zeaxanthin are accumulated in the retina and the macula of the eyes. Zeaxanthin predominates at the macula lutea while lutein predominates elsewhere in the retina (131–133).

The role of lutein and zeaxanthin in human health, in particular eye health and disease, is well established from experimental, clinical, and epidemiological studies (131–134). They constitute the main pigments found in the yellow spot of the human retina which protect the macula from damage by blue light, improve visual acuity, and scavenge harmful reactive oxygen species. They have also been linked to reduced risk of age-related macular degeneration (AMD) and cataracts (131–134). The relationship between lutein and zeaxanthin and visual and cognitive health is irrefutable because they are destinated selectively to eye and brain tissue. Moreover, their beneficial effects are thought to be attributable to their antioxidant and anti-inflammatory properties because they can neutralize free radicals engendered by blue light in the eye. In pediatric brains, lutein is found in twice greater amounts than in adult brains. It is suggested that lutein is needed for neural development. In adults, lutein is necessary for cognitive performance (132).

Structurally, the difference between lutein and zeaxanthin is in the type of ionone ring; lutein contains a β-ionone ring and a ε-ionone ring, whereas zeaxanthin has two β-ionone rings. Lutein and zeaxanthin are isomers, but not stereoisomers, which differ in the location of a double bond unsaturation in the end ring (134). Lutein can exist in eight possible stereoisomeric forms because of three chiral centers, but in nature it exists mainly in Z (*cis*)-form (R,R,R). Zeaxanthin, on the other hand, has two chiral centers but, because of symmetry, exists only in three stereoisomeric forms: (R,R), (S,S), and (R,S-meso) (134). The strong antioxidant activity of lutein and zeaxanthin is due to numerous conjugated double bonds in their lateral chain. Lutein and zeaxanthin are fat-soluble molecules and are generally insoluble in water.

In brief, lutein and zeaxanthin are strong antioxidants and are considered protector agents of eyes, especially the retina and its macula (131–134). They are also necessary for brain development in babies and cognitive function in adults. It has been suggested that six to eight mg of lutein per day, either through diet or supplements, is likely effective in protecting or reducing the risk of cataracts and age-related macular degeneration (AMD) in both healthy individuals or patients with eye disease (131–133).

3.3.1.2.2.2.3 Astaxanthin

Astaxanthin (AST) is a xanthophyll carotenoid like lutein and zeaxanthin which cannot convert to vitamin A. It is not a provitamin A. Astaxanthin, a red-orange pigment, is a strong biological antioxidant that occurs naturally in a wide variety of living organisms, primarily in marine organisms like microalgae, salmon, trout, shrimp, krill, krill oil, lobster, crab, prawn, crayfish, fish eggs, and so on (135–142).

Astaxanthin is synthetized by algae, bacteria, fungi, yeast, and some plants. Marine animals such as fish and crustaceans consume algae, therefore they accumulate astaxanthin in their body, giving them the reddish color which brightens the flesh, skin, or exoskeleton of animals, such as crabs, crayfish, krill, lobsters, salmon, shrimp, and trout (135). As AST is a red-orange pigment present in the shells of crustaceans and in the meat of some fishes, it provides the red color of salmon meat and cooked shellfish (142). AST may also be found in the feathers of birds, such as flamingoes and storks. It is also obtained by chemical synthesis and used as a colorant in aquaculture of salmon. The human body does not make astaxanthin, and ingested astaxanthin cannot be converted to vitamin A; excessive intake of astaxanthin will thus not cause hypervitaminosis A (135). Green microalgae comprise more than 7,000 species growing in a variety of habitats worldwide. The most known are *Haematococcus pluvialis*, *Chlorella zofingiensis*, *Chlorococcum sp.*, *Botryococcus braunii*, and the red yeast *Phaffia rhodozyma*. The unicellular microalga *Haematococcus pluvialis* is considered the richest source of astaxanthin and has the highest capacity to accumulate astaxanthin – up to 4–5% of cell dry weight (135–142).

Astaxanthin is a potent quencher of free radicals and reactive oxygen and nitrogen species. It is a powerful antioxidant and anti-inflammatory agent, and has potential health-promoting effects in the prevention and treatment of various human diseases (135–142). AST antioxidant activities toward peroxyl radicals are more potent than those of lutein, lycopene, α-carotene, β-carotene, α-tocopherol (vitamin E), and vitamin C. Precisely, AST is 65 times more powerful than vitamin C, 54 times stronger than β-carotene, ten times more potent than canthaxantin, zeaxanthin, lutein, and 100 times more effective than vitamin E (136–137).

Numerous studies have shown that astaxanthin may prevent and treat a large range of diseases, such as cancers, neurodegenerative diseases (Parkinson's disease, Alzheimer's disease, depression, aging), cardiovascular diseases (atherosclerosis, hypertension), chronic inflammatory diseases (asthma), liver diseases, eye diseases (cataract, glaucoma, age-related macular degeneration), gastrointestinal diseases, skin diseases, metabolic syndrome, diabetes, nephropathy, and male infertility (135–142). The anti-inflammatory activity of astaxanthin may also have a role in the prevention or treatment of asthma. It has been reported that ginkgolide B, astaxanthin, or their combination could suppress activation of T cells from asthma patients (136). In numerous animal trials in diverse species, natural AST in esterified form has demonstrated superior efficacy in extending lifespan, treating skin cancer, preventing the formation of gastric ulcers, improving resistance to stress, decreasing reactive oxygen species (ROS), increasing retinol conversion in the liver, augmenting enzyme levels, increasing growth rates, and improving exercise endurance (142). Astaxanthin has a wide range of applications in the food, feed, aquaculture (as food colorant), cosmetic, nutraceutical, and pharmaceutical industries.

Astaxanthin contains two chiral centers and can exist in three different stereoisomers: (3S, 3'S), (3R, 3'S), and (3R, 3'R) (137). Natural astaxanthin obtained from the microalga *Haematococcus pluvialis* biosynthesis contains about 100% S enantiomer, predominantly the 3S, 3'S stereoisomer, the most valuable one (137, 142). In contrast, artificial AST, prepared by chemical synthesis from asta-C15-triaryl-phosphonium salt and the C10-dialdehyde in a Wittig reaction, is a mixture of three different enantiomers with a ratio of 1:2:1. Precisely, artificial synthetic AST contains 25% 3S,3'S (the natural form), 50% meso-astaxanthin comprised of the 3R,3'S enantiomer and 25% pure 'R' enantiomer 3R,3'R (137, 142). Indeed, natural AST has 14 to 90 times greater antioxidant capacity than its synthetic counterpart (137, 142). In addition, there are concerns about the safety of using synthetic AST for direct human consumption due not only to the difference between stereoisomer forms of synthetic and natural compounds, but also to the presence of harmful synthesis intermediates or impurities. Currently, over 95% of the AST available in the market is produced synthetically; while natural AST sourced from microalgae corresponds to <1% of the commercialized sources, and is mainly used as nutrient supplement for humans (137). AST is a promising natural antioxidant for the prevention and treatment of numerous ailments; more epidemiological and clinical investigations are needed to confirm some preliminary results cited in the scientific literature. Although numerous health claims of AST appear in the literature, the therapeutic potential of this natural antioxidant in humans remains to be established (139). More controls by healthcare offices are necessary to avoid the use of synthetic AST for supplement preparation. It is of note that the therapeutic effects of AST supplement are still not approved by healthcare organizations like FDA or WHO.

3.3.1.2.2.2.4 Fucoxanthin   Fucoxanthin, a cousin of astaxanthin, is oil-soluble and is a red or orange-colored pigment belonging to tetraterpenoid of carotenoid group. It is isolated from edible brown seaweeds (algae), but is not found in green and red seaweeds (143–144). It is also found in diatoms (unicellular microalgae) and dinoflagellates (marine plankton). Some brown algae, such as wakame (*Undaria pinnatifida*) and kombu (*Laminaria japonica*), are commonly consumed in Japan and East Asia (144).

Recent studies have reported that fucoxanthin has many physiological functions and biological properties, such as antioxidant, anti-inflammatory, anticancer, anti-obesity, anti-diabetes activities, as well as hepatic, cardiovascular, and cerebrovascular protective effects (143–144). Due to being a strong scavenger of free radicals, fucoxanthin exerts tumor inhibitory effects in various cancer cells and mouse models such as colon, liver, prostate, or breast cancer (144). Many studies have demonstrated its anti-obesity and anti-diabetic effects in animals. Fucoxanthinol, a metabolite of fucoxanthin, also showed activity against colon and breast cancer cells *in vitro*. Therefore, fucoxanthin can be used as both a medicinal and a nutritional ingredient to prevent and treat chronic diseases. However, some studies have indicated that its structure can be unstable (143). More research is needed in the future regarding the promise of fucoxanthin. Consuming comestible brown algae may be helpful to the health.

3.3.1.2.2.3 Flavonoids   Flavonoids are polyphenolic compounds endowed with strong antioxidant properties. They are present in only plants, algae, and fungi (6, 145–158). Flavonoids are ubiquitous in various organs of most plants such as leaves, fruits, barks, peels, flowers, roots, and tubers.

Flavonoids belong to a large group of phenolic plant constituents. Phenolic compounds include mono-phenolic acids and polyphenolic compounds. Mono-phenolic acids or phenolic acids contain one phenol group and one carboxylic group in their chemical structure such as mono hydroxybenzoic acid – in food, mono hydroxycinnamic acid (147). In contrast, polyphenolics have many phenol groups in their chemical structure and are divided into two categories: flavonoids and non-flavonoid polyphenols in food.

Over 4,000 flavonoid structures have been identified among 8,000 to 10,000 phenolic compounds currently known in plant sources (145, 147–148). Among different secondary metabolites of plants, flavonoid and phenolic compounds represent the third largest group of natural products, following the alkaloids (12,000) and terpenoids (30,000–60,000) (149). These polyphenols have a wide variety of physiological functions in plants ranging from affecting plant pigmentation, flavor, growth, and reproduction, to providing an innate immunity and resistance against pathogens (bacterial, fungal and viral) and also protection against herbivores and insects. Flavonoids are also involved in electron transport during photosynthesis, acting as an antioxidant against the effects of air, ultraviolet light. Flavonoids are vital for almost all plants. Thanks to these compounds produced by plants for their self-defense, humans have discovered that natural flavonoids are also beneficial for their health by preventing or treating diseases. Recently, many studies have shown that flavonoids exhibit biological and pharmacological activities, including antioxidant, anticancer, antiviral, antibacterial, anti-parasitic, anti-malarial, anti-fungal, anti-inflammatory, anti-asthmatic, anti-allergic, antidiabetic, anti-gout, anti-angiogenic, anti-hypertensive, anti-histaminic, anti-obesity, anti-platelet, anti-spasmodic, antithrombotic, anti-arrhythmic, cardioprotective, hepatoprotective, neuroprotective, hypolipidemic, immunosuppressant, hypnotic, anxiolytic, and anti-steroidal properties(6, 145–162). The strong antioxidant properties of flavonoids are well-known due to their phenol groups and their specific chemical structures. Thanks to these properties, flavonoids can prevent cancer and inflammation and protect heart, brain, vessels, and the liver against oxidative stress (145–160). The antibacterial, antiviral, anti-fungal and anti-parasitic effects of flavonoids have been demonstrated by many recent experimental and clinical assays (145, 151–152, 155, 160–161). These properties may be used to prepare biopesticides that can protect plants against fungi, bacteria, and parasites, and at the same time can protect environmental and human health. All these effects depend on each flavonoid type and each plant variety. A plant organ can furnish one or many different flavonoid types.

Flavonoids are low molecular weight compounds composed of a three-ring structure with various substitutions (145–153). This basic structure is comprised of two benzene rings (A and B) linked through a heterocyclic pyran or pyrone (with a double bond) ring (C) in the middle. Flavonoids can be subdivided according to the presence of an oxy group at position 4, a double bond between carbon atoms 2 and 3, or a hydroxyl group in position 3 of the C (middle) ring. According to their chemical structures, flavonoids are usually subdivided into eight sub-groups: flavones, flavonols, flavanones, flavanonols, flavanols or flavan-3-ols, isoflavones, anthocyanidins, and chalcones (145–160). These compounds exist in plants usually as glycoside forms (e.g., glucosides, rhamnoglucosides, and rutinosides). They are found not only in our daily diet (fruits, vegetables, grains, seeds, bark, herbs, roots, flowers, stems, and spices) but also through drinking beverages such as honey, wine, chocolate, tea, and coffee (145–160).

Flavones include apigenin, chrysin, diosmin, luteolin, and tangeritin and are mainly found in apple skins, celery, carrot, honey, and propolis, to name a few.

Flavonols are derivatives of flavones with a hydroxyl (OH) group at C3 and include quercetin, kaempferol, myricetin, galangin, fisetin, robinin, rhamnetin, spirenoside, and rutin. They are mainly found in broccoli, grapes, olive, olive oil, honey, lesser galangal, onion, red wine, berries, grapefruit, walnut, caper, fennel, *Ginkgo biloba* leaves, and nuts. Flavonols are the most widespread compounds in the human diet. Some of these compounds are more predominant than others in each plant type. For example, galangin is mainly found in the rhizome of lesser galangal and not in broccoli, olive, walnut, or grapefruit, while quercetin levels are high in caper, fennel, and onion, low in broccoli and olive fruit, and absent in galangal rhizome.

Flavanones comprise naringenin, naringin, hesperetin, hesperidin, eriodictyol and are present in citrus fruit and peel, such as grapefruits, lemon, orange, mandarin, clementine.

Flavanonols are derivatives of flavanones with a hydroxyl (OH) group at C3 and include taxifolin or dihydroquercetin and aromadendrin or dihydrokaempferol. Taxifolin is found in some conifers in Russia, and the Chinese yew plant named *Taxus chinensis*. Taxifolin, extracted from *Taxus Chinensis*, is used against cancer. Aromadendrin is found in citrus fruits and some Siberian pines. Taxifolin is also found in citrus fruits, onion, and milk thistle (147, 151–152).

Flavanols or flavan-3-ols are often commonly called catechins. They are known as the major building blocks of tannins (150). They constitute a greatly complex group of polyphenols in the range from the monomeric flavan-3-ols (e.g., catechin, epicatechin, epigallocatechin, epigallocat-echin gallate) to oligomeric proanthocyanidins (OPC) known as condensed tannins, while theafla-vins and thearubigins are the dimers of gallocatechins and are formed during the preparation of black tea by fermentation. Flavanols are abundant in tea leaves, cocoa, chocolate, honey, red wine, grapes, apples, persimmon, apricots, peach, kiwi, blackberry and cereals (147–149, 162). Many *in vitro* animal and human studies have reported that green tea or its catechins may prevent cancer development, reduce cholesterol levels and hypertension, protect against neurodegenerative dis-eases, improve dental health, and more. Although the antioxidant potential of green tea is evident, the results from clinical and epidemiological studies of the relationship between green tea and pre-vention of these diseases in humans are mixed (162).

Proanthocyanidins are traditionally considered to be condensed tannins (147, 163). The building blocks of proanthocyanidins include catechin and epicatechin (163). Proanthocyanidins are oligo-mers or polymers of a basic flavan-3-ol unit, with an average degree of polymerization between 4 and 11 to form tannins (163–164). Oligomeric proanthocyanidins (OPCs) are also called condensed tannins, procyanidolic oligomers (PCOs), leucoanthocyanins, and pycnogenols. Pycnogenol is a trade name for an OPC extract from the pine bark isolated by French scientist Jacques Masquelier in 1953 (164). Oligomeric and polymeric proanthocyanidins are present in flowers, nuts, fruits, bark, and seeds of various plants, as a defense against biotic and abiotic stressors. Their astringency pro-tects the plants from pathogens and predators. They are mainly found in apples, grapes, grape seeds, wine, cranberries, and the leaves of bilberry, birch, ginkgo, hawthorn, and the barks of pine (163–164). Due to potent antioxidant activity, proanthocyanidins and OPCs have different pharmaco-logical properties such as antimicrobial, disinfection, anti-parasite, anti-obesity, anti-inflammation, anti-carcinogenicity, vasodilation, neuroprotection, for the prevention and eventual treatment of several diseases (163–164). They can inhibit lipid peroxidation and platelet aggregation. Plant tan-nins are also used to tan animal skins for leather production since antiquity.

Anthocyanidins are natural flavonoid pigments responsible for blue, red, purple, and orange colors present in many fruits and vegetables. Over 500 different anthocyanidins are known in dif-ferent plants (148, 150). The main anthocyanidins are cyanidin, delphinidin, pelargonidin, peonidin, malvidin, apigenidin, and petunidin. They are present in grapes, berries, cherries, apples, nuts, olive oil, cocoa, teas, honey, red wine, and more. Anthocyanins are the glycosides of anthocyanidins – of polyhydroxy and polymethoxy derivatives of flavilium salts – and are members of the flavonoid family (165). In plants, anthocyanins are more stable than anthocyanidins which are produced from proanthocyanidins. On heating in acidic media, proanthocyanidins generate anthocyanins (163). Plants typically produce anthocyanins as a protective mechanism against environmental stress fac-tors, such as UV light, cold temperatures, and drought (165). Anthocyanins are strong antioxidants and protect the body against oxidative stress. Epidemiological studies suggest that increased intake of anthocyanins lowers the risk of cardiovascular disease (165).

Isoflavones are a very distinctive subgroup of flavonoids and include genistein, daidzein, and glycetein. They are mainly found in beans, especially in soybean, tofu, apples, onions, peas, and leguminous plants (147–148, 151). They can act as phytoestrogens in mammals because of their estrogenic activity (147, 151).

Chalcones are aromatic ketone, in which two aromatic rings are linked by a three carbon α, β-unsaturated carbonyl system. They are precursors of flavanones and other flavonoids by chal-cone isomerase in plants. They include phloretin and phloridzin and are abundant in edible plants such as Chinese angelica (*Angelica sinensis* or Dong Quai), ashitaba (*Angelica keiskei koidzumi*) discovered in Japan, apples and peels, ciders, hops and beers. Ashitaba is a species of the celery family. Its stems have a thick yellow juice containing chalcones which is unique to this strain of angelica. Angelica herbs are considered to be anti-aging by Chinese and Japanese medicines (166). The chalcones in ashitaba are known as xanthoangelol, xanthoangelol-E, and 4-hydrooxyderricin, and were discovered by Japanese researchers. All chalcones are strong antioxidants and pos-sess a wide range of biological activities: anti-inflammatory, analgesic, antiviral, antimicrobial, anti-malarial, anti-leishmanial, antiplatelet, anticancer, anti-obesity, anti-platelet, hypo-lipidemic, cardio-protective agents, anti-fungal, and more (166).

3.3.1.2.2.4 Other Polyphenol Compounds Besides flavonoids, other phenol compounds are found in plants and do not have the flavonoid structure. They are classified as non-flavonoid compounds. There are about 5,000 to 6,000 non-flavonoid phenols among about 10,000 phenolic compounds currently known in plant sources. These natural phenols include resveratrol, ellagitannins, ellagic acid, xanthonoid or xanthone, curcumin, salicylic acid, eugenol, polyphenolic amides, and stilbenes. Polyphenol compounds are often present in our daily diet and have antioxidant and various pharmacological properties. Here we examine some main non-flavonoid phenol compounds such as resveratrol (a stilbene compound), ellagitannins, and xanthones. Curcumin and salicylic acid are described in Chapter 5 of this book.

3.3.1.2.2.4.1 Resveratrol Resveratrol (3,4',5-trihydroxystilbene) is a stilbenoid belonging to natural non-flavonoid polyphenols and mainly exists in plants in trans-isomer form which is more potent than cis-form. Resveratrol is synthesized by plants in response to infection, injury, stress, or UV radiations for their protection. It is present in a number of plants such as red grapes, peanuts, cocoa, soy, berries (blueberries, bilberries, mulberries, cranberries), and their products like red wine, grape juice, chocolate, and Itadori tea (consumed mainly in Japan). In grapes, resveratrol is mainly found in skins and seeds. Resveratrol is a strong antioxidant and phytoalexin (antimicrobial agent). Due to its antioxidant property, resveratrol is a cyclooxygenase (COX) inhibitor, peroxisome proliferator-activated receptor (PPAR) activator, endothelial nitric oxide synthase (eNOS) inducer, anti-inflammatory activator, gene regulator, silent mating type information regulation 2 homolog 1 (SIRT1) activator, and more (167–180). Numerous experimental studies have shown a broad range of biological activities of medicinal interest of resveratrol such as anticancer, anti-infection, anti-diabetic, anti-aging, anti-inflammatory, immunomodulator, cardiovascular protector, neuroprotector activities, and anti-obesity (167–180).

Since the 1939 discovery of resveratrol from the roots of the white hellebore (*Veratrum grandiflorum* O. Loes) by Japanese Dr. Michio Takaoka, over 20,000 research papers concerning the biological and pharmacological activities of resveratrol have been published worldwide (170, 173, 178). Pharmacological studies have shown that resveratrol is safe for humans – even at very high daily doses in humans, around five g/day, side effects are mild (178). However, resveratrol, especially resveratrol supplement, has poor bioavailability (absorption) in humans, due to its extensive hepatic metabolism and its total elimination in the urine within the first hours after consumption (167–180). Therefore, resveratrol has not translated well to treatment in humans. Several formulations of resveratrol are available as over the counter supplements which claim beneficial effects against various health conditions (177). However, clinical trials have shown mixed results for metabolic and cardiovascular diseases so far (179). In addition, results from a systematic review and meta-analysis of randomized controlled trials do not suggest any benefit of resveratrol supplementation on cardiovascular risk factors (176). However, many scientists observe that people in the Mediterranean region have lower cardiovascular incidence than people in other regions because they frequently consume natural foods and their byproducts rich in resveratrol, such as red grapes, berries, and red wine. This phenomenon may be due to the presence of other compounds present in these foods which can act synergistically with resveratrol to aid its efficacy in the prevention of CVD in humans.

In brief, results of resveratrol supplement assays in humans remain contradictory and controversial for the prevention of a number of diseases, although of those experimental assays are promising. Its use in therapy is still not approved by medical organizations. More research is needed about resveratrol in the future.

3.3.1.2.2.4.2 Ellagitannins (ETs) and ellagic acid (EA) are polyphenols present in some fruits (raspberry, blackberry, strawberry, pomegranate), nuts (walnut, almond), and seeds (181–182).

Ellagitannins (esters of hexahydroxydiphenoic acid and glucose) are slowly hydrolyzed in the digestive tract, releasing ellagic acid (EA). ETs and EA form a diverse group of bioactive polyphenols with antioxidant, anticancer, anti-inflammatory, and antimicrobial (antibacterial, antifungal and antiviral) activities. Moreover, they improve the health of blood vessels (181–182). ETs and EA are then gradually metabolized by the gut microbiota of different mammals to produce different types of urolithins (A, B, C, D) during the metabolism of non-absorbed nutrients containing ellagitannins and ellagic acid. Urolithins are then incorporated into enterohepatic circulation. Urolithins are important bioactive compounds which can play the role of hormone analogs (181). Urolithins could display estrogenic and/or anti-estrogenic activity and tissue disposition studies reveal that urolithins are enriched in prostate, intestinal, and colon tissues in mice, which could explain why urolithins inhibit prostate and colon cancer cell growth (182). Moreover, antiproliferative and apoptosis-inducing activities of EA and urolithins have been demonstrated by the inhibition of cancer cell growth (182). Urolithin A (UA) is a first-in-class natural food metabolite of ETs that stimulates mitophagy and prevents the accumulation of dysfunctional mitochondria with age, thereby maintaining mitochondrial biogenesis and respiratory capacity in cells (183). Recently, urolithin A (UA) is shown to stimulate mitophagy and improve muscle health in old animals and in preclinical models of aging. These observed effects on mitochondrial biomarkers show that UA induces a molecular signature of improved mitochondrial and cellular health following regular oral consumption of UA in humans (183). UA could be a promising anti-aging compound.

3.3.1.2.2.4.3 Xanthones   Xanthones, or xanthonoids, mainly found in mangosteen and canistel fruits, are natural phenolic compounds. Mangosteen fruit and canistel or egg fruit are native to Southeast Asia, Mexico, and South America. There are about 280 xanthones from natural sources, but mangosteen alone contains around 68 xanthone-type compounds, among which the best known are α-, β-, γ- mangostins (184–185). Several studies have shown that xanthones and mangosteen extracts possess antioxidant, antitumor, anti-inflammatory, anti-allergy, anti-asthmatic, antidiabetic, antidiarrheal, antiparasitic, antibacterial, antiviral, antifungal, anti-amebic, and analgesic activities (184–185). In laboratory experiments, they inhibited growth and proliferation of human leukemia cells and other cancer cells of the colon and bile duct (185). Xanthones are able to inhibit several molecular targets in the tumor cells, including cyclooxygenases, kinases, ribonucleotide reductase, and DNA polymerases (184). Xanthones may prevent cancer, heart attack, and inflammatory diseases (asthma) (184–185). Mangosteen extracts are a traditional remedy in many Asian countries for the treatment of ameba dysentery, diarrhea, cholera, and some local infections.

In summary, flavonoids and other phenolic antioxidants function as scavengers of free radicals by rapid donation of a hydrogen atom to radicals through the phenolic OH groups present in their chemical structures. Their radical-scavenging activity depends on the molecular structure and the number and location of the phenolic OH groups present in the flavonoid molecule as well as in other phenolic phytochemicals. The pharmacological, medicinal, and biochemical properties of flavonoids and other phenolic antioxidants in plants have been reported to have antioxidant, anti-carcinogenic, anti-aging, anti-neurodegenerative, anti-inflammatory, anti-allergic, antimicrobial, and immunostimulating effects. Therefore, they have been reported to prevent or delay a number of chronic and degenerative ailments. According to Leopoldini et al. (148), three main mechanisms through which the phenolic antioxidants in plants may play their protective roles are: the H atom transfer, the single electron transfer, and the metals chelation.

Every plant contains a unique combination of flavonoids, which is why different herbs, all rich in these substances, have very different effects on the body (6). Concerning the research strategy of phytochemicals such as polyphenols, epidemiological evidence is strong for the protective effects of consuming complex mixtures of polyphenols in food; it may be unjustified to expect single molecules to be as effective (186). The synergistic effects between plant polyphenols with each other or with other nutrients may be beneficial for the body in the treatment or prevention of diseases.

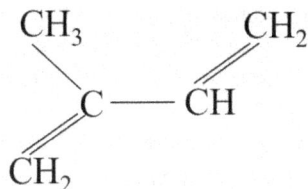

FIGURE 3.2   Isoprene unit.

3.3.1.2.2.5   Terpenoids   Terpenoids, also called 'isoprenoids', constitute one of the largest groups of natural products with important biological, pharmacological, medical and industrial properties (187–196). Most of the terpenoids are secondary metabolites of plants; however, a few of them are also synthesized by other organisms, such as bacteria and yeast. Terpenes and terpenoids account for 40,000 to 60,000 compounds according to each publication (188, 190, 193). Terpenes are simple hydrocarbons, while terpenoids are a modified class of terpenes with different functional groups (OH groups) and oxidized methyl group moved or removed at various positions (187). Terpenoids are composed of five-carbon 'isoprene' (C_5H_8) units or building blocks assembled and modified in thousands of ways (187–196).

Most natural terpenoid hydrocarbons have the general formula (C_5H_8) and are lipid compounds. Based on the number of isoprene building blocks, terpenoids are classified into several classes as C5 hemiterpenoids (1 isoprene unit), C10 monoterpenoids (2 isoprene units), C15 sesquiterpenoids (3 isoprene units), C20 diterpenoids (4 isoprene units), C25 sesterterpenoids (5 isoprene units), C30 triterpenoids (6 isoprene units), C40 tetraterpenoids or carotenoids (8 isoprene units), and C>40 polyterpenoids (187–188, 195). The most famous hemiterpenoid is the volatile hydrocarbon isoprene used in biofuel and the synthetic rubber industry (188). Some examples of monoterpenoids are myrcene from hops, linalool from lavender, menthol from mint, thymol from thyme, eucalyptol from eucalyptus leaves, and camphor from camphor trees. The most famous sesquiterpenoid is the antimalarial artemisinin. In the early 1970s, Chinese botanist Youyou Tu investigated plants used in traditional Chinese herbal medicine and discovered artemisinin, a sesquiterpenoid lactone naturally produced by the plant Artemisia annua L. for the treatment and the eradication of malaria caused by the *Plasmodium falciparum* parasite. Mrs. TU received a Nobel Prize in Medicine in 2015. Recently, it has been reported that artemisinin has anticancer effect where cancer cells, similar to the malaria parasites, possess high concentration of free iron (188). Another terpenoid recently discovered is Paclitaxel or Taxol[R]. It is a diterpenoid extracted from Pacific yew or *Taxus brevifolia* bark and is officially approved for the treatment of many cancer forms (ovary, breast, lung, pancreas), melanoma, and AIDS related Kaposi's sarcoma (188, 195–196). However, paclitaxel has many side effects. Some of the diterpenes also have cardiovascular activity, such as forskolin from the Indian Coleus plant, eleganolone from the French marine alga *Bifurcaria bifurcata*, and marrubenol from the plant *Marrubium vulgare* (white horehound) (187). Sesterterpenoids are naturally present in fungus, marine organisms, insects, sponges, lichens, and waxes of insects (187–188). These types of compounds are biologically active, having anti-inflammatory, anticancer, antimicrobial, and antifungal activities (187). Triterpenoids may be categorized into two major groups including steroidal triterpenoids such as sterols (cholesterol) and pentacyclic triterpenoid like saponin, hopane (188). As in animals, sterols are abundant membrane compounds in plants, with stigmasterol, sitosterol and campesterol being the major sterol constituents, and brassinosteroids constituting a class of hormones found in all plants (193). Triterpenoids are the metabolites of isopentenyl phosphate oligomers and constitute the largest group of phytochemicals, with more than 20,000 known compounds available in nature (195–196). A large number of triterpenoids have been shown to suppress the growth of a variety of cancer cells without exerting any toxicity in normal cells

(194–196). The most famous group of tetraterpenoids is the carotenoid pigments including alpha- and beta-carotene, lutein, lycopene, zeaxanthin, and astaxanthin. Carotenoids have important biological functions due to their antioxidant activity (187–188, 194–196). Alpha- and beta-carotene are precursors of essential vitamin A.

Plant terpenoids are used in food and traditional herbal therapy in Eastern and Western medicines due to their aroma, savor, and color. Eucalyptol is a monoterpenoid and an essential oil used in medicine as antiseptic and as mouthwash for the treatment of cold and cough. Other well-known terpenoids include some spices such as cineol in galangal root, gingerol in ginger tuber, menthol in peppermint, and eugenol in cinnamon and cloves. Terpenoids also include camphor in the wood of camphor laurel or the leaves of rosemary leaves, cannabinoids of cannabis (marijuana), ginkolide and bilobalide in *Ginkgo biloba* leaves, and beta-cryptoxanthin in persimmon fruits and leaves. In general, terpenoids occur widely in the leaves and fruits of higher plants, conifers, citrus, and eucalyptus. However, some terpenoids are toxic and inedible. They are used as drugs only such as artemisinin, paclitaxel, cannabinoids, camphor, and eucalyptol. Many terpenoids exert their effect on the nervous system and have psychoactive properties, such as tetrahydrocannabinol (THC), a cannabinoid in Cannabis (marijuana) (192).

Different terpenoid molecules have been reported to have antioxidant, antimicrobial, antifungal, antiviral, antiparasitic, antihyperglycemic, antiallergenic, anti-inflammatory, antispasmodic, immunomodulatory, and chemotherapeutic properties. They can also be used as natural insecticides and protective substances in storing agricultural products. The diverse array of terpenoid structures and functions has incited great interest in their medicinal use and commercial applications. Natural rubber or caoutchouc is a natural terpene (isoprene) polymer obtained mainly in the form of latex from the rubber tree (Hevea brasiliensis). Many terpenoids are essential oils and are used to prepare fragrances and flavor. Recently, plant terpenoids have been proposed for the fabrication of biofuel.

Briefly, almost all terpenoids possess antioxidant properties, especially tetraterpenes (carotenoids). Therefore, terpenoids have been found useful in the prevention and therapy of a variety of diseases from acute to chronic ailments since antiquity through today. Certain plants and spices containing terpenoids, flavonoids, and other phenolic compounds have been used for thousands of years in traditional Eastern medicine. However, Western medicine has not yet exploited these phytochemicals in the treatment of numerous chronic and bacterial diseases, although numerous non-exploited phytochemicals remain voluminous. Suggestions are made in search of the discovery of new drugs for the treatment of numerous dreadful diseases. Moreover, the synergistic effect between essential and non-essential exogenous antioxidants in the diet may enhance the efficacy of each component when used alone.

3.3.1.2.2.6 Trace Minerals Other potent antioxidants necessary for the maintenance of our health include trace elements such as selenium, zinc, copper, manganese, and iron. They are present in food, water, and soil and have antioxidant properties. They are vital for life and required from external supply in small quantities; hence, they are called essential micronutrients. However, high concentrations of these minerals become toxic for the body. Their antioxidant function intervenes in diverse processes and metabolic steps in the organism for the maintenance of health and prevention of disease (6, 15, 111).

3.3.1.2.2.6.1 Selenium As cited in Chapter 2 of this book, selenium (Se) is a trace metalloid (nonmetal) found in soil, water, vegetables (garlic, onion, grains, nuts, soybean, etc.), sea food, meat, liver, and yeast. Its primary source is in soil, where it is absorbed by plants and water. In food, Se compounds exist in two main forms: mineral or inorganic selenium and organic selenium (197–207). Inorganic compounds mainly include selenites containing Se(IV) (SeO_3^{2-}), and seleniates containing Se(IV) (SeO_4^{2-}). Main organic forms are selenoaminoacids (selenocysteine, selenomethionine), selenopeptides, selenoproteins, and selenoenzymes (antioxidant enzymes). The bioavailability, biological function, and toxicity of Se to human health depend on its different chemical forms. In general, organoselenium compounds have greater bioavailability and antioxidant activities than those of inorganic selenium and also are usually found to be less toxic than the inorganic forms (197–198). Se plays important roles in different biological processes such as antioxidant, anticancer, antiviral agent, immunomodulator, and so on. Due to their antioxidant activity, Se and its compounds are investigated in many studies for cancer chemoprevention, heart disease, infection, and immunity (197–208). Selenium insufficiency and gene mutations in selenoproteins are involved in the pathophysiology of many diseases, including CVDs, immune dysfunctions, cancer, thyroid gland, muscle and bone disorders, endocrine functions, and neurological disorders (199). However, Se deficiency in humans is rare because the normal diet can furnish Se in sufficient quantity to the body. However, in certain areas of the world such as the Keshan region in China, in Finland, New Zealand, or northern United States, where soil is poor in Se, people have developed different diseases such as cardiopathy, cancer, and infection, which are cured with Se supplement (111). To increase Se levels in soil of these regions, Se salts are added to chemical fertilizers and feed. Selenium deficiency can occur in patients on total parenteral nutrition and in patients with gastrointestinal disorders (6). Recommended Daily Allowance (RDA) of Se is 55 µg/day for men and 70 µg/day for women on lactation (119). Tolerable Upper Intake Level of Se is 400 µg/day (6). However, the narrow range between therapeutic and toxic doses of selenium, as well as the dependence of its effect on the applied form, dosage, and method of treatment, makes the choice of the most effective supplement a very complex issue (198). Excessive intake of Se can lead to selenosis which is a selenium poisoning characterized by gastrointestinal disorders, hair and nail loss, cirrhosis, pulmonary edema, and death (6).

3.3.1.2.2.6.2 Copper   Copper (Cu) is an essential trace element for the human body, which contains approximately 100 mg Cu (209–212). Copper is a redox active metal in aqueous solution. In biological systems copper can exist in two ionic forms: Cu^{2+} and Cu^{1+}, which are dominant in the extracellular oxidative and intracellular reductive environment, respectively (210). Copper is a cofactor of many copper redox enzymes such as ceruloplasmin, superoxide dismutase, and cytochrome C oxidase. Ceruloplasmin is a Cu-dependent ferroxidase enzyme, while superoxide dismutase is a strong antioxidant enzyme which is responsible for eliminating the superoxide anion, and cytochrome C oxidase is the terminal oxidase of cellular respiration (15, 111, 209). The ionic conversion between Cu^{2+} and Cu^{1+} provides a rich and potent redox reaction, acting as a reactive center for many critical enzymatic catalytic reactions which are important for numerous vital biological processes (211). Cu ions are delivered to the sites of utilization by special proteins called copper chaperones which are important components of the Cu metabolism (210).

Copper can act both as an antioxidant and as a pro-oxidant. As an antioxidant, Cu scavenges or neutralizes free radicals and may reduce or help prevent oxidative stress caused by free radicals. When copper acts as a pro-oxidant at times, it promotes free radical damage and may contribute to the development of chronic diseases such as Alzheimer's disease (212). Deficiency or excess of copper in the human body can cause diverse kinds of diseases. Excessive copper intake can cause nausea, vomiting, abdominal pain and cramps, headache, dizziness, weakness, and diarrhea. Since excess copper is excreted through bile, copper toxicity is most likely to occur in individuals with liver disease or bile disease (212). Maintaining the proper dietary balance of Cu, along with other minerals such as zinc and manganese, is important for maintaining good health. Beyond its role in iron metabolism, Cu also is involved in myriad biological processes, including antioxidant defense, neuropeptide synthesis, and immune function. It empowers the immune system, participates in the formation of enzymes, proteins, and brain neurotransmitters, and is an anti-inflammatory and anti-infectious agent. Similarly, it facilitates the synthesis of collagen and elastin (necessary constituents of the blood vessels, lungs, skin). In addition, it facilitates calcium and phosphorous fixation (15, 111, 209–212). The Tolerable Upper Intake Level (UL), and the recommended dietary allowances (RDAs), as well as the dietary source of copper are cited in Chapter 2 of this book.

3.3.1.2.2.6.3 Zinc   Zinc (Zn) is also a trace metal necessary for more than 200 human enzymes, including the cytoplasmic antioxidant Cu-Zn-superoxide dismutase (SOD), and it plays a role in immune function, wound healing, protein synthesis, DNA synthesis, and cell division (111, 212). In addition, zinc competes directly with copper and iron, thereby decreasing hydroxyl radical formation (15). It protects protein sulfhydryl groups from oxidation and stimulates the immune system. Zn deficiency is associated with lymphoid atrophy, decreased thymic hormone activity, decreased dermal delayed-hypersensitivity response, and delayed homograft rejection (15). Moreover, its deficit increases the production of oxidant species and oxidative stress (15, 111, 213). The ability of zinc to retard oxidative processes is well known. In general, the mechanism of antioxidation can be divided into acute and chronic effects. Chronic effects involve exposure of an organism to zinc on a long-term basis, resulting in induction of some other substance that is the ultimate antioxidant, such as the metallothioneins (213). Chronic zinc deprivation mainly results in increased sensitivity to some oxidative stress. The acute effects involve two mechanisms: protection of protein sulfhydryl or reduction of. OH free radical formation from H_2O_2 through the antagonism of redox-active transition metals, such as iron and copper (213). Zinc is capable of reducing postischemic injury to a variety of tissues and organs through a mechanism that might involve the antagonism of copper reactivity. Although the evidence for the antioxidant properties of zinc is convincing, the mechanisms are still unclear (213). Other biological roles of zinc as well as its dietary sources, UL doses, and RDAs are cited in Chapter 2 of this book.

3.3.1.2.2.6.4 Manganese   Manganese (Mn) is an essential micronutrient and a trace metal that intervenes in the activity of superoxide dismutase within the mitochondria (111, 214–215). Superoxide dismutase (SOD) is a metalloenzyme and antioxidant enzyme. SOD contains metal such as manganese, copper, zinc, or iron, used as cofactor for the enzyme's functioning. SOD protects cells from reactive oxygen species (ROS) by decomposing superoxide radical $O_2^{\cdot-}$ into molecular oxygen (O_2) and hydrogen peroxide (H_2O_2) by cyclic oxidation and reduction reactions with the active site metal (214–215). In humans, there are three forms of SODs: SOD-1, SOD-2, and SOD-3. SOD1 and SOD3 contain copper and zinc and are located in the cytoplam and the endoplasm, respectively. As for SOD-2, it contains manganese as cofactor and is located in the mitochondria. SOD-2 or Mn-SOD is of great interest to the medical field because of its protection against the deleterious effects of excessive superoxide in disease states (214). Decreased levels of SOD-2 may contribute to the development of certain diseases such as neurodegenerative diseases (Parkinson's disease and amyotrophic lateral sclerosis), diabetes, and cancer (214–215). Mn deficiency in the body leads to the inactivation of SOD-2 antioxidant enzyme. However, chronic exposure to Mn causes manganism, a manganese poisoning that is a classic 'pro-oxidant' disease.

3.3.1.2.2.6.5 Iron   Iron (Fe) is a trace metal essential to a variety of vital functions, including oxygen transport, antioxidant activity, DNA synthesis, metabolic energy, and cellular respiration (111, 216). It participates in the antioxidant system because it contributes to the elimination of the peroxide groups. However, its capacity to change valence with ease from 2^+ to 3^+ means that it can also intervene, depending on the environment, in the formation of free radicals (111). Iron homeostasis in mammals must be refined to avoid iron deficiency with a reduced oxygen transport and diminished activity of Fe-dependent enzymes, and also iron excess that may catalyze the formation of highly reactive hydroxyl radicals, oxidative stress, and programmed cell death (216–217). However, the ability of Fe to exchange single electrons with a number of substrates can lead to the generation of reactive oxygen species, as a result of Fe participation in the Fenton chemistry (216). Hence, maintaining iron homeostasis is essential for human health.

4   PRO-OXIDANTS

4.1   DEFINITION

Pro-oxidant refers to any endobiotic or xenobiotic that induces oxidative stress either by generation of harmful reactive oxygen species (ROS) or by inhibiting helpful antioxidant systems in the body (85–86). Pro-oxidants can damage cells and tissues. In general, the term 'pro-oxidant' is reserved for compounds that have antioxidant properties, but in certain conditions such as high dosage or prolonged use, they becomes harmful or toxic to the organism. For example, vitamin C is a strong antioxidant at low doses, and is used to fight or prevent diseases, but it becomes harmful to the body at high doses and can cause diseases. In this case, vitamin C becomes a pro-oxidant compound. Pro-oxidant is different from oxidant although these two compounds can both give oxidative stress and become toxic to the organism. Oxidant denotes a compound that produces an oxidation reaction and does not have antioxidant property in any dose or any physiological situation. For example, ozone O_3 and hydrogen peroxide H_2O_2 are oxidant compounds, and not pro-oxidants because they do not have antioxidant property, in contrast to vitamin C. Therefore, the term 'pro-oxidant' is reserved for compounds that have an antioxidant property.

4.2   MECHANISMS

Free radicals are considered pro-oxidants, but antioxidants can also have the potential to act as pro-oxidants under certain conditions. Some substances such as vitamins, carotenoids, and certain flavonoids, can serve as either antioxidants or pro-oxidants, depending on their concentrations and environment (17, 22, 85–86, 218–222). Generally, the higher doses of the substance and the presence of oxygen or transition metals (iron, copper, manganese, zinc) in its environment are the main factors transforming an antioxidant into a pro-oxidant (17, 85–86, 218–220). For example, vitamin C at high dose and in the presence of high concentration of ferric iron, is a potent potentiator of lipid peroxidation (17, 85, 218–219). Recent studies suggest that vitamin C sometimes increases DNA damage in humans (22). Recent mechanistic studies on the early stage of Low-density lipoprotein (LDL) oxidation show that the role of vitamin E is not simply that of a classical antioxidant. Depending on its concentrations and environment, vitamin E can have antioxidant, neutral, or pro-oxidant activity (17, 218–219). Beta-carotene in excess can become a pro-oxidant in the lungs of smokers and also produce significant increase in stroke incidence and cardiovascular diseases (17, 22, 218). Coenzyme Q10 can act as pro-oxidant in high concentrations, and may also cause severe hemorrhage if taken in very large quantities (22). Take note that some flavonoid antioxidants like myricetin, quercetin, hesperetin, naringenin, and catechins can behave, under certain circumstances (concentrations, transition metals, pH) like pro-oxidants and, hence, promote the oxidation of other compounds (86, 154, 219). Dietary phenolics can also act as pro-oxidants in systems that contain redox-active metals like iron and copper (218). Many antioxidants and natural flavonoids can become harmful to the body when used in excess in foods such as tea, coffee, chocolate, spices like chili, pepper, essential oils, or in dietary supplements. Briefly, high intake of dietary antioxidants, especially synthetic antioxidant supplements, is harmful to the body.

Indeed, oxidative stress results in a disturbance of the homeostasis (equilibrium status) between pro-oxidant and antioxidant levels in living organisms. Excess of free radicals like Reactive Oxygen Species (ROS) can damage cellular lipids, proteins, nucleic acids, and other macromolecules, inhibiting their normal functions (220). Although ROS are byproducts responsible for cellular damage, their contribution to aging is governed by cellular metabolic organization, protective systems, and the individual's genotype. Furthermore, oxidative damage could not represent the cause of aging (221).

However, it is misrepresenting to view pro-oxidant properties only as toxic ones. Other authors have also shown that the pro-oxidant effect of flavonoids might mitigate certain types of cancer (86, 154, 218–220). Some authors have postulated that pro-oxidants can have beneficial effects, since the imposition of a mild degree of oxidative stress might raise the levels of antioxidant defenses and xenobiotic-metabolizing enzymes, leading to increased cyto-protection (86, 220).

Briefly, pro-oxidants are considered toxic, except for pro-oxidants of some flavonoids that may be helpful in cell protection under certain conditions. Moreover, the transformation of a 'kind' antioxidant into a 'bad' pro-oxidant is mainly due to an 'overdose' of its external supply, like supplements and the presence of oxygen or transition metals (iron) in the environment.

5   DISCUSSION AND CONCLUSION

The roles of free radicals and antioxidants in diseases and health are now well established thanks to the investigations of enormous amounts of scientific research across the world over the past three decades. Our body is a homeostasis of all compounds; among them the equilibrium between antioxidants and free radicals plays an important role in the maintenance of our health. An excess of free radicals from internal sources or external origins may cause diseases. An unbalance of free radicals and antioxidants in the body is the origin of numerous chronic ailments such as cancer, cardiovascular, neurodegenerative, inflammatory diseases, immune disorder, diabetes, and more. Evidently, other causes can also engender these diseases such as gene, obesity, infection, and angiogenesis. However, it is of note that only 5–10% of cancer development is hereditary (38). To prevent or treat these diseases, the best way is to find the origin of unbalance between free radicals and antioxidants.

According to Li et al. (222), potent antiangiogenic molecules have now been identified in dietary sources, suggesting that a rationally designed antiangiogenic diet could provide a safe, widely available, and novel strategy for preventing cancer.

The implication of oxidative stress in the etiology of several chronic and degenerative diseases suggests that antioxidant therapy represents a promising avenue for future treatment or co-treatment with classical medicines. However, the use of artificial antioxidant supplements as adjuvant therapy must be carefully examined by a specialist because an excess of vitamins D, E, or C, as well as some flavonoids and terpenoids in dietary supplements may be harmful to the body. This phenomenon, known as the pro-oxidant effect, causes an imbalance between antioxidants and oxidants or free radicals because free radicals are also necessary to the body. To prevent these harmful pro-oxidant effects, the best choice is to consume a cocktail of natural plant and animal foods freshly prepared.

More research into new antioxidants in nature is necessary because several tens of thousands of natural beneficial antioxidants are still yet explored. Natural antioxidants exist not only in plants and animals, but also in mineral, soil, water, mushrooms, yeasts, molds, insects, and so on. Moreover, natural substances in different species are of great interest for the development of new drugs. The knowledge of different mechanisms of antioxidant activities as well as of free radical roles in the human body is necessary to resolve contradictory results found in clinical assays and also to find new therapies for many dreadful ailments.

6   REFERENCES

1. Gomberg M. (1900). An Instance of Trivalent Carbon: Triphenylmethyl. *J. Chem. Soc.*, **20**: 757–771.
2. Commoner B., Townsend J., Pake G.E. (1954). Free Radicals in Biological Materials. *Nature*, **174**: 689–691.
3. Schnell D.M., St Clair D. (2014). Redox Pioneer: Professor Joe M. McCord. *Antioxid. Redox Signal.*, **20**(1): 183–188.
4. Droge W. (2002). Free Radicals in the Physiological Control of Cell Function. Review. *Physiol. Rev.*, **82**: 47–95.
5. Valko M., Leibfritz D., Moncola J., Cronin M.D., Mazur M., Telser J. (2007). Free Radicals and Antioxidants in Normal Physiological Functions and Human Disease. Review. *Int. J. Biochem. Cell Biol.*, **39**: 44–84.
6. Pham-Huy A.L., He H., Pham-Huy C. (2008). Free Radicals and Antioxidants in Disease and Health. *Int. J. Biomed. Sci.*, **4**(2): 89–96.

7. Halliwell B., Gutteridge J.M.C. (2007). *Free Radicals in Biology and Medicine*. 4th edition. Oxford University Press, New York.

8. Halliwell B. (2007). Biochemistry of Oxidative Stress. *Biochem. Soc. Trans.*, **35**: 1147–1150.

9. Willcox J.K., Ash S.L., Catignani G.L. (2004). Antioxidants and Prevention of Chronic Disease. Review. *Crit. Rev. Food Sci. Nutr.*, **44**: 275–295.

10. Ozcan A., Ogun M. (2015). Biochemistry of Reactive Oxygen and Nitrogen Species, Chapter 3, pp. 37–58. In: *Basic Principles and Clinical Significance of Oxidative Stress*. Editor: S.J.T. Gowder. InTech, Rijeka, 328 pages.

11. Sharma N. (2014). Free Radicals, Antioxidants and Diseases. *Biol. Med.*, **6**(3): 1–6.

12. Young I.S., Woodside J.V. (2001). Antioxidants in Health and Diseases. *Clin. Pathol.*, **54**: 176–186.

13. Ifeanyi O.E. (2018). A Review on Free Radicals and Antioxidants. *Int. J. Curr. Res. Med. Sci.*, **4**(2): 123–133.

14. Kehrer J.P., Klotz L-O. (2015). Free Radicals and Related Reactive Species as Mediators of Tissue Injury and Disease: Implications for Health. *Crit. Rev. Toxicol.*, **45**(9): 765–798.

15. Knight J.A. (2000). Review: Free Radicals, Antioxidants, and the Immune System. *Ann. Clin. Lab. Sci.*, **30**(2): 145–158.

16. Halliwell B. (2012). Free Radicals and Antioxidants: Updating a Personal View. *Nutr. Rev.*, **70**(5): 257–265.

17. Devasagayam T.P.A., Tilak J.C., Boloor K.K., Sane K.S., Ghaskadbi S.S., Lele R.D. (2004). Free Radicals and Antioxidants in Human Health: Current Status and Future Prospects. *J.A.P.I.*, **52**: 794–804.

18. Genestra M. (2007). Oxyl Radicals, Redox-Sensitive Signalling Cascades and Antioxidants. Review. *Cell Signal.* **19**: 1807–1819.

19. Mathew B.B., Tiwari A., Jatawa S.K. (2011). Free Radicals and Antioxidants: A Review. *J. Pharm. Res.*, **4**(12): 4340–4343.

20. Kunwar A., Priyadarsini K.I. (2011). Free Radicals, Oxidative Stress and Importance of Antioxidants in Human Health. *J. Med. Allied Sci.*, **1**(2): 53–60.

21. Nimse S.B., Pal D. (2015). Free Radicals, Natural Antioxidants, and Their Reaction Mechanisms. *RSC Adv.*, **5**(35): 27986–28006.

22. Sen S., Chakraborty R. (2011). The Role of Antioxidants in Human Health, Chapter 1, pp. 1–37. In: *Oxidative Stress: Diagnostics, Prevention, and Therapy*. Editors: S. Andreescu, Hepel M. ACS Symposium Series, vol. 1083; American Chemical Society, Washington, DC.

23. He H., Pham-Huy A.L., Dramou P., Xiao D-L., Zuo P., Pham-Huy C. (2013). Carbon Nanotubes: Applications in Pharmacy and Medicine. *BioMed. Res. Int.*, ID 578290, 1–12.

24. He H., Xiao D-L., Pham-Huy A.L., Dramou P., Pham-Huy C. (2017). Carbon Nanotubes Used as Nanocarriers in Drug and Biomolecule Delivery, pp. 163–212. In: *Drug Delivery Approaches and Nanosystems, Volume 1. Novel Drug Carriers*. Editors: R.K. Keservani, A.K. Sharma, R.K. Kesharwani. Apple Academic Press Inc., New Jersey.

25. Shaikh N., Marri A., Pathan M., Qureshi B. (2015). Antioxidants Versus Free Radicals: An Informative Review. *Europ. Acad. Res.*, **2**(10): 13479–13493.

26. Pacher P., Beckman J.S., Liaudet L. (2007). Nitric Oxide and Peroxynitrite in Health and Disease. *Physiol. Rev.*, **87**(1): 315–424.

27. Levine A.B., Punihaole D., Levine T.B. (2012). Characterization of the Role of Nitric Oxide and Its Clinical Applications. *Cardiology*, **122**: 55–68.

28. Khazan M., Hdayati M. (2015). The Role of Nitric Oxide in Health and Diseases. *Scimetr* (or *Int. J. Med. Sci.*), **3**(1): e20987, 10 pages.

29. Tewari D., Sah A.N., Bawari S., Nabavi S.F., Dehpour A.R., Shirooie S., Braidy N., Fiebich B.L., Vacca R.A., Nabavi S.M. (2021). Role of Nitric Oxide in Neurodegeneration: Function, Regulation, and Inhibition. *Curr. Neuropharmacol.*, **19**(2): 114–126.

30. Repetto M., Semprine J., Boveris A. (2012). Chapter 1. Lipid Peroxidation: Chemical Mechanism, Biological Implications and Analytical Determination, pp. 3–30. In: *Lipid Peroxidation*. InTech, Rijeka.

31. Pourahmad J., Salimi A., Seyd E. (2016). Chapter 17. Role of Oxygen Free Radicals in Cancer Development and Treatment, pp. 347–362. In: *Free Radicals and Diseases*. InTech, Rijeka.

32. Valko M., Rhodes C.J., Moncol J., Izakovic M., Mazur M. (2006). Free Radicals, Metals and Antioxidants in Oxidative Stress-Induced Cancer. Mini-Review. *Chem Biol Interact.*, **160**: 1–40.

33. Deavall D.G., Martin E.A., Horner J.M., Roberts R. (2012). Drug-Induced Oxidative Stress and Toxicity. *J. Toxicol.*, Article ID 645460, 13 pages.

34. Nguyen A.L., He H., Pham-Huy C. (2006). Chiral Drugs. An Overview. *Int. J. Biomed. Sci.*, **2**: 85–100.

35. Klauning J.E., Kamendulids L.M., Hocevar B.A. (2010). Oxidative Stress and Oxidative Damage in Carcinogenesis. *Toxicol. Pathol.*, **38**: 96–109.

36. Fujiki H., Sueoka E., Suganuma M. (2013). Tumor Promoters: From Chemicals to Inflammatory Proteins. *J Cancer Res. Clin. Oncol.*, **139**: 1603–1614.

37. Benigni R., Bossa C., Tcheremenskaia O. (2013). Nongenotoxic Carcinogenicity of Chemicals: Mechanisms of Action and Early Recognition Through a New Set of Structural Alerts. *Chem. Rev.*, **113**: 2940–2957.

38. Rahner N., Steinke V. (2008). Hereditary Cancer Syndromes. *Dtsch Arztebl Int.*, **105**(41): 706–714.

39. Samadder N.J., Giridhar K.V., Baffy N., Riegert-Johnson D., Couch F.J. (2019). Hereditary Cancer Syndromes. A Primer on Diagnosis and Management, Part 1: Breast-Ovarian Cancer Syndromes. *Mayo Clin. Proc.*, **94**(6): 1084–1098.

40. Sudakin D.L., Stone D.L., Power L. (2011). Naphthalene Mothballs: Emerging and Recurring Issues and Their Relevance to Environmental Health. *Curr. Top Toxicol.*, **7**: 13–19.

41. Händel M.N., Cardoso I., Rasmussen K.M., Rohde J.F., Jacobsen R., Nielsen S.M., Christensen R., Heitmann B.L. (2019). Processed Meat Intake and Chronic Disease Morbidity and Mortality: An Overview of Systematic Reviews and Meta-Analyses. *PLoS One*, **14**(10): e0223883, 20 pages.

42. Pandiri A. (2015). Comparative Pathobiology of Environmentally Induced Lung Cancers in Humans and Rodents. *Toxicol. Pathol.*, **43**(1): 107–114.

43. Clapp R.W., Jacobs M.M., Loechler E.L. (2008). Environmental and Occupational Causes of Cancer New Evidence, 2005–2007. *Rev. Environ. Health.*, **23**(1): 1–37.

44. Truhaut R. (1967). *Potential Carcinogenic Hazards from Drugs. Evaluation of Risks*. UICC Monograph Series, Volume. 7. Editor: René Truhaut. Springer-Verlag, Berlin, 249 pages.

45. Schmahl D., Habs M. (1980). Drug-Induced Cancer, pp. 333–369. In: *Drug-Induced Pathology. Current Topics in Pathology*. Editor: E. Grundmann. Springer-Verlag, Berlin, Heidelberger, Germany.

46. Friedman G.D., Udaltsova N., Chan J., Quesenberry Jr. C.P., Habel L.A. (2009). Screening Pharmaceuticals for Possible Carcinogenic Effects: Initial Positive Results for Drugs not Previously Screened. *Cancer Causes Control*, **20**(10): 1821–1835.

47. Bahorun T., Soobrattee M.A., Luximon-Ramma V., Aruoma O.I. (2006). Free Radicals and Antioxidants in Cardiovascular Health and Disease. *Internet J. Med. Update*, **1**: 1–17.

48. Ceriello A. (2008). Possible Role of Oxidative Stress in the Pathogenesis of Hypertension. Review. *Diabetes Care*, **31** (Suppl. 2): S181–S184.

49. Halliwell B. (2001). Role of Free Radicals in Neurodegenerative Diseases: Therapeutic Implications for Antioxidant Treatment. *Drugs Aging*, **18**: 685–716.

50. Christen Y. (2000). Oxidative Stress and Alzheimer Disease. *Am. J. Clin. Nutr.*, **71** (Suppl.): 621S–629S.

51. Butterfield D.A. (2002). Amyloid Beta-Peptide (1–42)-Induced Oxidative Stress and Neurotoxicity: Implications for Neurodegeneration in Alzheimer's Disease Brain. A Review. *Free Radic. Res.*, **36**: 1307–1313.

52. Jenner P. (2003). Oxidative Stress in Parkinson's Disease. *Ann. Neurol.*, **53**: S26–S36.

53. Tretter L., Sipos I., Adam-Vizi V. (2004). Initiation of Neuronal Damage by Complex I Deficiency and Oxidative Stress in Parkinson's Disease. *Neurochem. Res.*, **29**: 569–577.

54. Liu Z., Zhou T., Ziegler A.C., Dimitrion P., Zuo L. (2017). Oxidative Stress in Neurodegenerative Diseases: From Molecular Mechanisms to Clinical Applications. *Oxid. Med. Cell Longev.*, **2017**, Article ID 2525967, 11 pages.

55. Park H.S., Kim S.R., Lee Y.C. (2009). Impact of Oxidative Stress on Lung Diseases. *Respirology*, **14**: 27–38.

56. Valavanidis A., Vlachogianni T., Fiotakis K., Loridas S. (2013). Pulmonary Oxidative Stress, Inflammation and Cancer: Respirable Particulate Matter, Fibrous Dusts and Ozone as Major Causes of Lung Carcinogenesis Through Reactive Oxygen Species Mechanisms. *Int. J. Environ. Res. Public Health*, **10**: 3886–3907.

57. Bowler R.P., Crapo J.D. (2002). Oxidative Stress in Allergic Respiratory Diseases. *J. Allergy Clin. Immunol.*, **110**(3): 349–356.

58. Repine J.E., Bast A., Lankhorst I. (1997). Oxidative Stress in Chronic Obstructive Pulmonary Disease. *Am. J. Respir. Crit. Care Med.*, **156**: 341–357.

59. Coppey L.J., Gellett J.S., Davidson E.P., Dunlap J.A., Lund D.D., Yorek M.A. (2001). Effect of Antioxidant Treatment of Streptozotocin-Induced Diabetic Rats on Endoneurial Blood Flow, Motor Nerve Conduction Velocity, and Vascular Reactivity of Epineurial Arterioles of the Sciatic Nerve. *Diabetes*, **50**(8): 1927–1937.

60. Mahajan A., Tandon V.R. (2004). Antioxidants and Rheumatoid Arthritis. *J. Indian Rheumatol. Ass.*, **12**: 139–142.

61. Galle J. (2001). Oxidative Stress in Chronic Renal Failure. *Nephrol. Dial. Transplant*, **16**: 2135–2142.

62. Sabolić I. (2006). Common Mechanisms in Nephropathy Induced by Toxic Metals. *Nephron Physiol.*, **104**: 107–114.

63. Sadeg N., Pham-Huy C., Martin C., Warnet J.M., Claude J.R. (1993). Effect of Cyclosporin A and Its Metabolites and Analogs on Lipid Peroxidation in Rabbit Renal Microsomes. *Drug Chem. Toxicol.*, **16**: 165–174.

64. Massicot F., Lamouri A., Martin C., Pham-Huy C., Warnet J.M., Claude J.R. (1997). Preventive Effects of Two PAF-Antagonists, PMS 536 and PMS 549, on Cyclosporin-Induced LLC-PK1 Oxidative Injury. *J. Lipid Mediat. Cell Signal.*, **15**: 203–214.

65. Massicot F., Martin C., Dutertre-Catella H., Ellouk-Achard S., Pham-Huy C., Warnet J.M., Claude J.R. (1997). Modulation of Energy Status and Cytotoxicity Induced by FK506 and Cyclosporin A in a Renal Epithelial Cell Line. *Arch. Toxicol.*, **71**: 529–531.

66. O'Connell S., Tuite N., Slattery C., Ryan M.P., McMorrow T. (2012). Cyclosporine A – Induced Oxidative Stress in Human Renal Mesangial Cells: A Role for ERK 1/2 MAPK Signaling. *Toxicol. Sci.*, **126**(1): 101–113.

67. Anderson R.E., Kretzer F.L., Rapp L.M. (1994). Free Radicals and Ocular Disease. Review. *Adv. Exp. Med. Biol.*, **366**: 73–86.

68. Nita M., Grzybowski A. (2016). The Role of the Reactive Oxygen Species and Oxidative Stress in the Pathomechanism of the Age-Related Ocular Diseases and Other Pathologies of the Anterior and Posterior Eye Segments in Adults. *Oxid. Med. Cell. Longev.* **2016**, Article ID 3164734, 23 pages.

69. Oduntan O.A., Mashige K.P. (2011). A Review of the Role of Oxidative Stress in the Pathogenesis of Eye Diseases. *S. Afr. Optom.*, **70**(4): 191–199.

70. Ferreira S.M., Lerner S.F., Brunzini R., Evelson P.A., Llesuy S.F. (2004). Oxidative Stress Markers in Aqueous Humor of Glaucoma Patients. *Am. J. Ophthalmol.*, **137**: 62–69.

71. Winkler B.S., Boulton M.E., Gottsch J.D., Sternberg P. (1999). Oxidative Damage and Age-Related Macular Degeneration. *Mol. Vis.*, **5**: 32–43.

72. Beatty S., Koh H.H., Phil M., Henson D., Boulton M. (2000). The Role of Oxidative Stress in the Pathogenesis of Age-Related Macular Degeneration. *Surv. Ophthalmol.*, **45**: 115–134.

73. Cheng A.C.K., Pang C.P., Leung A.T.S., Chua J.K.H., Fan D.S.P., Lam D.S.C. (2000). The Association Between Cigarette Smoking and Ocular Diseases. *HKMJ*, **6**: 195–202.

74. Harman D. (2001). Aging: Overview. *Ann. NY Acad. Sci.*, **928**: 1–21.

75. Junqueira V.B.C., Barros S.B.M., Chan S.S., Rodrigues L., Giavarotti L., Abud R.L., Deucher G.P. (2004). Aging and Oxidative Stress. *Mol Aspects Med.*, **25**: 5–16.

76. Kregel K.C., Zhang H.J. (2007). An Integrated View of Oxidative Stress in Aging: Basic Mechanisms, Functional Effects, and Pathological Considerations. *Am. J. Physiol. Regul. Integr. Comp. Physiol.*, **292**: R18–R36.

77. Dai D-F., Chiao Y.A., Marcinek D.J., Szeto H.H., Rabinovitch P.S. (2014). Mitochondrial Oxidative Stress in Aging and Health Span. *Longevity & Healthspan*, **3**(6), 22 pages.

78. Cui H., Kong Y., Zhang H. (2012). Oxidative Stress, Mitochondrial Dysfunction. *J. Signal Transduct.* **2012**, Article ID 646354, 13 pages.

79. Yan L-J. (2014). Positive Oxidative Stress in Aging and Aging-Related Disease Tolerance. *Redox Biol.*, **2**: 165–169.

80. Agarwal A., Makker K., Sharma R. (2008). Clinical Relevance of Oxidative Stress in Male Factor Infertility: An Update. *Am. J. Reprod. Immunol.*, **59**: 2–11.

81. Gharagozloo P., Aitken R.J. (2011). The Role of Sperm Oxidative Stress in Male Infertility and the Significance of Oral Antioxidant Therapy. *Hum. Reprod.*, **26**(7): 1628–1640.

82. Lobo V., Patil A., Phatak A., Chandra N. (2010). Free Radicals, Antioxidants and Functional Foods: Impact on Human Health. *Pharmacogn. Rev.*, **4**(8): 118–126.

83. Rahman K. (2007). Studies on Free Radicals, Antioxidants and Co-Factors. *Clin. Interv. Aging*, **2**(2): 219–236.

84. Lu J-M., Lin P.H., Yao Q., Chen C. (2010). Chemical and Molecular Mechanisms of Antioxidants; Experimental Approaches and Model Systems. *J. Cell. Mol. Med.*, **14**(4): 840–860.

85. Carocho M., Ferreira I.C.F.R. (2013). A Review on Antioxidants, Prooxidants and Related Controversy: Natural and Synthetic Compounds, Screening and Analysis Methodologies and Future Perspectives. *Food Chem. Toxicol.*, **51**: 15–25.

86. Rahal A., Kumar A., Singh V., Yadav B., Tiwari R., Chakraborty S., Dhama K. (2014). Oxidative Stress, Prooxidants, and Antioxidants: The Interplay. *BioMed. Res. Int.*, Article ID 761264, 19 pages.

87. Santos-Sánchez N.F., Salas-Coronado R., Villanueva-Cañongo C., Hernández-Carlos B. (2019). Chapter 2: Antioxidant Compounds and Their Antioxidant Mechanism. In: *Antioxidants*. Editor: Emad Shalaby. IntechOpen, London, 28 pages.

88. Boger R.H. (2007). The Pharmacodynamics of L-arginine. *J. Nutr.*, **137**: 1650S–1655S.

89. Yi J., Horky L.L., Friedlich A.L., Shi Y., Rogers J.T., Huang X. (2009). L-Arginine and Alzheimer's Disease. Review. *Int. J. Clin. Exp. Pathol.*, **3**: 211–238.

90. Raizner A.E. (2019). Coenzyme Q_{10}. *Methodist Debakey Cardiovasc J.*, **15**(3): 185–191.

91. Sharma A., Fonarow G.C., Butler J., Ezekowitz J.A., Felker G.M. (2016). Coenzyme Q10 and Heart Failure: A State-of-the-Art Review. *Circ. Heart Fail.*, **9**(4): e002639, 8 pages.

92. Garrido-Maraver J., Cordero M.D., Oropesa-Ávila M., Vega A.F., de la Mata M., Pavón A.D., de Miguel M., Calero C.P., Paz M.V., Cotán D., Sánchez-Alcázar J.A. (2014). Coenzyme Q10 therapy. *Mol. Syndromol.*, **5**: 187–197.

93. Aaseth J., Alexander J., Alehagen U. (2021). Coenzyme Q10 Supplementation – In Ageing and Disease. *Mech. Ageing Dev.*, **197**(111521): 1–7.

94. Mahto S.J.K., Ansari A.F.A.A., Singh P.P., Singh U.J., Chatur V. (2014). Benefits of Co-Enzyme Q10 – A Review. *Int. J. Pharm. Res. Scholars (IJPRS)*, **V-3**(I-4): 292–300.

95. Kawamukai M. (2009). Biosynthesis and Bioproduction of Coenzyme Q10 by Yeasts and Other Organisms. *Biotechnol. Appl. Biochem.*, **22**(53): 217–226.

96. Shay K.P., Moreau R.F., Smith E.J., Smith A.R., Hagen T.M. (2009). Alpha-Lipoic Acid as a Dietary Supplement: Molecular Mechanisms and Therapeutic Potential. *Biochim. Biophys. Acta*, **1790**(10): 1149–1160.

97. Goraca A., Huk-Kolega H., Piechota A., Kleniewska P., Ciejka E., Skibska B. (2011). Lipoic Acid – Biological Activity and Therapeutic Potential. *Pharmacol. Rep.*, **63**(4): 849–858.

98. Sautin Y.Y., Johnson R.J. (2008). Uric Acid: The Oxidant-Antioxidant Paradox. *Nucleos. Nucleot. Nucl. Acids*, **27**(6): 608–619.

99. de Oliveira E.P., Burini R.C. (2012). High Plasma Uric Acid Concentration: Causes and Consequences. *Diabetol. Metab. Syndr.*, **4**(12): 1–7.

100. Hardeland R., Pandi-Perumal S.R. (2005). Melatonin, a Potent Agent in Antioxidative Defense: Actions as a Natural Food Constituent, Gastrointestinal Factor, Drug and Prodrug. *Nutr. Metab.* (London), **2**(22), 15 pages.

101. Hardeland R. (2005). Antioxidative Protection by Melatonin: Multiplicity of Mechanisms from Radical Detoxification to Radical Avoidance. *Endocrine*, **27**(2): 119–130.

102. Tan D-X., Manchester L.C., Terron M.P., Flores L.J., Reiter R.J. (2007). One Molecule, Many Derivatives: A Never-Ending Interaction of Melatonin with Reactive Oxygen and Nitrogen Species? *J. Pineal Res.*, **42**: 28–42.

103. Stocker R., Yamamoto Y., McDonagh A.F., Glazer A.N., Ames B.N. (1987). Bilirubin Is an Antioxidant of Possible Physiological Importance. *Science*, **235**(4792): 1043–1046.

104. Kapitulnik J. (2004). Bilirubin: An Endogenous Product of Heme Degradation with Both Cytotoxic and Cytoprotective Properties. *Mol. Pharmacol.*, **66**(4): 773–779.

105. Wang A.M., Ma C., Xie Z.H., Shen F. (2000). Use of Carnosine as a Natural Anti-Senescence Drug for Human Beings. *Biochemistry (Mosc)*, **65**(7): 869–871.

106. Boldyrev A.A., Aldini G., Derave W. (2013). Physiology and Pathophysiology of Carnosine. *Physiol. Rev.*, **93**: 1803–1845.

107. Maninger N., Wolkowitz O.M., Reus V.I., Epel E.S., Mellon S.H. (2009). Neurobiological and Neuropsychiatric Effects of Dehydroepiandrosterone (DHEA) and DHEA Sulfate (DHEAS). *Front Neuroendocrinol.*, **30**(1): 65–91.

108. Rutkowski K., Sowa P., Rutkowska-Talipska J., Kuryliszyn-Moskal A., Rutkowski R. (2014). Dehydroepiandrosterone (DHEA): Hypes and Hopes. *Drugs*, **74**: 1195–1207.

109. Prough R.A., Barbara J., Clark B.J., Klinge C.M. (2016). Novel Mechanisms for DHEA Action. *J. Mol. Endocrinol.*, **56**(3): R139–R155.

110. Bentley C., Hazeldine J., Greig C., Lord J., Foster M. (2019). Dehydroepiandrosterone: A Potential Therapeutic Agent in the Treatment and Rehabilitation of the Traumatically Injured Patient. *Burn Trauma*, **7**(26): 13 pages.

111. Romero A.C., Olvera Hernández E.G., Cerón T.F., Chávez A.Á. (2013). Chapter 2. The Exogenous Antioxidants, pp. 33–57. In: *Oxidative Stress and Chronic Degenerative Diseases – A Role for Antioxidants*. Editor: José A. Morales-González. InTech Europe, Rijeka, Croatia, 512 pages.

112. Bouayed J., Bohn T. (2012). Dietary Derived Antioxidants: Implications on Health, pp. 1–22. In: *Nutrition, Well-Being and Health*. Editor: Dr. Jaouad Bouayed. InTech Europe, Rijeka, Croatia, 224 pages.

113. Brewer M.S. (2011). Natural Antioxidants: Sources, Compounds, Mechanisms of Action, and Potential Applications. *Compr. Rev. Food Sci. Food Saf.*, **10**: 221–247.

114. Marcadenti A., Assis Coelho R.C.L. (2015). Dietary Antioxidant and Oxidative Stress: Interaction Between Vitamins and Genetics. *J. Nutr. Health Food Sci.*, **3**(1): 1–7.

115. Liu R.H. (2004). Potential Synergy of Phytochemicals in Cancer Prevention: Mechanism of Action. *J. Nutr.*, **134**: 3479S–3485S.

116. Zhang Y-J., Gan R-Y., Li S., Zhou Y., Li A-N., Xu D-P., Li H-B. (2015). Antioxidant Phytochemicals for the Prevention and Treatment of Chronic Diseases. *Molecules*, **20**: 21138–21156.

117. Poljsak B., Ionescu J.G. (2009). Chapter V. Pro-Oxidant vs. Antioxidant Effects of Vitamin C, pp. 153–183. In: *Handbook of Vitamin C Research: Daily Requirements, Dietary Sources, and Adverse Effects*. Editors: Hubert Kucharski, Julek Zajac. Nova Science Publishers, Inc., New York, 415 pages.

118. Grosso G., Bei R., Mistretta A., Marventano S., Calabrese G., Masuelli L., Giganti M.G., Modesti A., Galvano F., Gazzolo D. (2013). Effects of Vitamin C on Health: A Review of Evidence. *Front Biosci.*, **18**: 1017–1029.

119. Jiang Q. (2014). Natural Forms of Vitamin E: Metabolism, Antioxidant, and Anti-Inflammatory Activities and Their Role in Disease Prevention and Therapy. *Free Radic. Biol. Med.*, **72**: 76–90.

120. Clarke M.W., Burnett J.R., Croft K.D. (2008). Vitamin E in Human Health and Disease. *Crit. Rev. Clin. Lab. Sci.*, **45**(5): 417–450.

121. Noh M.F.M., Gunasegavan R.D.N., Mustar S. (2019). Chapter 2. Vitamin A in Health and Disease. In: *Vitamin A*. Editors: Leila Queiroz Zepka, Eduardo Jacob-Lopes, Veridiana Vera de Rosso. IntechOpen, London.

122. Bushue N., Wan Y.J. (2010). Retinoid Pathway and Cancer Therapeutics. *Adv. Drug Deliv. Rev.*, **62**(13): 1285–1298.

123. Tan B.L., Norhaizan M.E. (2019). Carotenoids: How Effective Are They to Prevent Age-Related Diseases? *Molecules*, **24**(9): 1801, 23 pages.

124. Story E.N., Kopec R.E., Schwartz S.J., Keith Harris G. (2010). An Update on the Health Effects of Tomato Lycopene. *Annu. Rev. Food Sci. Technol.*, **1**: 1–24.

125. Holzapfel N.P., Holzapfel B.M., Champ S., Feldthusen J., Clements J., Hutmacher D.W. (2013). The Potential Role of Lycopene for the Prevention and Therapy of Prostate Cancer: From Molecular Mechanisms to Clinical Evidence. *Int. J. Mol. Sci.*, **14**: 14620–14646.

126. Van Breemen R.B., Pajkovic N. (2008). Multitargeted Therapy of Cancer by Lycopene. *Cancer Lett.*, **269**(2): 339–351.

127. Rao A.V., Agarwal S. (2000). Role of Antioxidant Lycopene in Cancer and Heart Disease. *J. Am. Coll. Nutr.*, **19**(5): 563–569.

128. Palozza P., Simone R.E., Catalano A., Mele M.C. (2011). Tomato Lycopene and Lung Cancer Prevention: From Experimental to Human Studies. *Cancers*, **3**: 2333–2357.

129. Basu A., Imrhan V. (2007). Tomatoes Versus Lycopene in Oxidative Stress and Carcinogenesis: Conclusions from Clinical Trials. *Eur. J. Clin. Nutr.*, **61**: 295–303.

130. Haseen F., Cantwell M.M., O'Sullivan J.M., Murray L.J. (2009). Is There a Benefit from Lycopene Supplementation in Men with Prostate Cancer? A Systematic Review. *Prostate Cancer Prostatic Dis.*, **12**: 325–332.

131. Eisenhauer B., Natoli S., Liew G., Flood V.M. (2017). Lutein and Zeaxanthin: Food Sources, Bioavailability and Dietary Variety in Age-Related Macular Degeneration Protection. *Nutrients*, **9**(2): 120, 14 pages.

132. Johnson E.J. (2014). Role of Lutein and Zeaxanthin in Visual and Cognitive Function Throughout the Lifespan. *Nutr. Rev.*, **72**(9): 605–612.

133. Koushan K., Rusovici R., Li W., Ferguson L.R., Chalam K.V. (2013). The Role of Lutein in Eye-Related Disease. *Nutrients*, **5**(5): 1823–1839.

134. Abdel-Aal el-S.M., Akhtar H., Zaheer K., Ali R. (2013). Dietary Sources of Lutein and Zeaxanthin Carotenoids and Their Role in Eye Health. *Nutrients*, **5**(4): 1169–1185.

135. Kidd M.P. (2011). Astaxanthin, Cell Membrane Nutrient with Diverse Clinical Benefits and Anti-Aging Potential. *Altern. Med. Rev.*, **16**(4): 355–364.

136. Yuan J.P., Peng J., Yin K., Wang J.H. (2011). Potential Health-Promoting Effects of Astaxanthin: A High-Value Carotenoid Mostly from Microalgae. *Mol. Nutr. Food Res.* **55**(1): 150–165.

137. Shah M.M., Liang Y., Cheng J.J., Daroch M. (2016). Astaxanthin-Producing Green Microalga Haematococcus pluvialis: From Single Cell to High Value Commercial Products. *Front Plant Sci.*, **7**, Art. 531: 1–28.

138. Fakhri S., Aneva I.Y., Farzaei M.H., Sobarzo-Sánchez E. (2019). The Neuroprotective Effects of Astaxanthin: Therapeutic Targets and Clinical Perspective. *Molecules*, **24**(14): 2640, 19 pages.

139. Kishimoto Y., Yoshida H., Kondo K. (2016). Potential Anti-Atherosclerotic Properties of Astaxanthin. *Mar. Drugs*, **14**(2): 35, 13 pages.

140. Fassett R.G., Coombes J.S. (2012). Astaxanthin in Cardiovascular Health and Disease. *Molecules*, **17**(2): 2030–2048.

141. Ambati R.R., Phang S.M., Ravi S., Aswathanarayana R.G. (2014). Astaxanthin: Sources, Extraction, Stability, Biological Activities and Its Commercial Applications-A Review. *Mar. Drugs*, **12**(1): 128–152.

142. Capelli B., Talbott S., Ding L. (2019). Astaxanthin Sources: Suitability for Human Health and Nutrition. *Funct. Foods Health Dis.*, **9**(6): 430–445.

143. Zhang H., Tang Y., Zhang Y., Zhang S., Qu J., Wang X., Kong R., Han C., Liu Z. (2015). Fucoxanthin: A Promising Medicinal and Nutritional Ingredient. *Evid. Based Complement Alternat. Med.*, **2015**, Article ID 723515, 10 pages.

144. Satomi Y. (2017). Antitumor and Cancer-Preventative Function of Fucoxanthin: A Marine Carotenoid. *Anticancer Res.*, **37**(4): 1557–1562.

145. Middleton Jr. E., Kandaswami C., Theoharides T.C. (2000). The Effects of Plant Flavonoids on Mammalian Cells: Implications for Inflammation, Heart Disease, and Cancer. *Pharmacol. Rev.*, **52**: 673–751.

146. Williamson G., Kay C.D., Crozier A. (2018). The Bioavailability, Transport, and Bioactivity of Dietary Flavonoids: A Review from a Historical Perspective. *Compr. Rev. Food Sci. Food Saf.*, **17**: 1054–1112.

147. Tsao R. (2010). Chemistry and Biochemistry of Dietary Polyphenols. *Nutrients*, **2**: 1231–1246.

148. Maniglia B.C., Rebelatto E.A., Zielinski A., de Andrade C.J. (2021). Chapter 1. Polyphenols. In: *Food Bioactives and Health*. Springer Cham, Switzerland. https://doi.org/10.1007/978-3-030-57469-7.

149. Santos E.L., Sales Maia B.H.L.N., Ferriani A.P., Teixeira S.D. (2017). Chapter 1. Flavonoids: Classification, Biosynthesis and Chemical Ecology, pp. 3–16. In: *Flavonoids – From Biosynthesis to Human Health*. IntechOpen, London.

150. Brodowska K.M. (2017). Natural Flavonoids: Classification, Potential Role, and Application of Flavonoid Analogues. *Eur. J. Biol. Res.*, **7**(2): 108–123.

151. Panche A.N., Diwan A.D., Chandra S.R. (2016). Flavonoids: An Overview. *J. Nutr. Sci.*, **5**: e47, 15 pages.

152. Kumar S., Pandey A.K. (2013). Chemistry and Biological Activities of Flavonoids: An Overview. *Sci. World J.*, Article ID 162750, 16 pages.

153. Kaurinovic B., Vastag D. (2019). Flavonoids and Phenolic Acids as Potential Natural Antioxidants. In: *Antioxidants*. Editor: Emad Shalaby. IntechOpen, London.

154. Procházková D., Boušová I., Wilhelmová N. (2011). Antioxidant and Prooxidant Properties of Flavonoids. *Fitoterapia*, **82**: 513–523.

155. Wang T-Y., Li Q., Bi K-S. (2018). Bioactive Flavonoids in Medicinal Plants: Structure, Activity and Biological Fate. *Asian J. Pharm. Sci.*, **13**(1): 12–23.

156. Lago J.H.G., Toledo-Arruda A.C., Mernak M., Barrosa K.H., Martins M.A., Tibério I.F.L.C., Prado C.M. (2014). Structure-Activity Association of Flavonoids in Lung Diseases. *Molecules*, **19**(3): 3570–3595.

157. Rodríguez-García C., Sánchez-Quesada C., Gaforio J.J. (2019). Dietary Flavonoids as Cancer Chemopreventive Agents: An Updated Review of Human Studies. *Antioxidants*, **8**(137): 23 pages.

158. Ayaz M., Sadiq A., Junaid M., Ullah F., Ovais M., Ullah I., Ahmed J., Shahid M. (2019). Flavonoids as Prospective Neuroprotectants and Their Therapeutic Propensity in Aging Associated Neurological Disorders. *Front. Aging Neurosci.*, **11**(155): 20 pages.

159. Figueira I., Menezes R., Macedo D., Costa I., Dos Santos C.N. (2017). Polyphenols Beyond Barriers: A Glimpse into the Brain. *Curr. Neuropharmacol.*, **15**(4): 562–594.

160. Górniak I., Bartoszewski R., Króliczewski J. (2019). Comprehensive Review of Antimicrobial Activities of Plant Flavonoids. *J. Phytochem. Rev.*, **18**(1): 241–272.

161. Arbia L., Chikhi-Chorfi N., Betatache I., Pham-Huy C., Zenia S., Mameri N., Drouiche N., Lounici H. (2017). Antimicrobial Activity of Aqueous Extracts from Four Plants on Bacterial Isolates from Periodontitis Patients. *Environ. Sci. Pollut. Res.*, **24**(15): 13394–13404.

162. Pham-Huy N.L.A., He H., Pham-Huy C. (2008). Green Tea and Health. An Overview. *J. Food Agric. Environ. (JFAE)*, **6**: 6–13.

163. Rauf A., Imran M., Abu-Izneid T., Ul-Haq I., Patel S., Pan X., Naz S., Silva A.S., Saeed F., Suleria H.A.R. (2019). Proanthocyanidins: A Comprehensive Review. *Biomed. Pharmacother.*, **116**: 108999, 6 pages.

164. Fine A.M. (2000). Oligomeric Proanthocyanidin Complexes: History, Structure, and Phytopharmaceutical Applications. *Altern. Med. Rev.*, **5**(2): 144–151.

165. Wallace T.C. (2011). Anthocyanins in Cardiovascular Disease. *Adv. Nutr.*, **2**: 1–7.
166. Chavan B.B., Gadekar A.S., Mehta P.P., Vawhal P.K., Kolsure A.K., Chabukswar A.R. (2016). Synthesis and Medicinal Significance of Chalcones. A Review. *Asian J. Biomed. Pharm. Sci.*, **6**(56): 1–7.
167. Pannu N., Bhatnagar A. (2019). Resveratrol: From Enhanced Biosynthesis and Bioavailability to Multitargeting Chronic Diseases. *Biomed. Pharmacother.*, **109**: 2237–2251.
168. Malaguarnera L. (2019). Influence of Resveratrol on the Immune Response. *Nutrients*, **11**(5): 946, 24 pages.
169. Vestergaard M., Ingmer H. (2019). Antibacterial and Antifungal Properties of Resveratrol. *Int. J. Antimicrob. Agents*, **53**: 716–723.
170. Espinoza J.L., Kurokawa Y., Takami A. (2019). Rationale for Assessing the Therapeutic Potential of Resveratrol in Hematological Malignancies. *Blood Rev.*, **33**: 43–52.
171. Wiciński M., Socha M., Walczak M., Wódkiewicz E., Malinowski B., Rewerski S., Górski K., Pawlak-Osińska K. (2018). Beneficial Effects of Resveratrol Administration-Focus on Potential Biochemical Mechanisms in Cardiovascular Conditions. *Nutrients*, **10**(11): 14 pages.
172. Xia N., Daiber A., Förstermann U., Li H. (2017). Antioxidant Effects of Resveratrol in the Cardiovascular System. *Br. J. Pharmacol.*, **174**(12): 1633–1646.
173. Nakata R., Takahashi S., Inoue H. (2012). Recent Advances in the Study on Resveratrol. *Biol. Pharm. Bull.*, **35**(3): 273–279.
174. Ramírez-Garza S.L., Laveriano-Santos E.P., Marhuenda-Muñoz M., Storniolo C.E., Tresserra-Rimbau A., Vallverdú-Queralt A., Lamuela-Raventós R.M. (2018). Health Effects of Resveratrol: Results from Human Intervention Trials. *Nutrients*, **10**(12): 1892.
175. Salehi B., Mishra A.P., Nigam M., Sener B., Kilic M., Sharifi-Rad M., Fokou P.V.T., Martins N., Sharifi-Rad J. (2018). Resveratrol: A Double-Edged Sword in Health Benefits. *Biomedicines*, **6**(3): 91.
176. Sahebkar A., Serban C., Ursoniu S., Wong N.D., Muntner P., Graham I.M., Mikhailidis D.P., Rizzo M., Rysz J., Sperling L.S., Lip G.Y., Banach M. (2015). Lack of Efficacy of Resveratrol on C-Reactive Protein and Selected Cardiovascular Risk Factors. Results from a Systematic Review and Meta-Analysis of Randomized Controlled Trials. *Int. J. Cardiol.* **189**: 47–55.
177. Singh C.K., Ndiaye M.A., Ahmad N. (2015). Resveratrol and Cancer: Challenges for Clinical Translation. *Biochim. Biophys. Acta*, **1852**(6): 1178–1185.
178. Pezzuto J.M. (2019). Resveratrol: Twenty Years of Growth, Development and Controversy. *Biomol. Ther. (Seoul)*, **27**(1): 1–14.
179. Bitterman J.L., Chung J.H. (2015). Metabolic Effects of Resveratrol: Addressing the Controversies. *Cell. Mol. Life Sci.*, **72**(8): 1473–1488.
180. Berman A.Y., Motechin R.A., Wiesenfeld M.Y., Holz M.K. (2017). The Therapeutic Potential of Resveratrol: A Review of Clinical Trials. *NPJ Precis. Oncol.*, **1**: 35, 9 pages.
181. Lipińska L., Klewicka E., Sójka M. (2014). Structure, Occurrence and Biological Activity of Ellagitannins: A General Review. *Acta Sci. Pol., Technol. Aliment*, **13**(3): 289–299.
182. Landete J.M. (2011). Ellagitannins, Ellagic Acid and Their Derived Metabolites: A Review About Source, Metabolism, Functions and Health. *Food Res. Int.*, **44**(5): 1150–1160.
183. Andreux P.A., Blanco-Bose W., Ryu D., Burdet F., Ibberson M., Aebischer P., Auwerx J., Singh A., Rinsch C. (2019). The Mitophagy Activator Urolithin a Is Safe and Induces a Molecular Signature of Improved Mitochondrial and Cellular Health in Humans. *Nat. Metab.*, **1**: 595–603.
184. Shan T., Ma Q., Guo K., Liu J., Li W., Wang F., Wu E. (2011). Xanthones from Mangosteen Extracts as Natural Chemopreventive Agents: Potential Anticancer Drugs. *Curr. Mol. Med.*, **11**(8): 666–677.
185. Negi J.S., Bisht V.K., Singh P., Rawat M.S.M., Joshi G.P. (2013). Naturally Occurring Xanthones: Chemistry and Biology. *J. Appl. Chem.*, **2013**, Article ID 621459, 9 pages.
186. Renaud J., Martinoli M.G. (2019). Considerations for the Use of Polyphenols as Therapies in Neurodegenerative Diseases. *Int. J. Mol. Sci.*, **20**(8): 1883, 25 pages.
187. Perveen S. (2018). Introductory Chapter: Terpenes and Terpenoids. In: *Terpenes and Terpenoids*. Editors: Shagufta Perveen, Areej Al-Taweel. IntechOpen, London.
188. Abdallah I.I., Quax W.J. (2017). A Glimpse into the Biosynthesis of Terpenoids. *KnE Life Sci.*, **3**(5): 81–98.
189. Jaeger R., Cuny E. (2016). Terpenoids with Special Pharmacological Significance: A Review. *Nat. Prod. Commun.*, **11**(9): 1373–1390.
190. Tholl D. (2015). Biosynthesis and Biological Functions of Terpenoids in Plants. *Adv. Biochem. Eng. Biotechnol.*, **148**: 63–106.
191. Bergman M.E., Davis B., Phillips M.A. (2019). Medically Useful Plant Terpenoids: Biosynthesis, Occurrence, and Mechanism of Action. *Molecules*, **24**: 3961, 23 pages.

192. Pichersky E., Raguso R.A. (2018). Why Do Plants Produce So Many Terpenoid Compounds? *New Phytol.*, **220**: 692–702.

193. Wang C., Liwei M., Park J-B., Jeong S-H., Wei G., Wang Y., Kim S-W. (2018). Microbial Platform for Terpenoid Production: Escherichia Coli and Yeast. *Front. Microbiol.*, **9**: 2460, 8 pages.

194. Wang G., Tang W., Bidigare R.R. (2005). Chapter 9. Terpenoids as Therapeutic Drugs and Pharmaceutical Agents, pp. 197–227. In: *Natural Products: Drug Discovery and Therapeutic Medicine.* Editors: Lixin Zhang, Arnold Demain. Humana Press, Totowa, NJ, 382 pages.

195. Thoppill R.J., Bishayee A. (2011). Terpenoids as Potential Chemopreventive and Therapeutic Agents in Liver Cancer. *World J. Hepatol.*, **3**(9): 228–249.

196. Grassmann J. (2005). Terpenoids as Plant Antioxidants. *Vitam. Horm.*, **72**: 505–535.

197. Perrone D., Monteiro M., Nunes J.C. (2015). Chapter 1: The Chemistry of Selenium, pp. 3–15. In: *Selenium: Chemistry, Analysis, Function and Effects.* 1st edition. Editors: Victor R. Preedy. Royal Society of Chemistry, London.

198. Kiełczykowska M., Kocot J., Aździor M., Musik I. (2018). Selenium – A Fascinating Antioxidant of Protective Properties. *Adv. Clin. Exp. Med.*, **27**(2): 245–255.

199. Zoidis E., Seremelis I., Kontopoulos N., Danezis G.P. (2018). Selenium-Dependent Antioxidant Enzymes: Actions and Properties of Selenoproteins. *Antioxidants (Basel)*, **7**(5): 66, 26 pages.

200. Tinggi U. (2008). Selenium: Its Role as Antioxidant in Human Health. *Environ. Health Prev. Med.*, **13**(2): 102–108.

201. Battin E.E., Brumaghim J.L. (2009). Antioxidant Activity of Sulfur and Selenium: A Review of Reactive Oxygen Species Scavenging, Glutathione Peroxidase, and Metal-Binding Antioxidant Mechanisms. *Cell Biochem. Biophys.*, **55**: 1–23.

202. Kurokawa S., Berry M.J. (2013). Selenium. Role of the Essential Metalloid in Health. *Met. Ions Life Sci.*, **13**: 499–534.

203. Fairweather-Tait S.J., Bao Y., Broadley M.R., Collings R., Ford D., Hesketh J.E., Hurst R. (2011). Selenium in Human Health and Disease. *Antioxid. Redox Signal.*, **14**(7): 1337–1383.

204. Guillin O.M., Vindry C., Ohlmann T., Chavatte L. (2019). Selenium, Selenoproteins and Viral Infection. *Nutrients*, **11**: 2101, 33 pages.

205. Wang N., Tan H-Y., Li S., Xu Y., Guo W., Feng Y. (2017). Supplementation of Micronutrient Selenium in Metabolic Diseases: Its Role as an Antioxidant. *Oxid. Med. Cell. Longev.* **2017**, Article ID 7478523, 13 pages.

206. Thomson C. (2004). Assessment of Requirements for Selenium and Adequacy of Selenium Status: A Review. *Eur. J. Clin. Nutr.*, **58**: 391–402.

207. Brown K.M., Arthur J.R. (2001). Selenium, Selenoproteins and Human Health: A Review. *Public Health Nutr.*, **4**(2B): 593–599.

208. Pham-Huy C., Nguyen P., Marchand V., Claude J.R., Duc H.T. (2001). Selenium and Tobacco Smoke Tars: In Vitro Effects on Different Immunocompetent Cells. *Toxicology*, **164**: 111–112. Presented in International Congress of Toxicology XI, Brisbane (Australia), July 7–12.

209. Bost M., Houdart S., Oberli M., Kalonji E., Huneau J-F., Margaritis I. (2016). Dietary Copper and Human Health: Current Evidence and Unresolved Issues. *J. Trace Elem. Med. Biol.*, **35**: 107–115.

210. Palumaa P. (2013). Copper Chaperones. The Concept of Conformational Control in the Metabolism of Copper. *FEBS Letters*, **587**: 1902–1910.

211. Li C., Li Y., Ding C. (2019). The Role of Copper Homeostasis at the Host-Pathogen Axis: From Bacteria to Fungi. *Int. J. Mol. Sci.*, **20**(175), 15 pages.

212. Osredkar J., Sustar N. (2011). Copper and Zinc, Biological Role and Significance of Copper/Zinc Imbalance. *J. Clinic. Toxicol.*, **S3**: 001, 18 pages.

213. Powell S.R. (2000). The Antioxidant Properties of Zinc. *J. Nutr.*, **130**: 1447S–1454S.

214. Jahaun Azadmanesh J., Borgstahl G.E.O. (2018). A Review of the Catalytic Mechanism of Human Manganese Superoxide Dismutase. *Antioxidants*, **7**: 25, 16 pages.

215. Houldsworth A. (2016). A Review of the Role of Mitochondrial Manganese Superoxide Dismutase in Human Disorders, Such as, Diabetes. *J. Endocrinol. Diab.*, **3**(3): 1–5.

216. Gozzelino R., Arosio P. (2016). Iron Homeostasis in Health and Disease. *Int. J. Mol. Sci.*, **17**(1): 130, 14 pages.

217. Fraga C.G., Oteiza P.I. (2002). Iron Toxicity and Antioxidant Nutrients. *Toxicology*, **180**(1): 23–32.

218. Alink G.M., Awad H.M., Boersma M.G., Cnubben N.H.P., De Haan L., Koeman J.H., Rietjens I.M.C.M., Spenkelink B., Van Der Woude H., Van Zanden J.J. (2002). The Prooxidant Chemistry of the Natural Antioxidants: Vitamin C, Vitamin E, Carotenoids and Flavonoids. *Environ. Toxicol. Pharmacol.*, **11**(3–4): 321–333.

219. Bouayed J., Bohn T. (2010). Exogenous Antioxidants – Double-Edged Swords in Cellular Redox State. Health Beneficial Effects at Physiologic Doses Versus Deleterious Effects at High Doses. *Oxid. Med. Cell. Longev.*, **3**(4): 228–237.

220. El-Ansary A.K., Kotb M., Rizk M.Z., Siddiqi N.J. (2014). Prooxidant Mechanisms in Toxicology. *BioMed Res. Int.*, **2014**, Article ID 308625, 2 pages.

221. Carocho M., Ferreira I.C.F.R., Morales P., Sokovic M. (2019). Antioxidants and Prooxidants: Effects on Health and Aging 2018. *Oxid. Med. Cell. Longev.*, **2019**, Article ID 7971613, 2 pages.

222. Li W.W., Li V.W., Hutnik M., Chiou A.S. (2012). Tumor Angiogenesis as a Target for Dietary Cancer Prevention. *J. Oncol.*, Article ID 879623, 23 pages.

4 Food Types, Dietary Supplements, and Roles

1 INTRODUCTION

Indeed, it is difficult to define and classify food into different 'food types'. In the literature, there are many different definitions of food types based either on their nutrients or on their preparation modes. Here, food is divided into different types based on their origin, production, preparation, and processing. The mode of food procurement varies with time, areas, and countries.

Historically, the type of food consumed by humans since antiquity was wild foods obtained by hunting and gathering. They then discovered the techniques of cultivation for plants and of farming for animals; this type of food is now known as natural foods. In the market nowadays, there are different food types such as natural foods, organic foods, industrial foods, functional foods, genetically modified foods, and fast foods. Moreover, there are different products obtained from food either by extraction or by biological or chemical synthesis; they are named dietary supplements and nutraceuticals. They are not considered a food or a drug, but they are classified as a complement of food. They are presented in drug forms such as capsule, tablet, liquid, or powder for oral use only. Therefore, dietary supplements and nutraceuticals can be sold over the counter. Recently, some new types of foods appear in the market such as alkaline diet and alkaline water. They are invented by some manufacturers who claim that the alkalinity of a food or a drink may protect the body against certain chronic diseases. Other types of foods named nano-foods are now prepared by nanotechnology for their long storage and preservation and also for enhancing the bioavailability and efficacy of their nutrients (antioxidants, phytonutrients).

2 CLASSIFICATION AND DESCRIPTION

The main food types described in this chapter include: wild foods, natural foods, organic foods, industrial foods, genetically modified foods, beverage types, food cooking types, functional foods, dietary supplements and nutraceuticals, alkaline diet, and nano-foods or food nanotechnology.

2.1 WILD FOODS

Wild foods may be defined as edible foods obtained from the wild or natural spaces such as hills, forests, lakes, rivers, seas, and oceans, by gathering or hunting, and without human care before. They are used directly for eating raw or cooking. They belong to animal, plant, and fungi species and they are nutritive and selected to be not dangerous for the health. 'Wild' foods are also defined as any uncultivated species, plant, or animal – procured without prior human care (1). Today, by Food and Agriculture Organization (FAO) estimate, around one billion people still use wild foods in their diet (2). Forests provide livelihoods and food for some 300 million people in the form of non-timber forest products (2). Wild aquatic foods including saltwater and freshwater fish and shellfish are the preferable foodstuffs for a large number of people worldwide because they are rich in nutrients and abundant in the environment. A number of wild vegetable and animal foods are now cultivated or farmed, then processed by different techniques to become other food types like natural foods, organic foods, industrial foods, functional foods, and genetically modified organism foods. Most edible wild plants and animals living in forests, mountains, prairies, seacoasts, lakes, ponds, and so on are consumed as food mainly in developing countries; some of them are now domesticated

DOI: 10.1201/9781003220817-4

or cultivated, and called farmed foods. Wild edible plants are species that are neither cultivated nor domesticated but growing wild and are, however, edible (3). Poor countries throughout the world are dependent on these wild plants for their food, nutrition, and subsistence needs (3). Nutritional superiority of some of the wild edible plants has also been reported over cultivated ones (3). The list of wild edible plants and fruits is long. Here are some species most appreciated throughout the world: amaranth, angelica, arrowhead, balsamroot, blueberry, wild blackberry, black raspberry, bamboo shoot, cattail, maple, mulberry, oak, nettle, sea buckthorn, butternut, chickweed, chicory, clover, gooseberry, hawthorn, licorice, lotus, milkweed, mint, spearmint, peppermint, salsify, sarsaparilla, thistle, pepper elder, and more (3–7).

Wild plant and animal source foods are the most consumed by local populations in developing countries, especially when famine occurs. Wild land animal meats are rarely found in the markets of developed countries, but are still present in developing communities. In contrast, nowadays, wild seafood (fish and shellfish), as well as wild freshwater fish and some wild algae, are the most consumed worldwide, especially in countries near sea or ocean. Wild seafood harvested in large oceans are better than farmed fish because they contain less contaminant compounds like mercury and industrial waste than farmed fish. In the recent past, thousands of wild plants have been used for food and other purposes by Native Americans. Many were still used by autochthonous people living in different regions of this planet such as in Mediterranean countries, Spain, Russia, New Zealand, the America continents, and Asia (4–10).

In brief, wild plant and animal foods are food items obtained directly from nature and they do not content artificial chemicals like pesticides and insecticides; therefore, they are safer than cultivated and farmed foods. However, be careful with some poisonous wild plants such as mushrooms and algae, because their appearance can be similar to other edible varieties. Do not eat wild plants and fruits if you are not sure. Purchase them in a professional store.

2.2 NATURAL FOODS

In general, natural foods come from plants and animals naturally obtained by farming, cultivation, harvesting, fishing or catch, and are not modified chemically or obtained by synthesis. They are different from wild foods because they are obtained from cultivated plants and farmed animals. For example, a wild fruit gathered in the forest may be different in nutrients from the same fruit cultivated in the garden; a cultivated manioc may be healthier than a wild manioc; a sea fish captured by fishing may be richer in nutrients than the same sea food by farming or aquaculture, and so on. In general, natural foods do not contain artificial food additives such as hormones, antibiotics, sweeteners, food colors, or flavorings (11). However, in some countries, plants treated by fertilizers, pesticides, preservatives are considered natural foods. Plants exempt from these chemicals are called organic foods.

Natural foods are also the raw material of other types of food recently marketed as organic foods, industrial or processed foods, functional foods, genetically modified organism (GMO) foods, and so on. Therefore, the term 'natural food' may be defined as food obtained from natural origin without any ulterior chemical or physical processing.

Many natural plant foods vary in their nutrient composition due to their different cultivars and geographic culture. Many cultivated plant species have several distinct cultivars. A cultivar (cultivated variety) is a variety or race of plant that has been selected by the cultivator and maintained through cultivation. Plant variety and cultivar identification is one of the most important aspects in agricultural systems (12). For example, different cultivars of the same crop may differ in nutrient composition, which can also vary depending on fertilizer regimen, growing conditions, season, climate, country, soil, and other factors. An apple may have many varieties with different nutrients, savors, odors, colors, health effects, and so on. Turmeric, a spice, can have different levels of its antioxidant, curcumin, depending on its cultivar and the region where it is cultivated. For animal foods, the nutrient composition of livestock products can similarly be affected by factors such as age and breed of the animal, feeding regimen, and season. The choice and combination of different natural foods for consumption play an important role in health maintenance and disease prevention.

2.3 ORGANIC FOODS

The term 'organic' refers to the process used for the production of vegetal and animal foods. It is denotes foods that have been grown or farmed without the use of artificial chemicals such as chemical fertilizers, pesticides, insecticides, preservatives, hormones, antibiotics, or genetically modified organisms (GMO) (13–19). The other foods are called non-organic, natural, industrial, or conventionally-grown products. In general, organic foods are originated from natural foods exempt of artificial chemicals. In order to be labelled organic by an official organization such the USDA (United States Department of Agriculture) with a special certification, a food product must be free of artificial food additives. This includes artificial sweeteners, preservatives, natural coloring, flavoring, and monosodium glutamate (MSG). Organically grown crops tend to use natural fertilizers like manure to improve plant growth. Animals raised organically are also not given antibiotics or hormones. Organic farming tends to improve soil quality and the conservation of groundwater. Although organic fruits and vegetables are slightly more expensive than ordinary species and have shorter storage periods, they are beneficial not only for human health, but also for the environment, such as water, air, birds, fish, and bees. In summary, organic foods preserve human and animal health and reduce air and water pollution. The most commonly purchased organic foods are fruits, vegetables, grains, dairy products, and meat.

Indeed, a wild food may be called an organic product if it is certified by an official institution because wild foods come from nature and do not contain artificial chemicals like pesticides and preservatives. Otherwise, they are labelled with the mention of wild products, such as wild trout fishing, wild bolete, wild blackberry, and so on. A natural food may also be named an organic food if this natural food is obtained from a cultivated plant or a farmed animal exempt of all artificial chemicals. In general, organic foods are issued from natural foods or wild foods grown without preservatives or pesticides, and are certified by an official organization.

Actually, many questions are often posed about the difference in nutrients (carbohydrates, proteins, fats, vitamins, antioxidants, minerals) between organic foods and non-organic foods. The responses are found mixed in the literature. According to Dangour et al. (13) and some other authors (17), there is no evidence of a difference in nutrient quality between organically and conventionally produced foodstuffs after a systematic review of studies of satisfactory quality. The small differences in nutrient content detected are biologically plausible and mostly relate to differences in production methods. However, some studies have recently concluded that organic production methods lead to increases in nutrients, particularly organic acids and polyphenolic compounds, many of which are considered to have potential human health benefits as antioxidants (14–16, 18–19). According to a recent systematic literature review and meta-analysis (16), there is evidence that higher antioxidant concentrations and lower toxic cadmium metal concentrations are linked to specific agronomic practices (e.g., non-use of mineral nitrate and phosphate fertilizers) prescribed in organic foods. These authors concluded that organic crops, on average, have higher concentrations of antioxidants and lower concentrations of cadmium than non-organic crops (16).

Two major hypotheses explaining the higher quantities of organic acids and polyphenolics in organic versus conventional foods have been proposed (14). One hypothesis considers the impacts of different fertilization practices on plant metabolism. In conventional agriculture, synthetic fertilizers such as nitrates frequently make nitrogen more available for the plants than do the organic fertilizers and may accelerate plant growth and development. Therefore, plant resources are allocated for growth purposes, resulting in a decrease in the production of compounds non-essential to the life of the plant such as organic acids, polyphenolics, chlorophyll, and amino acids. The second hypothesis considers the responses of plants to stressful environments such as attacks from insects, weeds, and plant pathogens. The reaction of plant to this situation results is the fabrication of new compounds such as vitamins, antioxidants, and minerals in order to resist this invasion (14). This phenomenon is comparable to the immune defense in humans and animals. Other studies using organically and conventionally cultivated strawberries demonstrated that extracts from organic strawberries showed higher anti-proliferative activity against colon cancer and breast cancer cells *in vitro* than did extracts from conventional strawberries (15). A comparative study of crops produced by an organic farming system to crops produced using a conventional farming system reported that organic crops contained 27% more vitamin C, 21.1% more iron, 29.3% more magnesium, and 13.6% more phosphorus than did conventional crops (14). Moreover, other factors that influence the nutrient content in plants are soil, climate, and which cultivars (plant varieties) are chosen.

In summary, contrary to conventional foodstuffs, organic foods are now more widely appreciated by a lot of people worldwide thanks to the absence of harmful chemicals (pesticides, insecticides, hormones, preservatives), despite their higher price and their shorter preservation time (19). It is preferable to eat organic products when consuming entire fruits and vegetables such as berries, grapes, apples, apricots, pears, plums, celery, broccoli, lettuce, tomato, cabbage, and green beans, as well as mushrooms. However, fruits with thick peel such as grapefruit, mangosteen, jackfruit, watermelon, and coconut may be used as nonorganic entities, except if the producer has injected preservatives into the fruits.

2.4   Food Industry or Food Processing

The term 'food industry', also called 'food processing' or 'processed foods', pertains to all foods obtained or processed by different manual and mechanical techniques in industry in order to preserve food for a long time, present ready-to-use, or to create other products with more attractive forms and/or delicious tastes (20–25). Food processing requires several operations such as cleaning, peeling, cutting, drying, evaporation, freezing, grinding, filtration, cooking, baking, roasting, toasting, frying, boiling, grilling, sterilization, lyophilization, pasteurization, canning, packaging, and so on. Therefore, processed foods are more practical and appealing than natural foods, but their effects on human health leave much to be desired. The food production in industry takes fruits, vegetables, and grains in their harvested forms as well as meat directly after the butchering process and transforms these into the types of food products that are available for sale in supermarkets. Food production ranges from minimal processing, like cleaning and packaging, to complicated processing involving lots of additives and ingredients. A few examples of industrial foods include: packaged foods (fresh fruits, fresh meat, etc.), dairy foods (milk, cheese, yogurt, etc.), frozen foods (fish, meat, vegetable, etc.), dried foods (cake, chip, chocolate, pasta, rice, flour, sugar, etc.), conserved foods (jam, jelly, marmalade, etc.), canned foods (sardine, mushroom, orange juice, etc.), and fast foods (sandwiches, pizza, etc.). On the other hand, the term food industry covers a series of industrial activities directed at the processing, conversion, preparation, preservation, vacuum cooling, and packaging of foodstuffs such as in the agriculture industry, frozen food factories, wine manufacture, corn production, and so on. (26–27). Concerning the advantages and disadvantages of industrial foods in human health and life, there are different approaches depending on the processing chosen for a type of natural food. For example, a fresh food conserved by freezing or pasteurization contains nutrient and antioxidant levels higher than the same food prepared by boiling, grilling, or drying. Similarly, a ready-to-eat food like dried food (biscuit, cake) or fast food is often less nutritious than a frozen or a fresh food. A number of industrial foods are rich in calories due to the addition of sugar, fat, chemical additives, preservatives, artificial savor and flavor, in order to make them delicious and appealing, such as cake and canned fruit juice. Recently, five systematic reviews have concluded that there is an association between soft drink intake and increased energy intake, excess body weight, and diabetes (28–29). Moreover, some beneficial nutrients like vitamins C and E, as well as antioxidants in fresh foods, can be destroyed by heat, air, or time during preparation and conservation. For example, polyphenol antioxidants (catechins) are not found in canned tea, contrary to the same tea freshly prepared by infusion. However, canned tomato juice is an exception because lycopene, an antioxidant in tomato fruit, is stable with heat, air, and time (30). Additionally, some snack foods and fast foods contain unhealthy ingredients and preservatives such as saccharine, glutamate, and sulfite. The advantages of industrial foods are their long preservation, hygienic property, practicability, and savings on time and money.

2.5 GENETICALLY MODIFIED FOODS OR TRANSGENIC FOODS

Genetic modification is a biological technique that effects alterations in the genetic machinery of all kinds of living organisms. Genetically modified organisms (GMO) are defined as follows by WHO (World Health Organization): 'Organisms (i.e., plants, animals or microorganisms) in which the genetic material (DNA) has been altered in a way that does not occur naturally by mating and/or natural recombination' (31). The definition seeks to distinguish the direct manipulation of genetic material from the millennial-old practice of improvement in the genetic stock of plants and animals by selective breeding. With DNA recombinant technology, genes from one organism can be transferred into another, usually unrelated, organism (31–32). In genetic modification (or engineering) of food plants, scientists remove one or more genes from the DNA of another organism, such as a bacterium, virus, animal, or plant, and 'recombine' them into the DNA of the plant they want to alter. By adding these new genes, genetic engineers hope the plant will express the traits associated with the genes (31–33). Actually, the use of genetically modified organisms (GMO) in foods, also called GM foods, is a controversial subject regarding their effects on human health and environment (31–38). However, advantages and disadvantages of genetically modified foods in human health and environment are still under hot debate worldwide. Some main advantages are: insect resistance, high harvest yield, increase of food production, and incorporation of new nutrients in plants (31–35) For example, Golden Rice is rice incorporated with a gene for vitamin A production, thereby improving food quality. Some GMO plants (cereal, canola, tomato, potato) have showed more resistance to insects and other pests, thereby reducing the use and propagation of pesticides and insecticides in the environment and also increasing production yield. However, for the consumers, the debates over GM foods focus mostly on uncertainties concerning the potential adverse effects of GM foods on human health and environmental safety. Three major health risks potentially associated with GM foods are: toxicity, allergenicity, and genetic hazards (31–38). These arise from three potential sources: the inserted gene and its expressed proteins per se, secondary or pleiotropic effects of the products of gene expression, and the possible disruption of natural genes in the manipulated organism (31). Other negative effects are: cross-pollination (pollen from the GMO crop may carry to a non-GMO one by pollen dissemination in air), the creation of new diseases by using virus and bacterium genes for the GMO plants, and antibiotic resistance due to the use of antibiotics as a genetic modifying agent (31, 35–37). According to a recent review concerning the toxicity study of GM plants and food worldwide, the author concluded that the number of research studies was surprisingly limited and incomplete; where is the scientific evidence showing that GM plants and food are toxicologically safe? (38). A total of 38 countries worldwide have officially banned the cultivation of GM crops, and only 28 actually grow GM crops (39). These are the European countries which have a ban on GMO crops: Austria, Azerbaijan, Bosnia and Herzegovina, Bulgaria, Croatia, Cyprus, Denmark, France, Germany, Greece, Hungary, Italy, Latvia, Lithuania, Luxembourg, Malta, Moldova, The Netherlands, Northway, North Ireland, Poland, Russia, Scotland, Serbia, Slovenia, Switzerland, Ukraine, and Wales (37, 39). In contrast, few countries fervently grow GM crops including: USA, Argentina, Brazil, China, Canada, South Africa, Australia, India, and Pakistan (39). For a number of countries, their opinions are unknown or mitigated.

Briefly, it is evident that GMO protects crops of some cereal plants like corn, wheat, and rice against insects and give them higher production outputs; however, their noxious effects are still unknown, regarding genetic inheritance of humans in the long term, and on genes of other plants or animals, due to the recent discovery of transgenic plants. More toxicological and genetic studies in the long term are needed to ensure the safety to consumers worldwide.

2.6 BEVERAGE TYPES

A beverage or drink is an artificial liquid designed for human consumption. Beverages do not include natural water such as tap or municipal water, source water, spring water, distilled water, and so on. Natural water and its different varieties are described in Chapter 7 of this book.

Most beverages contain a great deal of water. This does not add many nutrients to the diet, but it does play an important role in maintaining body balance by preventing dehydration (40). Beverages are used to satisfy thirst and also to give some sensation to the consumer through the flavor of the product added in this liquid. Beverages are divided into two types: non-alcoholic and alcoholic beverages. Non-alcoholic drinks include non-carbonated drinks and carbonated drinks. Non-carbonated drinks include tea, coffee, pure or diluted fruit or vegetable juices, and syrups, while carbonated drinks or gazed drinks contain carbon dioxide (CO_2) gas, sugar, or saccharine with other ingredients (40). In general, drinks do not provide enough energy to the body. However, beverages rich in sugar and fruits can be a good source of energy. In addition, pure fruit juices provide a supply of vitamins and minerals (40). Certain drinks contain artificial flavorings, colorings, and preservatives. The use of such additives is governed by legal requirements and it is vital to abide by these regulations in order to protect the consumer from any undesirable side effects (40). Some flavoring, coloring and preservative agents may cause hypersensitivity such as asthma and rhinitis in some allergic people, especially in children, and are therefore to be avoided.

Beverages can be prepared on the spot (home, coffee shop) like tea or coffee, or already industrially processed and sold in bottles, like juices, soft drinks, energy drinks, alcoholic drinks, alkaline water, and so on. Aside from pure water, the types of beverages most consumed include tea, coffee, fruit juices, soft drinks, and alcoholic drinks.

2.6.1 Soft Drinks

Soft drinks, also called sparkling soft drinks, are in general sweet water and sweet carbonated water containing some artificial or natural flavors, colorings, and preservatives (40). The sweet taste is either due to sugar, fruit juice or saccharine, a synthetic sugar substitute reserved for diet consumer. These soft drinks, with gas or without, can refresh you and give you some energy, but the presence of sugar or equivalent and preservatives is not good for your health if taken regularly.

Recently, many scientific reviews have reported that regular soft drink intake in young people is linked to obesity, diabetes, and other diseases (28–29, 41). Soft drink consumption has become a highly visible and controversial public health and public policy issue (41). Soft drinks are viewed by many as a major contributor to obesity and related health problems, and have consequently been targeted as a means to help curtail the rising prevalence of obesity, particularly among children. Soft drinks have been banned from schools in Britain and France, and in some states of the United States (41). Many studies found clear associations of long-term soft drink consumption with increased energy intake and body weight. The fact is that soft drinks offer energy with little accompanying nutrition, they displace other nutrient sources, and are linked to several key health conditions such as diabetes, obesity, cardiovascular diseases, tooth decay. In children and adults, frequent soft drink intake has also been associated with lower intakes of milk and other foods rich in calcium, as well as other nutrients which are necessary for health maintenance and disease prevention, all along with an increased risk of several medical problems (41).

2.6.2 Energy Drinks

Other soft beverages most consumed by young people are energy drinks. Recently, a number of scientists have raised alarm about the harmful effects of energy drinks in young people (42–44). 'Energy drinks' are non-alcoholic beverages containing high levels of caffeine (>150 mg/L) in combination with other ingredients such as taurine, vitamins, herbal supplements, and sugar, or sweeteners known to have stimulant properties (42–43). They are marketed explicitly as a way to relieve fatigue and improve mental alertness and to improve energy, weight loss, stamina, athletic performance, and concentration (42–43). According to some report surveys, energy drinks are con-sumed by 30 to 50% of adolescents and young adults (42). Frequently, these drinks have been reported in association with serious adverse effects such as seizures, cardiac abnormalities, dia-betes, and mood disorders, especially in children, adolescents, and young adults. Energy drinks have no therapeutic benefit, and many ingredients are understudied and not regulated (42). The known and unknown pharmacology of agents included in such drinks, combined with reports of toxicity, raises concern for potentially serious adverse effects in association with energy drink use. Educating adolescents and increasing the community's awareness of the hazards of energy drinks is of paramount importance (42).

2.6.3 Fruit Juice Drinks

Fruit juice drinks are divided into two groups: those that are drunk as pure fruit juice without the addition of other ingredients, and those that are diluted with sugar syrup. The former group should not need any preservatives if processed and packaged properly. However, the latter must contain certain amounts of permitted preservatives to have a long shelf-life after opening (40). It is also noteworthy that some labile vitamins (like C and E) and some antioxidants like polyphenols and flavonoids present in fruit or legume juices could be lost with heat, air, and time during preparation and conservation.

2.6.4 Alcoholic Drink

Alcoholic drinks are aqueous liquids that contains ethanol or ethyl alcohol, an organic chemical molecule obtained by fermentation. The products used for fermentation must contain plant sugars or carbohydrates (starch, disaccharides, or monosaccharides) often present in fruits, tubers, grains, stems, and saps. Two main plant materials used for fermentation are fruits and cereal grains. To obtain alcoholic beverages by fermentation, sugar (glucose, sucrose, or fructose) present in fruits or cereals is converted to alcohol and gases ($CO2$) by the action of yeasts such as some varieties of the yeast *Saccharomyces cerevisiae*. This reaction occurs within the yeast cell by anaerobic process and under certain conditions of temperature and time (45–46).

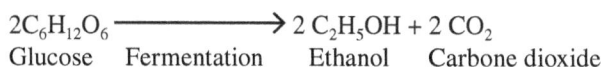

$$2C_6H_{12}O_6 \xrightarrow{\text{Fermentation}} 2\,C_2H_5OH + 2\,CO_2$$

Glucose   Fermentation   Ethanol   Carbone dioxide

The most common examples of alcoholic beverages are wines and beers. Beer is usually made from cereals (mainly malt and sometimes corn, rice, and hops), whereas wine can be produced from fruits (especially grapes, and sometimes plum, cherry, pomegranate, etc.) and cereals (rice). Alcohol has been produced from antiquity about seven thousand years ago, firstly in China, and then spread to Middle East and Europe. Nowadays, the most widely consumed alcoholic drinks are wines and beers. Other alcoholic beverage types include liquor, cider, whisky, vodka, tequila, brandy, sake, rice alcohol, rum, and absinthe. All these drinks contain ethanol in different degrees, called alcohol by volume (abv), and expressed in ml of pure ethanol per 100ml (%). Cider and beer have the low-est degree of alcohol among alcoholic drinks, in general 5% abv (usually between 4–6% for beer and 2–8% for cider). Red wine and white wine have about 12–14% abv. Light liqueurs, sake, rice alcohol, rice wine or Mijiu, and vermouth have about 20% abv. Spirits vary between 20–70% abv, in which whisky, rum, vodka, brandy, gin, all contain about 40% abv, while absinthe varies between 55–90% abv (45).

Alcoholic drinks are judged in terms of flavor and the stimulant effect they produce. Owing to these attractive effects, alcohol drinks can bring the consumer to a situation of alcohol dependence called alcoholism, a form of addiction. In many countries, alcohol production is strictly controlled by government agencies and it may be difficult to obtain the necessary permits to produce these bev-erages legally. Alcohol is a psychoactive substance with dependence-producing properties that has been widely used in many cultures for centuries. The harmful use of alcohol causes vast disease as well as social and economic burden in societies. According to World Health Organization (WHO), about three million deaths every year worldwide, or 5.3% of all global deaths, result from harmful use of alcohol (46). Alcohol consumption is a causal factor in more than 200 disease and injury conditions. Drinking alcohol is associated with a risk of developing health problems such as mental and behavioral disorders, including alcohol dependence, liver cirrhosis, neurodegenerative diseases, cardiovascular diseases, gastro-intestinal diseases, and some cancers, as well as injuries resulting from violence and road clashes and collisions (46). A significant proportion of the disease burden attributable to alcohol consumption arises from unintentional and intentional injuries, including those due to road traffic crashes, violence, and suicides, and fatal alcohol-related injuries tend to occur in relatively younger age groups (46). Therefore, the problems of alcoholic drinks in health and disease are mainly linked to the quantity and the frequency of alcohol consumed in each individual per day. The phrase 'drink with moderation' makes no sense because it is not the volume of alcoholic drink that counts, but it is the quantity of pure alcohol intake that is important. For example, a cup of beer is less toxic than a cup of wine or whisky. Moreover, the origin of the alcoholic beverage also plays an important role in health and disease. For example, two mL of pure ethanol in red wine is less toxic than the same volume of pure alcohol in rice wine, because red wine has many flavonoid antioxidants present in red grapes, while rice wine does not. In brief, do not drink alcoholic beverages regularly, even it is a light alcoholic drink, because you could become alcohol dependent. However, some scientists have observed that among men, consumption of alcohol at least three to four days per week was inversely associated with the risk of myocardial infarction (47). Recently, a review has reported that a number of studies have consistently linked alcoholic beverage consumption with the development of several chronic disorders, such as cancer, immune diseases, cardiovascular diseases, diabetes mellitus, and obesity. The impact of drinking is usually dose-dependent, and light to moderate drinking tends to lower risks of certain diseases, while heavy drinking tends to increase the risks. Besides, other factors such as drinking frequency, genetic susceptibility, smoking, diet, and hormone status can modify the association. The amount of ethanol in alcoholic beverages is the determining factor in most cases (48). However, for the same degree of alcohol, red wine is better than white wine because red wine is prepared from red grapes which contain more strong antioxidants, like resveratrol, than white grapes.

The metabolism of alcohol is essential to human life. Alcohol metabolism takes place mainly in the liver and relies on two major nicotinamide adenine dinucleotide (NAD)-dependent enzymes, alcohol dehydrogenase (ADH), and aldehyde dehydrogenase 2 (ALDH2). Alcohol is first converted into acetaldehyde by ADH and cytochrome p450 2E1 (CYP2E1) via oxidative degradation, and the acetaldehyde is then oxidized to nontoxic acetate by ALDH and the coenzyme NAD or NADP for excretion (49). These two enzymes help break apart the alcohol molecule in order to eliminate it from the body. First, alcohol dehydrogenase (ADH) metabolizes alcohol to acetaldehyde, a highly toxic substance and known carcinogen (50). Acetaldehyde is generally short-lived; it is quickly broken down to a less toxic compound called acetate (CH_3COO^-) by another enzyme called aldehyde dehydrogenase (ALDH). Acetate then is broken down into carbon dioxide gas (CO_2) and water, mainly in tissues other than the liver for easy elimination (49–51).

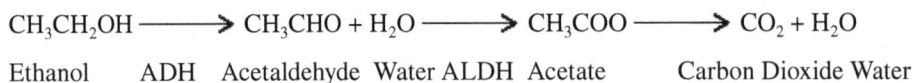

$$CH_3CH_2OH \longrightarrow CH_3CHO + H_2O \longrightarrow CH_3COO \longrightarrow CO_2 + H_2O$$

Ethanol   ADH   Acetaldehyde   Water   ALDH   Acetate   Carbon Dioxide   Water

The balance between the various ADH and ALDH isoforms regulates the concentration of acetaldehyde, which is important as a key risk factor for the development of alcoholism (49–50). Acetaldehyde dehydrogenase 2 (ALDH2) is the key enzyme responsible for metabolism of the alcohol metabolite acetaldehyde in the liver (49). Certain individuals, usually of Asian origin (China, Japan, Korea, Vietnam), have an inactive mitochondrial ALDH2 because of a genetic ALDH deficiency. Of note, approximately 8% of the world's population, and approximately 30–40% of the population in East Asia, carry an inactive ALDH2 gene (49). Thus, when these individuals consume ethanol, blood levels of acetaldehyde are 5-to 20-fold higher than those found in individuals with the active ALDH allele. Individuals with the inactive ALDH show marked vasodilator (facial flushing or red face), nausea, headaches, and palpitation when consuming alcohol (50). Acetaldehyde is poorly eliminated by these individuals and as a consequence, little alcohol is consumed. ALDH2 deficient individuals are at lower risk for alcoholism. In contrast, they may have possibly increased risk for liver damage and esophageal cancer if alcohol continues to be consumed due to the accumulation of acetaldehyde in these organs (49–51).

It is important to remember that light alcohol drinks such as beer, wine and cider contain sulfites which are used as preservative (52–53). Sulfites have been used since Roman times to preserve food flavor and color, inhibit bacterial growth, reduce spoilage, stop fresh food from spotting and turning brown, and help preserve medication and increase shelf life. Sulfites release sulfur dioxide, which is the active component that helps preserve food and medication (53). Sulfur dioxide (SO_2) is a colorless gas at room temperature, with a pungent odor which is readily soluble in water. Sulfur dioxide in aqueous solution gives a mixture of sulfur dioxide, sulfurous acid (H_2SO_3), bisulfite ion (HSO_3^-), and sulfite ion (SO_3^{2-}) which all have bactericide properties (52). Sulfites can occur naturally in a number of foods and beverages as a result of fermentation, such as those that occur in beer and wine (52). Sulfites can cause allergy-like reactions (intolerances) – most commonly asthma, rhinitis, wheezing, occasionally urticaria (hives), and very rarely, anaphylaxis (53). By law, the presence of sulfites must be indicated on the label of all foods by code numbers 220 to 228, or the word 'sulfite' (53). Red wine contains fewer sulfites than white wine because red wine contains many polyphenol antioxidants which are bactericide. Therefore, red wine is better than white wine.

2.6.5 Coffee

Coffee is an infusion of milled roasted coffee bean. This infusion is prepared on the spot, at home or at a coffee shop by mixing instant coffee powder with boiling water in a cup or by using a tool such as filter jug, plunger, or espresso machine containing coffee powder soaked with boiling water. Coffee is generally taken hot and pure or mixed with sugar, cream, or milk due to its slightly bitter taste. Although coffee is lauded for its aroma and flavor, coffee and its caffeine content play a role in its ability to help avoid somnolence, stimulate mood, and maintain alertness (54–57). With a history that began in 800 A.D. in the Ethiopian highlands, coffee is now one of the most popular beverages in the world, mostly in Western and Arab countries (54). There are different species of coffee plants, and the most common ones are *Coffea arabica* and *Coffea robusta* (56). *Coffea arabica* is originally from the eastern African region (Ethiopia, South Sudan, Yemen). It is now cultivated in many tropical countries and accounts for 70% of the global coffee production. *Coffea robusta* is originally from central and western sub-Saharan Africa, and is now cultivated in Vietnam and Brazil. In fact, coffee is a complex chemical mixture reported to contain more than a thousand different chemicals, including carbohydrates, lipids, nitrogenous compounds, vitamins, minerals (magnesium), alkaloids, and phenolic compounds (55–56). Coffee contains two main compounds: chlorogenic acids and caffeine. Caffeine or trimethylxanthine is a bitter purine alkaloid; while chlorogenic acids, which belong to a group of phenolic compounds, are a family of esters formed between the 3-hydroxyl position of quinic acid and caffeic acid (cinnamic acid). Other bioactive compounds in coffee are the pentacyclic diterpenes known as cafestol and kahweol, trigonelline, and melanoidins (54–56). Caffeine is also present in tea, kola, cacao, and more.

According to the review article of Higdon and Frei (55), the results of epidemiological research suggest that coffee consumption may help prevent several chronic diseases, including type 2 diabetes mellitus, Parkinson's disease and liver disease (cirrhosis and hepatocellular carcinoma). Most prospective cohort studies have not found coffee consumption to be associated with significantly increased cardiovascular disease risk. However, coffee consumption is associated with increases in several cardiovascular disease risk factors, including blood pressure, tachycardia, palpitation, and plasma homocysteine. At present, there is little evidence that coffee consumption increases the risk of cancer. For adults, consuming moderate amounts of coffee (3–4 cups/d providing 300–400 mg/d of caffeine), there is little evidence of health risks and some evidence of health benefits. However, some groups, including people with hypertension, children, adolescents, and the elderly, may be more vulnerable to the adverse effects of caffeine. In addition, currently available evidence suggests that it may be prudent for pregnant women to limit coffee consumption to 3 cups/day providing no more than 300 mg/day of caffeine to exclude any increased probability of spontaneous abortion or impaired fetal growth (55). Overall, the health benefits clearly outweigh the risks of moderate coffee consumption in adult people for the majority of health outcomes considered (57). This finding is largely based on observational data and, moreover, major interactions were noted between coffee consumption and other lifestyle habits (such as smoking, alcoholism). More additional clinical trials are needed about coffee, particularly in relation to sex, age, genetic polymorphisms, cardiovascular and gastrointestinal disorders, and the preparation type of coffee (57).

2.6.6   Tea

Tea infusion is the most widely consumed beverage in the world, aside from water (58–61). Tea is primarily consumed in Asia, but is becoming increasingly common in Western countries, due not only to its aromatic flavor and thirst-quenching property, but also to its perceived health benefits. Tea plant (*Camellia sinensis*), an evergreen shrub, originates from China and is now cultivated in about 30 countries, mainly in East and South Asia. In the market, three main tea types are found: green, black and oolong, are all prepared from the leaves of the same *Camellia sinensis* plant. The difference among them is due to the processing method called fermentation. Green tea is unfermented tea, produced by steaming or pan-frying the fresh-cut tea leaves at moderated temperatures (58–61). Black tea is fermented tea, obtained by allowing the leaves to oxidize at ambient temperature in certain time. During fermentation, enzymes in leaves oxidize many polyphenolic compounds, giving it the strongest flavor, darkest color, and lowest content of antioxidants. Oolong tea, a semi-fermented tea, is obtained by partial auto-oxidation process, giving oolong its unique flavor, and also its partial loss of antioxidants. The heating process used in green tea preparation inactivates the enzymes present in tea leaves, thereby avoiding the oxidation of tea polyphenolic antioxidants (58, 60). Several chemical components of green tea have been identified and determined. The most abundant constituents of green tea are catechins belonging to the flavan-3-ol class of flavonoids. The major four catechins in green tea leaves are: (-)-epigallocatechin gallate (EGCG), (-) epigallocatechin (EGC), (-)-epicatechin gallate (ECG), and (-)-epicatechin (EC) (58–61). They are all polyphenolic compounds and account for 78% of the antioxidant potential of green tea. Caffeine, theobromine and theophylline, the principal alkaloids, account for about 4% of the dry weight, of which 3.5% is caffeine. Green tea has about 1/10–1/6 as much caffeine as coffee, about 1/3 as black tea and about 1/2 as oolong tea. Tea is also rich in fluoride, an essential micro-mineral, for bone and tooth formation.

These green tea polyphenols/catechins are promising compounds in exhibiting antiviral activities. They show antiviral activity against a wide range of human viruses including influenza, hepatitis B, hepatitis C, herpes simplex virus, and HIV (human immunodeficiency viruses) (59). Recently, some scientists found that tea polyphenols might be potential inhibitors in vitro against the main protease (Mpro) of SARS CoV-2, a coronavirus (59). Coronavirus disease 2019 (Covid-19) is a viral respiratory disease which caused pandemic disease in 2019–2021 (59). In addition, tea polyphenols/catechins may prevent numerous pathologies such as cancer, cardiovascular disorders, neurodegenerative diseases, dental caries, obesity, and diabetes (58, 60–61). Amongst the proposed benefits are the prevention of breast and prostate cancers in humans and the maintenance of endothelial function and vascular homeostasis and an associated reduction in CVD risk and atherogenesis (58, 61). Green tea can prevent dental caries and some oral infections thanks to its catechins and fluoride content. Several human studies have shown that bacteria present in dental plaque stopped growing when people rinsed their mouths with tea many times in a day (58, 61–62). Moreover, green tea can inhibit the bacteria of periodontal disease (62). However, due to the presence of caffeine and polyphenols, some side effects have been reported with long-term or excessive use of green and black tea: insomnia, nervousness, anxiety, stomach ulcers, constipation, palpitation, vertigo, headache, iron deficiency anemia, and kidney disorders (58). It is recommended that children, breastfeeding and pregnant women also avoid consumption of tea. Tea infusion must be taken as soon as possible (within a couple of hours) and becomes darker with time because of the oxidization of polyphenols with air and eventually with light (58). Although the antioxidant potential of green tea is evident, the results from epidemiological and clinical studies of the relationship between green tea or black tea and prevention of cancer, arthritis, diabetes, and cardiovascular diseases in humans are mixed. Briefly, the health benefits of green tea may be primarily preventive, still not therapeutic (58).

2.6.7 Plant-Based Milk Products

Plant-based or non-dairy milk alternative is a fast-growing segment in newer food product development category of functional and specialty beverages across the globe. Plant-based milk products are fluids resulting from the breakdown of plant material (cereals, legumes, oilseeds, nuts) extracted in water and further homogenization of such fluids (63). These products resemble cow's milk in appearance and consistency. The most well-known plant milk products are soy milk, coconut milk, and almond milk.

2.6.7.1 Soy Milk

Soy milk was the first plant-based milk which serves the purpose of providing nutrients to the population where the milk supply was inadequate. It is also popular among populations who are allergic to milk proteins and are lactose intolerant (63). Soy milk is a good source of essential unsaturated fatty acids (omega-3) which are considered good for cardiovascular health. It serves as an inexpensive, refreshing, and nutritional beverage for consumers. Isoflavones appear to be the functionally active component responsible for the beneficial effects of soybean. Isoflavones are well-known for their protective effect against cancer, cardiovascular disease, and osteoporosis (63). Genistein is the most abundant isoflavone in soybean and is proposed to be the most biologically active. Apart from isoflavones, soy proteins are also known to provide protective and therapeutic benefits against several diseases (63). Soy milk is naturally free of cholesterol and lactose and low in saturated fat.

2.6.7.2 Coconut Milk

Coconut milk plays an important part in the cuisine of Southeast Asia. It is not only consumed as a beverage but used as an ingredient in a number of sweet and savory recipes. Coconut milk has high fat content. Coconut milk is rich in fiber, vitamins C and E, and minerals such as iron, calcium, potassium, magnesium, and zinc (63). The use of coconut milk is associated with health benefits such as anti-carcinogenic, anti-microbial, anti-bacterial, and anti-viral. It contains a saturated fat, lauric acid which is present in mother's milk and has been related to promote brain development (63). Lauric acid is also helpful in boosting the immune system and maintaining the elasticity of blood vessels. Coconut milk helps digestion, nourishes the skin, and has cooling properties. In spite of all health benefits, presence of saturated fats limits its consumption (63).

2.6.7.3 Almond Milk

Almond milk contains approximately 25% protein, the majority of which is present in the form of amandin (63). Compared to other plant-based milks, almond milk is naturally a good source of vitamins, especially vitamin E and manganese. It is also rich in calcium, magnesium, zinc, selenium, potassium, phosphorus, and copper, and possesses potential prebiotic properties contributed by arabinose present in cell wall pectic substances which may lower serum cholesterol level (63).

2.6.8 Alkaline Water

The pH is a measure of the acid-base balance of a solution or a water. The pH (potential Hydrogen) measures the concentration of free hydrogen ions in a solution. The pH scale ranges from 0 (the most acidic) to 14 (the most basic), with 7 as the neutral mid-point. Most tap water and a number of spring and natural mineral waters have a pH around 7. Human blood has a pH of approximately 7.4 ± 0.05. It is essential for our bodies to maintain our blood pH within a tight range. Even a small fluctuation of as little as .05 in our blood pH can have severe health risks. However, the pH of the organs throughout the rest of the body can vary widely. In our stomach, the pH is acidic and varies from 1.5 to 3.5 during food digestion, while the pH of pancreatic juice is alkaline from 7.5–8.0.

There are two types of alkaline water: artificial alkaline water and natural alkaline water (64). Artificial alkaline water, also known as alkaline ionized water, is generally tap water run through an electrical ionizer to make the pH more alkaline – between eight and ten, on average nine. This alkaline water can be prepared at home or bought as a bottle in markets from some makers. An electrical water ionizer with platinum electrodes also known as an alkaline ionizer uses electrolysis to separate the incoming water stream into acidic and alkaline ions. The obtained water from this ionizer is named alkaline water because its original pH of seven now becomes between eight and ten (64). Moreover, some companies add alkaline minerals to the water to make it more basic and also to call it alkaline water. When you purchase artificial alkaline water in the market, you should pay attention to its pH, its salt levels, and its possible contaminants.

Natural alkaline water is water obtained from natural sources such as spring water; natural mineral water that has a pH in alkaline range. These natural waters pass through rocks and soil and picks up various minerals, which generally increase their pH between 7.4 and 9.0, on average 8.2. Naturally-occurring mineral water contains alkalizing compounds, such as calcium, silica, potassium, magnesium, and bicarbonate. Spring water with naturally occurring minerals seems to be the healthiest type of alkaline water source. According to a specialist of nutrition, a good source of alkaline water is spring water, with pH of 8 to 8.5 that naturally becomes alkaline by acquiring minerals as it passes over rocks (64). Therefore, natural alkaline water is generally better than artificial. Different types of natural water are spring water and mineral source water, and their detailed composition and obtention are developed in Chapter 7 of this book.

The use of artificial alkaline water for health and diseases is a controversial subject through today. Some people believe it has many health benefits. In contrast, scientific evidence is sparse to back this up. The benefits people claim include decreased risks for diseases, like cancer, preventing aging, and boosting metabolism. However, none of these claims have been verified in scientific studies (64–65). Since alkaline water has a higher pH, there is some empirical evidence for benefits of alkaline water. Preliminary studies have shown possible results for treating acid reflux disease in the stomach and some benign acidosis, a decrease of pH in blood, such as respiratory insufficiency (emphysema, bronchitis, asthma, etc.) that results from an accumulation of carbon dioxide in the blood. It is also used to treat metabolic acidosis caused by the accumulation of lactic acid and other acids in the body due to diabetes or renal insufficiency (64). Aside from these diseases, the abuse of artificial alkali water in long term may be harmful to the body. However, there isn't enough scientific evidence to support the use of alkaline water as a treatment for any health condition. Medical experts warn against believing all the marketing claims (64). Also keep in mind, drinking too much artificial alkaline water may leave you deficient in minerals (64). It should be noted that lowering stomach acid is not beneficial for most people. Stomach acid or gastric acid, mainly composed of hydrochloric acid (HCl) with pH from 1.5–3.5, is secreted to digest foods. Moreover, the other role of gastric acid is to kill bacteria and other unwanted pathogens present in foods so they don't pass into the bloodstream. Acidity is also essential to properly digest vitamin B-12 and protein. Some studies reported that the protein-based enzyme needed to digest protein in the stomach was completely deactivated by alkaline water (64). Therefore, regular consumption of artificial alkaline water or drinking water with a high pH may disrupt the normal pH in the body. This can lead to a condition called metabolic alkalosis, which may cause confusion, nausea, vomiting, hand tremors, muscle twitching, and tingling in the face, hands, or feet. Until today, no scientific research nor health organizations recommend the use of alkaline water for cancer and CVD prevention (64–65). The pH of an organ or tissue is not the cause of cancer as many people think. If cancer cells cannot survive in high alkaline environments, the other cells in our body cannot live also. It has been observed that tumors grow faster in acidic environments because cancer cells often liberate acidic compounds in their environment, in their tissue or organ; that's why their environment becomes acidic. This explains why it is not the acidic environment that causes the cancer. It would be remembered that cancer cells can also grow in alkaline environments such as alkaline water. No scientific studies have yet proven alkaline water to prevent cancer and aging in humans, except for some preliminary experiments in mice. The promotion of an alkaline diet and alkaline water to the public for cancer prevention or treatment is not justified (65). Briefly, there is no link between acidic water and cancer and the intake of alkaline water has no role in the prevention of cancer. The treatment of acidosis caused by different diseases must be done by healthcare professionals with the aid of medicines and not only by alkaline water. The abuse of artificial alkaline water in the long term may be harmful to the body because it neutralizes our gastric acid necessary for the digestion of foods as well as for the destruction of microbes eventually present in foods. In contrast, drinking natural alkaline water is generally considered safe, since it contains natural minerals. Natural alkaline water may be helpful for treating acid reflux disease and bone loss in some cases. Supporting evidence exists that natural alkaline water and alkaline diet with sufficient protein intake can support bone mineralization, whereas consumption of excess fruits, vegetables, and natural alkaline water has shown a significant promotion of health, especially for people of an older age (66).

Briefly, among all beverages cited here, natural mineral water is considered the safest, healthiest, and cheapest drink for everybody. Other beverages such as soft drinks, energy drinks, fruit juices, tea, coffee, beer, wine, liquor, and alkaline ionized water have some benefits, but they also may engender some or many harmful effects. Alcohol can cause dependence and is the source of many dramatic problems not only for the consumer but also for the family and society. Although some beverages are more beneficial than the others, there is no drink safer than natural water. Besides natural water, you could choose other beverages such as pure fruit juices, tea, coffee, and soy milk, but their consumption must be taken from time to time and in moderation. The choice of a good drink for your health requires some thought. Keep in mind that your health is not only in your plate, but also in your cup.

2.7 ALKALINE DIET

Human life requires a tightly controlled pH level in the serum of about 7.4 (a slightly alkaline range of 7.35 to 7.45) to survive. The alkaline diet is based on the idea that certain types of foods after digestion can modify the pH value of the body or can make certain organs or tissues more alkaline or more acidic (67). Alkaline diets result in a more alkaline urine pH and may result in reduced calcium in the urine, however, as seen in some recent reports, this may not reflect total calcium balance because of other buffers such as phosphate. There is no substantial evidence that an alkaline diet alone improves bone health or protects from osteoporosis (67). However, alkaline diets may result in a number of health benefits as outlined below:

Increased fruits and vegetables in an alkaline diet would improve the K/Na ratio and may benefit bone health, reduce muscle wasting, as well as mitigate other chronic diseases such as hypertension and stroke (65–67). The resultant increase in growth hormone with an alkaline diet may improve many outcomes from cardiovascular health to memory and cognition. An increase in intracellular magnesium, which is required for the function of many enzyme systems, is another added benefit of the alkaline diet. Available magnesium, which is required to activate vitamin D, would result in numerous added benefits in the vitamin D apocrine/exocrine systems. Alkalinity may result in added benefits for some chemotherapeutic agents that require a higher pH (67). From the evidence outlined above, it would be prudent to consider an alkaline diet to reduce morbidity and mortality of chronic disease that are plaguing our aging population (67).

So, alkaline foods are considered to be good for the body, while neutral foods have no effect, and acidic foods are harmful. According to the classification of this food conception, acidic foods include meat, poultry, fish, dairy, eggs, grains, and alcohol, while alkaline foods comprise fruits, nuts, legumes, and vegetables, and neutral foods are formed by natural fats, starches, and sugars (67). If this classification of foods based on their pH is true, it affects the blood pH of 7.4 ± 0.05 only very weakly, if at all, thanks to the body's acid-base homeostasis mechanism. Therefore, foods cannot change the pH value of the blood. If not, you would be in trouble after each meal. In reality, foods can only change the pH of urine by excreting the excess of acidic or alkaline compounds present in blood into the urine. That being said, urine pH is actually a very poor indicator of overall body pH and general health. It can be influenced by many factors other than diet. According to a recent systematic review of the literature, promotion of an alkaline diet and alkaline water to the public for cancer prevention or treatment is not justified (65). The use of vegetables, fruits, nuts and legumes for health promotion and disease prevention is well known due to their abundance in vitamins, antioxidants, and minerals, and not due to their alkaline pH, as this conception promotes. According to this classification, certain processed foods or fast foods are considered acidic and must be avoided. In reality, the noxiousness of these foods is due to the presence of some toxic compounds such as polycyclic aromatic hydrocarbons and acrolein formed during food cooking or food processing and not due to their acidity. Despite the promotion of the alkaline diet and alkaline water by the media and salespeople, there is almost no actual research to either support or disprove the promotion of these alkaline foods because of the lack of evidence (65). Therefore, the promotion of alkaline foods is still a 'hypothesis' and their explanations from some promoters have no scientific values in theory as well as in practice (65–67). A mixed diet composed of fruits, vegetables, animal foods, and dairy products is the ideal diet for the maintenance of good health.

2.8 FUNCTIONAL FOODS, FORTIFIED FOODS, AND ENRICHED FOODS

2.8.1 Functional Foods

Recently, a new type of food called functional foods has been introduced in the market. The term 'functional foods' was first introduced in Japan in the mid-1980s and refers to processed foods containing ingredients such as vitamins and minerals that aid specific bodily functions in addition to being nutritious (68–71). Functional foods are produced by the food industry to make them more attractive to consumers by adding healthy nutrients to classic foods. The Institute of Medicine's Food and Nutrition Board (IOM/FNB, 1994) in the United States defined functional foods as 'any food or food ingredient that may provide a health benefit beyond the traditional nutrients it contains' (68–69). Other definitions of functional foods are found in the scientific literature as follows. Functional foods are designed to have physiological benefits and/or reduce the risk of chronic disease beyond basic nutritional functions, and may be similar in appearance to conventional food and consumed as part of a regular diet (70). 'Food similar in appearance to conventional food that is intended to be consumed as part of a normal diet, but has been modified to sustain physiological roles beyond the provision of simple nutrient requirements' is another definition of functional foods (71). According to the European Commission's Concerted Action on Functional Food Science in Europe, and coordinated by International Life Science Institute in Europe, functional food is defined as follows: "a food product can only be considered functional if together with the basic nutritional impact it has beneficial effects on one or more functions of the human organism thus either improving the general and physical conditions or/and decreasing the risk of the evolution of diseases (71–74). The amount of intake and form of the functional food should be as it is normally expected for dietary purposes. Therefore, it could not be in the form of pill or capsule just as normal food form" (71, 72).

Functional foods are usually similar to foods that are consumed as part of our typical diet, like yogurt, drinks, bread, rice, eggs, and so on. Indeed, most natural foods that we eat daily such as fishes, vegetables, and fruits, are functional in some way. Therefore, the definition of functional foods is still a contentious issue. Regulatory agencies do not recognize 'functional food' as a nutritional entity. In other words, functional foods are branded foods, which claim, explicitly or implicitly, to improve health or well-being. These regulations often allow manufacturers to imply that a food promotes health without providing proper scientific evidence. At the same time, regulations may ban claims that a food prevents disease, even when it does (75). Although of course at some level all foods are functional, these foods would additionally have the potential to promote long-term health, improving both physical and mental health and well-being (76). In spite of attractive health claims, these products do not have legal or regulatory status in most countries. Moreover, health risks and side effects of functional foods are not studied and may exist.

In brief, most of the functional foods are derived from existing traditional foods by adding ingredients like vitamins, minerals, antioxidants, and probiotics, or by modifying the composition. The added ingredients are usually common food components. Functional foods have been developed in virtually all food categories: probiotics, prebiotics, functional drinks, functional cereals, functional eggs, functional meats, bakery products, dairy products, spreads, and more. Some main ingredients often added in functional foods are: probiotics, prebiotics, synbiotics, plant stanols and sterols, omega-3 fatty acids, vitamins, and minerals (71–77). The roles of probiotics, prebiotics, and synbiotics are described in Chapter 9 of this book.

Omega-3 unsaturated fatty acids including alpha-linoleic acid (ALA), docosahexaenoic acid (DHA), and eicosapentaenoic acid (EPA) are essential nutrients for the human body and found mainly in flaxseed, fish oil, and sea algae. As hen eggs contain a small amount of omega-3s, farmers now produce functional eggs by feeding hens with seeds and grains rich in omega-3s, mainly ALA. (68–69, 71–72, 77).

Other functional foods or drinks can be foods fortified with a nutrient that would not usually be present, such as bread or breakfast cereals fortified with folic acid (vitamin B9). Often, a food is termed functional because it contains high amounts of fibers such as oatmeal and pea fiber-fortified breads and pasta because they contain soluble fiber (beta-glucan) that can help lower cholesterol levels in blood for the prevention and treatment of atherosclerosis. Some foods are modified to have health benefits. An example is orange juice that has been fortified with calcium for bone health (69). Some components in plants, called 'phytochemicals' or 'secondary metabolites' such as catechins in tea, flavonoids in fruits, stanols and sterols in plants, terpenoids in turmeric, or ginger are added in foods for the prevention of some chronic diseases (68, 72, 74, 77). Functional foods and drinks may provide some health benefits but should not be seen as an alternative to a varied and balanced diet and a healthy lifestyle. Therefore, functional foods may be 'designed to have physiological benefits and/or reduce the risk of chronic disease beyond basic nutritional functions, and may be similar in appearance to conventional food and consumed as part of a regular diet' (69–70). However, not all foods in the market today that are claimed to be functional foods are supported by enough solid data to merit such claims (68). Though functional foods represent one of the most intensively investigated areas in the food and nutrition sciences today, it must be emphasized that these foods and ingredients are not magic bullets or panaceas for poor health habits (68).

2.8.2   Fortified Foods and Enriched Foods

Some definitional attempts have been made to distinguish between a functional food, a fortified food, and an enriched food. As previously cited, a functional food is any food or food ingredient that may provide a health benefit beyond the traditional nutrients it contains. A fortified food is a food that has nutrients added to it to boost the levels that are naturally present in this food; for example, salt fortified with iodine, water fortified with fluorine, and milk fortified with vitamin D. An enriched food is a food in which some micronutrients lost during processing are now restored by adding these micronutrients into the processed food (78). For example, a number of vitamins B and minerals are added to white bread by law as they are removed when the wheat is milled to make flour. During the processing of white rice from brown rice, many vitamins have been lost because they are in the brown bran of rice; white rice with added vitamins is called enriched rice. Fortified foods and enriched foods are subclasses of functional foods. Therefore, functional foods could be called fortified foods, and vice versa.

Concerning the roles of fortified foods in health and diseases, many international organizations such as World Health Organization (WHO) and Food and Agriculture Organization (FAO) have recognized that there are over two billion people worldwide who suffer from a variety of micronutrient deficiencies caused largely by a dietary deficiency of vitamins and minerals (78). The deficiency of iodine, iron, fluorine, selenium, vitamin A, and others, can be resolved by food fortification of these micronutrients. For example, salt fortified with iodine, tap water with fluorine, and soil enriched by fertilizer containing selenium have resolved the outbreak of many diseases due to deficiency of these micronutrients in certain areas of this planet. However, there are limitations to food fortification because of the toxicity of these micronutrients. When they are added in food with adequate quantity and used in case of micronutrient deficiency, they are useful for the health. However, they may become harmful at incorrect levels. Therefore, the addition of fluorine in tap water or of selenium in soil must be done by a competent public or private service. Although it is recognized that food fortification alone will not combat nutrient deficiency, it is a step towards reducing the prevalence of these deficiencies and their associated health conditions (78). Moreover, fortified foods or enriched foods are more costly than natural foods. For example, brown rice is cheaper than white rice enriched with vitamins B, and also, the vitamins in brown rice are in natural form, in contrast to synthetic vitamins added in white rice. In brief, food fortification must be used wisely in order to obtain expected results and also to avoid side effects. Therefore, the consumption of natural foods is the best way.

2.9 Nutraceuticals and Dietary Supplements

2.9.1 Definitions

In the literature there are many definitions about nutraceuticals and dietary supplements, and also many explanations concerning the differences between nutraceuticals and functional foods.

The term nutraceutical, a syncretic neologism of the words nutrient and pharmaceutical, was originally coined in 1989 by Stephen DeFelice, who defined nutraceuticals as 'food or part of a food that provides medical or health benefits, including the prevention and/or treatment of a disease' (79). According to Gupta (80), a nutraceutical is a substance that is cultivated/produced/extracted or synthesized under optimal and reproducible conditions and, when administered orally to patients, would provide the nutrient(s) required for bringing altered body structure and function back to normal, thus improving the health and well-being of the patients. Therefore, nutraceuticals fall somewhere between food nutrients and drugs (80). In the United States, nutraceutical and dietary supplements are considered the same product and the term dietary supplement is officially used. Regulation of nutraceuticals varies widely around the world. For example, China allows health claims for a nutraceutical if it has been approved by a Chinese regulatory body; whereas the United States does not allow any health claims for nutraceuticals because there is no formal review and approval process for the marketing authorization of nutraceuticals. In USA, they are classified as foods, not drugs, allowing them to be sold without proof of safety and effectiveness (80).

The similarity between dietary supplements, nutraceuticals and functional foods is that they are all products designed to supplement the human diet by increasing the intake of bioactive agents that are thought to enhance health and fitness. However, dietary supplements or nutraceuticals are sold in pill, capsule, tablet, or liquid form, while functional foods are whole natural foods in which some vitamins or antioxidants are added, such as functional eggs.

In summary, the term nutraceutical or dietary supplement is reserved only for ingredients (vitamins, amino acids, antioxidants, etc.) obtained from the extraction of natural foods and presented as drug forms (pill, tablet, capsule, powder, liquid) for oral use only. For example, fish oil, cod liver oil, and krill oil are products obtained from simple extraction of fresh fish – fresh cod liver and krill and are called nutraceuticals. In dietary supplements, the ingredients may be obtained from artificial chemical synthesis, or biosynthesis or natural food extraction. In a dietary supplement, a mixture of these three previous forms of ingredients may be present, for example, in capsules of multivitamins and antioxidants.

2.9.2 Benefits and Risks of Dietary Supplements

If the beneficial effects of different ingredients (vitamins, minerals, antioxidants, fibers) in natural foods are well admitted by many healthcare organizations or researchers worldwide, the main problems of dietary supplements reside in their absence of controls concerning their efficacy and their preparation by different health services in many countries. In the United States, the FDA does not require manufacturers of dietary supplements to prove safety or efficacy (80). Most supplements have not been rigorously studied. For most, evidence suggesting safety or efficacy comes from traditional use, in vitro studies, case reports, animal studies, and often based on the claims of the furnishers (80). Moreover, the difference between their preparation such as extraction, biosynthesis or chemical synthesis and their required conditions also lend to their efficacy and safety (81). Therefore, opinions are divided over whether or not dietary supplements offer the same health benefits as micronutrients in natural foods (82). Even while dietary supplementation is receiving enthusiastic debate and is increasingly adopted in many industrial countries, supporting evidence is still ambiguous. Despite many cohort studies suggesting that vitamins and antioxidants may have a beneficial effect on many chronic diseases, the systematic use of supplements is hindered by several factors: the lack of prospective and controlled studies, especially regarding the long-term effects and the dosages necessary for each type of disease. Indeed, most people who use dietary supplements assume that they are good for health generally, are safe and effective for treating and/ or preventing specific diseases (80). Therefore, the use of dietary supplements must be done with caution because some ingredients (vitamins, minerals, antioxidants) added in the pill or powder are not universally recognized as benefic and/or safe for human health, contrary to natural foods.

Like conventional medicines, dietary supplements may cause side effects, or interaction with another medication or supplement, that may make the health worse. This is the case of vitamins A, E, D, selenium, fluorine, iodine, folic acid, iron, and more. Vitamins A, E, and D are fat-soluble compounds, stocked long-term in the body; in the case of prolonged supplementation in high doses, they become harmful to the body. Therefore, they must be managed by a healthcare professional and their levels in the blood need a therapeutic control in order to avoid excess as well as to find optimal efficacy. Recently, one large clinical study observed that prolonged use of vitamin E supplement was associated with a higher risk of hemorrhagic stroke (83–84). In contrast, vitamin E from foods, not supplements, may reduce the risk of death from stroke in postmenopausal women (83). Also, antioxidant supplements can act as pro-oxidants – as oxidative stress inducers – if they are consumed at levels significantly above the recommended dietary intakes (RDI) (82). This is the case of vitamin C supplements when dosage exceeds 1,000 mg/day. Pro-oxidants are also toxic as oxidants and free radicals and can induce oxidative stress, a phenomenon that can lead to inflammatory diseases (rheumatism, asthma) and even cancer in our body. Selenium (Se), fluorine (F), and iodine (I) are essential micro-minerals and commonly present in foods. However, these elements are absent or in very low levels in soil and water of some areas of this planet, hence their absence in foods. The supplementation of these minerals (Se, F, I) in soil, water or table salt respectively has resolved many diseases caused by their deficiency in foods. However, direct intake of these micro-minerals in tablet form may induce toxicity due to the narrow window between toxicity levels and therapeutic levels of these elements. Therefore, the indirect supplementation of these minerals in soil, water or table salt allows both the prevention of their deficiency and their toxicity in the human body. Indeed, taking supplements in high doses or in the long term may be harmful; always consult a healthcare professional about combining a dietary supplement with a conventional medical treatment (82). In addition, some dietary supplements can exert negative effects on cardiovascular health

(CVH). Certain supplements such as β-carotene, calcium, and vitamin E may even be harmful to CVH. In short-term trials, calcium and magnesium supplements also modestly lowered blood pressure (BP), although with substantial heterogeneity among studies. However, calcium supplements with or without vitamin D may significantly increase risk of myocardial infarction in long-term randomized trials (85). Observational studies demonstrate links between higher plasma vitamin D obtained by sun exposure, and lower CVD risk; however, large trials of vitamin D supplements have shown no benefits (85).

Concerning the benefits of dietary supplements, there are some citations in the scientific literature. This is the case of some supplements such as fish oil, cod liver oil, chondroitin-glucosamine tablets, St. John's wort capsules, and ginkgo extract. They are now proven to be safe and useful complements for the prevention and treatment of some chronic diseases (80). For example, fish oil may be considered a supplement for CVD prevention, especially among patients with prevalent cardio-heart diseases (CHD), based on reduction of cardiac death (85). These dietary supplements are often prepared by simple extraction from natural foods. Moreover, dietary supplements can become necessary and useful in some particular situations, such as people living in soils poor in some essential micronutrients, soldiers on the front-line, sailors in ships, patients with gastrointestinal disorders, or people with low incomes – people who cannot afford a variety of vegetables, fruits, and/or sea foods. In these cases, taking one or two mineral multivitamin tablets and fish oil capsules in RDI concentrations may be helpful to maintain good health (82). In general, the best way to prevent diseases is to consume a mixed natural diet composed of fresh fruits, vegetables, spices, seafoods, white meat, milk, cheese, yogurt, vegetable oils, and a small amount of red meat. For example, for the growth of children, or the prevention of rickets in children or osteoporosis in the elderly, the best way is to consume dairy products, especially milk and hard cheese, as well as exposure to sunlight. The use of nutraceuticals or dietary supplements is reserved for special cases such as people living in areas poor in micronutrients like vitamins and minerals, people with gastrointestinal diseases, and the elderly. The combination of medicines and supplements are also proposed by many healthcare professionals in some chronic diseases such as simultaneous use of fish oil and drugs for cardiovascular diseases, of niacin and statins in hypercholesterolemia, and so on. However, the uses of these supplements alone or in combination with drugs must be controlled by a healthcare professional because their long-term use or high dosage can cause severe side effects. The abuse of dietary supplements is harmful to health.

2.9.3 Choice of Supplements

There are three main preparations of dietary supplements in the market: simple extraction from natural foods, biosynthesis, and chemical synthesis or semi-synthesis. In general, extraction from natural foods (plants, animals, fungi) is the simplest technique and can make dietary supplements chemically identical to those previously present in natural foods. This technique is easy to do, but it is applied only when the levels of these micronutrients are high in the natural foods. Fish oils, krill oils, curcumin in turmeric rhizomes, eucalyptol in eucalyptus leaves, and ginkgo extract from *Ginkgo biloba* leaves are some examples of products obtained by this extraction technique. However, many micronutrients exist in low or very low quantities in natural foods, hence they cannot be extracted. Therefore, other techniques of preparation have been employed such as biosynthesis from yeasts or from bacteria, chemical synthesis, and semi-synthesis – a mixture of biosynthesis and chemical synthesis. Some antioxidants such as astaxanthin and coenzyme Q-10 can be prepared by two or three different methods. Natural astaxanthin obtained from the alga *Haematococcus pluvialis* contains predominantly the 3S, 3′S stereoisomer – the most valuable one. In contrast, artificial astaxanthin, prepared by chemical synthesis, is a mixture of these three stereoisomers with a ratio of 1:2:1 and has 20 times lower antioxidant capacity than its natural counterpart (86). Therefore, depending on the technique used, the efficacy and the safety of the same supplement astaxanthin can vary enormously. It is the same for coenzyme Q-10 which is prepared by biosynthesis from yeast fermentation or by semi-synthesis. In general, the extraction method from natural foods is the best way, while biosynthesis is safer than chemical synthesis. Unfortunately, chemical synthesis is the most widely used because it gives high yield at low expense. When you search a supplement in the market, pay attention to its label to find its fabrication mode. Moreover, when a dietary supplement is registered in a national pharmacopeia, choose the product that mentions 'conform to USP' (US Pharmacopeia) or an equivalent mention, and do not take the same supplement without this mention, which indicates the validity of its fabrication. However, a number of supplements are still not examined by different pharmacopeias; therefore, this mention cannot be found in the labels of these supplements, even if they are well-made.

2.9.4   Chemical Structures of Dietary Supplements

The bioavailability of a micronutrient in food is generally higher than that in supplement tablets or pills due to the synergistic effect of other compounds such as coenzymes and cofactors present in food. Keep in mind that many micronutrients in supplements are less absorbed in the body than their corresponding natural compounds in foods. For example, calcium in tablets is less absorbed than calcium in milk by the gut because calcium in tablets is generally in insoluble salt form, while the same mineral in milk is a soluble organic compound. Iodine in fortified salt is more toxic than iodine in sea foods when it is used in doses higher than the Tolerable Upper Intake Level because iodine in table salt is mineral form, while iodine in sea foods is an organic compound. Moreover, some vitamins and antioxidants are easily deteriorated with time, air, light, or heat; hence, their efficacy also decreases when they are stored long-term. This is also a reason why artificial supplements are less effective than their natural forms.

Most antioxidants and vitamins in animal and plant organisms are chiral compounds, and exist under single stereoisomer form only. The same chiral artificial products obtained by chemical synthesis are often under racemic form – a mixture of two stereoisomers such as d-isomer and l-isomer, S- and R-enantiomers, or cis- and trans-isomers. Our body is a great factory of chiral selectors, and can well distinguish the stereoform of a biological compound (87). That means our organism is smart enough to differentiate the 'good' and the 'bad' isomer present in our body, although both isomers have the same apparent chemical structure. For example, alpha-lipoic acid, a chiral endogenous antioxidant, exists only under R-isomer in humans, animals, and plants, while its dietary supplement is a racemic (R,S) form. When alpha-lipoic acid supplement is introduced in our body, only the 'good' R-isomer is selected for use, while the 'bad' S-form is eliminated. We must ask if this is the reason why artificial products are less effective than natural ones. More research is needed to perform the synthesis of bio-compounds so that synthetic antioxidants, vitamins, or drugs may become more effective and safe for use in therapy with one isomer form only as natural chiral compounds.

However, dietary supplements containing phytochemicals or micronutrients that are extracted from foods or plants, are also helpful and necessary for the treatment of many diseases because of their high doses used and the commodity of their galenic form (capsule, tablet). Moreover, some toxic compounds present in whole leaves, tubers, fruits, stems, or bark are eliminated during the preparation of dietary supplements. Their conservation also lasts longer. In general, for disease prevention, whole food consumption is better than dietary supplements. But, for the treatment of a specific disease, a single phytochemical or micronutrient may become more potent and practical than whole food. The supplementation of some micronutrients used alone is also necessary in the case of the absence of this compound in the diet; compounds such as iodine, fluorine, iron, vitamin B12, and so on.

In summary, dietary supplements can be helpful in some situations, but eating a balanced diet rich in macro and micronutrients is the best way to promote better health and to prevent some chronic diseases, mostly in elderly people. Many nutritionists and healthcare organizations such as WHO, FAO, and FDA have recommended food first because foods provide a large range of vitamins, antioxidants, minerals, and macronutrients in natural forms that are often not found in dietary supplements. However, when a deficiency of some micronutrients occurs in your body due to illness or old age, a supply of these micronutrients through supplements may be necessary.

Supplements can be used as co-treatment with drugs in some specific diseases under the control of a doctor. When an essential micronutrient is not found in foods of your locality, the supplementation of this compound becomes useful. In contrast, the abuse of dietary supplements may be not only harmful to your body, but also a useless waste of your money. Keeping your money for buying natural healthy food may be the best way to prevent disease and to be in good health.

2.10   NANO-FOODS OR FOOD NANOTECHNOLOGY

At the beginning of the twenty-first century, the development of nanotechnology in general and of nanomaterials in particular, has attracted a number of scientists worldwide for their applications in different areas including medicine, pharmacy, food technology, electronics, optics, and plastics. Nanomaterials the most used in medicine, pharmacy and food nanotechnology are: carbon nanotubes (CNTs), carbon nanofibers, carbon nanoparticles, polymeric micelles, polymers, superparamagnetic Fe_3O_4 nanoparticles, liposomes, and more (88–97). A nanoparticle is usually considered to be a single particle of material with sizes of diameter between one and 100 nanometers (nm) (88–94). A nanocarrier is a nanomaterial being used as a vehicle to transport drug, nutrient, antibody, DNA, and so on to the target cell or organ (93–94).

Food nanotechnology uses different nanomaterials cited earlier for the processing of foods (88–92). The major food sectors for nanotechnology applications include food safety, biosecurity, product traceability, and the efficacious delivery of nutraceuticals (91). The most common abilities of nanotechnology are: removal of fat, enhanced taste, and adding nutrients such as vitamins, antioxidants, enzymes, coenzymes in different nanocarriers for their absorption and transportation in the body. Nano food packaging materials may extend food life, improve food safety, alert consumers that food is contaminated or spoiled, repair tears in packaging, and even release preservatives to extend the life of the food in the package. Nanotechnology applications in the food industry can be utilized to detect bacteria in packaging or produce stronger flavors and color quality, as well as bolstering safety by increasing the barrier properties (88).

In food engineering field, two major applications related to nanotechnology, that is, food nanosensing and food nanostructured ingredients, are expected to come. Advances in technologies such as DNA microarrays, microelectromechanical systems, and microfluidics will enable the realization of the potential of nanotechnology for food applications. In the latter, food processing can be largely improved in the aspects of smart delivery of nutrients, bio-separation of proteins, rapid sampling of biological and chemical contaminants, nanoencapsulation of nutraceuticals, solubilization, delivery, and color in food systems; these being some of the emerging topics of nanotechnology for food and agriculture (90).

In medicine and pharmacy, the use of different nanocarriers for the transport of drugs in the body in order to enhance drug efficacy and to avoid toxicity is now exploited to treat many dreadful diseases such as cancer, infection, and more (92–95) The important characteristics of nanotechnology in pharmaceutics are to revolutionize the methods of drug delivery, since traditional drug administration cannot resolve the problems of toxicity and/or bioavailability of numerous effective drugs, thereby limiting their use in therapeutics. The applications of these research have been recently extended to the transportation of many labile and unabsorbed nutraceuticals or dietary supplements for their bioavailability and their treatment efficacy. For example, curcumin, a water insoluble polyphenol of turmeric spice, has multiple biological and pharmacological *in vitro* and *in vivo* activities, including antioxidant, anti-carcinogenic, anti-inflammatory, antiangiogenic, and antimicrobial activities (92–97). Fortunately, no obvious toxicity or side effects of curcumin were found when used for a long period in animals (92). However, its widespread application in clinic tumor therapy is greatly hindered by its water-insolubility, instability, and especially its very low bioavailability in the human body (95–97). To resolve the problem of low bioavailability of curcumin, different nanoparticles, liposomes, micelles, and phospholipid complexes have been used as nanocarriers to overcome this obstacle of curcumin use in therapy. Nanoparticle-based delivery systems like superparamagnetic Fe3O4 nanoparticles have been assayed by many researchers in order to circumvent the poor bioavailability of curcumin (95–96). Yallapu et al. demonstrated that their conjugate magnetic nanoparticle-curcumin induced potent anti-cancer effects on human pancreatic cancer cells *in vitro* and *in vivo* in mice (96). Other researchers investigated the *in vitro* and *in vivo* antitumor activity of liposomal curcumin against human pancreatic carcinoma cells and demonstrated that liposomal curcumin inhibits pancreatic carcinoma growth and in addition, exhibits antiangiogenic effects (97). The preclinical anticancer activity of a liposomal curcumin formulation in colorectal cancer was also recently evaluated. Nevertheless, these novel findings are still not applied in clinical study because the toxicity of many nanocarriers is still not evaluated in long-term use (93–94). It would be remembered that many nanoparticles are cytotoxic and some of this toxicity has been linked to free radicals and oxidative stress. These nanomaterials include metals, metal oxides (Fe3O4), carbon nanoparticles and fullerenes (93).

The applications of nanotechnology in the food sector are only newly emergent, but they are predicted to grow rapidly in the coming years (89). In fact, nanotechnology introduces new chances for innovation in the food industry at immense speed, but uncertainty and health concerns are also emerging (88). Concerning their applications in disease prevention and health promotion, conjugates of nanomaterials with nutraceuticals (vitamins, antioxidants) and phytonutrients (terpenoids, alkaloids, glycosides) could be used in clinical study in the future, as long as they have shown to be devoid of toxicological effects.

2.11 FOOD COOKING TYPES

Cooking can be defined as the art and the techniques of preparing food for eating with or without the use of heat. A cuisine is a characteristic style of cooking practices in order to give food savor, taste, and odor according to individual preference or collective tradition of a country or establishment. The main materials of cooking are foods and their byproducts primarily obtained from animal and vegetable origins.

2.11.1 Raw Food Cooking

Some natural foods can be directly consumed in raw form without the aid of heat, such as fruits and certain vegetables used for salad (lettuce, Batavia, celery, tomato, algae, onion, garlic, chili, pepper, etc.). Some animal dishes like raw oyster, Italian beef carpaccio, French beef steak tartare, Japanese fish sashimi, Vietnamese duck blood soup, and so on are prepared without heat. The advantage of eating raw natural foods is that they keep all nutrients intact, including antioxidants and vitamins that are sensitive to heat. However, there are some risks of bacterial or parasitic contamination when eating raw foods. It is necessary to carefully wash raw vegetables and fruits before consumption. For raw meat or seafood, they must be guaranteed without microbial contamination by an authorized food shop, then immediately prepared. In general, cooking with the aid of heat is the most used method since antiquity.

2.11.2 Heat Cooking Methods

Heat cooking makes food edible and delicious, and gives it new flavors, fragrances, and colors. It also guarantees food safety in terms of hygiene, by destroying heat-sensitive microbes and parasites, and in terms of nutrition levels, transforming some inactive compounds in raw foods into digestible nutrients (98). For example, rice must be boiled in water in order to transform insoluble starch into digestible form. Heat also dissolves the chitin of mushroom cell walls to liberate all its nutrients into the food dish, because the human digestive system is unable to destroy the cell wall.

Heat cooking methods are divided into two general groups: moist-heat cookery and dry-heat cookery (98–102). Moist-heat methods such as boiling, simmering, steaming, braising, and stewing, are those in which the heat is conducted to the food product by water or water-based liquids such as broth and sauces, or by water steam. Dry-heat methods such as grilling, barbecuing, roasting, and baking are those in which the heat is conducted by open flame, broiling, grilling or pan frying, hot air, hot metal, radiation, or hot fat without the use of water moisture. Frying is a heat cooking method that use vegetal oils or animal fats heated at high temperatures between 170 °C–200 °C to cook foods (98–99). There are three kinds of frying: deep-frying, pan-frying, and stir-frying. Deep-frying means to cook food submerged in hot fat; pan-frying means to cook food in moderate hot fat and, stir-frying or sautéing involve cooking foods quickly in small amounts of oil (98–99).

Microwave ovens are often used for heating up or defrosting food. The heating by microwave is generally rapid and can reduce the loss of nutritional substances in foods, but this type of heating is rarely used to prepare food (98). Remember never to microwave heat a processed food, fast food, or liquid like milk or tea in a plastic container, but in a porcelain or glass plate or bowl, because heated plastic can release carcinogenic toxicants such as bisphenol A into foods. The more the plastic is soft or thin like a plastic bag, the higher the level of liberated toxicants.

2.11.2.1 Heat Cooking Methods and Nutrient Contents

However, some heat cooking methods can alter the nutrient composition of foods, leading to the loss of some beneficial nutrients like labile vitamins and antioxidants, or to the formation of toxic compounds by the direct action of heat on foods. Food safety depends not only on the choice of cooking methods, but also on the personal habits, the cuisine traditions, and the time available for the cooker. Generally, every food cooking method more or less reduces the amount of nutrients in food. In particular, processes that expose foods to high levels of heat, time, and air cause the greatest nutrient loss (98–102). By boiling, water-soluble vitamins in vegetables such as vitamins C, B1, B2, B6, B12, folic acid could lose about 50% of their original contents. However, these vitamins could be recovered if you consume this liquid or you keep it to prepare a soup. However, fat-soluble vitamins such as vitamins A, D, E, and K, as well as carotenes, zeaxanthin, lutein, and minerals (calcium, magnesium, iron, copper, zinc, sodium, potassium, phosphorous) are more resistant to boiling water, with percentage losses of around 25% only (99–102). Exceptionally, lycopene in tomato can resist heat and its level may be unchanged or slightly higher after boiling due to the liberation of lycopene from tomato cell walls (30). To avoid the loss of these essential nutrients in vegetables and some tubers, reduce the time of cooking or replace boiling by steaming (102). In contrast, cereals (rice, corn, wheat, etc.) and tubers (sweet potato, manioc, etc.) need a longer cooking time to make them digestible. In general, moist-heat cookery methods like boiling, steaming, braising, simmering, and stewing are the safest mode to cook all vegetable and animal foods (102).

2.11.2.2 Dry-Heat Cooking and Health Risks

Dry-heat methods such as barbecuing, roasting, grilling, frying, baking, and so on are generally used to make food delicious and to give it new flavor, fragrance, and color. However, the foods obtained could contain toxic compounds formed during their preparation by dry-heat methods.

High temperature cooking methods such as grill and barbecue may produce heterocyclic amines (HCAs) and polycyclic aromatic hydrocarbons (PAHs) (103). When a meat of beef, pork, fish, or poultry, is cooked using high-temperature methods, such as barbecuing, grilling, broiling, pan-frying and griddling, fats, proteins and juices in meat directly exposed to a flame or very high-temperature surface can produce potentially harmful substances such as PAHs and HCAs (98–99, 103–105). Meat smoked or charred or burned over an open fire or heated surface also contains toxic PAHs. Exposure to high temperatures even for a short period of time can also generate in meat high levels of advanced glycation end-products (AGEs), which have been shown to increase oxidative and inflammatory processes in the body (106). The formation of HCAs and PAHs varies by meat type, cooking method, and 'doneness' level (rare, medium, or well-done). These toxic compounds adhere to the surface of food; the more intense the heat, the more they are present. Whatever the type of meat, meats cooked at high temperatures, especially above 300 °F (149 °C) as in grilling or pan frying, or meats that are cooked for a long time, tend to form more HCAs (106). For example, well-done, grilled, or barbecued chicken and steak all have high concentrations of HCAs. Cooking methods that expose meat to smoke contribute to PAH formation (104–105). Heterocyclic amines (HCAs) and polycyclic aromatic hydrocarbons (PAHs) have been found to be mutagenic – they cause changes in DNA (gene) that may increase the risk of cancer in humans (104–106). It has been shown that the prostate gland can metabolize these chemicals (HCAs, PAHs) into activated carcinogens which in turn can induce DNA damage, thereby contributing to prostate cancer formation (103, 106). They are widely believed to play a significant role in human cancers such as stomach, colon, rectal and breast cancers (101). The fumes produced by these cooking methods are also carcinogens and can cause lung cancer in cookers. Eating rare steak or medium-rare beefsteak causes less stomach cancer than eating medium-well or well-done steak because the former contains less toxins (HCAs and PAH) than the latter. Roast pork, roast chicken, and roast duck (Peking duck) also contain HCAs and PAH, mainly in their skin. Some practices could reduce the amounts of HCAs and PAHs formed during barbecuing such as marinating meats or adding rosemary to meats before heating. Grilling at lower temperatures and selecting leaner meats are other ways to reduce toxic compounds.

Frying is a complex cooking process that uses vegetable oils heated at high temperatures for the cooking of foods in order to give them savor and flavor and also to destroy microbes and parasites. Frying modifies the composition of foods and oils through oxidation, polymerization, and hydrogenation (107–113). During frying by vegetable oils, foods can lose water and absorb fat, and the frying oils deteriorate, especially when reused. This degradation of oil with food at high temperatures lends to the formation of numerous toxic compounds such as toxic aldehydes, lipid hydroperoxides, and their degradation products (107–108). These toxic products are present not only in frying oil, but also in fried food and cooking oil fumes (108). The formation of these toxic compounds depends on the temperatures of boiling vegetable oils, the frying duration, and the chemical nature of vegetable oil used. The choice of frying oil is dependent on a number of factors, including cost, stability and the resistance of oil and fried food products to oxidation. At high temperatures (150–200 °C), vegetable oils high in polyunsaturated fatty acids (PUFAs) have a short frying life due to their susceptibility to oxidation (112). Oils rich in saturated fatty acids (SFAs) and partially hydrogenated oils have improved stability profiles for prolonged frying. Palm oil is a good frying oil, but contains 45%–50% SFA (bad fat). Partially hydrogenated sunflower, rapeseed, and soybean oils contain <20% SFA, but have high amounts of trans-fatty acid (TFA), a bad fat – up to 20% (113). Olive oil is highly resistant to oxidation; therefore, it is suitable for food cooking, but it is costly. In addition, virgin olive oil significantly reduces the risk of CVD clinical events (113). Choice of oils also varies with location where fried food is consumed. Most people in Spain use olive oil for frying at home. In contrast, the most common oil used for frying away from home, especially in national chain fast food restaurants, is corn oil (112).

Smoke point temperatures of some vegetable oils are: 160–190°C (320–374°F) for extra virgin olive oil, 234°C (453°F) for soybean oil, 160°C (320°F) for unrefined peanut oil, 160°C (320°F) for unrefined sunflower oil, and 178°C (352°F) for unrefined corn oil (114). The ideal temperature for frying food in oil is 170–180°C. The most suitable oils for frying are olive oil, corn oil, sunflower oil, and peanut oil; margarine and butter are to be avoided (98). Finally, it is also recommended to avoid frying food in oil that has already been used for cooking because this used oil can contain acrolein and other toxic products formed in previous cooking. In addition, the formation of toxic compounds during frying foods also depends on the duration of this cooking mode. Results showed the highest total aldehyde emissions in cooking methods were produced by deep frying, followed by pan frying then by stir frying (108). This study suggests that using gentle cooking methods (e.g., stir frying) and using oils low in unsaturated fatty acids (e.g., olive oil, palm oil, rapeseed oil) can reduce the production of aldehydes in cooking oil fumes, especially long-chain aldehydes (108). Frying is the method that causes the highest loss of amino acids in fish samples (101).

Frying has always been regarded as 'fairly unhealthy' because of not only the amount of oil absorbed by the food but also the formation of harmful substances such as acrylamide and acrolein by the Maillard reaction when oil burns (99, 111). Acrylamide or acrylic amide (CH_2=CHC(O)NH_2)

is formed by condensation of the amino acid asparagine and glucose in meat or starch food such as potato at high temperature, about 310°F (154°C), and in absence of water. This condensation is called the Maillard reaction. Acrolein is an unsaturated aldehyde with an acrid smell due to the breakdown of burnt fat. The result is that food turns brown on the dry surface and develops richer flavors (99). Acrolein has been associated with higher risk of all-cause, cardiovascular, and cancer mortality (111). In addition, frying makes food crunchy and more appetizing, which can lead to excess intake. Dietary acrylamide is often formed during frying in oil or roasting. French fries and potato chips are two processed foods mainly consumed in Western countries. French fries contain a small amount of acrolein that may be not harmful to the body if eaten moderately. But frequent consumption of French fries and chips can cause obesity. It is of note that regular consumption of fried foods, especially fried chicken and fried fish/shellfish, was associated with a higher risk of all-cause and cardiovascular mortality in women in the United States (111). There is strong evidence suggesting a higher risk of developing chronic disease when fried foods are consumed more frequently (i.e., four or more times per week) (112). It may be advisable to the public to consume fried foods in moderation while emphasizing an overall healthy diet. However, another study did not recognize the myth that frying foods is generally associated with a higher risk of CVD and only accepted that high intake of fried foods is probably related to a higher risk of weight gain, though the type of oil may perhaps modify this association (113).

In summary, cooking meat below 212 °F (100 °C) or microwaving meat before cooking may reduce toxic compounds formed during frying or barbecuing. Eating raw meat may avoid toxic heterocyclic amines fully, but this eating mode is also dangerous for health due to microbial or parasitic contamination. Boiling in a liquid (soup or sauce) or steaming may be the best process of cooking to avoid both microbial contamination and toxic compound formation. For roasted foods and fried foods, the best way is to consume them with moderation, about two to three times a week. Frequent consumption of barbecued or fried foods may lead to obesity, CVDs, and cancer formation.

2.11.3   Cooking at Home, Fast Foods, Packaged Foods

There are two forms of eating: eating at home and eating out of the home. Based on popular definition, cooking at home means a domestic cooking process; in contrast, eating out of the home means eating at restaurant or in a fast-food shop. Fast foods also include 'foods to go' or packaged foods. Indeed, these foods can be taken away, economize time and money to eat, and give necessary energy to work, but they are harmful for health if consumed in the long term. It is well known that both fast foods and packaged foods are notoriously high in calories including meat, carbohydrates (bread, French fries), sugars, fats, and salt, and poor in vegetables that are the sources of antioxidants and vitamins. Therefore, consuming these foods everyday could cause obesity, diabetes, and cardiovascular diseases (CVDs). Regarding food quality and nutritive value, eating at restaurants is generally better than eating at fast food shops (flavor, savor, etc.). However, concerning food safety, eating at restaurants cannot be compared to cooking at home. Eating at home or home cooking is still preferable worldwide because you are in control of the food you choose and cook. Cuisine at home allows you to distinguish the 'good' and the 'bad' foods – organic or non-organic foods, wild fishes or farmed fishes, and so on, and also to choose your own cooking methods. This choice plays an important role in health and disease. However, cooking at home in the United States has declined steadily over the last 40 years, decreasing by almost a quarter (23%) from 1965 to 2008 (115). It is important to promote the advantages of cooking at home and the disadvantages of eating fast foods and packaged foods concerning health protection to all people, mostly in industrialized countries.

Although some cooked foods are delicious and attractive by their savor and flavor, such as French fries, barbecued meat, packaged food, and fast food, there is always the other side of this 'coin'. Remember that 'every rose has its thorn'; the consumption of these seductive foods for long periods could induce obesity, diabetes, cardiovascular diseases, and cancer. Let your mind choose the good way for the sake of your health.

3   DISCUSSION AND CONCLUSION

Different food types have been developed by humans since antiquity through today. Nowadays, about 12 food types have been listed including primitive wild foods until recent nano-foods. Dietary supplements and nutraceuticals are considered derivatives of foods and not whole foods. Thanks to the progress of technology, foods now become healthier and safer than the past, and therefore the mode of food procurement varies with time, area, and country. However, this progress resembles a double-edged sword. For example, the use of pesticides, herbicides, and insecticides can increase the output of cereal, fruit, vegetable production, on the one hand, but these products are harmful for human and animal health, on the other hand. Hence, it is preferable to choose organic products that are exempt from toxic pesticides and insecticides, especially fruits and vegetables such as strawberry, grape, lettuce, broccoli, and so on. It is the same for industrial foods and foods obtained by genetically modified organisms (GMO). For the food industry, the benefits of this food type include hygienic property, practicability, time saving, long-term preservation of foodstuffs and sometimes money saving. Their disadvantages are due to the production of many foods ready-to-eat such as packaged foods, snack foods, tonic drinks, and alcohol, that are rich in calories and stimulants, but poor in essential nutrients. It is reported that eating these food types regularly may be the source of some chronic diseases such as obesity and diabetes, mostly in young people.

Concerning dietary supplements, these complements of food have also a double face. On the one hand, they are beneficial when the deficiency of some essential nutrients such as vitamins, antioxidants, or minerals due to diseases, aging, or other situations manifests in the body. In these cases, the use of dietary supplements is necessary. On the other hand, their abuse can become harmful to health due to their side effects and their accumulation in the body, such as many fat-soluble vitamins including A, D, E, and K. Flooding the body with antioxidant supplements (vitamins C, A, and E, for example) may be just as detrimental as excessive exposure to free radicals present in cigarette smoke, air pollution, fast foods, snack foods, and pesticides. More and more evidence suggest that the health benefits of fruits, vegetables, whole grains, and other natural foods (seafood, meat, dairy products) are attributed to the synergy or interactions of bioactive compounds and other nutrients in whole foods. Therefore, consumers should obtain their nutrients, antioxidants, bioactive compounds, and phytochemicals from a balanced diet composed of a variety of natural foods for optimal nutrition, health, and well-being – not from dietary supplements (116).

Beverages are also a type of foods. There are also 'good drinks' and 'bad drinks'. Tea, coffee, pure fruit juice, and ginseng tea are considered good for health, while tonic drink and strong alcohols like rum, cognac, whisky, and rice alcohol may be harmful to the body. Light alcohol drinks such as red wine, beer, and cider are not dangerous if taken in moderation. Alcoholism is not only harmful to individual health, but also to the family and society. The alkaline diet, alkaline water and nano-foods have recently been introduced to the market since about 15 years ago. Their benefits and risks are still difficult to evaluate. Their usage needs caution.

Choice of cooking modes also plays an important role not only in the preservation of essential macro and micronutrients in your foods to cook, but also in the avoidance of toxic compounds formed during cooking such as frying, grilling, or barbecuing. Moist-heat cookery methods like boiling, steaming, or braising are the safest modes for cooking all vegetable and animal foods. Eating at home is the wise way to preserve your health because you can choose not only the cooking mode, but also the type of foods such as organic vegetables, wild seafood, and so on. Selecting between 'good' foods and 'bad foods' is not always simple, owing to the temptation of many attractive foods in the market such as packaged food, fast food, snack food, tonic drink and alcohol. Think carefully about these choices surrounding buying, cooking and eating food to bolster your health and prevent disease.

The decisions about your diets are surely important not only for you today, but also for you and your family tomorrow. A lot of patience and determination are required to change some wrong eating habits for the sake of your health. With this knowledge in mind, humans should be able to develop a base of food consumption that is beneficial to the health and well-being of humankind.

4 REFERENCES

1. Powell B., Maundu P., Kuhnlein H.V., Johns T. (2013). Wild Foods from Farm and Forest in the East Usambara Mountains, Tanzania. *Ecol. Food Nutr.*, **52**(6): 451–478.
2. Bharucha Z., Pretty J. (2010). The Roles and Values of Wild FOODS in Agricultural Systems. Review. *Phil. Trans. R. Soc. B (Philosophical Transactions of the Royal Society B)*, **365**: 2913–2926.
3. Chakravarty S., Bhutia K.D., Suresh C.P., Shukla G., Pala N.A. (2016). A Review on Diversity, Conservation and Nutrition of Wild Edible Fruits. *J. Appl. Nat. Sci.*, **8**(4): 2346–2353.
4. Elias T.S., Dykerman P.A. (2009). *Edible Wild Plants: A North America Field Guide to Over 200 Natural Foods*. 10th edition. Sterling Publishing Company, Inc., New York, April 7, 288 pages.
5. Tardío J., Pardo-de-Santayana M., Morales R. (2006). Ethnobotanical Review of Wild Edible Plants in Spain. *Bot. J. Linn. Soc.*, **152**: 27–71.
6. Ceccanti C., Landi M., Benvenuti S., Pardossi A., Guidi L. (2018). Mediterranean Wild Edible Plants: Weeds or "New Functional Crops"? *Molecules*, **23**(9): 2299, 15 pages.
7. Shikov A.N., Tsitsilin A.N., Pozharitskaya O.N., Makarov V.G., Heinrich M. (2017). Traditional and Current Food Use of Wild Plants Listed in the Russian Pharmacopoeia. *Front Pharmacol.*, **8**: 841, 15 pages.
8. Bharucha Z., Pretty J. (2010). The Roles and Values of Wild Foods in Agricultural Systems. *Phil. Trans. R. Soc. B*, **365**: 2913–2926.
9. Guil-Guerrero J.L., Torija-Isasa M.E. (2002). Chapter: Edible Wild Plants, pp. 431–466. In: *Recent Progress in Medicinal Plants*, Volume 8. Editors: D.K. Majundar, J.N. Govil, V.K. Singh. Sci. Tech Publishing LLC, Austin.
10. King N.J., Lake R.J., Kerr G.N. (2013). Wild Foods, pp. 287–299. In: *Ecosystem Services in New Zealand – Conditions and Trends*. Editor: J.R. Dymond. Manaaki Whenua Press, Lincoln.
11. Johnson J. (2008). It's Only Natural, pp. 1–17. In: *Food Regulation in United States*. Editor: Pr. Neal Fortin, November 26. www.iflr.msu.edu/uploads/files/Student%20Papers/It_s_Only_Natural.pdf.
12. Korir N.K., Han J., Shangguan L., Wang C., Kayesh E., Zhang Y., Fang J. (2013). Plant Variety and Cultivar Identification: Advances and Prospects. *Crit. Rev. Biotechnol.*, **33**(2): 111–125.
13. Dangour A.D., Dodhia S.K., Hayter A., Allen E., Lock K., Uauy R. (2009). Nutritional Quality of Organic Foods: A Systematic Review. *Am. J. Clin. Nutr.*, **90**(3): 680–685.
14. Winter C.K., Davis S.F. (2006). Organic Foods. *J. Food Sci.*, **71**(9): R117–R124.
15. Olsson M.E., Andersson C.S., Oredsson S., Berglund R.H., Gustavsson K.E. (2006). Antioxidant Levels and Inhibition of Cancer Cell Proliferation in Vitro by Extracts from Organically and Conventionally Cultivated Strawberries. *J. Agric. Food Chem.*, **54**(4): 1248–1255.
16. Baranski M., Srednicka-Tober D., Volakakis N., Seal C., Sanderson R., Stewart G.B., Benbrook C., Biavati B., Markellou E., Giotis C., Gromadzka-Ostrowska J., Rembiałkowska E., Skwarło-Sonta K., Tahvonen R., Janovska D., Niggli U., Nicot P., Leifert C. (2014). Higher Antioxidant and Lower Cadmium Concentrations and Lower Incidence of Pesticide Residues in Organically Grown Crops: A Systematic Literature Review and Meta-Analyses. *Br. J. Nutr.*, **112**: 794–811.
17. Smith-Spangler C., Brandeau, M.L. Hunter G.E., Bavinger J.C., Pearson M., Eschbach P.J., Sundaram V., Liu H., Schirmer P., Stave C., Olkin I., Bravata D.M. (2012). Are Organic Foods Safer or Healthier Than Conventional Alternatives? A Systematic Review. *Ann. Intern. Med.*, **157**: 348–366.
18. Robinson L., Segal J., Segal R. (2019). Organic Foods: What You Need to Know About Eating Organic. The Benefits and Basics of Organic Food and How to Keep It Affordable, June. www.helpguide.org/articles/healthy-eating/organic-foods.htm.
19. Hughner R.S., McDonagh P., Prothero A., Shultz C.J., Stanton J. (2007). Who Are Organic Food Consumers? A Compilation and Review of Why People Purchase Organic Food. *J. Consumer Behav.*, **6**: 1–17.
20. Knorr D., Watzke H. (2019). Food Processing at a Crossroad. *Front Nutr.*, **6**(85): 1–8.
21. Weaver C.M., Dwyer J., Fulgoni V.L. 3rd, King J.C., Leveille G.A., MacDonald R.S., Ordovas J., Schnakenberg D. (2014). Processed Foods: Contributions to Nutrition. *Am. J. Clin. Nutr.*, **99**(6): 1525–1542.
22. Monteiro C.A., Levy R.B., Claro R.M., Ribeiro de Castro I.R. (2010). A New Classification of Foods Based on the Extent and Purpose of Their Processing. *Cad. Saúde Pública*, **26**(11): 2039–2049.

23. Amit S.K., Uddin M.M., Rahman R., Islam S.M.R., Khan M.S. (2017). A Review on Mechanisms and Commercial Aspects of Food Preservation and Processing. *Agric. & Food Secur.*, **6**(51), 22 pages.

24. Singh R. (2015). Different Types of Food Processing Techniques in Industry and Their Significance. *R.R.J.F.D.T (Research & Reviews: Journal of Food and Dairy Technology)*, **3**(1): 9–20.

25. Chemat F., Rombaut N., Meullemiestre A., Turk M., Périno-Issartier S., Fabiano-Tixier A-S., Abert-Vian M. (2017). Review of Green Food Processing Techniques. Preservation, Transformation, and Extraction. *Innov. Food Sci. Emerg. Technol.*, **41**: 357–377.

26. Floros J.D., Newsome R., Fisher W., Barbosa-Canovas G.V., Chen H., Dunne C.P., German J.B., Hall R.L., Heldman D.R., Karwe M.V., Knabel S.J., Labuza T.P., Lund D.B., Newell-McGloughlin M., Robinson J.L., Sebranek J.G., Shewfelt R.L., Tracy W.F., Weaver C.M., Ziegler G.R. (2010). Feeding the World Today and Tomorrow: The Importance of Food Science and Technology. An IFT Scientific Review. *Compr. Rev. Food Sci. Food Saf.*, **9**: 572–599.

27. Malagié M., Jensen G., Graham J.C., Smith D.L. (2012). Chapter 67. Food Industry. In: *Encyclopaedia of Occupational Health and Safety*. 4th edition. Editor: International Labor Organization. www.ilocis.org/documents/chpt67e.htm.

28. Monteiro C.A., Levy R.B., Claro R.M., Ribeiro de Castro I.R., Cannon G. (2010). Increasing Consumption of Ultra-Processed Foods and Likely Impact on Human Health: Evidence from Brazil. *Public Health Nutr.*, **14**(1): 5–13.

29. Dunford E.K., Ni Mhurchu C., Huang L., Vandevijvere S., Swinburn B., Pravst I., Tolentino-Mayo L., Reyes M., L'Abbé M., Neal B.C. (2019). A Comparison of the Healthiness of Packaged Foods and Beverages from 12 Countries Using the Health Star Rating Nutrient Profiling System, 2013–2018. *Obesity Rev.*, **20** (Suppl. 2): 107–115.

30. Alda L.M., Gogoaşa I., Bordean D-M., Gergen I., Alda S., Moldovan C., Niţa L. (2009). Lycopene Content of Tomatoes and Tomato Products. *J. Agroaliment. Proc. Technol.*, **15**(4): 540–542.

31. Zhang C., Wohlhueter R., Zhang H. (2016). Genetically Modified Foods: A Critical Review of Their Promise and Problems. *Food Science and Human Wellness*, **5**: 116–123.

32. Kramkowska M., Grzelak T., Czyżewska K. (2013). Benefits and Risks Associated with Genetically Modified Food Products. *Ann. Agric. Environ. Med.*, **20**(3): 413–419.

33. Wilson D.R., Barrell A. (Medical News Today). (2019). What Are the Pros and Cons of GMO Foods? February 27. www.medicalnewstoday.com/articles/324576.php.

34. Key S., Ma J.K-C., Drake P.M.W. (2008). Genetically Modified Plants and Human Health. *J.R. Soc. Med.*, **101**(6): 290–298.

35. Prakash D., Verma S., Bhatia R., Tiwary B.N. (2011). Risks and Precautions of Genetically Modified Organisms. *ISRN Ecol.*, **2011**, Article ID 369573, 13 pages.

36. Peterson G., Cunningham S., Deutsch L., Erickson J., Quinlan A., Raez-Luna E., Tinch R., Troell M., Woodbury P., Zens S. (2000). The Risks and Benefits of Genetically Modified Crops: A Multidisciplinary Perspective. *Conserv. Ecol.*, **4**(1), Art. 13, 10 pages.

37. Lisowska K. (2011). Genetically Modified Crops and Food: Pros and Cons. *Chemik*, **66**(11): 1193–1203.

38. Domingo J.L. (2007). Toxicity Studies of Genetically Modified Plants: A Review of the Published Literature. *Crit. Rev. Food Sci. Nutr.*, **47**(8): 721–733.

39. Journey E. (GMO Watch). (2019). Where Are GMOs Banned? November 12. https://gmowatch.com/where-are-gmos-banned/.

40. Food and Agriculture Organization (FAO) of the United Nations. (2008). Chapter 7. Beverages, July 24. www.fao.org/WAIRdocs/x5434e/x5434e0b.htm.

41. Vartanian L.R., Schwartz M.B., Brownell K.D. (2007). Effects of Soft Drink Consumption on Nutrition and Health: A Systematic Review and Meta-Analysis. *Am. J. Public Health*, **97**: 667–675.

42. Seifert S.M., Schaechter J.L., Hershorin E.R., Lipshultz S.E. (2011). Health Effects of Energy Drinks on Children, Adolescents, and Young Adults. *Pediatrics*, **127**: 511–528.

43. Visram S., Cheetham M., Riby D.M., Crossley S.J., Lake A.A. (2016). Consumption of Energy Drinks by Children and Young People: A Rapid Review Examining Evidence of Physical Effects and Consumer Attitudes. *BMJ Open*, **6**: 1–23.

44. Gunja N., Brown J.A. (2012). Energy Drinks: Health Risks and Toxicity. *Med. J. Aust.*, **196**(1): 46–49.

45. Wine Folly. (2020). Alcohol Content in Wine and Other Drinks (Infographic), March 12. http://winefolly.com/tutorial/alcohol-content-in-wine/.

46. World Health Organization (WHO). (2018). Alcohol, September 21. www.who.int/news-room/fact-sheets/detail/alcohol.

47. Mukamal K.J., Conigrave K.M., Mittleman M.A., Camargo C.A. Jr., Stampfer M.J., Willett W.C., Rimm E.B. (2003). Roles of Drinking Pattern and Type of Alcohol Consumed in Coronary Heart Disease in Men. *N. Engl. J. Med.*, **348**: 109–118.

48. Zhou Y., Zheng J., Li S., Zhou T., Zhang P., Li H-B. (2016). Alcoholic Beverage Consumption and Chronic Diseases. *Int. J. Environ. Res. Public Health*, **13**(522): 1–27.

49. Wang W., Wang C., Xu H., Gao Y. (2020). Aldehyde Dehydrogenase, Liver Disease and Cancer. *Int. J. Biol. Sci.*, **16**(6): 921–934.

50. National Institute of Health (NIH). National Institute on Alcohol Abuse and Alcoholism. (2007). Alcohol Alert. Published: July 2007. Number 72. https://pubs.niaaa.nih.gov/publications/AA72/AA72.htm.

51. Cederbaum A.I. (2012). Alcohol Metabolism. *Clin. Liver Dis.*, **16**(4): 667–685.

52. Guido L.F. (2016). Sulfites in Beer: Reviewing Regulation, Analysis and Role. *Sci. Agric.*, **73**(2): 189–197.

53. ASCIA (Australasian Society of Clinical Immunology and Allergy). (2019). Sulfite Sensitivity. Content Last Updated 2019. www.allergy.org.au/patients/other-allergy/sulfite-allergy.

54. Whayne T.F. (2015). Coffee: A Selected Overview of Beneficial or Harmful Effects on the Cardiovascular System? *Curr. Vasc. Pharmacol.*, **13**(5): 637–648.

55. Higdon J.V., Frei B. (2006). Coffee and Health: A Review of Recent Human Research. *Crit. Rev. Food Sci. Nutr.*, **46**(2): 1001–1023.

56. Messina G., Zannella C., Monda V., Dato A., Liccardo D., De Blasio S., Valenzano A., Moscatelli F., Messina A., Cibelli G., Monda M. (2015). The Beneficial Effects of Coffee in Human Nutrition. *Biol. Med. (Aligarh)*, **7**(4): 240–244.

57. Pourshahidi L.K., Navarini L., Petracco M., Strain J.J. (2016). A Comprehensive Overview of the Risks and Benefits of Coffee Consumption. *Compr. Rev. Food Sci. Food Saf.*, **15**: 671–684.

58. Pham-Huy N.L.A., He H., Pham-Huy C. (2008). Green Tea and Health. An Overview. *J. Food Agric. Environ. (JFAE)*, **6**: 6–13.

59. Ghosh R., Chakraborty A., Biswas A., Chowdhuri S. (2020). Evaluation of Green Tea Polyphenols as Novel Corona Virus (SARS CoV-2) Main Protease (Mpro) Inhibitors – An *in Silico* Docking and Molecular Dynamics Simulation Study. *J. Biomol. Struct. Dyn.*: 1–13.

60. Chen Z-M., Lin Z. (2015). Tea and Human Health: Biomedical Functions of Tea Active Components and Current Issues. *J. Zhejiang Univ-Sci. B (Biomed. & Biotechnol.)*, **16**(2): 87–102.

61. Reygaert W.C. (2017). An Update on the Health Benefits of Green Tea. *Beverages*, **3**(6): 14 pages.

62. Arbia L., Chikhi-Chorfi N., Betatache I., Pham-Huy C., Zenia S., Mameri N., Drouiche N., Lounici H. (2017). Antimicrobial Activity of Aqueous Extracts from Four Plants on Bacterial Isolates from Periodontitis Patients. *Environ. Sci. Pollut. Res.*, **24**(15): 13394–13404.

63. Sethi S., Tyagi S.K., Anurag R.K. (2016). Plant-Based Milk Alternatives an Emerging Segment of Functional Beverages: A Review. *J. Food Sci. Technol.*, **53**(9): 3408–3423.

64. Marengo K., Goldman R. (2019). Alkaline Water: Benefits and Risks, May 30. www.healthline.com/health/food-nutrition/alkaline-water-benefits-risks#takeaway.

65. Fenton T.R., Huang T. (2016). Systematic Review of the Association Between Dietary Acid Load, Alkaline Water and Cancer. *BMJ Open*, **6**: e010438, 5 pages.

66. Mousa H.A-L. (2016). Health Effects of Alkaline Diet and Water, Reduction of Digestive-Tract Bacterial Load, and Earthing. *Altern. Ther. Health Med.*, **22** (Suppl. 1): 24–33.

67. Schwalfenberg G.K. (2012). The Alkaline Diet: Is There Evidence That an Alkaline pH Diet Benefits Health? *J. Environ. Public Health*, **2012**, Art. 727630, 7 pages.

68. Hasler C.M. (2002). Functional Foods: Benefits, Concerns and Challenges. A Position Paper from the American Council on Science and Health. *J. Nutr.*, **132**(12): 3772–3781.

69. Hasler C.M., Brown A.C. (2009). Position of the American Dietetic Association: Functional Foods. *J. Am. Diet. Assoc.*, **109**(4): 735–746.

70. US Department of Agriculture, Agricultural Research Service. (2010). Basics About Functional Food, June 25. www.ars.usda.gov/ARSUserFiles/00000000/NPS/FinalFunctionalFoodsPDFReadVersion6-25-10.pdf.

71. Siro I., Kapolna E., Kapolna B., Lugasi A. (2008). Functional Food. Product Development, Marketing and Consumer Acceptance. A Review. *Appetite*, **51**: 456–467.

72. Ozen A.E., Pons A., Tur J.A. (2012). Worldwide Consumption of Functional Foods: A Systematic Review. *Nutr. Rev.*, **70**(8): 472–481.

73. Crowe K.M., Francis C. (2013). Position of the Academy of Nutrition and Dietetics: Functional Foods. *J. Acad. Nutr. Diet.*, **113**(8): 1096–1103.

74. Pang G., Xie J., Chen Q., Hu Z. (2012). How Functional Foods Play Critical Roles in Human Health. *Food Science and Human Wellness*, **1**: 26–60.
75. Katan M.B., De Roos N.M. (2004). Promises and Problems of Functional Foods. *Crit. Rev. Food Sci. Nutr.*, **44**: 369–377.
76. Howlett J. (2008). Functional Foods from Science to Health and Claims. In: *ILSI (The International Life Sciences Institute)*. Europe Concise Monograph Series, 36 pages. http://ilsi.eu/wp-content/uploads/sites/3/2016/06/C2008Func_FoodEng.pdf.
77. Guiné R., Lima M.J., Barroca M. (2010). Role and Health Benefits of Different Functional Food Components. *Int. J. Med. Biol. Front.*, **17**(9): 31 pages.
78. Allen L., de Benoist B., Dary O., Hurrell R. (2006). Guidelines on food fortification with micronutrients. Published by World Health Organization (WHO), 341 pages. www.who.int/nutrition/publications/guide_food_fortification_micronutrients.pdf
79. Santini A., Cammarata S.M., Capone G., Ianaro A., Tenore G.C., Pani L., Novellino E. (2018). Nutraceuticals: Opening the Debate for a Regulatory Framework. *Br. J. Clin. Pharmacol.*, **84**(4): 659–672.
80. Gupta R.C. (2016). Introduction. In: *Nutraceuticals Efficacy, Safety and Toxicity*. Editor: Ramesh C. Gupta. Elsevier, Amsterdam, the Netherlands, 1042 pages.
81. Keservani R.K., Kesharwani R.K., Sharma A.K., Vyas N., Chadokar A. (2010). Nutritional Supplements: An Overview. *Int. J. Curr. Pharm. Rev. Res.*, **1**(1): 59–75.
82. Pham-Huy A.L., He H., Pham-Huy C. (2008). Free Radicals and Antioxidants in Disease and Health. *Int. J. Biomed. Sci. (IJBS)*, **4**(2): 89–96.
83. Yochum L.A., Folsom A.R., Kushi L.H. (2000). Intake of Antioxidant Vitamins and Risk of Death from Stroke in Postmenopausal Women. *Am. J. Clin. Nutr.*, **72**: 476–483.
84. Schürks M., Glynn R.J., Rist P.M., Tzourio C., Kurth T. (2010). Effects of Vitamin E on Stroke Subtypes: Meta-Analysis of Randomised Controlled Trials. *BMJ*, **341**: c5702.
85. Mozaffarian D. (2016). Dietary and Policy Priorities for Cardiovascular Disease, Diabetes, and Obesity. A Comprehensive Review. *Circulation*, **133**: 187–225.
86. Shah M.M., Liang Y., Cheng J.J., Daroch M. (2016). Astaxanthin-Producing Green Microalga Haematococcus pluvialis: From Single Cell to High Value Commercial Products. *Front Plant Sci.*, **7**, Art. 531, 1–28.
87. Nguyen A.L., He H., Pham-Huy C. (2006). Chiral Drugs. An Overview. *Int. J. Biomed. Sci.*, **2**: 85–100.
88. Sekhon B.S. (2010). Food Nanotechnology. An Overview. *Nanotechnol. Sci. Appl.*, **3**: 1–15.
89. Chaudhry Q., Scotter M., Blackburn J., Ross B., Boxall A., Castle L., Aitken R., Watkin R. (2008). Applications and Implications of Nanotechnologies for the Food Sector. *Food Addit. Contam. Part A Chem. Anal. Control Expo. Risk Assess.*, **25**(3): 241–258.
90. Ravichandran R. (2010). Nanotechnology Applications in Food and Food Processing: Innovative Green Approaches, Opportunities and Uncertainties for Global Market. *Int. J. Green Nanotechnol.: Phys. Chem.*, **1**(2): P72–P96.
91. Gunasekaran S. (2014). Nanotechnology for Food: Principles and Selected Applications. Chapter 8, pp. 171–205. In: *Food Processing: Principles and Applications*. 2nd edition. Editors: Stephanie Clark, Stephanie Jung, Buddhi Lamsal. John Wiley & Sons, New Jersey.
92. Dias-Souza M.V., dos Santos R.M. (2017). Chapter 9. Drug and Food Applications of Liposomes and Nanoparticles: From Benchmark to Bedside? pp. 299–326. In: *Drug Delivery Approaches and Nanosystems, Volume 1. Novel Drug Carriers*. Editors: R.K. Keservani, A.K. Sharma, R.K. Kesharwani. Apple Academic Press Inc., New Jersey.
93. He H., Xiao D-L., Pham-Huy A.L., Dramou P., Pham-Huy C. (2017). Chapter 6. Carbon Nanotubes Used as Nanocarriers in Drug and Biomolecule Delivery, pp. 163–212. In: *Drug Delivery Approaches and Nanosystems, Volume 1. Novel Drug Carriers*. Editors: R.K. Keservani, A.K. Sharma, R.K. Kesharwani. Apple Academic Press Inc., New Jersey.
94. He H., Pham-Huy A.L., Dramou P., Xiao D-L., Zuo P., Pham-Huy C. (2013). Carbon Nanotubes: Applications in Pharmacy and Medicine. *BioMed. Res. Int.* **2013**, ID 578290, 1–12.
95. Qi M., Zhang K., Li S., Wu J., Pham-Huy C., Diao X., Xiao D-L., He H. (2016). Superparamagnetic Fe3O4 Nanoparticles: Synthesis by a Solvothermal Process and Functionalization for a Magnetic Targeted Curcumin Delivery System. *New J. Chem.*, **40**: 4480–4491.
96. Yallapu M.M., Ebeling M.C., Khan S., Sundram V., Chauhan N., Gupta B.K., Puumala S.E., Jaggi M., Chauhan S.C. (2013). Novel Curcumin Loaded Magnetic Nanoparticles for Pancreatic Cancer Treatment. *Mol. Cancer Ther.*, **12**: 1471–1480.

97. Anand P., Kunnumakkara A.B., Newman R.A., Aggarwal B.B. (2007). Bioavailability of Curcumin: Problems and Promises. *Mol. Pharmaceutics*, **4**(6): 807–818.

98. Canada's Food Guide. (2019). Healthy Cooking Methods, December 11. https://food-guide.canada.ca/en/tips-for-healthy-eating/healthy-cooking-methods/.

99. Gisslen W. (2011). Chapter 4. Basic Principles of Cooking and Food Science, pp. 63–91. In: *Professional Cooking*. Editor: Wayne Gisslen. John Wiley & Sons Inc., Copyright 2011. http://standring.weebly.com/uploads/2/3/3/5/23356120/4_-_basic_cooking__food_science.pdf.

100. Yong W., Amin L., Dongpo C. (2019). Status and Prospects of Nutritional Cooking. *Food Qual. Saf.*, **3**(3): 137–143.

101. Sobral M.M.C., Cunha S.C., Faria M.A., Ferreira I. (2018). Domestic Cooking of Muscle Foods: Impact on Composition of Nutrients and Contaminants. *Compr. Rev. Food Sci. Food Saf.*, **17**: 309–333.

102. Fabbri A.D.T., Crosby G.A. (2016). A Review of the Impact of Preparation and Cooking on the Nutritional Quality of Vegetables and Legumes. *Int. J. Gastron. Food Sci.*, **3**: 2–11.

103. John E.M., Stern M.C., Sinha R., Koo J. (2011). Meat Consumption, Cooking Practices, Meat Mutagens, and Risk of Prostate Cancer. *Nutr. Cancer*, **63**(4): 525–537.

104. National Cancer Institute. (2017). Chemicals in Meat Cooked at High Temperatures and Cancer Risk. July 11. www.cancer.gov/about-cancer/causes-prevention/risk/diet/cooked-meats-fact-sheet.

105. Sugimura T., Wakabayashi K., Nakagama H., Nagao M. (2004). Heterocyclic Amines: Mutagens/Carcinogens Produced During Cooking of Meat and Fish. *Cancer Sci.*, **95**(4): 290–299.

106. Wolk A. (2017). Potential Health Hazards of Eating Red Meat. *J. Intern. Med.*, **281**(2): 106–122.

107. Moumtaz S., Percival B.C., Parmar D., Grootveld K.L., Jansson P., Grootveld M. (2019). Toxic Aldehyde Generation in and Food Uptake from Culinary Oils During Frying Practices: Peroxidative Resistance of a Monounsaturate-Rich Algae Oil. *Sci. Rep.*, **9**(1): 4125.

108. Peng C.Y., Lan C.H., Lin P.C., Kuo Y.C. (2017). Effects of Cooking Method, Cooking Oil, and Food Type on Aldehyde Emissions in Cooking Oil Fumes. *J. Hazard Mater.* **324**(Pt B): 160–167.

109. Guillén M.D., Uriarte P.S. (2012). Aldehydes Contained in Edible Oils of a Very Different Nature After Prolonged Heating at Frying Temperature: Presence of Toxic Oxygenated α, β Unsaturated Aldehydes. *Food Chem.*, **131**(3): 915–926.

110. Grootveld M., Silwood C.J.L., Addis P., Claxson A., Serra B.B., Viana M. (2001). Health Effects of Oxidized Heated Oils. *Foodservice Res. Intern.*, **13**: 41–55.

111. Sun Y., Liu B., Snetselaar L.G., Robinson J.G., Wallace R.B., Peterson L.L., Bao W. (2019). Association of Fried Food Consumption with All Cause, Cardiovascular, and Cancer Mortality: Prospective Cohort Study. *BMJ.*, **364**: k5420, 9 pages.

112. Gadiraju T.V., Patel Y., Gaziano J.M., Djoussé L. (2015). Fried Food Consumption and Cardiovascular Health: A Review of Current Evidence. *Nutrients*, **7**(10): 8424–8430.

113. Sayon-Orea C., Carlos S., Martínez-Gonzalez M.A. (2015). Does Cooking with Vegetable Oils Increase the Risk of Chronic Diseases? A Systematic Review. *Br. J. Nutr.* **113** (Suppl. 2): S36–S48.

114. Gunstone F., Editor (2011). *Vegetable Oils in Food Technology: Composition, Properties and Uses.* Blackwell Publishing Ltd, New Jersey.

115. Raber M., Chandra J., Upadhyaya M., Schick V., Strong L.L., Durand C., Sharma S. (2016). An Evidence-Based Conceptual Framework of Healthy Cooking. *Prev. Med. Rep.*, **4**: 23–28.

116. Liu R.H. (2013). Health-Promoting Components of Fruits and Vegetables in the Diet. *Adv. Nutr.*, **4**(3): 384S–392S.

5 Plant Source Foods

1 PLANT PRESENTATION

To understand the role of plants in our health, it is important to know first their origin, morphology, biology, and physiology. Plants have been living on earth from millions of years and are everywhere on this earth, from land or mountains to fresh or marine waters. The kingdom Plantae includes a diverse group of complex photosynthetic organisms ranging from mosses to flowering plants such as algae (green algae, seaweeds), bryophytes (mosses, liverworts), pteridophytes (horsetails, ferns), gymnosperms (Cycas, Pinus, Ginkgo, etc.) and angiosperms, including the monocotyledons (cereals, crops, wolffian, etc.) and the dicotyledons (beans, oaks, teak, Eucalyptus, etc.) (1–2). Their life span can also vary enormously from a few months, like some mosses, grasses, to many centuries like teak, Ginkgo.

According to Christenhusz and Byng, there are about 374,000 plant species of which approximately 308,312 are vascular plants (3). However, scientists believe that there are millions more to be discovered. Like animals, plants are living things that are made up of cells. Unlike animals, plants only need air, water, nutrients in soil, sunlight, and the right temperature to live, except for about 600 angiosperm species that are recognized as carnivorous (4). A typical carnivorous plant is sundews (Drosera) (4).

The immune system of plants shares similarities with the innate immune system of animals (5). But as plants lack an adaptive immune system, they rely solely on innate immunity to recognize microbial pathogens and pests. Conceptually, plant immunity can be divided into cell-surface and intracellular immunity (5). Since plants are immobile, they have a whole arsenal of defense substances to protect themselves from being eaten (6–8). Most of these defense substances are secondary metabolites including antioxidants, alkaloids, and glycosides. Some of them are used for the preparation of drugs such as quinin, salicylic acid, artemisinin, morphine, digitoxin and so on (6–8).

Plants in nature are divided into two categories: edible and inedible (non-edible, toxic). Edible plants exist in wild and cultivated forms. Plant agricultural production is the basis for human nutrition. Plants that produce grain, tuber, fruit, and vegetables are the main source of human foods because they are rich in macro and micronutrients, especially carbohydrates, lipids, proteins, vitamins, and antioxidants. Grass, fruits, leaves, and straw are feeds for many domestic and wild animals. Flowers are the main foods for insects, especially bees. Besides, plants are also an important medicine source for the prevention and/or treatment of numerous human diseases. However, most wild medicinal plants are toxic. A number of plants possess both nutritive and medicinal activities. Additionally, plants through their different parts like trunk, leaves, bark, flowers, and their byproducts such as oil, essence, resin, have been used since antiquity for the well-being of humans, in the construction of houses, manufacture of furniture, paper, textiles, perfume and rubber, production of fuel for machine called green energy – to name a few ways. Green plants are very necessary for the environment because their photosynthesis absorbs carbonic gas (CO_2) from the atmosphere and liberates oxygen (O_2) to their surroundings. They are the basis of most of Earth's ecosystems.

1.1 PLANT CLASSIFICATION

As cited above, the plantae kingdom is classified under algae, bryophytes, pteridophytes, gymnosperms, and angiosperms (2).

DOI: 10.1201/9781003220817-5

Algae are chlorophyll-bearing simple, thalloid, autotrophic and largely aquatic organisms such as seaweeds and green algae. Bryophytes including mosses and liverworts are plants which can live in soil but are dependent on water for sexual reproduction. Pteridophytes include horsetails and ferns. However, in pteridophytes, the main plant body is a sporophyte which is differentiated into true root, stem, and leaves and produces spores (2).

The gymnosperms are non-flowering or seed-producing plants such as Cycas, Pinus, Ginkgo in which ovules are not enclosed by any ovary wall; hence they are called naked-seeded plants. In angiosperms or flowering plants, the male sex organs (stamen) and female sex organs (pistil) are borne in a same flower. The anther produces pollen grains (male gametophyte). The pistil consists of an ovary enclosing one to many ovules. Within the ovule is the female gametophyte or embryo sac which contains the egg cell. The angiosperms are divided into two classes: the monocotyledons or monocots (seed with a single cotyledon or one embryonic leaf) and the dicotyledons or dicots (seed having two cotyledons or two embryonic leaves) (2). They range in size from tiny, aquatic Wolffia to tall trees of Eucalyptus (over 100 m). Plants provide us with food, fodder, fuel, medicines, and several other commercially important products (2).

It should be noted that fungi or mushrooms do not belong to the plant and animal kingdoms; they are classified as a separate kingdom of eukaryotic organisms.

1.2   PLANT PARTS USED BY HUMANS

Different parts of edible plants used as food are leaf, fruit, root, tuber, stem, seed, bean, shoot, and flower.

Plants that produce grain, fruit, and vegetables are the basic human foods and have been cultivated since antiquity. They are the fundamental components of agriculture. Other byproducts of plants such as oil, essence, resin, and sap are also utilized in cuisine, medicine, perfumery, and industry. Seeds of cereals like wheat, rice, corn, and oat are considered staple foods for many populations in the world. Vegetables, fruits, tubers, beans, seeds, and shoots are the main sources of vitamins, minerals, and antioxidants necessary to maintain health. Some other constituents of plants are used as drugs.

1.3   PLANT BIOLOGY

Like animals, all plants are multicellular and eukaryotic; their cells contain a nucleus and other organelles enclosed within membranes. However, the two main differences between plant cells and animal cells are that plant cells have a cell wall and many chloroplasts (6, 7).

1.3.1   Cell wall, Cellulose and Insoluble Fibers

Cell walls play different roles in plant cells. They aid in providing the overall form, growth, and development of the plant body (9). Despite the fact that the contents of plant cell walls differ from those of fungi and animals, certain functional aspects are similar. These include roles in cell protection, intercellular communication, cell adhesion and proliferation, and also in plant-microbe interactions for the defense against potential pathogens (9). Plant cell walls are usually divided into two categories: primary walls that surround growing cells or cells capable of growth, and secondary walls that are thickened structures containing lignin and surrounding specialized cells such as vessel elements or fiber cells. Plant cell wall is made up of about 90% carbohydrates and 10% proteins (6). The main constituent of plant cell walls is cellulose, which gives cells rigidity and strength, offering protection against mechanical stress (6, 9).

Cellulose is a type of fiber called insoluble fiber comprised of long, linear polymers of hundreds of glucose molecules (polysaccharides), and plays an important role in human and animal digestion and nutrition (6, 9–10). These fibers aggregate into bundles of about 40, which are called microfibrils (6). In the diet, cellulose fibers are mainly present in green vegetables (stems, leaves), fruits, and whole grains. For humans, although cellulose is not digested, it plays important roles in digestion for health maintenance and disease prevention. Cellulose is used as a broom for the intestines, especially for the colon. Its benefits include helping food move through the digestive system more quickly, thus preventing constipation, and reducing the risk of developing a condition called diverticular disease (9–11). Cellulose or insoluble fibers can also bind toxins and cholesterol to avoid the risks of colon cancer development and cardiovascular diseases, and might reduce the risk of developing Type 2 diabetes (9–11). In industry, cellulose around the seeds of the cotton plants *Gossypium* has been used to make textiles since prehistoric times (2). Cellulose pulp obtained from wood or grasses is used to fabricate paper after pressing and drying processes. In trees, a secondary cell wall is constituted by a thicker additional layer of cellulose which increases wall rigidity. Both wood and bark cells of trees and leaf stalks have secondary walls (6, 9).

Other major constituents of the cell wall are hemicellulose and pectin. Hemicelluloses are polysaccharides that contain, in addition to D-glucose, other carbohydrates such as D-mannose, D-galactose, D-fucose, D-xylose, and L-arabinose. Pectin is a mixture of polymers from sugar acids, such as D-galacturonic acid (6).

1.3.2 Soluble Fibers

Some plants contain significant amounts of soluble and insoluble fibers. For example, plums and prunes have a thick skin covering a juicy pulp. The skin is a source of insoluble fiber, whereas soluble fiber is in the pulp. Prunes are super fruits that relieve constipation due to high contents of fibers and sorbitol, a laxative sugar. Grapes also contain a fair amount of soluble and insoluble fibers. Some soluble fiber products are inulin, a polysaccharide of fructose polymers and other oligosaccharides like oligofructose and oligomannose (10–12). These soluble fibers are found in a number of fruits and vegetables (legumes, bananas, berries, broccolis, apples, etc.), but they are not the constituents of plant cell walls, contrary to insoluble cellulose and semi-cellulose. They are also called prebiotics, and may contribute to relieving symptoms of irritable bowel syndrome, such as diarrhea, constipation, and abdominal discomfort (10–12). Individuals with high intakes of dietary fiber appear to be at significantly lower risk for developing coronary heart diseases (hypercholesterolemia, stroke, hypertension), obesity, cancer, and certain gastrointestinal diseases. Increased intake of soluble fiber improves glycemia and insulin sensitivity in non-diabetic and diabetic individuals. Fiber supplementation in obese individuals significantly enhances weight loss. Increased fiber intake benefits a number of gastrointestinal disorders including the following: gastroesophageal reflux disease, duodenal ulcer, diverticulitis, constipation, and hemorrhoids. Prebiotic fibers appear to enhance immune function (10). However, a diet high in soluble and insoluble fibers can produce significant intestinal gas (flatulence) like belching and bloating due to the fermentation of these carbohydrates in the digestive tract. In summary, soluble and insoluble fibers in fruits and vegetables are necessary to the health of the digestive system, liver, and heart. Dietary fiber intake provides similar benefits for children as for adults (10–12).

1.3.3 Chloroplast and Chlorophyll

1.3.3.1 Chloroplasts

Another characteristic of plants is the presence of a number of chloroplasts in cells. Chloroplasts are organelles named plastids found exclusively in plant and algal cells for the major conversion of the sun's radiation energy to chemical energy-rich molecules that is usable by organisms – like solar panels. A chloroplast is a green plastid that contains chlorophylls and is responsible for light-powered photosynthetic reactions and carbon assimilation in the plant cell (6, 13–14).

The main role of chloroplasts is to perform photosynthesis, where the chlorophylls capture the energy from sunlight and converts it in ATP (Adenosine triphosphate) and NADPH (reduced form of Nicotinamide adenine dinucleotide phosphate), which are both chemical molecules rich in energy. The photosynthesis is accompanied by freeing oxygen from the water into the air, which plays an important role in the ecosystem (6, 14). They then use the ATP and NADPH to synthesize a number of organic molecules like carbohydrates (sugars, starch), amino acids, fatty acids, and other nutrients such as vitamins, antioxidants from carbon dioxide in the atmosphere, or from water, minerals in the soil under the action of sunlight (6, 13–14). A majority of the nutrients obtained are transported from the leaves through the stem via the vascular system into other regions of the plant such as roots, trunk, stem, and fruits, supplying them with energy. Chloroplasts can produce around 3,000 proteins; however, their functions are still not well-known (14). They have their own DNA. They also have a critical role in plant immunity as they are the site for the production of secondary metabolites like alkaloids and glycosides which are important mediators of plant immune response.

1.3.3.2   Chlorophylls

Chlorophylls are unique pigments with green color and are found in the chloroplasts of diverse plants, algae, and cyanobacteria (15). Chlorophyll is a chelate made up of carbon, nitrogen, oxygen, and hydrogen atoms along with a magnesium metal ion in the central position. The whole chemical structure of chlorophyll is a porphyrin (6, 15). The porphyrin of chlorophyll contains four pyrrole-like rings (tetrapyrrole ring) bonded to a magnesium ion via their four nitrogen atoms in a square planar arrangement. Porphyrin structures of chlorophyll molecules are similar to those of hemoglobin and myoglobin in humans and of vitamin B12. The main difference is the presence of an iron ion in the central position of hemoglobin and myoglobin structures, and of a cobalt ion in vitamin B12 (6, 15). The numbers of naturally occurring chlorophylls may not yet be fully known. However, five classes of chlorophylls are well-known, namely a, b, c, d, and f (15). Chlorophyll a and chlorophyll b are the main components of photosystems in all photosynthetic organisms (6–7, 15–16). In green plants, most chloroplasts have three times more chlorophyll a than b (7). The green chlorophyll pigments are the source of magnesium, an essential mineral of human cell activity after calcium. Indeed, the consumption of green vegetables containing chlorophylls is indispensable for our health maintenance and for the prevention of some chronic diseases such as cancer and cardiovascular diseases due to their antioxidant activity.

In addition to chlorophylls, chloroplasts also contain carotenoids. These include the orange carotenes and yellow xanthophylls (7). Carotenoids are called accessory pigments, and the light energy absorbed by these pigments is transferred to chlorophyll for photosynthesis. Although present in all leaves, the orange color of carotenoids is normally masked by the green color of chlorophylls (7).

1.3.3.3   Photosynthesis

Photosynthesis is a reaction between carbon dioxide (CO_2) and water (H_2O), under the action of sunlight, to produce glucose ($C_6H_{12}O_6$) and oxygen (O_2), inside the chloroplast with the aid of chlorophylls (6, 15–16). The chemical equation is as follows:

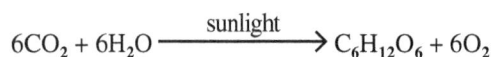

$$6CO_2 + 6H_2O \xrightarrow{\text{sunlight}} C_6H_{12}O_6 + 6O_2$$

Glucose obtained from photosynthesis is used to provide energy for plant growth, or can be converted to starch as stock for plant consumption later. Oxygen liberated is used to clean the atmosphere, and also for the respiration of animals, plants, and other organisms (6, 15–16).

Photosynthesis sustains virtually all life on planet Earth and is the ultimate source of all of humankind's food and oxygen, whereas fossilized photosynthetic fuels provide about 87% of the world's energy (16). Photosynthesis converts about 200 billion tons of CO_2 into complex organic compounds annually and produces about 140 billion tons of oxygen into the atmosphere (16). Nearly all living organisms use the complex organic compounds derived from photosynthesis as a source of energy. The O_2 produced as a byproduct of photosynthesis allows the formation of the ozone layer, the evolution of aerobic respiration, and thus, complex multicellular life (16). Therefore, protecting plants and forests means protecting all living beings on this planet, which is becoming more and more polluted by excessive industrialization and deforestation.

1.3.3.4   Mechanism of Color Change in Leaves

Remember that in addition to green chlorophylls, chloroplasts also contain carotenoids that include orange carotenes and yellow xanthophylls (7). Although present in all leaves, the yellow color of carotenoids is normally masked by the predominant green color of chlorophylls. These carotenoids become apparent in autumn in temperate latitudes, when chlorophyll degrades (7). Some plants produce anthocyanins, which are red pigments, turning some leaves red in autumn. Thanks to the abundance of sunlight during spring and summer, plants make more chlorophyll in leaves to capture this natural energy by transforming it into food for plant life. This green pigment is predominant in leaves and masks the yellow carotenoid pigment; hence, leaves are green. Due to the decrease of sunlight during autumn and winter, the production of chlorophylls becomes low; the green color is not predominant, therefore, the yellow or orange color of carotenoids is now visible on the leaves and gives a beautiful spectacle of autumn. The dropping of leaf is also an economic way for plants to preserve their food during winter.

Contrary to deciduous plants with leaves that change color during autumn and winter, some evergreens like conifers (pine, cedar, cypress, hemlock), live oak, eucalypt, sequoia, and so on, can maintain their leaves green and intact throughout the year, especially during autumn and winter (17). Evergreens that have adapted to grow in climatic zones with marked annual temperature changes between summer and winter have developed physiological mechanisms that enable them to alternate their growth and dormant periods in concert with seasonal climatic changes (18–19). Conifers have special leaves in the form of needles that are adapted to survive in harsher and colder conditions compared to broad leaves. Evergreens may continue to photosynthesize during winter, but the reactions are slower and undergo a process of acclimation to the cold season (18–19). Another explanation for evergreens is an adaptation of plants to low nutrient levels in soil or to a higher soil acidity and lower soil nitrogen content. In cool temperate climates, fewer plants are evergreen, except some evergreens cited previously with a predominance of conifers. Leaf persistence in evergreen plants varies from a few months to several decades (18–19). However, in tropical areas, most plants are considered to be evergreens, due to permanent sunlight and heat. Plants in tropical areas replace their leaves gradually throughout the year.

1.3.4   Pigments and Flavors of Plant

The plant kingdom gives us a marvelous diversity of color, flavor, taste, and aroma through their different parts like flowers, fruits, leaves, tubers, or stems. These varying appearances result from different chemical compounds formed in plants under certain conditions. In general, the color, flavor and taste of these natural compounds are due to the presence of double bond conjugated systems in their chemical structures. In other words, a conjugated system is formed by means of alternating single and double bonds. For example, the green chlorophyll pigment of leaves, the yellow β-carotene of carrot tuber, or the red lycopene of ripe tomato fruit is formed by many single and double bonds in their chemical structure. It is the same for the spicy taste of piperine in black pepper, the umami taste of catechins in tea leaves, the foul odor of allicin in garlic, the yellow color and the astringent savor of turmeric, and so on (20–21). The formation of these colors, savors, odors, depends on the variety of each species, but their intensity can vary under certain natural or artificial conditions such as climate, soil, fertilizers, and cultivation mode. The number of double bonds in a molecule plays an important role in its antioxidant activity; the higher the number of double bonds, the better the activity.

1.3.4.1   Pigments

The main plant pigments in leaves, flowers, fruits, and vegetables include chlorophylls, carotenoids, flavonoids, anthocyanins, and betalains (20, 22). All biological pigments selectively absorb certain wavelengths of sunlight while reflecting others, giving different colors to different parts of plants (22). The principal colors of these pigments are green, orange, yellow, red, blue, and violet, though brown and black are also present in some fruits, seeds, and leaves. However, in fruits and vegetables, colors derived from these natural pigments can change as the plant proceeds through maturation and ripening.

Chlorophylls a and b are the primary green pigments in leaves and stems of plants and vegetables and also the most abundant in plant kingdom including green algae. Chlorophylls absorb yellow and blue wavelengths of light and reflect green color. They are fat-soluble pigments and strong antioxidants (23). The chlorophylls are sensitive to heat and acid, but stable to alkali.

Carotenoids, also called tetraterpenoids, are fat-soluble and share the same global chemical isoprenoid structure, with different quantities of conjugated double bonds and isolated double bonds. More than 700 carotenoids have been identified in nature (20, 22, 24). The most abundant carotenoids in plants are: alpha-carotene, beta-carotene, lycopene, canthaxanthin, astaxanthin, zeaxanthin, and lutein. Their colors are yellow for carotenes and zeaxanthine, orange for lutein, pink for canthaxanthin, and red for lycopene and astaxanthine (20, 22, 24). Carotenoids are also divided into two classes: xanthophylls and carotenes. The difference between them is the presence of oxygen in xanthophyll chemical structure such as canthaxanthin, zeaxanthin, and astaxanthin, while carotenes like α-carotene, β-carotene, and lycopene are purely hydrocarbon compounds. Due to the presence of numerous conjugated double bonds or isolated double bonds in their chemical structures, all carotenoids are strong antioxidant compounds and also play an important role in human nutrition and health, providing provitamin A for eye health and having anti-cancer activities. However, only 10% of carotenoids show provitamin A activity. The most important ones have the property to produce vitamin A are β-carotene, as well as some xanthophylls including β-cryptoxanthin (22, 24).

Carotenoids are present in a variety of fruits and vegetables like carrots, tomatoes, pumpkins, melon, watermelon, paprika, chili pepper, yellow sweet potatoes, mango, microalgae, gac fruit, Brussels sprouts, saffron, and more (22, 24). Carotenoids are sensitive to light and oxidation but relatively stable to heat. Therefore lycopene, a red pigment and strong antioxidant in ripe tomato fruit, is not destroyed by heat; in contrast, its levels may be higher when heating tomatoes. Natural lycopene in fresh ripe tomato is all in trans-isomer form. It is transformed into all cis-isomer form by heating (25). The absorption of cis-lycopene is higher than its natural trans-isomer. Therefore, lycopene bioavailability of processed tomato foods like tomato juice is higher than that in unprocessed fresh tomatoes (25). Intake of processed tomato products is the best way to prevent oxidative stress and carcinogenesis in healthy and Type 2 diabetic patients, as well as prostate cancer patients.

Flavonoids belong to the class of phenylpropanoids containing phenolic compounds, and have the widest color range, from pale-yellow to blue (22). Depending on their structures, flavonoids may be classified into about a dozen groups, such as chalcones, flavones, flavonols, and anthocyanins, and each group has its specific color. In particular, anthocyanins, a class of flavonoids, give colors from orange to blue and are found in many flowers, leaves, fruits, seeds, and other tissues (22). Anthocyanins are water-soluble pigments belonging to the phenolic group. They appear red, purple, or blue, depending to pH of plant part. They provide color in leaves, plant stem, roots, flowers, and fruits. Berries, currants, grapes, and some tropical fruits have high anthocyanin content (22, 26). Anthocyanin and its aglycone anthocyanidin possess antioxidative and antimicrobial activities, improve visual and neurological health, and protect against various chronic diseases (cardiovascular diseases, diabetes, cancer) (26).

Betalains are classified into red (crimson) betacyanins and yellow betaxanthins that are water-soluble pigments (22, 27–28). Betalains are unique nitrogen-containing pigments found exclusively in families of the Caryophyllales order and some higher order fungi, where they replace anthocyanin pigments (27–28). Anthocyanins and betalains have never been detected jointly in plant tissues. Betalains show brilliant color in edible fruits and roots, flowers, stems and bracts of species belonging to the families of Caryophyllales, except for Caryophyllaceae and Molluginaceae (27–28). Edible sources of betalains consist primarily of red beetroots (*Beta vulgaris*) and prickly pears (fruit of the Opuntia genus of cacti) (28). It seems that treatment with betalains and betalain-rich diets is not only nontoxic but could also prove to be a promising alternative to supplement therapies in some chronic diseases such as atherosclerosis, hypertension, and cancer (28). Besides some main plant pigments previously cited, there is another pigment named melanin that is also present in certain fruits, seeds, and leaves.

Melanin represents a group of high molecular weight black and brown pigments produced from oxidation and polymerization of polyphenols. Melanin is produced by different organisms such as animals, plants, fungi, and bacteria (29–31). Melanin is classified into three groups: eumelanin, pheomelanin in the animal kingdom, and allomelanin in the plant kingdom. Melanin of the nervous system is known as neuromelanin which is a mixture of pheomelanin and eumelanin and is found in the substantia nigra of the brain. Colors of eumelanin and allomelanin are black or brown, while those of pheomelanin are reddish-brown, and of neuromelanin, dark-brown (30–31). Melanin is a highly insoluble pigment with various biological and pharmacological properties (29–31). These pigments found in animals and plants are not essential for their development, but rather have a defensive role. Light absorption by melanin has several biological functions, including photoreceptor shielding, photoprotection, thermoregulation, camouflage, and display. Melanin is a powerful cation chelator and may act as a free radical scavenger (29–31). Its antioxidant, anti-inflammatory, immunomodulatory, hypoglycemic, hepatic, gastrointestinal and radioprotective benefits have only recently been recognized and studied. The loss of neuromelanin is the cause of certain disorders of the nervous system such as Parkinson's disease (31). In animals, melanin is found in the skin and hair, as well as in the eyes, like the iris, in various quantities. In plants, melanin is mostly present in the outer layers of fruits such as the brown spots in banana peels. Dates and prunes are rich in melanin, hence their colors are black or dark brown. Browning is a serious quality defect in fresh-cut fruits.

In summary, the color of fruits and vegetables plays important roles in human health. Keep in mind that more the pronounced color, the better the antioxidant activity. For the same species, colored fruits and vegetables contain larger amounts of antioxidants than their less colorful counterparts. For example, blackberry is richer in antioxidants than strawberry; black or red grapes provide more flavonoids than white grapes; yellow or blue potatoes contain carotenoids or/and flavonoids, while white potatoes do not. For some fruits such as apple, grape, and kiwi, antioxidants are mainly present in their peel. So, eating these fruits with the peel is better for the health. Nevertheless, it is of note that the color of a plant part (fruit, leaf, tuber, etc.) is responsible for its antioxidant or vitamin properties and does not interfere in its nutrient values. For example, white sweet potato contains the same quantity of carbohydrates (sugars) as colorful sweet potato; it means that both give you the same caloric content, but not the same quantity of antioxidants. The Table 5.1 covers the biological properties of different plant pigments.

TABLE 5.1

Major Plant Pigments and Their Sources and Properties

Pigments	Colors	Fruits and Vegetables	Properties
Chlorophylls a and b	Green	Lettuce, kale, broccoli, celery, parsley, etc.	Antioxidant, rich in Magnesium and fibers
Carotenes (β-carotene, lycopene)	Orange, yellow, pink, red	Carrot, watermelon, fig, pumpkin, melon, chilly,	Antioxidant, anticancer For eye and skin health
Xanthophylls (lutein, lycopene, astaxanthin)	Red, red purple, rose	Tomato, grape, berries, orange, cherry, etc.	Antioxidant, anticancer, anti-inflammatory
Anthocyanins (peonidin cyanidin, pelargonidin)	Red purple, dark violet, violet	Grape, mango, bilberry, raspberry, cauliflower	Antioxidant, anticancer, anti-inflammatory
Flavonoids (flavonols, catechins, chalcones,)	Yellow, purple, brown, blue, red, pale-green	Citrus, apple, shallot, tea, eggplant, papaya	Antioxidant, anticancer, antibacterial properties
Betalains (betacyanins, betaxanthins)	Red, yellow, violet	Red beetroot, prickly pear, dulce potato, etc.	Antioxidant, anticancer, hypertension
Melanins (allomelanin)	Black, dark brown	Prune (dried plum), date	Antioxidant, anti-UV-B

1.3.4.2   Flavors: Aroma and Taste

Flavor is defined as the combination of taste and aroma (odor) (20–21). It is, however, influenced by other sensations such as pain, heat, cold, and tactile sensations, often referred to as the 'texture' of foods (21).

Aroma compounds or odorants are volatile chemical compounds and primarily perceived with the nose, while taste receptors exist in the mouth and are impacted when the food is chewed (20–21). Taste is mainly composed of five primary sensations: sweetness, sourness, bitterness, saltiness, and umami. Umami, a Japanese name, is a savory taste associated with salts of amino acids (glutamates) and nucleotides (20). More than 700 flavor chemicals have been identified and catalogued (21).

The main flavor compounds present in herbs and spices are: piperine in black pepper; capsaicin in chili; eugenol in clove; gingerol in ginger; turmerone, zingiberene in turmeric; galangol in galangal; menthol in mint, peppermint; thymol, carvacrol in thyme; and apiol in parsley (32). These flavors are usually aromatic and pungent due to the presence of varying types of essential oils. In plants, essential oils are derived from terpenoids and/or flavonoids that are often strong antioxidants. Flavor compounds are used as flavoring and seasoning to enhance the quality of foods and beverages. They also have medicinal properties.

The use of aromatic plants and their natural essential oils in the treatment of diseases is well known since antiquity and called aromatherapy. For example: mint is stimulant, carminative, and antispasmodic. Garlic is antimicrobial, diuretic, diaphoretic, antiflatulence, cholesterol lowering, and anti-inflammatory. Chili is carminative, antirheumatic. Ginger is carminative, anti-nausea, antiflatulence, antihistaminic, aphrodisiac, and cholesterol lowering. Galangal is antiseptic, antimicrobial, aphrodisiac, anti-inflammatory, and anti-emetic. Turmeric is carminative, antiflatulence, anti-inflammatory, anticarcinogenic, and antiseptic (32). And so on.

1.3.5   Plant Metabolites

Plants use different raw materials in air and soil such as carbon dioxide, oxygen, nitrogen, water, temperature, and sunlight through enzyme-mediated chemical reactions to synthetize their necessary nutrients. This enzymatic synthesis is called metabolism and its products obtained are named metabolites (33). This metabolism produces two kinds of biological compounds synthesized by plants including primary metabolites and secondary metabolites that are both necessary for their life and defense (8, 33–35).

1.3.5.1   Primary Metabolites and their Roles

In the plant kingdom, primary metabolites have functions that are essential to growth and development and are therefore present in all plants. Primary metabolites in plants include carbohydrates (sugars), polysaccharides, amino acids, proteins, nucleic acids, fatty acids (saturated and unsaturated fatty acids), organic acids, and water-soluble vitamins (B group and C) (33–35). Primary metabolites are produced using the same (or nearly the same) biochemical pathways (33). Plant primary metabolites are generally obtained by photosynthesis, a process that needs sunlight, water, and air. All primary metabolites are essential to life because they provide energy for plants to survive and spread and consequently, for humans and animals also. Humans knew how to use plant primary metabolites as food since antiquity and then how to select them for cultivation. Humans and herbivore animals use these primary metabolites of plants as their food. Most of them are essential for human life. In the synthesis of plant metabolites, if any of the raw materials, such as water, is in shortage, all living things in this area could die together. Besides their main uses as energy sources, some primary metabolites also have medicinal properties for the prevention of some chronic diseases. For example, unsaturated fatty acids in vegetable oils are used for the prevention of CVDs; or β-glucan, a polysaccharide, present in oat and barley, for the lowering of hypercholesterolemia (33).

1.3.5.2   Secondary Metabolites and their Roles

Secondary plant metabolites are numerous chemical compounds produced by the plant cell through metabolic pathways derived from primary metabolic pathways (8, 33–34). Secondary plant metabolites do not participate directly in growth and development of plants, but are required for the plant to interact with its environment for adaptation and defense (8, 33–35). Secondary metabolites determine the colors and flavors of each plant part (fruit, flower, leaf, tuber) and are used as signal molecules in the protection of plants; hence, their functions are multiple. For example, they are needed in plant defense against herbivores and pathogens like microbes, parasites, and fungi. Contrary to essential primary metabolites in plants, secondary metabolites are non-essential to plant life but contribute to the species' fitness for survival and act as signal molecules under stress conditions (33, 35). Their roles are vast and varied according to each plant type; many of which remain unknown and are being elucidated. Sometimes it is hard to discriminate primary and secondary metabolites (35). For example, both primary and secondary metabolites are found among the terpenoids and the same compound may have both primary and secondary roles (35). Vitamins are classified as plant primary metabolites because they are essential for life, but some vitamins, such as vitamin E (tocopherols and tocotrienols) and vitamin K1 (phylloquinone), are ranked as secondary metabolites due to their chemical structures. According to the nomenclature adopted by the British Nutrition Foundation, different plant secondary metabolites include: phenolic and polyphenolic compounds (about 8,000 compounds), terpenoids (about 25,000 compounds), alkaloids (about 12,000 compounds), glycosides, and sulfur-containing compounds (33–34).

Phenolic and polyphenolic compounds are secondary metabolites that contain a phenol group in their structures and include flavonoids, phenolic acids, tannins, coumarins, xanthones, chromones, stilbenes, and lignans (33–34). Many of the phenolic molecules are also effective antioxidants, especially flavonoids. They are widespread in plants and give color, taste, and flavor to many herbs, foods, and drinks. They are found in many plants and their byproducts such as tea, coffee, chocolate, grape, red wine, lettuce, parsley, thyme, celery, endives, broccoli, soy, artichokes, chicory, spinach, plum, cherry, berry, prune, and in many edible oils such as olive, peanut, almond, sunflower oils, and more (33–34).

Terpenoids also called 'isoprenoids', are a large family of chemical compounds derived from 5-carbon isoprene units assembled in different ways (33–36). According to the number of isoprene units in the molecule, terpenoids are classified into monoterpenes (C10), sesquiterpenes (C15), diterpenes (C20), triterpenes (C30), tetraterpenes (C40), and polyterpenes (34, 36). Major plant dietary terpenoids include carotenoids, quinones (vitamins K), and sterols (β-sitosterol, campesterol, brassicasterol, stigmasterol, and ergocalciferol or vitamin D2) (33). The side chains of these compounds contain isoprene units. Carotenoids are tetraterpenoids and have been described above. Tocopherols and tocotrienols, or vitamin E, are monophenols with an isoprene side chain. Phylloquinone, known as vitamin K1, is a quinone with a terpene side chain. Ergocalciferol or vitamin D2 is a sterol present in plant and mushrooms. Many terpenoids have a wide range of biological activities against cancer, inflammation, malaria, and infectious diseases, and are used for the treatment of a number of human diseases (36). Recently, the discovery of artemisinin, a sesquiterpene lactone isolated from *Artemisia annua*, has saved millions of lives suffering from dreadful malaria around the world. Paclitaxel, a terpenoid obtained from bark of the Pacific yew, *Taxus brevifolia*, has been used for the treatment of diverse cancer forms in humans (36). In addition, many terpenes in plants have antioxidant property and are the source of many flavors, colors, and spices used in the industries of food additives, perfumery, and cosmetic products (36). Limonen, a monoterpene essential oil, is found in different fruits and herbs such as mint leaves, citronella grass, orange, citrus, or lemon peels (36).

Alkaloids are organic compounds containing at least one nitrogen atom in a heterocyclic ring and mainly derived from amino acids. In other words, they are named all nitrogen-containing compounds (33–35). Some well-known alkaloids are: caffeine in coffee, tea, kola, and cocoa; nicotine in tobacco leaves; cocaine in coca leaves; morphine, codeine in opium poppy; quinine in the bark of cinchona tree; and atropine in belladonna leaves. Most alkaloids are very toxic and, therefore, have potential functions in the chemical defense against herbivores and microorganisms (33–34). Some of them are used in therapeutics; for example, quinine against malaria, morphine as analgesic, codeine as cough medicine, caffeine as stimulant, atropine as antispasmodic and mydriatic (pupil dilatator) (37). Nicotine, cocaine, and morphine are psychotropic drugs and can cause addiction. Nicotine is used as a green insecticide because it does not harm the environment (34).

Glycosides are natural organic compounds, usually of plant origin, formed by a sugar (carbohydrate) named glycone linked to a non-sugar compound named aglycone or genin (37). By hydrolysis, glycosides yield one or more sugars. The aglycon may be a terpene, a flavonoid, a coumarin, or any other natural product. Among the sugars found in natural glycosides, D-glucose is the most abundant one, L rhamnose and L-fructose also occur quite frequently (37). Based on the chemical properties, glycosides can be classified into Cardiac glycosides, Phenolic glycosides (flavonoids, lignans and other phenolic compounds), Aldehyde glycosides, Cyanogenic glycosides, Anthraquinone and and Saponin glycosides (37). The aglycones of cardiac glycosides or digitalis glycosides are: digitoxin, digoxin, and gitoxin, and they have a direct effect on myocardial contraction. They are cardiotonic. Saponins are compounds that possess a lipid soluble aglycone consisting of either a sterol or a triterpenoid attached to a water-soluble sugar unit (monosaccharide or oligosaccharide) (33–34, 37). Saponins are found in peas, beans, tomatoes, spinach, asparagus, onions, garlic, potatoes, and ginseng (33).

Cyanogenic glycosides are found in bitter cassava roots and bitter almond (37). They are decomposed by an enzyme present in situ and release toxic hydrogen cyanide (HCN) or salt cyanide when plant tissue is crushed or chewed. Cyanide in high doses can cause death.

Sulfur-containing secondary metabolites include glucosinolates (GSL), glutathione (GSH), alliin, thionin, and defensins, which have been linked directly or indirectly with the defense of plants against microbial pathogens (35). Glucosinolates are plant organic compounds containing sulfur (S) and nitrogen (N) and are derived from glucose and an amino acid. In plants, glucosinolates belong to the glucosides and act as natural pesticides and as a defense against herbivores and parasites because their break down products release volatile defensive substances exhibiting toxic or repellent effects (33, 35). They are found in red radish, horseradish, cabbage, Brussels sprouts, cauliflower, broccoli, and mustard (33). Glutathione (GSH) is sulfur tripeptide and antioxidant in plants, animals, fungi. Alliin is a cysteine sulfoxide in fresh garlic and is rapidly broken down to form different organosulfur compounds such as allicin when garlic is broken down. Allicin is responsible for the heady, pungent garlic smell. Thionin is a protein with disulfide bonds. Plant defensins are proteins rich in cysteine, a sulfur amino acid, and are used to defend plants against parasites.

In summary, secondary metabolites are often issued from primary metabolites and are designed by different chemical names like flavonoids, terpenoids, carotenoids, sterols, phenolic acids, alkaloids, glycosides, and so on. They protect plants against microorganisms and herbivores, and attract pollinators and seed-dispersing animals. They act as signal molecules under stress conditions and are often colored, fragrant, or flavorful compounds. There are about some hundred thousand secondary metabolites in different plants around the world; most of them have not yet been exploited for therapeutic and dietary purposes.

2   PLANT SOURCE FOODS

Plants are considered the most complete foods for human life. Different parts of plants used as food are: cereals (wheat, rice, corn), vegetables, fruits, tubers, leaves, stems, barks, seeds, algae, and their byproducts such as oil, resin, essence, and juice.

Herein, we examine some ten edible plants regularly used as food. They include staple foods, fruits, vegetables, tubers, beans, nuts, seeds, and spices.

2.1   STAPLE FOODS RICH IN CARBOHYDRATES

A staple food is a food that is regularly consumed by a large community in a region and is rich in energy such as carbohydrates, mostly in forms of starch (insoluble sugar). The most consumed staple foods in the world are wheat, rice, corn, potato, sweet potato, cassava, and yam.

2.1.1   Wheat

Wheat belongs to the *Triticum* genus of the grass-like family Gramineae or Poaceae. Among many varieties of wheat, common wheat (*Triticum aestivum*) is the most cultivated since antiquity and is the staple food in most populations of this planet from Middle East to Europe, America, North Africa, Australia, and a part of Asia (38). A wheat grain is divided into three main parts: the bran, endosperm, and germ. The bran, the outer layer, is composed of fibers (50%), antioxidants, B vitamins, and 50–80% of minerals are composed of selenium, iron, copper, zinc, and magnesium (38–39).

Wheat grain is comprised mainly of starch, proteins, and cell wall polysaccharides (dietary fiber). These components in combination account for 90% of the grain composition on dry weight basis (38–39). Wheat grain is composed of starch, about 60–70% of the total dry weight of the grain. Additionally, it contains proteins and some amino acids. Proteins are mainly composed of about 75% gluten formed by two proteins: gliadins and glutenins; the remaining 25% are albumins and globulins (40). Storage proteins in wheat are unique because they are technologically active. They have no enzyme activity, but they have a function in the formation of dough as they retain gas, producing spongy baked products (39). Wheat proteins naturally occur as oligomers of different polypeptides containing more than 35% hydrophobic amino acid residues (isoleucine, leucine, tryptophan, tyrosine, valine, phenylalanine, and proline) (40). Among many minerals present in wheat, selenium (Se) is an essential micronutrient for humans and animals, with antioxidant, anti-cancer, and anti-viral effects. Indeed, wheat constitutes an important dietary source of Se (39). Soils are frequently low in available Se, and hence the food systems of many countries are deficient in Se. For example, in Australia, wheat is estimated to supply nearly half the Se intake of most people. However, Se concentration in wheat grain is highly variable. Published values range from 0.02–0.60–1 mg.kg for most of the world's wheat (39). Remember that excess of Selenium is also toxic to the organism. Other minor components present in wheat are lipids, terpenoids, phenolics, and vitamins. The fat-soluble nutrients that include vitamin E (tocopherols) and the carotenoids (precursors of vitamin A) are located in wheat flour (38–39).

The gluten proteins in wheat consist of monomeric gliadins and polymeric glutenins. Gluten is also present in barley and rye, but not in oat, maize, rice, and glutinous rice (40). Glutenins and gliadins are recognized as the major wheat storage proteins, constituting about 60–85% of total grain proteins. They tend to be rich in asparagine, glutamine, arginine, or proline, but very low in nutritionally important amino acids lysine, tryptophan, and methionine (40). The gliadins are a polymorphic mixture of proteins soluble in 70% alcohol. Glutenins can be broadly classified into two groups: the high molecular weight and the low molecular weight subunits. Generally, it is believed that gliadin controls the viscosity of dough and glutenin controls the elastic or strength properties. The precise balance between viscosity (extensibility) and elasticity (dough strength), or the glutenin to gliadin ratio, is important for bread making and other processed foods such as pizza, biscuits, cakes, pastries, and so on (40). However, gluten can cause allergy to some people. Among the different gluten subunits, the α-gliadins are considered the most immunogenic, while γ-gliadins and glutenins are much less responsible for gluten intolerance. The most well-known form of gluten intolerance is celiac disease, an autoimmune disease at the small intestine that affects about 1% of the population when ingesting foods containing gluten (39–40). The chronic gastrointestinal disorder called irritable bowel syndrome is another condition also affected by gluten (40). To avoid this allergy that affects about 5–10% of the population, mostly in children, the only effective therapy is to avoid exposure by strictly following a gluten-free diet.

Apart from the starch, cereals such as oats and barley contain in their cell walls a soluble fiber called beta-glucan that is used in the prevention or the co-treatment of some chronic diseases like hypercholesterolemia, Type 2 diabetes, immune system deficiency, and cardiovascular diseases (38–39, 41). Wheat is not a good source of beta-glucan; its levels are usually less than 1 %, commonly about 0.6% (39). However, oat and barley are good sources of β-glucans and contain around 4.5% β-glucans for each cereal (41). Beta-glucans in oat and barley have several positive effects on health, including lowering the postprandial glucose response and the improvement of blood cholesterol levels. Due to their particular structure, cereal beta-glucans generate viscosity within the intestinal tract, which is thought to be the main mechanism of action responsible for their positive health effects. Cooking and processing methods generally will modify the physicochemical characteristics of beta-glucans, such as molecular weight, extractability, and the resulting viscosity (41). Cooked oat porridges or oat meals, generally rich in beta-glucans, are good foods for the prevention of hypercholesterolemia. Therefore, the health benefits of beta-glucans in the prevention and treatment of diabetes and hypercholesterolemia will depend not only on the dose administered, but also on the ways they are processed or converted into food products. Cereal beta-glucans also exert favorable effects on intestinal function and gut health through activity on intestinal microflora and bacterial metabolites (41).

2.1.2 Rice

Rice (*Oryza*) belongs to the family Poaceae or Gramineae. Rice is the main staple food for nearly two-thirds of the world's population, especially in Asia such as Japan, Vietnam, China, Korea, Thailand, India, and so on. Among more than 8,000 varieties of rice, *Oryza sativa* is the variety the most cultivated in the world (42–44). Rough rice or paddy can be separated into husk and brown rice through a threshing process. The components in brown rice that are hulled from rough rice are bran layers (6–7%), embryo or rice germ (2–3%), and an endosperm or rice grain (about 90%) (44). There are two main kinds of rice in the market: white rice and brown rice. Brown rice is a whole-grain rice without the outer husk, while white rice is the same grain without the husk, bran, and germ. Brown rice can be further separated into polished rice, commonly called white rice, which is obtained by removing the bran. The color of whole-grain rice is due to the presence of different antioxidant pigments in bran that give different colors like brown, red, or black to whole grain. White rice is the most consumed type in the world, but brown rice or colored rice is becoming increasingly popular due to its health benefits. Another variety of rice is glutinous or sticky rice (*Oryza sativa var. glutinosa*). Glutinous rice differs from other types of rice in that the grain starch contains essentially no amylose (0–2%) and a high amount of amylopectin, which is responsible for the sticky quality of cooked glutinous rice (43). It is mainly used to prepare many kinds of traditional Asian desserts such as rice cakes, rice plates, sushi, and rice wine. Take note that not all rice varieties contain gluten, contrary to wheat.

Rice is primarily composed of carbohydrates. It contains 80% carbohydrates, 7–8% protein, 3% fat, and 3% fiber (42). About 90% of carbs in rice are mainly in the form of starch which is metabolized in the digestive tract into glucose for furnishing energy to cell activity. White rice is richer in carbs than wheat grain, brown rice and glutinous (sticky) rice, but lower in proteins and micronutrients (vitamin, minerals, antioxidants). Bran in brown rice is rich in fibers, vitamins of group B, especially B1, B2, B3, vitamin E (tocopherol, tocotrienol), many essential amino acids, and many minerals, especially calcium, magnesium, selenium, iron, and zinc, as well as oils including γ-oryzanol, triacylglycerols, fatty acids (linoleic, oleic, palmitic acids), and so on. (42, 44). Brown rice also contains gamma aminobutyric acid (GABA), an amino acid that plays a role as inhibitory neurotransmitter in the central nervous system. In addition, the bran of brown, red, and purple rice is rich in antioxidants, especially anthocyanins, proanthocyanins, tannins, flavonoids, polyphenols and γ-oryzanol, which all possess antioxidant and anti-inflammatory properties for the prevention of cancer, cardiovascular diseases, and infection (42, 44).

Brown rice or colored rice is less consumed than white rice because its cooking is more difficult than white rice due to its slow water absorption, and the palatability of brown rice is often found to be inferior to white rice (44). Brown rice has a nutty flavor, chewier than white rice, but more easily goes rancid. The removal of rice bran from brown or colored rice by milling leads to a loss of nutrients. During milling and polishing, about 85% of essential fatty acids, 15% of protein and amino acid, 50–75% of phosphorus, 90% of calcium and magnesium, 50% of manganese, 70% of B vitamins, and all fibers are removed (42, 44). There are two types of brown rice: germinated and non-germinated. Germinated brown rice is obtained by immersing brown rice grain in water to initiate germination. The benefits of germinated brown rice are that the nutrients found in brown rice are more easily digested and the texture of brown rice is better (44).

Several population-based studies have shown increased risk of Type 2 diabetes associated with the high intake of white rice or glutinous rice, while higher dietary intake of brown rice in the diet may decrease the risk of this disease (44). Other studies showed rice bran and brown rice to lower cholesterol (42, 44). Bran and brown rice may help lowering incidences of some chronic diseases such as cancer, cardiovascular disorders, hypercholesterolemia, inflammation, aging, and obesity. Therefore, bran and brown rice are becoming increasingly popular nowadays in the world due to their health benefits. However, bran and brown rice contain phytic acid (inositol polyphosphate), an antioxidant that impairs absorption of iron and zinc from the digestive tract (44). This problem is not significant because the quantity of phytic acid in rice is not enough to neutralize all the minerals in the diet of omnivorous people, except vegans. Rice husk can be used as a fuel, and in paper manufacturing (42). Because rice needs a lot of water to grow, different rice varieties can accumulate higher amounts of toxic minerals in the bran, like arsenic, lead, cadmium, and mercury, more than other cereals (wheat, oat, corn) grown in the same polluted areas. Therefore, a control of rice composition is necessary before going to market.

2.1.3 Corn (Maize)

Corn or maize grain (*Zea mays*, family: Poaceae or Gramineae), is considered a staple food in many parts of the world. Maize grain (kernel) is an edible and nutritive part of the plant. It is the third leading crop of the world, after wheat and rice, in providing nutrients to humans and animals. Maize plant is used for animal feed, while maize silk or maize stigma (*Maidis stigmata*) is reserved for medicinal purposes (45–46). Maize is also used for production of starch, oil, alcoholic beverages, nutraceuticals, food sweeteners and recently, biofuel. Corn flour is used to make flat breads and other dishes for different populations in the world.

Maize grain (kernel) has a high nutritional value. Its composition per 100 g of the total dry weight of the grain is the following: carbohydrate 71.9 g, protein 8.8 g, fat 4.5 g, fiber 2.1 g, phosphor 348 mg, sodium 16 mg, sulfur 114 mg, riboflavin 0.10 mg, thiamine (B1) 0.4 mg, vitamin C 0.12 mg, amino acids 1.8 mg, minerals 1.5 g, calcium 10 mg, iron 2.3 mg, potassium 286 mg, magnesium 139 mg, copper 0.14 mg, ash 2.3 g, and moisture 10.2 g (45–46). In comparison with wheat and rice, its energetic value is between that of wheat and rice. Its carbohydrate and protein contents are between those of wheat and rice. However, its lipid levels are the highest, hence, corn can give oil. Maize germ contains about 45–50% of oil that is used in cooking or salad preparation. The oil contains 14% saturated fatty acids, 30% monounsaturated fatty acids, and 56% polyunsaturated fatty acids. The refined maize oil contains linoleic acid 54–60%, oleic acid 25–31%, palmitic acid 11–13%, stearic acid 2–3%, and linolenic acid 1% (45). Maize grain is an essential source of various major phytochemicals such as carotenoids, phenolic compounds, and phytosterols (45). Maize flour is nutritious, tasty, and easy to digest. Regularly consumed, it cleanses the colon and aids digestion by reducing stomach acid. Consumed as popcorn, it helps avoid constipation (46).

Corn silk or maize stigma contains various constituents essential for medicinal and nutritive purposes. Corn stigmata have the form of silky filaments, slightly bent, yellow-gold or brown-red, and are used fresh or dried and mildly anodyne. They have a pleasant, specific, sweet-mucilaginous taste. The stigmata contain flavonoids (0.1–6.3%), saponins (3%), volatile oils (0.2%), potassium and calcium salts, vitamins C, E, and K, carbohydrates, and allantoin (46). Moreover, corn silk contains fixed oils, resin, sugar, mucilage, salt, and fibers (45). Used as infusion with water (about one in ten), corn silk has diuretic action, helping eliminate water from tissues, increasing bile secretion for heart diseases and obesity, and acting favorably in cases of vesical pain, urinary tract (45–46). In the traditional medicine of some countries such as India, China, Romania, Spain, France, and Greece, corn silk is used to treat kidney stones, urinary tract infections, jaundice, and fluid retention (45–46). It may improve blood pressure and support liver function. It acts as a good antioxidant due to the high content of phenols and flavonoids like maysine, maizenic acid (46). Maysine, an important flavonoid contained in maize silk, may have the potential to prevent prostate cancer (46).

2.1.4 Millets

Millets are a group of cereal crops or grains for human foods and fodder and mainly found in the semiarid tropics of Asia (India, China) and West Africa. Millets secure the sixth position in terms of world agricultural production of cereal grains, and are still a staple food in many regions of the world (47). The main millets include pearl millet (*Pennisetum glaucum*), finger millet (*Eleusine coracana*), foxtail millet (*Setaria italica*), and proso millet (*Panicum miliaceum*). They belong to the family Poaceae and are important crop species. Millets abode vital nutrients and the protein content of millet grains are considered to be equal or superior in comparison to wheat, rice, maize, and sorghum grains. Millets are gluten-free cereal products and high in B-vitamins (B1, B2, B6, B9), minerals (calcium, iron, zinc, iodine), amino acids (methionine, valine, lysine), antioxidants (phenolic acids, flavonoids, tannins), essential fatty acids, and fibers (47). Due to the richness of millets in polyphenols and other phytochemicals, they can lower fat absorption and slow down sugar release, thus reducing risk of heart disease, diabetes, high blood pressure, and maybe cancer (47). Millet grains are staple food in arid areas of the world and ingredients in cake, porridge, cookie, and alcohol recipes of many Asian countries.

2.1.5 Potato

Potato (*Solanum tuberosum*, Solanaceae) is the fourth most important food crop worldwide, after rice, wheat, and maize, and is the starchy vegetable that is a tuber. Potatoes were domesticated between 7,000–10,000 years ago, likely in the Andes between Peru and Bolivia (48–51). Potato tuber is a rich source of energy due to the high levels of starch. Fresh potato tuber contains about 80% water and 20% solids. Potato dry matter consists of 75–80% starch. Of the 20 grams of solids in 100 grams tuber, about 18 grams are carbohydrate and 2 grams protein. The major proteins present in potato tubers are albumin, globulin, prolamine, and glutenin (49–51). Another protein fraction is made up of glycoproteins (patatin, lectin), metaloprotein, and phosphoproteins. Patatins account for 40% of the soluble protein content. Potatoes contain high levels of essential amino acids like methionine, lysine, threonine, and tryptophan (49–51). The lipid content of potatoes is very low and is mainly composed of free fatty acids such as linoleic acid, linolenic acid, oleic acid, palmitic acid, and stearic acid (50). Lecithins are the most important phospholipids of potatoes. The predominance of unsaturated fatty acids like oleic acid, linoleic acid, and linolenic acid confers easy oxidation of dehydrated potato products. Therefore, this presents a problem in the manufacture and storage of potato tubers (51). Beside their high levels of starch, potatoes tubers are a valuable source of dietary vitamins, antioxidants, and essential minerals (48–51). Vitamin C (about 100–250 mg/kg) is the most abundant vitamin in potatoes (51). Wounding can substantially increase vitamin C levels in potato tubers. For example, a 400% increase in vitamin C in sliced tubers was observed compared to intact potatoes for 2 days of storage, but a 347% decrease was noted in bruised tubers (49). Potatoes are an important source of several B vitamins, especially vitamin B6, vitamin B9 (folic acid) and different minerals (potassium, iron, phosphorus, magnesium, calcium and zinc). Potatoes are rich in antioxidants such as vitamin E, carotenoids, flavonoids, phenolic acids, and anthocyanins (49–50). They also contain some alkaloids such as glycoalkaloids, calystegines (tropane alkaloids), and some polyamines like kukoamines (phenolic-polyamine conjugates) (48). There are about 5,000 potato varieties, but the potato *Solanum tuberosum* is the species most cultivated throughout the world (48). The factor variety plays an important role in nutrient content. The differences in color between varieties of potatoes are due to antioxidant pigments such as carotenoid, anthocyanin, phenolics (chlorogenic acid, flavonoid), and so on. (48). Chlorogenic acid, a polyphenol antioxidant, may be implicated in prevention of Type 2 diabetes and cardiovascular disease (50). White-fleshed potato varieties contain lower amounts of phenolic antioxidants as compared to purple-fleshed wild species. Potato cultivars with flesh that is purple, red, or blue are particularly high in anthocyanin content (51). The most abundant tuber carotenoids which have yellow and orange flesh colors, are usually lutein, zeaxanthin, violaxanthin, and antheraxanthin. Both blue potatoes (rich in flavonoids) and yellow potatoes (rich in carotenoids) are found to promote good health. Indeed, colorful potato tubers are generally better for the health than white ones due to the presence of colored antioxidants, although both white and colored potatoes give the same energy content.

Beside many phytonutrients cited above, potato tubers naturally contain some types of alkaloids such as glycoalkaloids and calystegines. Glycoalkaloids are nitrogenous compounds and include α-chaconine and α-solanine (49–51). Their effects in humans can be both deleterious and beneficial (50). Glycoalkaloids are capable of causing vomiting, intestinal inflammation, teratogenicity, and cholinesterase inhibition, if ingested in high enough amounts (49–50). On the other hand, glycoalkaloids have some health-promoting effects like hypocholesterolemia, hypoglycemia, bactericide, and anti-inflammation (50). Glycoalkaloids (GAs) are concentrated in the outer region of the tuber; therefore, peeling reduces the GA content substantially. Glycoalkaloids are not destroyed during cooking and frying (51). In addition, potato tubers also contain small quantities of calystegines, which are nortropane alkaloids with glycosidase inhibitory activity (51). Potatoes are not a source of allergens. However, patatin, a glycoprotein rich in potato, may induce allergic symptoms during potato peeling or after eating raw potatoes (48, 51). Cooking or processing potatoes greatly improves the digestibility of potato starch. In general, unpeeled potatoes have better nutrient retention than peeled potatoes after cooking. Baking, roasting, and frying generally result in lower losses of vitamins than boiling. The fiber content of potatoes is reduced greatly by peeling. However, tuber peel is rich in pesticides and insecticides and sometimes may contain bacteria and parasites. Organic potatoes are preferable in case of unpeeled tuber boiling. Microwave cooking may produce the smallest losses of ascorbic acid (50). Concerning the formation of toxic acrylamide levels reported in fried potatoes like French fries and chips, there is general consensus that asparagine, a free amino acid present in potato, reacts with sugars at temperatures greater than 120°C to form acrylamide (50, 52). Until today, no significant correlation between the acrylamide content in food and the occurrence of cancer has been found (52). However, the International Agency for Research on Cancer (IARC) and the European Scientific Committee on Food (SCF) have classified acrylamide as a probable human carcinogen and genotoxic carcinogen, respectively (52). Moreover, eating fried potatoes and chips every day is not good for the health because they may cause obesity, diabetes, or hypercholesterolemia. Consuming them moderately is the best choice.

2.1.6 Sweet Potato

Sweet potato, *Ipomoea batatas* (L.) Lam, is a perennial crop which belongs to the family Convolvulaceae. The sweet potato is not the same species as the potato (*Solanum tuberosum*), which belongs to the family Solanaceae. Sweet potato is mostly harvested for its tubers. It is also a staple food source for many indigenous populations of the tropical and subtropical areas such as in Central and South Americas, Africa, the Caribbean, Okinawa Island, the Maori people, Hawaiians, and Papua New Guineans, because of its good source of energy, its high nutrient content, its easy cultivation, and its low costs of production (53–57). The leaves are also sometimes consumed as an alternative to other leafy vegetables. It is the sixth most important food crop in the world and it contains phytochemicals which are important for human health (54). The sweet potato root provides significant amounts of carbohydrates when compared to other starchy crops such as rice, maize, and sorghum porridge, although the protein content is slightly lower than in potatoes and other grain crops (54). In comparison with potatoes of white and red varieties, sweet potato is richer in energy and carbohydrates than the two potato varieties and constitutes an important source of vitamin A

(56). Protein contents of sweet potato leaves and roots range from 4.0% to 27.0% and 1.0% to 9.0%, respectively (53). Sporamin or ipomoein is a soluble protein without glycan and is the main storage protein in sweet potato roots and accounts for about 60–80% of its total proteins. Moreover, sweet potato contains a number of antioxidants and phytochemicals such as flavonoids, terpenoids, carotenoids, tannins, and phenolic acids (53–57). These constituents may vary with varieties depending on flesh and skin colors. Orange varieties are particularly rich in beta-carotene, while purple or blue-violet sweet potato contains higher anthocyanin content than other varieties of sweet potato (53–57). Orange-fleshed and yellow-fleshed sweet potato cultivars have been recognized as good sources of beta-carotene, a precursor of vitamin A, and are promoted across the developing world. The antioxidant activities of sweet potato are due to anthocyanins and beta-carotenes. Peonidin and cyanidin are anthocyanins only present in purple sweet potato, but absent in white and orange varieties (57). Luteolin, a flavonoid, is found in orange and purple varieties but is absent in the white ones. Phenolic acids such as chlorogenic, isochlorogenic, hydroxycinammic, cinammic, and caffeic acids are also present and have antioxidant properties (55). Sweet potato leaves also contain anthocyanins and polyphenolic compounds. Indeed, colored sweet potatoes are healthier than white ones. Additionally, many studies have reported different medicinal potentials of sweet potato tubers and leaves in humans such as cardiovascular protector, immunomodulatory, hypoglycemic, and anti-ulcerative effects (55). Fresh sweet potato roots are often eaten after cooking by boiling in water, steaming, or baking with peel or without peel. They can be cut into thin chips and then dried in the sun. Dried chips can be milled into flour used alone or mixed with other flours like wheat. Sweet potato flour is used to make bread, noodles, donuts, and cakes. It is also used as feed for farmed animals and makes an excellent source for the functional food market. Indeed, sweet potato could be considered as an excellent novel source of natural health-promoting compounds (53).

2.1.7 Cassava

Cassava or manioc (*Manihot esculenta*) belonging to the family Euphorbiaceae, is a perennial shrub native to South America. It is one of the most important staple food crops in tropical and subtropical parts of the world (58–59). The genus *Manihot* comprises 98 species and *M. esculenta* is the most widely cultivated member (58). Production of this crop plays a role in the maintenance of food security in much of the developing world, including Africa, the Asian Pacific, and South America. More than 750 million people, including 45% of sub-Saharan Africans, currently rely on cassava as their primary food source (59).

The root is a physiological energy reserve with high carbohydrate content, which is mostly constituted of starch. About 83% of starch is in the form of amylopectin and the rest (17%) is amylose (60). Roots contain small quantities of sucrose, glucose, fructose, and maltose. Cassava has bitter and sweet varieties. In sweet cassava varieties, up to 17% of the root is sucrose with small amounts of dextrose and fructose. Raw cassava root has more carbohydrate than potatoes and less carbohydrate than wheat, rice, yellow corn, and sorghum. The fiber content in cassava roots is about 1.5% in fresh root and 4% in root flour (60). The lipid content in cassava roots is relatively low compared to maize and sorghum, but higher than potato and comparable to rice. The contents of protein and of some essential amino acids, like cysteine, methionine, and tryptophan, are also very low. However, the roots contain an abundance of arginine, glutamic acid, and aspartic acid. Cassava roots also contain some minerals such as calcium, phosphorus, potassium, magnesium, copper, iron, zinc, and manganese (61). The vitamin content of the roots is low, except for vitamin C. Thus, cassava roots are rich in calories given by starch, but low in protein, fat, and some minerals and vitamins except calcium, phosphorus, and vitamin C (61). Their nutritional value is lower than those of some cereals (maize, sorghum) and some other root and tuber crops. Tapioca is a commercial starch product of cassava roots in form of dried powder (60). It is used to make many processed foods such as chips, crisp cakes, cassava bread, and so on. However, cassava contains antinutrients and toxic substances namely cyanogenic glucosides, oxalates, nitrates, and phytates. The cyanogenic glucosides are decomposed by an enzyme naturally present in cassava, releasing toxic hydrogen cyanide (HCN) or salt cyanide, when plant tissue is crushed or chewed (58–61). Cyanide is present in both sweet and bitter varieties, but its content is much higher in bitter cassava, in the root as well as in the leaves (58, 60). The highest concentrations of cyanide are in the peel of the tuberous root. The flesh tuber contains less cyanide. Cyanide is the most toxic factor restricting the intake of cassava roots and leaves. Cassava, particularly bitter varieties, has a cyanide level higher than the FAO recommendations, which is less than ten mg cyanide /kg, to prevent acute toxicity in humans (60). Consumption of 50 to 100 mg of cyanide leads to acute poisoning and can cause death in adults (60). For sweet varieties, cooking peeled tubers in boiling water is sufficient to eliminate all toxicity. For bitter varieties, cyanogenic glycosides can be reduced or removed by processing. Processing methods include drying, roasting, boiling, soaking, wetting, and fermentation because hydrogen cyanide (HCN) becomes volatile when heating (59–61). Detoxification processes can be used singularly or in combination. In general, the combined process gives better nutrient quality (61). The intake of lower cyanide amounts is not lethal but long-term use could cause neuropathy like ataxia, partial paralysis (60). Cassava-eating populations ingesting cyanide and high amounts of nitrates and nitrites have the risk of developing stomach cancer (61). Apart from some toxic compounds in the cassava plant, its tuber root plays an important role in supplying energetic food for people living in arid areas, such as with low rainfall and high temperatures, due to its ease of cultivation in poor soils.

2.1.8 Yam

Yam (*Dioscorea sp.*) is an herbaceous perennial plant of the monocotyledonous family Dioscoreaceae. There are many different varieties of yams. They are cultivated for the consumption of their starchy tubers and are the staple food in West Africa, Southeast Asia, Oceania, and the Caribbean regions (62). Yam is considered to be the most nutritious of the tropical root crops. It contains about four times as much protein as cassava, and is the only major root crop that exceeds rice in protein content (62). Yam is rich in amino acids especially sulfur-containing amino acids like cysteine and methionine. Overall, essential amino acid content is higher in yam than in sweet potato. Yam is also a good source of vitamins A and C, and of fiber and minerals, except calcium. Yam is low in antinutrients such as oxalate, phytate and trypsin inhibitor (62). Yam tubers have various bioactive components, namely, mucin, dioscin, dioscorin, allantoin, polyphenols, choline, diosgenin, and vitamins such as carotenoids and tocopherols (58). Mucilage of yam tuber contains soluble glycoprotein and dietary fiber.

Yam is consumed as raw yam, cooked soup, and powder or flour in food preparations. Yam extracts may have hypoglycemic, antimicrobial, antidiabetic, and antioxidant activities (58). Yam stimulates the proliferation of gastric epithelial cells and enhances digestive enzyme activities in the small intestine. Diosgenin, a steroidal saponin of yam, has antioxidative and hypolipidemic activities *in vivo*. The anti-hypercholesterolemic effect of yam saponin is due to its inhibitory effects against cholesterol absorption (58). Yam may reduce the risk of cancer and cardiovascular diseases in postmenopausal women. Regular consumption of yam may enhance bone strength in osteoporosis during menopause (58). Indeed, yam is a safe and good energizing food and may prevent some chronic diseases cited above.

2.1.9 Sugarcane

Sugarcane or sugar cane (*Saccharum officinarum* Linn.) is a perennial grass of the family Poaceae (63). It was first grown in Southeast Asia and western India. It is now cultivated in the tropical and sub-tropical regions from Australia, India, South Asia to South Africa, South America, Cuba, Mexico, and the United States. Approximately 70% of crystal sugar production worldwide comes from sugarcane and 30% from sugar beet. The most important constituent in whole sugarcane is sucrose which is typically measured in the plant stalk (64). Sugarcane juice is the extracted liquid mainly used for the production of crystalline sugar or white sugar and other products like raw sugar, brown sugar, molasses, jaggery, candies, and ethanol. Fresh sugarcane juice is a common drink in Southeast Asia. The main byproducts of the sugar industry are bagasse, molasses, and sugar wax

(64). After treatment of sugarcane juice by evaporation, concentration and centrifugation, crystalline raw sugar is settled down, then refined to give table sugar or white sugar, while the viscous supernatant liquid is called molasses. Jaggery is generally produced in developing countries from sugarcane juice after filtration and boiling, but without sugar refining. Hence, jaggery sugar has a natural dark brown color (63–64).

Sugarcane juice has a high water content (75–85%) and contains mainly sucrose (13–15%) and reducing sugars like glucose, fructose, and fiber. The protein and the vitamin contents in sugarcane juice are insignificant. The most abundant amino acids are aspartic acid, glutamic acid, and alanine. Several color components in sugarcane juice are: chlorogenic acid, cinnamic acid, flavones, and flavone glycosides (63–64).

The composition of molasses is highly variable. It is primarily influenced by the processing technology used rather than differences in plant composition. All grades of molasses contain significant amounts of sugars with a majority of sucrose. Yet, molasses has no fat or fiber, and very little protein. Molasses products are low in phosphorus, but are high in calcium and potassium. Molasses is used for preparation of brown sugar by mixing white sugar with molasses. It is also the main raw material for industrial alcohol production of rum, after fermentation and distillation. Sugarcane molasses contains some polyphenolic compounds which have antibacterial activity (63–64). Sugarcane bagasse typically contains approximately 40–50% moisture, and 1–3% sugar, with the remainder as fiber. The fiber fraction includes cellulose, hemicellulose, and lignin. Bagasse has also been recognized as a potential feedstuff for large ruminants. Bagasse can be used as combustible fuel for power generation and the manufacture of pulp and paper products (63–64). Sugarcane tops are usually left in the field after harvest, but are used for feed purposes in some countries.

Sugarcane wax is a whitish to dark-yellowish powdery deposit on the surface of stalks and leaves of *S. officinarum*, which appears as a cuticle layer (63). The amount of wax in sugarcane ranges between 0.1 and 0.3%, depending upon its variety. Sugarcane wax is rich in policosanols that are a mixture of long chain primary aliphatic alcohols (63). Some reports have found that human policosanol consumption is safe and is effective at lowering blood cholesterol and lipids (65). It is a dietary supplement marketed in some countries for the prevention of CVDs (63). However, some other scientists reported no effects of policosanols on hypercholesterolemic persons (66). It is noteworthy that there is no important difference between white sugar, brown sugar, and raw sugar in terms of human health benefits. Theoretically, brown sugar and raw sugar contain about 10% more molasses than white sugar, therefore, the variation of some essential nutrients like minerals and vitamins mainly present in the molasses between white and brown sugars is insignificant in the consumer body. However, overconsumption of soluble sugars like sweet drinks, fruit syrups, and snacks, is unhealthy and may lead to obesity, CVDs, hypercholesterolemia, and hyperlipidemia. The American Heart Association recommends six teaspoons of sugar a day for women, and about nine teaspoons a day for men (64).

2.1.10 Sugar Beet

Sugar beet (*Beta vulgaris*, var. *Altissima Doell*, Family Amaranthaceae) is a plant rich in sucrose that is now cultivated worldwide for sugar production, though primarily in temperate climates such as France, Germany, and the northern United States (67). It is a plant with a swollen round root with white flesh which is eaten or used to make sugar. Sugar beet provides about 20% of the global demand for sugar and occupies a second place after sugarcane (67–69). Processing of sugar beet is similar to that of sugarcane. Sugar is extracted from beet roots using hot water followed by concentration as a syrup form, then washing and finally drying (68–69). In general, sugar beets have around 20% sucrose by weight. Once extracted, sucrose can be directly fermented into ethanol using traditional or industrial methods (68). The non-crystallized syrup from this extraction is called beet molasses which has upwards of 50% by weight of sugar (68). Vinasses results from fermentation of molasses and is used as soil conditioner or animal feed. Beet molasses is usually fermented into alcohol. The leftover molasses is rich in nitrogen and is used either as animal feed or as a fertilizer (69). Sugar beet pulp also contains cell wall polysaccharides including pectin and dietary fiber. Pectin is a cell-wall polysaccharide consisting of galacturonic acid with rhamnose sidechains in varying proportions. Pectin is best known for its gelling properties in fruit products. Beet pectin exhibits better emulsifying properties than other sources of pectin (68). The non-sucrose substances in sugar beet roots include other soluble saccharides, cell wall components, saponins, proteins, free amino acids, and betaine. Minerals include nitrates, phosphates, chlorides, sulfates, potassium, sodium, calcium, magnesium, and ammonium (69). Fiber products from sugar beet pulp are recognized as safe, containing around 8% protein (by weight) and 67% carbohydrates such as hemicelluloses (28%), cellulose (19%), and pectin (18%) (68). Fiber products from sugar beets are used as prebiotic in the human gut. Adverse effects to human or animal health due to sugar beet intake have not been observed (69).

Other varieties of sugar beet are called beetroots. Although they have culinary and medicinal uses, they cannot produce sugar. Beetroot varieties have red, violet, or yellow flesh.

2.2 FRUITS

Fruit is a component of flowering plants (angiosperms). Fruit results from the mature ovary of a flower and refers to the edible part of a plant that consists of the seeds and surrounding tissues called flesh (70). Some fruits without seeds are called seedless fruits such as bananas and pineapples. Fruits are generally eaten in their fresh form or also after processing such as pressure, drying, or cooking. Most cultivated fruits are edible, but some wild fruits are toxic and inedible. Depending upon their regional temperature, fruits are classified into sub-tropical fruits, tropical fruits, and temperate fruits. Tropical regions product more fruits than temperate climate because fruits need sunlight and heat. In temperate climates, fruits are abundant from spring to autumn. Most fruits contain various macro and micronutrients such as sugars, oils, proteins, soluble and insoluble fibers, unsaturated and saturated fatty acids, amino acids, minerals, vitamins, and antioxidants. Moreover, they have numerous phytochemicals like polyphenols, flavonoids, terpenoids, alkaloids, and glycosides, and can be used as plant medicines (70–71). Most phytochemicals are stocked in the peel. In general, colored fruits are better than uncolored fruits. Many experimental studies have supported the protective role of fruits against cancer, cardiovascular diseases (CVDs), chronic inflammatory diseases (rheumatoid arthritis, osteoarthritis, asthma), diabetes, and aging (70–71). The involved mechanisms in CVDs included protecting vascular endothelial function, regulating lipid metabolism, modulating blood pressure, inhibiting platelet function, suppressing thrombosis, reducing oxidative stress, attenuating inflammation, and alleviating ischemia injury (71). In addition, fruits such as prune, date, plum, and apricot contain a good amount of dietary fiber that aids digestion, prevents constipation, ensures good bowel movement, and cleanses the colon (70). Fruits are an important part of the balanced diet for humans. Daily consumption of five servings of fruits is recommended to obtain most of the health benefits. However, for some particular people, some fruits can cause allergy or incompatibility with some diseases. An excessive intake of fruits, although they are delicious or healthy, is also to be avoided. Some of the main fruits are summarily described as follows.

2.2.1 Apple

Apple is the fruit of the apple tree (*Malus pumila or domestica*) of the family Rosaceae. It is native to Central Asia and is grown all over the world. There are about 7,000 varieties of apples in the world with different colors, savors, flesh, and aromas. Apples are among the most popular types of fruit in the world – mostly in Western countries. The old English proverb originated in Wales (UK) and emitted in 1860s: '*an apple a day keeps the doctor away*' is now scientifically justified. Recently, many scientists in the world have found that regular consumption of apples can contribute to improve heart health and to reduce the risk of cancer, CVDs, hypercholesterolemia, asthma, diabetes, infection, cognitive decline, bone diseases, obesity, and gastrointestinal troubles (72–74). In the laboratory, apples have been found to have very strong antioxidant activity, inhibit cancer cell proliferation, decrease lipid oxidation, lower cholesterol, and prevent infection.

Apples are high in fibers, vitamin C and various antioxidants with different beneficial properties for health. Apples also rank second for total concentration of antioxidant phenolic compounds, with the highest portion of free phenolics when compared to other fruits (72–73). Apples are a good source of several antioxidants including flavonoids (quercetin, catechins, oligomeric proanthocyanidins), and chlorogenic acid (73). The phytochemical composition of apples varies greatly between different varieties of apples, and there are also small changes in phytochemicals during the maturation and ripening of the fruit. Apples contain fructose, sucrose, glucose, and water. They are also high in soluble and insoluble fibers (about four g/apple), mainly formed of pectin, a soluble fiber. Soluble fiber promotes gut health by stimulating good bacteria in the colon and may also prevent colon cancer, lower blood cholesterol and blood sugar levels, and cause weight loss for obese individuals. Storage has little effect on apple phytochemicals, but processing can greatly affect apple phytochemicals.

Various colors and flavors are due to the antioxidants mainly formed in the apple peels which are used for protecting the fruit against bacteria, parasites, molds, and so on. Apples are usually eaten raw, but they are also used in the preparation of various recipes, juices, and drinks like ciders. Seeds contain amygdalin, a cyanogenic glycoside that can liberate toxic cyanide in the body. Ingesting some apple seeds may have no noxious effect; however, eating a large amount is dangerous for the health. Allergy to apple is rare but can exist. Anthocyanin is a red pigment mainly found in some red apples. Apples with red or green peels are better than apples with pale yellow peels. Because the apple peels contain more antioxidant compounds, especially quercetin and ursolic acid (a terpenoid described below). Apple peels contain from two to six times more flavonoids and terpenoids than the apple flesh (72–73). So, do not discard the peel.

Beside its high antioxidant and nutrient content, apple could also be beneficial for the human gut flora or intestinal microbiota because an apple contains on average 100 million good bacterial cells (74). Fruit pulp and seeds are rich in beneficial bacteria, while the peel is less colonized. Among bacterial phyla in apple, Proteobacteria dominated with 80%, followed by Bacteroidetes (9%), Actinobacteria (5%), and Firmicutes (3%) (74). They are probiotics. Organic apples contain more good bacteria than non-organic ones.

2.2.2 Banana

Banana is a tropical edible fruit of the herbaceous flowering plants belonging to two main species, *Musa acuminata* and *Musa balbisiana* (family Musaceae). All edible banana fruits are seedless (75–76). More than 300 types of bananas are cultivated throughout the world (75). Banana is a very popular fruit in the world market and is consumed as staple food in many countries. It is either eaten raw or processed, and also as a functional ingredient in various food products. Banana is known to be rich in carbohydrates (23 g/100), dietary fibers (2.6 g/100), soluble sugars (12.2 g/100), proteins (1.1 g/100), and lipids (0.33 g/100) (76). Starch in banana flesh changes into sugars (fructose and sucrose) when ripe. Banana is rich in calories. A single banana provides 90 Kcal energy, but low in fat, making it the best food to give quick energy supply for athletes during competition. In addition, the fruit also prevents muscular contractions as it contains significant amounts of vitamins and minerals (76).

Moreover, banana is also a good source of resistant starch that is an indigestible compound available in banana fruit. Resistant starch escapes absorption in the small intestine and is transported to the large intestine where digestion takes place. This occurrence makes banana a preferred fruit for consumers suffering from diabetes (75–76). Banana contains many bioactive compounds, such as carotenoids, flavonoids, phenolics, biogenic amines, phytosterols, vitamin C, and vitamin E, with antioxidant activities providing many human health benefits (75–76). It is also high in magnesium, phosphorus, sodium, potassium, calcium, iron, copper, zinc, and manganese (75).

As banana is rich in magnesium and vitamins, it may relieve stress. Well-ripened fruit can mitigate intestinal diseases (constipation, flatulence) and improve digestion and absorption (75–76). Green banana has antidiarrheal activity in children. Bananas have some potential health benefits for cancer (kidney cancer), stomach ulcer, cholesterol metabolism, and some cardiovascular diseases like hyperlipidemia, high blood pressure, and atherosclerosis (75–76).

Banana pulp and peel can be used as natural sources of antioxidants and pro-vitamin A. Banana peel is reported to have higher antioxidant capacity than banana pulp (76). In brief, banana is a good fruit rich in energy, vitamins, antioxidants, and minerals.

2.2.3 Grape

A grape is a berry fruit of the vines (Vitis) originally from the Mediterranean region. There are a few thousand varieties of *Vitis vinifera* grapes; some of them have commercial values. Grape is eaten fresh or processed to make wine, jam, juice, jelly, raisins, grape seed extract, grape seed oil, and vinegar. Grape berries contain three major types of tissue: skin, flesh, and seeds (77–78). Grapes have high soluble healthy sugar, fiber, and water content. They are a rich source of vitamins: B1, B2, B5, B6, C, K, and minerals (calcium, magnesium, potassium) (77–78). Grape berries are very rich in potassium (78). Grapes also contain a variety of colored phenolic antioxidants such as anthocyanidins and resveratrol which are responsible for the color of purple grapes and red wines (72, 77–78). Grapes grow in clusters, and their colors vary from yellow, green, orange, pink to crimson, dark blue, and black. The darker the colors, the richer the grapes are in antioxidants.

Resveratrol (3,4',5-trihydroxystilbene) is a polyphenolic antioxidant, and has been reported to protect cardiovascular and nervous systems, prevent cancer, improve diabetes, and extend lifespan. Resveratrol is only found in different red or black grape varieties, primarily in their skins and seeds. For example, levels of resveratrol in skins and seeds of muscadine grapes are about one hundred times higher than those in pulp (78). Resveratrol in fruit is more potent than its supplement because its bioavailability (absorption) in red grape is higher than that of its supplement. Tannins, including the monomeric catechins, are present in the skin and seed tissues but nearly absent in the flesh (78). Grapes also contain tartaric acid and malic acid. Tartaric acid is accumulated during the initial stages of berry development and its concentration is highest at the periphery of the developing berry. By contrast, malic acid is accumulated in the flesh cells at the end of the first growth phase. These acids confer acidity to the wine, and are therefore critical to its quality (78). Flavor that builds in grapes is mostly the result of the acid/sugar balance and the synthesis of flavor and aromatic compounds (78). Briefly, red grapes and red wines are better than white grapes and white wines in the prevention of CVDs and cancer, due to numerous polyphenol antioxidants cited above. The quality of a wine depends on the variety of the vine, its cultivation mode, and its environment.

2.2.4 Berries

Beside grape berry cited above, the most consumed berries belong to two families: Rosaceae (blackberry, raspberry, strawberry), and Ericaceae (blueberry, cranberry) (79). Some other berries like goji berry are considered exotic berries. These berries are among the best dietary sources of many antioxidant compounds such as phenolic acids, flavonoids, anthocyanins, tannins, and ascorbic acid. They are colored fruits with delicious taste and flavor (79–80). These compounds, either individually or combined, are responsible for various health benefits of berries, such as prevention of inflammation disorders, cardiovascular diseases, or protective effects to lower the risk of various cancers (72, 79–80).

2.2.4.1 Blackberry

Blackberries belonging to the genus *Rubus* in the family Rosaceae, are aggregate fruits consisting of many drupelets. The most common cultivated variety is *Rubus fruticosus* (79). They are cultivated mainly in Europe and North America (USA); while wild blackberries make a significant contribution to worldwide production (79). Blackberries are one of the healthiest fruits on this planet due to the presence of different minerals (iron, magnesium, calcium, zinc), phytonutrients, fats, carbohydrates, dietary fiber, vitamin C, vitamin K, vitamins of group B, and more. (79–81). Blackberries are also a rich source of polyphenolic antioxidants including anthocyanins, procyanidins, ellagitannins, ellagic acid, flavonols, flavan-3-ols, flavones, isoflavones, and so on (79–81). Blackberry phenolic compounds have protective effects on age-related neurodegenerative diseases and bone loss in vivo and can inhibit low-density lipoprotein and liposomal oxidation in vitro. Polyphenol extracts from blackberry also possess anti-inflammatory properties (79–81). Blackberries are known for curing and preventing a wide variety of ailments, such as colitis, in folk medicine. Blackberry extracts have also exerted antimutagenic effects in vitro and in vivo by modifying cell signaling pathways and suppressing tumor promotion factors. Some studies suggested that blackberries may help to fight diseases like cancer, heart diseases, and gout, as well as slow down aging. They also promote healthy skin, bone development, weight loss and improve memory, eye vision, immune system, and digestion (79–81). However, these medicinal properties of blackberry are still preliminary and need more investigation (81). Blackberries are consumed raw or made in jam or jelly.

2.2.4.2 Raspberries

The raspberry is the edible fruit of many plant species in the genus Rubus of the Rosaceae family. Raspberries are available in many varieties that include red raspberries (the most abundant), purple raspberries, black raspberries, and blue raspberries. Raspberries are called bramble fruit and are an aggregate of drupelets (79). Raspberries are among the healthiest fruits due to their high nutrient content including polyphenolic antioxidants (anthocyanins, ellagitannins, ellagic acid), phytonutrients, soluble vitamins such as vitamin C, fiber, magnesium, potassium, iron, manganese, zinc, and so on (79–80). They are low in sugar. The fruits have been used in traditional and alternative medicine for a long time to cure wounds, colic, diarrhea, and renal illnesses (79). Raspberries could be helpful for managing early stages of Type 2 diabetes and hypertension. Raspberry extracts could inhibit proliferation of cancer cells in vitro (79). As they are rich in antioxidants and flavonoids, raspberries can prevent DNA damage in cells from free radicals; thereby protecting from many health problems like cancer, CVDs, and premature aging (79–80). Recent human clinical trials utilizing black raspberry have demonstrated chemo-preventive effects in the oral cavity, esophagus, and colon (82). However, raspberry, especially black raspberry, contains a high amount of oxalates which are dangerous for the health. So, people with kidney or gallbladder diseases must avoid consuming black raspberry. Raspberries could be consumed fresh, but due to their short storage life, are limited by rot and loss of firmness. More often they are utilized as processed products, such as jams, jellies, purees, juices, ice creams, or as ingredients for yogurts, smoothies, and so on (79).

2.2.4.3 Strawberries

Strawberry (genus: *Fragaria*, cultivated variety: *F. ananassa*, wild variety: *F. virginiana*, family: Rosaceae) is native to Europe and is now cultivated worldwide. Its fruit is bright red on the exterior and white in interior with a sweet taste and an attractive aroma (79, 83). Botanically, strawberry is not a berry, but it is an aggregate fruit with many one-seeded achenes to form a large fleshy receptacle. Among the fruits, fresh strawberries are considered to have one of the highest contents of vitamin C (79–80, 83). Strawberries are also an excellent source of fibers, folate (vitamin B9), potassium and manganese. Iron, copper, magnesium, phosphorus, vitamin B6, vitamin K, and vitamin E are present in moderate levels. Strawberries are very rich in antioxidants and phytochemicals, such as pelargonidin (a colored anthocyanin), ellagic acid (a polyphenol antioxidant), and ellagitannins and procyanidins (two flavonoids) (79–80, 83). As they are rich in antioxidants and vitamins, strawberries may prevent heart disease by lowering blood pressure and cholesterol profile and reducing inflammation and oxidative stress (79–80, 83). Strawberries can cause allergies like asthma and swelling of lips and face to some sensitive persons, especially young children. It is better to consume organic berries and wash them carefully before eating. Strawberries are usually consumed raw and fresh, but can be used as prepared foods (jams, jellies, desserts).

2.2.4.4   Blueberries

Blueberries, blue colored fruits, belong to the genus *Vaccinium*, family Ericaceae, are sweet, tasty, and nutritious fruits. Blueberries are high in dietary fibers (3–3.5% of their fruit weight) and vitamins, such as vitamin C, B complex, E, and β-carotene (provitamin A). Blueberries also provide high amounts of selenium, zinc, iron, and manganese, and contain lutein and zeaxanthin (79–80, 83). In addition, the levels of antioxidants like flavonoids, especially anthocyanidins, flavonols, phenolic acids, in blueberries are much higher than those in other berries mentioned previously (79, 83). Blueberries have become more popular due to their well-known health benefits, nutritional value, and excellent sensory evaluation. Blueberries might prevent cataract and macular degeneration and diabetes. They could also be used for decreasing blood pressure and blood cholesterol, therefore lowering CVDs and atherosclerosis risks (72). In addition, blueberries might ameliorate cognitive function and mental health and could prevent Parkinson's and Alzheimer's diseases (79, 83). Generally, blueberries are sold in fresh, frozen, and processed forms (dried and canned fruits, juices, and jams, in beverages, yogurts) for various food applications (79).

2.2.4.5   Cranberries

There are two major species of cranberry: the American cranberry (*Vaccinium macrocarpon*) and the European cranberry (*V. oxycoccos*), both belonging to the Ericaceae family. The European cranberry fruit is smaller (0.6–1.2 cm) and only half the size of the American fruit. The American cranberry is a red berry when ripe with acidic taste. The United States and Canada together account for more than 90% of the world's cranberry production (79, 84). Cranberries contain a lot of biologically active substances, such as vitamins (especially vitamin C), phenolic antioxidants (flavonoids, quercetin, proanthocyanidins, anthocyanins), and minerals (calcium, magnesium, potassium) (79, 84). Cranberries could prevent and treat urinary tract infections and stomach ulcers. They might prevent or reduce cardiovascular disease risks and protect against lipoprotein oxidation (79, 84). Cranberry fruit and juice can reduce the oxidation of low-density lipoprotein (LDL) or 'bad' cholesterol and, thus, reduce the atherosclerotic process. In the last decade, *in vitro* anti-cancer activity, anti-mutagenic effects and anti-tumorigenic activities of cranberries have been examined (79, 84). About 90% of cranberries are usually consumed as dried fruits, and products such as juices or food ingredients in cereals, meat, milk products, and sauces. The rest (10%) is consumed via fresh fruits (79).

2.2.4.6   Wolfberry or Goji Berry

Goji berry or wolfberry has two main species: *Lycium barbarum* and *Lychium chinense*, both belonging to the Solanaceae family. The species *L. barbarum* is widely cultivated for food and traditional medicine in China. Goji berry is native to Northwest China. The fruit has an ovoid shape with about 0.6–2 cm in length and 0.3–1 cm in diameter with deep orange-red waxy skin. The fruit contains 20–50 seeds and has a sweet and fruity taste and a creamy-white flesh (85). Harvested fresh goji berries are sun-dried for several days before marketing for culinary or medicinal uses. Dried goji can store well for up to one year. Dried goji berries are an excellent source of energy and essential nutrients (sugars, proteins, dietary fibers, vitamins). They contain several potentially bioactive components arabinogalactanproteins (AGPs), the carotenoid zeaxanthin, and the vitamin C precursor: β-D-glucopyranosyl ascorbic acid (85). AGPs are soluble glycoconjugates or soluble polysaccharides or a type of glycans. The main biological properties of AGPs are: modulation of the immune system, antitumor activity, and antioxidant activity (85).

It is noteworthy that wolfberry is rich in a number of potent antioxidants that are not polysaccharides, such as zeaxanthin, lutein, quercetin, and polyphenols, and vitamin C. The dried goji berries are employed in traditional Chinese medicines (TCM) to treat inflammation, to relief nervousness, to improve memory, and to stimulate eyes and skin. Although the benefits of dried wolfberry are well-known and thought highly of in TCM, scientific evidence regarding its benefits is unclear (85). Eating raw goji berry could be toxic and therefore, should be avoided. Goji berries are only consumed as dried fruits, or as different culinary or medicinal preparations. Dried goji can store well for up to one year. Do not consume dried goji berries for patients on anticoagulant medications such as warfarin because these berries may potentiate the anticoagulant effect of warfarin and increase the risk of bleeding.

2.2.5 Citrus Fruits: Oranges, Grapefruits, Lemon, Lime

Citrus fruits are produced by the genus Citrus, a flowering plant, belonging to the family Rutaceae. The main citrus fruits are orange, grapefruits, mandarin, pomelo, citron, Lemon, clementine, and tangerine. The three ancestors in the genus *Citrus* are the mandarin, pomelo, and citron. Almost all the citrus fruits cited here are hybrids of these three ancestors, or with their main progenies. Citrus fruits are rich in vitamin C, vitamins B1, B5, folic acid, calcium, potassium, fibers, soluble sugars, and water. They are also high in phytochemicals such as beta-carotene, lutein, flavanones, flavonoids (naringenin), terpenes, citric acid, volatile acids, and so on. Citrus fruits have a wide range of biological activities such as antioxidant, anti-inflammatory, immunomodulatory, metabolic, cardiovascular, and neuroprotective effects (86–87). In general, citrus fruit is globose to oval, and comprises two distinct parts: the pericarp also called the peel, skin or rind, and the endocarp, or pulp and juice sacs. Citrus peels are subdivided into the epicarp or flavedo (colored peripheral surface with numerous small aromatic oil glands) and mesocarp or albedo (white soft middle layer). Citrus peel, the primary waste, is a good source of molasses, pectin and limonene, and is usually dried, mixed with dried pulps and sold as cattle feed (88). As citrus peel is rich in polyphenols, fibers, vitamins, and essences, it can be used for the preparation of low-cost nutritional dietary supplements (88).

2.2.5.1 Oranges

Sweet orange (*Citrus sinensis*) is a small evergreen tree 7.5 m high and in some cases up to 15 m. It originated from southern China (89). Sweet orange is a cross between a mandarin and a hybrid pomelo. The fruit, which may be globose to oval is 6.5 to 9.5 cm wide, and ripens to orange or yellow. The peel consists of an epidermis of epicuticular wax with numerous small aromatic oil glands that gives it its particular smell (89). Sweet oranges also contain a phytochemical called hesperidin, which may lower blood cholesterol and triglyceride levels. Due to being high in antioxidants and other phytonutrients, oranges fight free radicals, enhance immunity, reduce cancer development, and CVDs (89). Vitamin C levels in orange juice decrease over preservation time. The mesocarp or albedo (edible white part of the orange rind) is also rich in vitamin C and other nutrients, so eat this white part too.

Blood orange or sanguine orange is a natural mutation of *Citrus sinensis*, and contains high levels of anthocyanin which is responsible for their dark red color in the flesh, juice, and rind. Blood orange is also healthy as classic orange and generally consumed as juice or marmalade. Other varieties of oranges are: bitter orange, mandarin, clementine, and tangerine. Bitter orange (*Citrus aurantium*), also known as Seville orange, contains many essential oils used as a flavoring for food or in the production of marmalade. It is also used in folk medicines as a stimulant, but can cause side effects (90). Mandarin (*Citrus reticulata*) is the natural ancestor of orange and many hybrid citrus cultivars. Tangerine (*Citrus tangerina*) is an artificial hybrid of mandarin orange, while clementine (*Citrus clementina*) is a hybrid between a sweet orange and a mandarin. Tangerine and clementine come from Morocco and Algeria, respectively, while mandarin is originated of China. Mandarin, tangerine and clementine have thin peels rich in volatile oils. Peels are used fresh or dried as a spice for cuisine or as traditional medicine for treatment of flatulence (gas in the digestive tube). The nutrients of these three fruits are similar to those of orange.

2.2.5.2 Grapefruit

The grapefruit (Citrus paradisi) is a cross between an orange and a pomelo (shaddock) and its flesh varies in color from white and yellow to pink and red depending on its variety. Its taste ranges from acidic and even bitter to sweet and sugary. It is a healthy fruit and contains all nutrients for our daily requirement (91–95). It provides up to 69% of the RDA for vitamin C along with as many as 250 mg of potassium (93). It is also rich in calcium, magnesium, vitamins of B group, citric acid, natural sugars, essential oils, and antioxidants including carotenoid, flavonoid, terpenoid groups such as beta-carotene, lycopene, naringin, naringenin, lutein, and xanthine (91–95). Thanks to its high content of flavonoids such as naringin and its aglycone naringenin, medical research has observed that grapefruit and its juice may reduce hypercholesterolemia, atherosclerotic plaque formation and inhibit breast cancer cell proliferation in vitro and mammary cell tumorigenesis (92). Grapefruit juice has been found to contain antioxidant, antiseptic, cardiotonic, hypocholesterolemic, detoxicant, and stomachic activities (91–93). Grapefruit essential oil (EO) is extracted from grapefruit peel and has been used for a long time as a valuable ingredient for its characteristic aroma in flavor and fragrance (94). Similar to most citrus EOs, its major components are terpenes and terpene oxides. Grapefruit essential oil has been reported to have a wide range of bioactivities such as inhibitory effects against bacteria and fungi, and antioxidant activity, which is important for food preservation and disease prevention. Grapefruit peel extracts could also inhibit the growth and proliferation of cancer cells such as neuroblastomas, leukemias, and prostate, and lung cancer lines (94).

Briefly, grapefruit juice has been traditionally indicated throughout time for anorexia, bacteria, benign prostatic hypertrophy, cancers (breast, colon, prostate), candida, cold, diabetes, dysuria, high cholesterol, infection, mycosis, insomnia, mycobacterium, nervousness, pseudomonas, and rheumatism (93).

Grapefruit juice has however, been found to be an inhibitor of the intestinal cytochrome P-450 3A4 system, which is responsible for the first pass metabolism of many drugs (93). The P-glycoprotein pump, found in the brush border of the intestinal wall which transports many of these cytochrome P-450 3A4 substrates, has also been shown to be inhibited by grapefruit juice. By inhibiting these enzyme systems, grapefruit juice alters the pharmacokinetics of a variety of medications, leading to elevation of their serum concentrations and thereby their toxicity. It has potential interactions with anti-hypertensive drugs (calcium channel blockers, nifedipine), lipid lowering agents (atorvastatin, simvastatin), tranquilizers (diazepam, carbamazepine), drugs used in erectile dysfunction (sildenafil or Viagra*), antidepressants, antimalarials, immunosuppressors (cyclosporine, tacrolimus), and more (91, 93). Therefore, always ask your doctor or pharmacist when you consume grapefruit with drugs or supplements.

2.2.5.3 Lemon and Lime

Lemon is the yellow sour fruit of the species *Citrus limon*, an evergreen tree, while lime fruit is the green citrus of the species *Citrus aurantifolia*. Both are more acidic than other citrus fruits of the family Rutaceae, but lime is more acidic and aromatic than lemon. They are rich in citric acid, vitamin C, vitamin B6, volatile terpenes, and flavanones (a group of flavonoids). For lemons, total flavanones are 26 mg/100 g and for limes, 17 mg/100 g (95). The flavanone profiles of both lemons and limes are dominated by eriocitrin and hesperidin, the two flavonoid glycosides (95). Hesperidin and eriocitrin are antioxidant pigments with certain benefits for health. The flesh and peel of both fruits are edible, aromatic, and healthy because they contain a number of vitamins and polyphenol antioxidants, cited previously (95). Therefore, do not discard the peel when eating lemon or lime. Lemon and lime strengthen immunity, protect from common diseases like cold and flu, aid weight loss, regulate blood pressure, improve digestion, and brighten skin tone. Their flesh, skin, and juice are often used to prepare drink, sauce, and plate (soup) due to their aroma and flavor. They are not consumed as dessert because of their strong acid savor.

2.2.6 Prunus Fruits: Peach, Nectarine, Apricot, Plum, Cherry

The genus *Prunus* belongs to the *Rosaceae* family and consists of about 430 species of deciduous or evergreen trees and shrubs naturally widespread throughout temperate regions of the Northern hemisphere (96–97). Main prunus fruits include peaches, nectarines, apricots, plums, and cherries. The fruit of these species is botanically defined as a drupe. The main bioactive compounds in prunus fruits are: carotenoids, vitamin C, vitamin E, phenolic compounds (phenolic acids, flavonoids, anthocyanins, pro-anthocyanidins or condensed tannins and tannins), terpenoids, and steroids (96–97). However, unlike citrus fruits, prunus fruits are not particularly rich in vitamin C (96). Due to the presence of many bioactive compounds cited above, prunus fruits have strong antioxidant, anti-inflammatory, and anti-cancer activities.

2.2.6.1   Peaches and Nectarines

Peaches and nectarines differ primarily in that nectarines have a smooth skin whereas peaches possess a downy skin, but both may be freestone (98). Peach (*Prunus persica*) and nectarine (*P. persica* var. *nectarina* or var. *nucipersica*) are native to northwest China. Peach and nectarine have an important place in human nutrition, and can be used as fresh, dried, or processed fruit. Peach and nectarine are good sources of antioxidants due to high levels of carotenoids (provitamin A), vitamin C, and phenolic compounds (98). They are also rich in dietary fibers and volatile compounds. More than one hundred volatile compounds have been identified. The most abundant volatile compounds are linalool, benzaldehyde, ester terpinoids, nor-isoprenoids, ketones, and lactones (98). Peach oil is an excellent moisturizer for skin. Peach and nectarine have many anti-disease properties such as anticancer, anti-allergic, antibacterial, anti-inflammatory, and so on (98). They are also a natural diuretic and a good immunomodulator.

2.2.6.2   Plum and Prune

Plum fruits (*Prunus domestica*) are consumed fresh or dried and used for desserts and processing. Fresh plum fruits are quite similar to peaches and nectarines with their similar carbohydrate, organic acid, calorie and cellulose contents, and they all qualify as energy fruit foods (99). Plums are rich in antioxidant substances including high contents of phenolic compounds, with the predominance of derivatives of caffeic acid, mainly neochlorogenic and chlorogenic acids, and smaller amounts of anthocyanins and flavonols (100). Fresh plums and processed plums like jams may improve glucose and lipid metabolism, reduce bile acid levels, and inhibit osteoporosis (99, 100).

Prunes are dried plums. After harvest, prune-making plums are dehydrated in hot air at 85 to 90°C for 18 h, then further processed into prune juice, puree, or other prune products. Most dried prunes are produced from the plum cultivar Agen, which originated in France and California. Dried prunes contain about 6.1 g of dietary fiber per 100 g, while prune juice is devoid of fiber due to filtration before bottling (101). The laxative action of both prune and prune juice could be explained by their high sorbitol content (14.7 and 6.1 g/100 g, respectively). Three to six dried prunes a day may prevent constipation. Prunes are a good source of energy in the form of simple sugars, but do not cause diabetes because of high fiber, fructose, and sorbitol content. Prunes contain large amounts of phenolic compounds (184 mg/100 g), mainly as neochlorogenic and chlorogenic acids, which may aid in laxative action and delay glucose absorption (101). Phenolic compounds in prunes have been found to inhibit human LDL (bad cholesterol) oxidation *in vitro*, and thus might serve as preventive agents against heart disease and cancer. Additionally, the high potassium content of prunes (745 mg/100 g) might be beneficial for cardiovascular health. Dried prunes are an important source of vitamin K and boron. Boron, a metalloid, is postulated to play a role in the prevention of osteoporosis (101).

2.2.6.3   Apricot

Apricot (*Prunus armeniaca*) is a drupe, like peach, plum, and cherry, in which the outer fleshy part (exocarp and mesocarp) surrounds a hard stone (endocarp) with a seed inside. Its color ranges between orange to orange-red, and some cultivars are cream white to greenish-white (102). Apricot is rich in sugars (more than 60%), proteins (8%), crude fiber (11.50%), crude fat (2%), total minerals (4%), vitamins (vitamin A, C, K and B complex), and reasonable quantities of organic acids (citric acid and malic acid), on a dry weight basis (102). In addition, there are appreciable amounts of total phenolic compounds and flavonoids in the fruit which make them more valuable as a functional food. The fruit is reported to contain polysaccharides, polyphenol, fatty acid, sterol derivatives, carotenoids, cynogenic glycosides, and volatile components (102). In very small amounts, the hydrogen cyanide present in apricot kernels has been traditionally prescribed in traditional Chinese medicine for treating asthma, cough, and constipation (102). Apricot is reported to have some pharmacological activities; it may be effective against chronic gastritis, oxidative intestinal damage, hepatic steatosis, atherosclerosis, coronary heart disease, and tumor formation. The oil of apricot was also used in England during the seventeenth century to treat ulcers and tumors (102).

2.2.6.4 Cherry

There are two main species of cherry fruit: sweet cherry (*Prunus avium*) and sour cherry or tart cherry (*Prunus cerasus*), both belonging to the genus Prunus of the Rosaceae family. The sour cherry varieties are divided in three main groups, depending on tree habit and fruit characteristics: Kentish cherries, morellos, and marasca (103). The cherry fruit is a nutrient dense food with relatively low caloric content and significant amounts of important nutrients and bioactive food components including fiber, polyphenols, carotenoids, vitamin C, and potassium. In addition, cherries are also a good source of tryptophan, serotonin, and melatonin (104). The majority of sweet cherries are consumed fresh with the remaining 20–25% processed as brined, canned, frozen, dried, or juiced. In contrast, 97% of sour cherries are processed primarily for cooking and baking (104). Both sweet and sour cherries contain several antioxidants and polyphenols that possess many biological activities, such as antioxidant, anticancer, and antiinflammation properties (103–104). Sour cherries commonly used in pie and jam, have more vitamin C and polyphenols than sweet cherries do, but much of it is lost when they are heated. The higher levels of total phenolics in sour cherries have been attributed to higher concentrations of anthocyanins and hydroxycinnamic acids (103). However, fresh sweet cherries are preferred over sour cherries. Red cherries are healthier than rose ones because red cherries contain more anthocyanins than rose ones. Results from published animal and human studies suggest that consumption of cherries may reduce the risk of several chronic inflammatory diseases including, arthritis, cardiovascular disease, diabetes, and cancer. Furthermore, cherry consumption may improve sleep, cognitive function, and recovery from pain after strenuous exercise (104).

2.2.7 Pear

Pears come from genus *Pyrus* belonging to the Rosaceae family, and are often called pome fruits. There are several thousand varieties of pears in the world, but only about 100 varieties are grown commercially (105).

Pears contain phytochemicals, especially antioxidants and provide between 27 and 41 mg of phenolics per 100 g (105). Pears are also a source of vitamin C and potassium. Animal studies with pears suggest that pears may regulate alcohol metabolism, protect against ulcers, and lower plasma lipids (105). Pears are high in fructose, sorbitol, and dietary fiber; this may explain their laxative properties. Many recent studies reported that fresh mature pears consumed alone or in combination with prunes can be used to treat constipation and to prevent colon cancer in humans (105). Pears have been used as a traditional folk remedy in China for more than 2,000 years because of their reported anti-inflammatory, diuretic, and antihyperglycemic activities. Other traditional uses of pears include usage as remedies for alcohol hangovers, to relieve cough, and constipation (105).

2.2.8 Avocado

Avocado is the fruit of the avocado tree, called *Persea Americana*, family Lauraceae. It is native to Mexico and Central America and is now cultivated in tropical and subtropical climates (Mediterranean area, Central America, South Asia). There are many varieties of avocado; among them, the Hass cultivar is the most commercially popular avocado worldwide (106). The fruits are egg-shaped or spherical and have a dark green skin and a fleshy and creamy body. One-half an avocado (68 g), is a nutrient and phytochemical dense food consisting of the following: dietary fiber

(4.6 g), total sugar (0.2 g), potassium (345 mg), sodium (5.5 mg), magnesium (19.5 mg), vitamin A (5.0 μg RAE), vitamin C (6.0 mg), vitamin E (1.3 mg), vitamin K_1 (14 μg), folate (60 mg), vitamin B-6 (0.2 mg), niacin (1.3 mg), pantothenic acid (1.0 mg), riboflavin (0.1 mg), choline (10 mg), lutein/ zeaxanthin (185 μg), cryptoxanthin (18.5 μg), phytosterols (57 mg), and high-monounsaturated fatty acids (6.7 g), and 114 kcals or 1.7 kcal/g, all of which may support a wide range of potential health effects (106). Avocado oil consists of 71% monounsaturated fatty acids, 13% polyunsaturated fatty acids, and 16% saturated fatty acids, which help to promote healthy blood lipid profiles and enhance the bioavailability of fat-soluble vitamins and phytochemicals from the avocado or other fruits and vegetables, naturally low in fat, which are consumed with avocados (106). Avocado consumption protects the cardiovascular system and eyes, promotes digestion, prevents oxidative stress, slows down age-related degenerative diseases, helps weight management, and supports healthy aging.

2.2.9   Pineapple

Pineapple is a multiple fruit built-up of coalesced berries from the tropical plant *Ananas comosus* belonging to the family of *Bromeliaceae*. Pineapple is grown in several tropical and subtropical countries including Philippines, Vietnam, Thailand, Indonesia, Malaysia, Kenya, India, and China (107). Pineapple is a rich source of dietary fiber along with vitamin B1, B6, B9 (folate), vitamin C and minerals like manganese and copper. Pineapple fruit contains a natural proteolytic enzyme called bromelain that digests food by breaking down protein (107). Bromelain is obtained commercially from the fruit or stem of pineapple. Fruit bromelain and stem bromelain are prepared differently and they contain different enzymatic composition. 'Bromelain' refers usually to the 'stem bromelain'. Bromelain is a mixture of different thiol endopeptidases and other components like phosphatase, glucosidase, peroxidase, cellulase, escharase, and several protease inhibitors (107). In vitro and in vivo studies demonstrate that bromelain exhibits various fibrinolytic, antiedematous, antithrombotic, and anti-inflammatory activities (107). Bromelain is absorbable in the body without losing its proteolytic activity and without producing any major side effects. Bromelain accounts for many therapeutic benefits like the treatment of angina pectoris, bronchitis, sinusitis, surgical trauma, and thrombophlebitis, debridement of wounds, and enhanced absorption of drugs, particularly antibiotics. It also relieves osteoarthritis, diarrhea, and various cardiovascular disorders such as hypertension. Bromelain also possesses some anti-cancerous activities and promotes apoptotic cell death for cancer prevention (107). It may increase the absorption and the anti-inflammatory effects of curcumin in turmeric. However, pineapple may cause uterine bleeding during pregnancy if eaten in excess. Only pineapple flesh is edible, while the skin, 'eyes', crown, and base of the fruit must be discarded. It is eaten raw or prepared as juice or salad.

2.2.10   Date

Dates are the fruits of the palm tree called *Phoenix Dactylifera* (Arecaceae) and have origin in Middle East.

Dates are high in energy, sugar, protein, dietary fiber, minerals (calcium, sulfur, phosphorous, potassium, copper, manganese, iron, selenium and magnesium), and some vitamins such as vitamin B5 (pantothenic acid) and B6 (pyridoxine) (108). A high percentage of sugar in the date fruit provides a good source of rapid energy. In addition, date fruit contains significant amounts of flavonoid glycosides including quercetin, apigenin, p-coumaric acid, ferulic acid, and sinapic acids (108). High-fiber diets are associated with the prevention and treatment of some diseases such as constipation, diabetes, coronary heart disease, hypercholesterolemia, diverticular disease, and colon cancer (108). Some of the most profound benefits of consuming dates is that they prevent constipation, control diarrhea, and are useful for curing many gastrointestinal disorders. Rich in iron, dates prevent anemia. The minerals found in dates make them the best food to avoid bone diseases such as osteoporosis (108). Allergic reactions and seasonal allergies reduce by half when dates are consumed. Moreover, dates may help with sex development. The fruit is eaten fresh or dried, as well as prepared as pudding, syrup and other desserts.

2.2.11 Melon (Cantaloupe)

Also known as muskmelon or honeydew, cantaloupe (*Cucumis melo*) in the Cucurbitacea family is a very fragrant and sweet fruit. Its flesh is orange, flavored, and sweet. It is eaten fresh after peeling or used to prepare dessert and salad. It is well-recognized for culinary and medicinal purposes (109).

Cantaloupe is an excellent source of vitamin A, vitamin C, and microelements such as potassium and magnesium (109). In recent years, it has been shown to possess useful medicinal properties such as analgesic, anti-inflammatory, antioxidant, antiulcer, anticancer, antimicrobial, diuretic, and antidiabetic properties (109). Furthermore, it has shown a hepato-protective effect, activity against hypothyroidism, and immune-modulator action (109). Melon protects health of the eyes and rejuvenates skin.

2.2.12 Watermelon

Watermelon (*Citrullus lanatus*) is a tropical fruit in the Cucurbitacea family (110). It is very rich in water (92%) and soluble sugar fruit. It is a very safe fruit for children and adults and is often eaten fresh after peeling. Citrullus lanatus (watermelon) is known to contain bioactive compounds such as citrulline, vitamins, minerals, lycopene, cucurbitacin, triterpenes, sterols, and alkaloids (110). Only lycopene and vitamin C are high in quantity. Lycopene, a strong antioxidant, gives the red color of its flesh when the fruit is ripe and has anti-cancer activity, especially for the prostate gland. Citrulline is an amino acid first isolated from *Citrullus lanatus* in 1930, hence its name. It is a non-essential amino acid for humans. Traditionally, *Citrullus lanatus* had been reportedly used as purgative and emetic in high doses. It is also a vermifuge, demulcent, diuretic, and tonic (110). The seed is used in the treatment of urinary tract infections, renal stones, hypertension, diabetic, diarrhea, and gonorrhea (110). Watermelon is both a refreshing fruit and a medicinal agent.

2.2.13 Kiwi

There are two main varieties of kiwifruit or kiwi fruit: *Actinidia deliciosa* or green kiwifruit and *Actinidia chinensis* or gold kiwifruit, both belonging to the Actinidiacea family. Kiwifruit is native to northern China, India, and Siberia. The green cultivar is an oval-shaped berry with a dull brown hairy skin and a bright translucent green flesh interspersed with several rows of small black seeds; while the gold variety has a bright yellow flesh surrounded by a smooth, hairless, bronze-colored skin. The flesh of the green kiwi is described as a tangy, sweet, and sour combination providing a unique flavor combination, whereas the gold cultivar is described as having a sweet and tropical taste (111).

Kiwifruits are exceptionally high in vitamin C and contain an array of other nutrients, notably dietary fibers, potassium, magnesium, vitamin E, and folate, as well as various antioxidants, phytonutrients, and enzymes, that act to provide functional and metabolic benefits. Of particular interest are the digestive benefits for healthy individuals as well as for those with constipation and other gastrointestinal disorders, including symptoms of irritable bowel syndrome. The mechanisms of action behind the gastrointestinal effects, such as changes in fecal (stool) consistency, decrease in transit time, and reduction of abdominal discomfort, relate to the water retention capacity of kiwifruit fiber, favorable changes in the human colonic microbial community and primary metabolites, as well as the naturally present proteolytic enzyme actinidin, which aids protein digestion both in the stomach and the small intestine (111). Moreover, kiwifruit alleviates symptoms of asthma, controls diabetes, lowers blood triglyceride levels, maintains cardiovascular health, and prevents macular degeneration. Kiwi skin is also rich in vitamins and antioxidants. Most people remove the fuzzy skin, but kiwis can be eaten whole with the skin after carefully scrubbing the skin with water. Kiwi is eaten fresh or prepared as juice or dessert.

2.2.14 Persimmon

Persimmon (*Diospyros kaki*) belongs to the Ebenaceae family. It is widespread in China, Japan, and Korea, where it is traditionally used for medicinal purposes. The whole fruit is edible, with the exemption of its seed and calyx. The color of the fruit varies from yellow or orange to deep

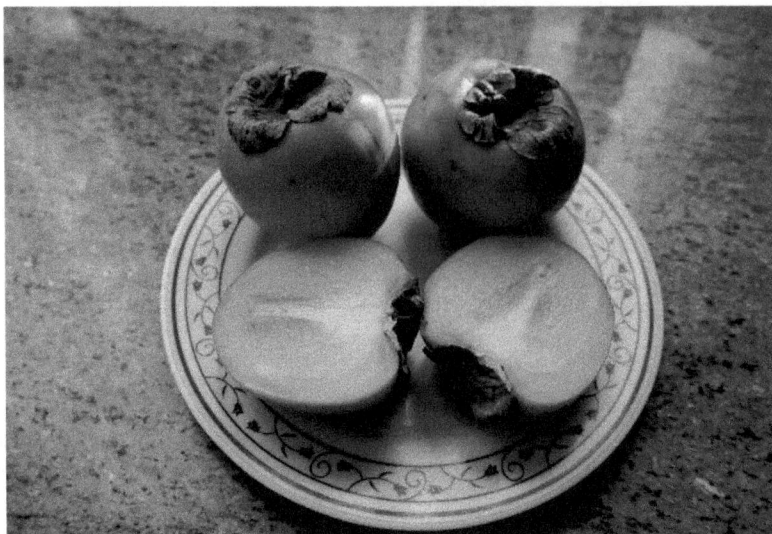

FIGURE 5.1 Persimmon.

red (Figure 5.1), (112). Persimmon fruits are usually classified into astringent and non-astringent varieties depending upon their taste. Persimmon is rich in carbohydrate (sugar), dietary fiber and is low in fats. It is also high in manganese and vitamins A, B6, and C. Persimmon contains many bioactive phenolic compounds such as ferulic acid, p-coumaric acid, gallic acid, β-cryptoxanthin, lycopene, β-carotene, zeaxanthin, and lutein, which are important antioxidants with high therapeutic potential (112). They prevent oxidation of low-density lipoproteins, safeguard beta cells of the pancreas, and reduce cardiovascular diseases, cancer, diabetes mellitus, and damage caused by chronic alcohol consumption (112). Persimmon might promote weight loss, protect eyes, improve digestion, lower hypertension, delay aging, and boost immune function. Persimmons are flavored, eaten fresh with peel or dried and used in traditional Chinese medicine. However, some vitamins and antioxidants in dried persimmons can be lost after drying and storage.

2.2.15 Jujube Fruit

Jujube or Chinese date is the fruit of *Ziziphus jujube* belonging to the Rhamnaceous family. It grows mostly in Europe, southern and eastern Asia, especially the inland region of northern China, and Australia. Jujube fruit is consumed all around the world because of its health benefits, as both food and herbal medicine (113–114). Its main biologically active components include vitamin C, phenolics, flavonoids, triterpenic acids, cyclic adenosine monophosphate (cAMP), jujuboside, and polysaccharides. Recent phytochemical studies of jujube fruits have shed some light on their biological effects, such as the antioxidant, anticancer, anti-inflammatory, anti-obesity, immunostimulating, hepatoprotective, and gastrointestinal protective activities (113). Jujube also possesses neuroprotective activities, including protecting neuronal cells against neurotoxin stress, stimulating neuronal differentiation, increasing expression of neurotrophic factors, and promoting memory and learning (114). In herbal medicine, one of the main functions of jujube is to calm the mind and to improve quality of sleep (114). More clinical studies of jujube fruits will be necessary for future therapeutic applications.

2.2.16   Mango

Mango (*Mangifera indica*), family Anacardiaceae, is a tropical fruit with a distinctive phytochemical and nutritional composition. The plant is native to India and Southeast Asia and is now cultivated in Central America, Africa, Australia, and the Mediterranean area (Spain, Israel, Sicily). Mango is a supremely tasty fruit. Its flesh is flavored, sweet, and yellow, when it is well ripened. Mango fruit has a large stone and is often eaten fresh without peel or is processed for chutney, pickles, curries, dried products, puree, nectar, and canned or frozen slices that are popular worldwide (115).

Mango is high in sugar, dietary fiber, vitamins: A, E, B6, B9 (folate), and C, and is an important source of potassium, but other minerals are in moderate levels. Mango is also rich in antioxidants, lutein, and zeaxanthin, which may improve eye health. It lowers cholesterol, improves digestion if taken in moderation, and boosts immunity. Furthermore, an extract of mango mesocarp has been reported to exert antitumor activity in a human colon adenocarcinoma cell line, as well as in a rodent model of colorectal cancer (115). Many studies provided evidence that many of the anti-scavenging properties of mango can be ascribed to mangiferin. Mangiferin is a plant natural polyphenol of xanthone structure that has antioxidant and anti-inflammatory effects (115). More research is needed to discover the therapeutic properties of this fruit which have not yet been elucidated.

2.2.17   Mangosteen

Mangosteen (*Garcinia mangostana*) belonging to the Clusiaceae or Guttiferae family, is a tropical tree originated in Southeast Asia. Mangosteen fruit is round, six to eight cm (2.4–3.1 in) in outside diameter. The thick peel or rind (pericarp or exocarp) of mangosteen fruit when ripe is dark brown or violet and inedible. Inside is the endocarp which has an edible white juicy pulp with a slightly acidic and sweet flavor (Figure 5.2) (116–118). Mangosteen is a healthy fruit, which is rich in energy, protein, and carbohydrates. Its flesh is white, soft, delicious, and rich in antioxidants, vitamins, minerals, and fibers, but low in calories. The pericarp of this fruit contains several families of bioactive compounds such as xanthones, flavonoids, triterpenoids, and benzophenones (116–118). Xanthone is a family of tricyclic isoprenylated polyphenols. At least 68 derivatives of xanthones have been identified in different parts of the *G. mangostana* plant with 50 being present in the fruit's pericarp at higher concentrations than in the aril or edible portion of the fruit. The majority of xanthone derivatives are α- and γ-mangostin which are natural phenolic compounds and strong antioxidants (116–118).

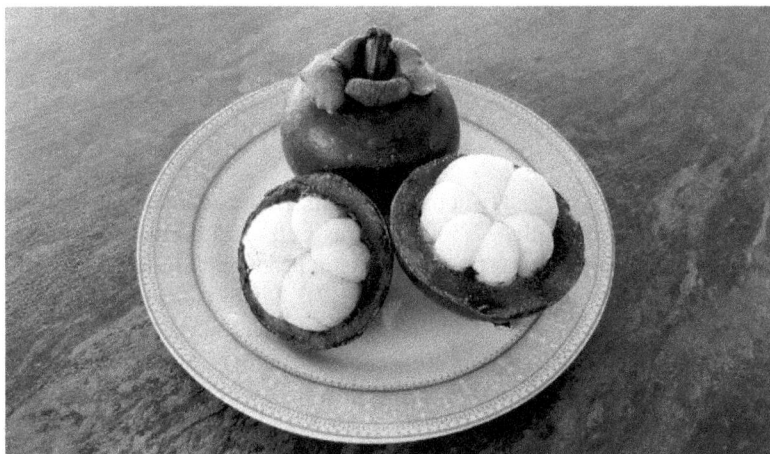

FIGURE 5.2 Mangosteen.

The pericarp has been used in traditional medicine in Southeast Asia for centuries to treat infection, wounds, inflammation, dysentery, and diarrhea (116–118). Nowadays, mangosteen extract is known to possess important anti-inflammatory and anti-tumor properties through different in vitro and in vivo studies. By far, the most studied xanthone is α-mangostin (α-MG) for which antioxidant, anti-proliferative, pro-apoptotic, anti-inflammatory, anti-carcinogenic, and anti-microbial activities have been reported (116). Despite the numerous *in vitro* and *in vivo* studies on the bioactivities of mangosteen xanthones, more research is needed to evaluate their safety and health benefits before they can be recommended for preventive or therapeutic purposes. There is insufficient scientific evidence at this time to support the use of mangosteen containing supplements as enhancers of health and useful adjuvants for treatment of various pathophysiological illnesses (116). More research is needed about this promising fruit.

2.2.18 Papaya

Papaya (*Carica papaya*) is the sole species in the genus Carica of the family Caricaceae. It is native to southern Mexico and Central America. It is a renowned nutritious and medicinal plant. Each part of the papaya – fruit, root, stem, flower, seed, rinds, and latex – has its own nutraceutical properties. It serves as food as well as ethnomedicine to prevent and treat a wide range of diseases and disorders (119). Papaya fruit is low in fat, but high in carbohydrate and fiber. The ripe fruit has orange flesh and is rich in vitamin A, vitamin C, folate, and magnesium. Orange papaya fruit contains carotenoids (zeaxanthin, beta-carotene) and a variety of polyphenol antioxidants, while green papaya fruit (unripe fruit) is rich in papain, a protease used for protein digestion. Papaya has also been traditionally used as appetite enhancer, purgative, vermifuge, abortifacient, medicine for acne, and meat tenderizer (119). Over decades, a series of scientific attempts were made to authenticate the nutraceutical properties of papaya. Recent scientific studies validated that papaya has anti-plasmodial, antitrichomonal, anti-dengue, and anti-cancer activities, and also possesses antiseptic, antiparasitic, anti-inflammatory, antidiabetic, and contraceptive features. Moreover, it helps in the management of sickle-cell anemia, HIV, heart diseases and digestive disorders (119). Recently, some researchers found that papain extracted from Carica papaya leaves exhibited anti-tumor activity and immunomodulatory effects in different tumor cell lines and human peripheral blood mononuclear cells (120). However, papaya powder can cause allergy to some people because it contains enzymes called papain and chymopapain that can induce allergy (119). In addition, the ingestion of unripe and semi-ripe papaya could be unsafe during pregnancy because it induces miscarriage in susceptible pregnant women (119). In these cases, papaya consumption must be avoided because crude papaya latex contains papain and chymopapain which are strong inducers of uterine contraction (119).

Further pharmacological and clinical research on different parts of papaya plant is necessary to confirm some preliminary results previously cited and to explain their mode of actions.

2.2.19   Litchi (Leechee)

Litchi or leechee (*Litchi chinensis*) is a fruit tree belonging to the Sapindaceae family. It was originally cultivated in China for more than 2,300 years, as well as in northern Vietnam (121). Litchi fruits, which are similar in volume to a strawberry, are in pendulous clusters, roundish, green, and, once mature, become pinkish or reddish (Figure 5.3) (121). Litchi fruits have a thin, stiff skin that peels off easily to show a pearly white jelly pulp with excellent flavor due to the combination of acids and sugars. Litchi is a tasty fruit used for food consumption and nutritional benefits in various parts of the world. Due to its biological activities, the fruit is becoming increasingly known and deserves attention not only for its edible part, the pulp, but also for its peel and seed that contain beneficial substances with antioxidant, cancer preventive, antimicrobial, and anti-inflammatory functions (121). Although literature demonstrates the biological activity of Litchi components in reducing tumor cell viability in *in vitro* or *in vivo* models, data about the biochemical mechanisms responsible for these effects are quite fragmentary (121).

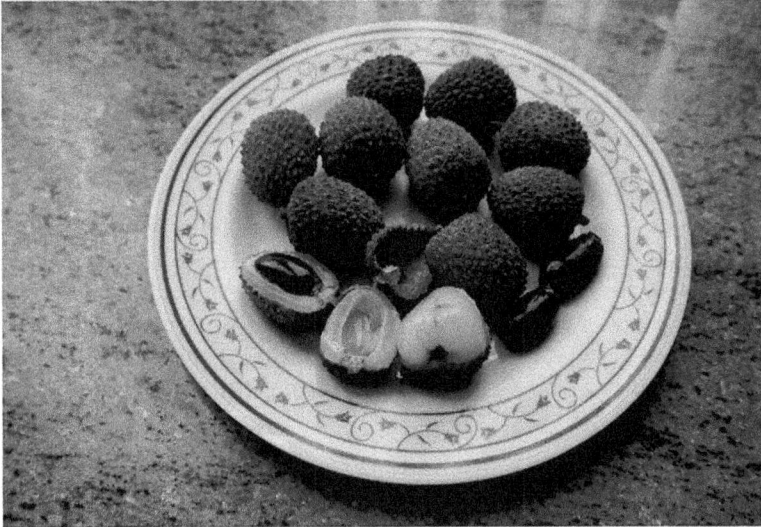

FIGURE 5.3 Litchi (Leechee).

2.2.20 Olive Fruit

The olive tree (*Olea europaea*, family Oleaceae) is native to the Mediterranean region, tropical and central Asia, and various parts of Africa. It is widely cultivated for its fruit and oil (122). There are three kinds of olive fruits: green olive, black olive, and brown semi-ripe olive. Raw or fresh olives are bitter and rarely consumed. They are often prepared by fermentation in order to remove the bitter taste caused by a phenolic compounds present in the raw fruit. Fermented olive fruits are called table olives and become flavored and tasty. However, they are rich in salt, which is not good for people with high arterial blood pressure. In contrast, pure olive oil extracted from fresh fruit is good for health.

The major components of olive fruit and oil consist of oleic acid (monounsaturated omega-9 fatty acid). Minor components include α-tocopherol (vitamin E), linoleic acid, phenolic antioxidants (flavonols, flavonones, anthocyanins), squalene, and sterols (122). Both major and minor components have strong antioxidant activity and are beneficial to human health. Many studies have proven its protector potential through oil, whole fruit and leaf extract in cardiovascular disorders, cancer, degenerative diseases, viral and microbial infections (122). Regular olive consumption may decrease bad cholesterol levels, aid weight loss, delay degenerative diseases, and improve fertility in women (122).

2.2.21 Coconut

Coconut is a fruit of the *Cocos nucifera* tree (family Palmaceae or Arecaceae), mainly found in Southeast Asia and Pacific islands. It is used as food for inhabitants in these areas. The coconut fruit comprises an outer epicarp, a mesocarp, and an inner endocarp. The epicarp, which is the outer skin of the fruit, and the mesocarp, which is heavy, fibrous, and tanned when dry, have many industrial uses. The endocarp is the dark and hard core. Inside is an edible white kernel (meat) which is a solid white albumen of varied thickness, depending on the age of the fruit, and with an oily pulp consistency and a liquid albumen called coconut water that is thick, sweet, and slightly acidic (123).

Fresh coconut fruits contain some amount of sweet water inside the central hollow cavity. Coconut flesh and water are edible, sweet, tasty, and rich in nutrients. Coconut water and coconut kernels contain microminerals and nutrients which are essential to human health, and hence coconut is used as food by many peoples across the globe, mainly in the tropical countries (124). White kernel is rich in saturated fats mainly constituted of lauric acid, which supports blood vessels by increasing good HDL cholesterol, contrary to other saturated fatty acids found in animal fats (123). The kernel is also an excellent source of minerals such as copper, iron, manganese, magnesium, calcium, zinc, and B-complex vitamins. It is also rich in proteins which make it a good source of energy.

Coconut water is rich in simple sugar, cytokinin, and enzymes (catalase, phosphatase, peroxidase, dehydrogenase) which aid digestion (123). Coconut water and coconut kernel might have numerous medicinal properties such as antibacterial, antifungal, antiparasitic, anti-dermatophytic, antiviral, anti-helminthic, antidiarrheal, hypoglycemic, hepatoprotective, immunostimulant, antiarthritic, analgesic, antipyretic, and antioxidant activities (123–124). In addition, other properties such as vasodilation, anti-hypertensive, cardioprotective, hepatoprotective, nephroprotective, anti-inflammatory, antiseizure, and anti-osteoporosis effects have also been also reported (123–124). Coconut oil extracted from the dry kernel is an excellent emollient agent for hair nourishment and is used in cooking. Some people are allergic to kernel and coconut oil. Food containing coconut as an ingredient must mention it in its label.

2.2.22 Sea Buckthorn

Sea buckthorn (Hippophae rhamnoides), belonging to the family Elaeagnaceae, has recently gained world-wide attention, mainly for its medicinal and for the nutritional properties of its super fruits and leaves. Sea buckthorn (SBT) is a wild deciduous shrub of cold arid regions from Europe to Central Asia (125–127). It is now domesticated in several parts of the world due to its nutritional and medicinal potential.

Its super fruits (berries) are orange-yellow to red color. They are a rich source of all nutrients, vitamins, and antioxidants such as multiple vitamins (C, B6, E, and K), carotenoids (carotenes, lycopene, lutein and zeaxanthin), flavonoids (isorhamnetin, quercetin, isorhamnetin-3-beta d-glucoside; isorhamnetin-3-beta-d-glucosaminide; kaempferol, etc.) organic acids, amino acids, micro and macronutrients (125). The berries are also rich in fatty acids (saturated 13.7% and 86.3% unsaturated) including palmitic acid, oleic acid (omega-9), palmitoleic acid (omega-7), linoleic acid (omega-6), and linolenic acid (omega-3); and phytosterols (125). Since ancient times, sea buckthorn has been used extensively in oriental traditional medicine for treatment of asthma, skin diseases, gastric ulcers, and lung disorders (125–126). Nowadays, sea buckthorn has emerged as an important plant, which has been investigated for numerous biochemical and pharmacological studies and shown to be beneficial in a number of therapeutic areas. Various pharmacological activities such as cytoprotective, anti-tumor, immunomodulatory, hepatoprotective, anti-stress, anti-atherogenic, anti-microbial, radioprotective, and tissue regeneration have been reported. Recently, various *in vitro* studies have demonstrated that sea buckthorn has anticancer activity (127). It was found that sea buckthorn berry juice, like blackberry and black chokeberry juices, has anti-proliferative properties (127). Several clinical trials have demonstrated the therapeutic potential of sea buckthorn for the treatment of many diseases including cardiovascular diseases, inflammation, diabetes, platelet inhibition, and more (125–127). More clinical research is needed to evaluate the safety and health benefits of sea buckthorn, especially its fruit, for preventive or therapeutic purposes.

The list of fruits cited herein is not exhaustive; there are still some hundreds of different edible fruits in the world. In general, it is better to eat fresh and ripe fruits than canned and dried fruits because vitamins and antioxidants can be lost with time and heat. Moreover, canned and dried fruits contain preservatives. Remember that the darker the color of a fruit the more nutrients it contains.

Be careful with some fruits which can cause allergy in certain hypersensitive people or incompatibility with some drugs or diseases. It is better to eat organic fruits, mostly fruits with thin peel like strawberry, blackberry, grapes, etc. In addition, it is preferable to consume local fruits rather imported fruits because many antioxidants can be destroyed with time.

2.3 Vegetables

Vegetables are certain parts of plants such as leaves, stems, flowers, tubers, and beans. They are eaten raw or cooked. As fruits, they contain a large range of vitamins, minerals, antioxidants, and other phytochemicals necessary to human health. Different parts of plants used as vegetables are:

- Leaves: cabbage, kale, celery, lettuce, spinach, Brussels sprouts, endive, watercress, pepper elder, gai lan (Chinese kale), parsley, mint, water spinach, etc.
- Fruits: tomato, cucumber, eggplant, calabash, wax gourd, gac (*Momordica cochinchinensis*), etc.
- Beans, seeds, or nuts: kidney beans, green beans, butter beans, soybeans, mung beans, peas, sesame, chia seed, sunflower seed, chestnut, peanut, walnut, cashew nut, chestnut, pistachio, almond, macadamia, etc.
- Roots or tubers: carrot, onion, garlic, leek, shallot, radish, turnip, etc.
- Sprouts, shoots, or stems: asparagus, bamboo shoots, bok choy, etc.
- Flowers: broccoli, cauliflower, etc.

Some vegetables rich in good nutrients and healthy properties are described below.

2.3.1 Cabbage, Kale

Cabbage and kale are two closely cruciferous vegetables and belong to the same species *Brassica oleracea* of the Brassicaceae or Cruciferae family (order Brassicales), but not the same variety. Cabbage belongs to the variety 'capitate', while kale belongs to 'acephala' (128). Cruciferous vegetables of this family include several important vegetable crops such as cabbage, kale, broccoli, radish, horseradish, rocket, watercress, cauliflower, Brussels sprouts, Kai Lan, Chinese cabbage, and more (128–129). Cabbage leaves form a head and have different colors (white, green, red, or purple); while the central leaves of kale do not form a head (128). Cabbage and kale are rich in glucosinolates (128–129). Glucosinolates are a group of sulfur- and nitrogen-containing glycosides found in the plant order Brassicales. They are considered the stronghold in the plant defense system as they can deter pest and pathogen attacks (128–129). Unlike most defense compounds of the plant, glucosinolates are not toxic per se (129). For human health, glucosinolates have been associated with many beneficial effects against cancer, diabetes, heart diseases, obesity, bacteria, and fungi, as well as antioxidant and antimutagenic properties (129). Cabbage and kale are also rich in fibers, vitamins, and minerals.

2.3.2 Broccoli

Broccoli (*Brassica oleracea* var. *italica*) belongs to the cruciferous family and is native to the Mediterranean region. It has large green flower heads with a big, edible stalk surrounded by leaves. Vitamin C is more abundant in broccoli than similar crucifers tested (Brussels sprout, cabbage, cauliflower) (129, 130). Broccoli is rich in β-caroten, lutein, zeaxanthin, folate, potassium, and sulforaphane (a glucosinolate), which has anti-cancer activity (130, 131). Broccoli is one of the top 20 healthiest foods in the world.

2.3.3 Cauliflower

Cauliflower, like broccoli and cabbage, belongs to the cruciferous (Brassicaceae) family of vegetables, which has been shown to be effective in fighting certain forms of cancer. Cauliflower is so closely related to broccoli that both are designated as the same variety of the cruciferous family, which not only share wonderful phytochemicals such as glucosinolates, but also contain the nutritive values of vitamin A, thiamine, riboflavin, niacin, vitamin C, calcium, iron, phosphorous, and fat to help fight diseases (132). Cauliflower has a wide variety of uses directly as a vegetable or as an ingredient in salads, soups, and condiment.

2.3.4 Watercress

Watercress (*Nasturtium officinale*), of the family Brassicaceae or Cruciferae, is an aquatic plant native to Europe and Central Asia. The leaves are dark green with 4–12 cm long. Watercress is rich in glucosinolates (sulforaphane), carotenoids, and polyphenols, as well as Vitamin C, Vitamin K, Vitamin A, lutein, zeaxanthin, α-tocopherol (vitamin E), and folic acid. It is a good source of iron, calcium, and iodine (133). It provides a reservoir of flavonoids, terpenoids, tannins, and many other glycosides. In traditional medicine, the leaves are used as diuretic, stomachic, depurative, expectorant, hypoglycemic, odontalgic, and stimulant (133). Consumption of watercress may lower arterial blood pressure and prevent diabetes. Rich in vitamin K, watercress can interfere with blood-thinners like warfarin when taken in excess. Recent scientific studies have reported that watercress might delay or impede some forms of cancer like breast, prostate, melanoma, esophageal, pancreatic cancers, because watercress is rich in glucosinolates (sulforaphane) (133).

The list of cruciferous vegetables is long. Some of the most widely consumed are: Brussels sprouts, Kai Lan (Chinese kale), Bok Choy (Chinese cabbage), radish, horseradish, rocket, and turnip. They are all rich in vitamins (C, K), phytochemicals (glucosinolates, antioxidants), and minerals (calcium, magnesium). They may prevent cancer, diabetes and heart diseases. Their regular consumption is good for the health.

2.3.5 Celery

Celery is also known as *Apium graveolens* and belongs to the Apiaceae family. Celery stems and leaves can be eaten raw or cooked, and lose very little of their nutrients when steamed. Celery contains many of the following phytonutrients: carbohydrates, flavonoids, steroids, alkaloids, glycosides, phenols, furocoumarins, volatile oils, and sesquiterpene alcohols (134–136). It is also a good source of fatty acids, vitamins like K, β-carotene, C, B9 (folic acid), and minerals such as potassium, magnesium, calcium, and sodium. Celery is also rich in chlorophyll, silica, and dietary fibers (134–136). Moreover, celery seeds contain several substances, including volatile essential oils, coumarins, and linoleic acid (an omega-6 fatty acid) (134–135).

In traditional medicine, celery has been used to treat spasm and stomach problems and as a diuretic, laxative, and sedative. It is also used to lower blood pressure and to treat inflammation (arthritis, gout), muscle spasms, and joint problems (134–136). Pharmacologically, celery leaves, stems and seeds exerted antioxidant, anti-inflammatory, gastrointestinal, cardiovascular, cytotoxic, antimicrobial, anti-helminthic, hypolipidemic, and central nervous effects. Celery may prevent hypercholesterolemia and some cancer forms (134–136). However, no official documents have yet recognized these therapeutic effects in humans. A few animal studies suggest that celery and its seed extract may help lower blood pressure and cholesterol, as well as reduce pain. Celery and its seed can cause a severe allergic reaction called anaphylaxis, which can be fatal for some people (136). Avoid celery and its seed for pregnant women and hypersensitive people. Take note that it can also interfere with some drugs (anticoagulants, thyroid medications, lithium, and sedatives).

2.3.6 Lettuce

Lettuce (*Lactuca sativa*) is a plant of the family Asteraceae. There are many cultivars of lettuce in the world. However, nutrient composition and bioactive compounds vary within lettuce types and cultivars. Crisp head lettuce, popularly consumed in the United States, is comparatively low in bioactive compounds. Romaine is a more nutritious lettuce, with folate and antioxidant contents comparable to other rich leafy vegetable sources (137–139). Batavia, also known as French crisp, Summer Crisp Lettuce or summer crisp, is a cultivar of lettuce in Europe. The large leaves of lettuce and Batavia are usually green, but sometimes red or purple depending on the variety. Red lettuce varieties are rich in bioactive compounds and antioxidants mainly due to higher total phenols and flavonoid compounds (139). The levels of phenolic antioxidants are higher in red lettuce than in green lettuce. Lettuce is low in calories and fat but high in chlorophyll and dietary fiber. Moreover, lettuce is high in potassium but low in sodium. Lettuce contains minerals (calcium, iron, magnesium, potassium, phosphorous, zinc), vitamins (B1, B2, B3 or niacin, B6, B9, C, A, E, and K) and antioxidants (137–139). Lettuce is often eaten raw or lightly cooked. In vitro and in vivo pharmacological studies of lettuce have shown anti-inflammatory, cholesterol lowering, and anti-diabetic activities (137–139). Briefly, lettuce is a good source of beneficial bioactive compounds. However, excessive consumption of lettuce can interfere with anticoagulant drugs like warfarin because it is rich in vitamin K.

2.3.7   Spinach

Spinach (*Spinacia oleracea*) is an edible plant in the family Amaranthaceae. Spinach leaves and stems can be eaten raw or cooked. Fresh spinach is rich in fibers and contains many nutrients and phytochemicals such as magnesium, iron, calcium, potassium, and a number of vitamins: A (from β-carotene), C, K, and folate (140–141). The major active components of spinach are carotenoids (β-carotene, lutein, zeaxanthin) and phenolic compounds (flavones, flavanols). Some epidemiological and laboratory studies have found that consuming spinach or spinach extracts may prevent some eye diseases like macular degeneration, and protect against cancer through various different mechanisms. Spinach is also used for ethnomedical therapy of obesity, inflammation of lungs, lumbago, flatulence, and treatment of urinary calculi (140).

2.3.8   Pepper Elder

Pepper elder (*Peperomia pellucida*) also called shining bush plant belongs to the family Piperaceae. It is used as a food item as well as a traditional medicinal herb in many countries from Asia to America. The entire plant is edible and can be eaten raw, cooked, or drunk as tea by infusion. Pepper elder has potential bactericide property for some pathogen germs and anti-fungal activity in some *in vitro* tests. Its analgesic and anti-inflammatory activities have been scientifically proven in rats and mice (142). In traditional medicine, pepper elder herbs and teas can treat gastrointestinal disorders including dysentery, diarrhea, stomachache; respiratory tract disorders including asthma, nasopharyngeal infections, cough; skin diseases including eczema, wounds, abscess, acne, boils, scabies, dermatitis; and other ailments such as arthritis, gout, headache, rheumatic pain, hypertension, and kidney disorders (142). Pepper elder contains various active chemicals including tannins, flavonoids (acacetin, apigenin, isovitexin, and pellucidatin), cardiac and xanthone glycosides, alkaloids (secolignans, tetrahydrofuranlignans, peperomins, isoswertisin, sesamin), saponins, inulins, terpenes, phenolic compounds, phytosterols (sitosterol, stigmasterol, and campesterol) and other steroids, as well as resins. Pepper elder also contains several essential oils, like dillapiole, β-caryophyllene, and carotol. Moreover, pepper elder might be considered a nontoxic plant (142). Much additional work is needed to confirm preliminary biomedical results of these compounds.

2.3.9   Tomato

Tomato vegetable is the red fruit of the plant *Solanum lycopersicum* belonging to the family Solanaceae. It is botanically a fruit and only considered a vegetable during culinary purposes, often causing confusion (143). Tomato is consumed raw, cooked in many dishes or processed industrially as sauce, juice, ketchup, paste, and so on (143–145). The major phytochemicals in tomato are the carotenoids consisting of 60–65% lycopene, and the rest of carotenes (α-carotene, β-carotene, γ-carotene), phytoene, and neurosporene (143). Lycopene is an antioxidant that is not destroyed by heat, contrary to other antioxidants and vitamins. In addition, tomato is rich in vitamin C, vitamins of group B, and minerals like potassium, magnesium, and calcium (143–144). Multiple studies have shown that lycopene from thermally processed tomato products (sauce, paste, juice, and ketchup) is more bioavailable than lycopene from fresh tomatoes (145). Greater than 90% of the lycopene found in processed tomato products is in the all-*trans* conformation (145). In vivo studies demonstrate that the *cis*-isomers of lycopene appear to be more bioavailable than the all-*trans* isomer (145). Antioxidant properties of lycopene may prevent atherogenesis and carcinogenesis by protecting DNA, lipids, low density lipoprotein (LDL), and proteins (143–145). Tomato and tomato products may also have anti-inflammatory, antithrombotic, and lipid-lowering effects (143–145). In brief, tomatoes in the diet may help protect against cancer, especially prostate and breast cancers, maintain healthy blood pressure, and prevent diabetes and eye diseases. Tomato fruits can contain high levels of pesticide residue. Therefore, wash tomatoes carefully before eating or cooking. The best way is to select organic tomatoes.

2.3.10 Pumpkin

Pumpkin belongs to the family *Cucurbitaceae*, genus *Cucurbita*. It is found in tropical and sub-tropical countries, with its three varieties being *Cucurbita maxima*, *Cucurbita moschata*, and *Cucurbita pepo* (146). Pumpkin fruit is composed of pulp and seeds. Pumpkin pulp contains polysaccharides, carotenoids, amino acids, active proteins, and minerals. Pumpkin fruit and seeds are high in lipids and proteins, and they are a good source of potassium, copper, manganese phosphorus, and magnesium (146). Pumpkins are rich in macro- and micronutrients and antioxidants that promote immunity against cancer and other diseases (146). Pumpkins are consumed in various ways, whether fresh, canned, frozen, or dried. Preservation of pumpkin by drying is an important way to prevent postharvest losses. Pumpkin fruit can be processed into flour which has a longer shelf-life, highly desirable sweet flavor, and deep yellow-orange color. Pumpkin flour contains high levels of carbohydrates, starch, dietary fiber, protein, and low levels of lipids and crude fiber, and is an ideal food for diabetes patients, cardiovascular disease patients, and the elderly (146). Many countries, such as India, China, Brazil, Argentina have been using different species of this fruit as a medicine. The various health benefits of pumpkin include antioxidant, anti-diabetic, anti-carcinogenic, and possible anti-fatigue effects (146). Pumpkin may protect eye health and lower blood cholesterol.

2.3.11 Gac Fruit (*Momordica Cochinchinensis*)

Gac fruit (*Momordica cochinchinensis*), of the Cucurbitaceae family – also known as Cochinchin gourd, baby jackfruit, and spiny bitter gourd – is a bright orange spikey fruit found in Southeast Asia – mostly in Vietnam, hence its name (147). The fruit is ovoid and usually large (10–13 cm). It is orangey-red when ripe, with spines on the outside, red fleshy pulp, and black flat seeds inside. Gac is often eaten cooked with other vegetables or rice and has a mild taste. Gac fruit is reputed to be an exceptional source of phytochemicals. Nutritionally, gac contains extraordinarily elevated levels of carotenoids (particularly β-Carotene, lycopene, and lutein), α-tocopherol, and essential fatty acids available in all parts of the fruit (i.e., peel, pulp, aril, and seeds). Both carotenoids (lycopene and β-Carotene) from gac fruit were found to be at least eight times higher than the carotenoids found in carrot root and tomato fruit (147). The concentrations of phenolics and flavonoids found in gac fruit were also high and found about 26.08 and 1.32 mg/100 g, respectively (147). Unsaturated fatty acids in gac fruit were found to be relatively high. Oleic, palmitic, and linoleic acids were found to be predominant in gac aril (32.3%, 29.2%, and 28.1% respectively), while the predominant fatty acid found in gac seed was stearic acid (60.5%) with small levels of linoleic (20.3%), oleic (9%), and palmitic acids (5.6%) (147). Additionally, gac oil after being extracted from the aril has also been traditionally used as a tonic and given to lactating or pregnant women. It is also given to children to treat xerophthalmia (dry eyes) and night-blindness. In Chinese medicine, the gac seed has been used to treat inflammation, swelling, scrofula, tinea, diarrhea, and skin infections such as sores, carbuncles, furuncles, and boils in humans and animals (147). The entire potentiality surrounding the health benefits of gac fruit is not well-known. Several parts of the gac fruit such as the skin, the outer rind, and the seeds, are toxic and inedible. Only the cooked red pulp is edible and very healthy. More research is needed for this promising plant.

2.3.12 Beans

Beans or Legumes are fruits or seeds of plants from the Fabaceae family or Leguminosae. Beans are eaten fresh or dried. A bean generally has many seeds. Bean is the term used to designate the seed belonging to the Fabaceae family. Dried beans or grain legumes can be stored long-term at room temperature and are often used to prepare pastry, dough, and sprouts. Most beans must be cooked to be safe to eat. Some common bean varieties include soybean, kidney bean, cannellini bean, Great Northern bean, navy bean, fava bean, cranberry bean, black bean, green bean, red bean, pinto bean, black-eyed pea, chickpea, and lentil (148–150). Beans are a good source of protein, carbohydrate, fiber, amino acids, B vitamins, and minerals (iron, copper, potassium, magnesium, manganese, zinc, phosphorous). Beans are important sources of protein in vegetarian diets. In particular, they are among the only plant foods that provide significant amounts of the indispensable amino acid lysine. They are naturally low in fat and are practically free of cholesterol and saturated fat. They also provide large amounts of polyphenols, many of which are potent antioxidants (148–150). An expanding body of research suggests that beans promote good health and reduce risk for, or improve outcomes of, various diseases such as cardiovascular disease, hypercholesterolemia, diabetes, constipation, cancer risk, obesity, and hypertension (148–150). However, for some people, beans can cause flatulence, stomach pain, or bloating (149–150). Some beans such as red kidney beans, fava beans, also contain several antinutrients, which are compounds that can interfere with the digestion and utilization of nutrients. These include protease inhibitors, lectins, phytates, and oxalates (150). However, high temperatures such as boiling can inactivate most lectins and protease inhibitors. Mineral absorption is adversely affected by both phytates and oxalates, although the latter affects only calcium. Phytate is an example of an antinutrient that may exert beneficial effects. It is an antioxidant that may reduce the risk of certain cancers and kidney stones (150). Except for some harmful beans, most cooked beans are highly nutritious and healthy.

2.3.12.1 Soy Bean or Soybean

Soy, Glicine max (L.), is a plant of Asian origin belonging to the Fabaceae family or Leguminosae. Soybean is a basic food ingredient of traditional Asian cuisine (China, Japan, Korea), used for thousands of years (151–152). Dry soybean contains 36% protein, 35% carbohydrate (17% of which dietary fiber), 19% oil, 5% minerals and several other components including vitamins (152). Soybean is an abundant source of protein. Contrary to other beans and vegetables, proteins in soybean are similar to those in animal meat, because they contain all nine essential amino acids, especially indispensable amino acid lysine. Therefore, soybean and soy foods are common nutritional solutions for vegetarians, due to their high protein content and versatility in the production of meat analogues and milk substitutes. High protein content, together with lower carbohydrate content, characterizes soy as a unique vegetable protein source compared to other beans (151–152). Some main byproducts of soybean are: soy milk, soy sauce, soy meat, tofu, natto, and tempeh. The soy components that have stimulated the most research interest are isoflavones, which are polyphenols with estrogenic properties highly contained in soybeans (151). Isoflavones belong to a functional class of non-steroidal phytochemicals called phytoestrogen that possess a chemical structure and functions similar to animal endogenous estrogens. The main isoflavones contained in soybeans are genistein, and daidzein. This phytoestrogen raises doubts about safe use, especially at high dose (151). Several studies have reported the ability of soybeans to lower cholesterol levels and to decrease the risk of osteoporosis and carcinogenesis in humans (151–152). However, there are some doubts about the potential effects of soybeans on health, such as its effectiveness in reducing risk of cardiovascular issues, or, conversely, its possible disruption of thyroid function and sexual hormones (151). More studies are needed to confirm some preliminary results about the therapeutic effects and the side effects of soybean in long-term use, especially for vegans and Asian people. Asians consume about 20–80 g daily of customary soy foods, while Western people consume only about one to three g daily soy foods (152). Moderate consumption of soybean and its byproducts (soy milk, soy meat, tofu, natto, tempeh) may contribute to the maintenance of good health.

2.3.13 Seeds

Seeds are small embryonic plants enclosed in a coat, the product of the ripened ovule of flowering plants after pollination and the completion of the reproduction process (153). Seeds are made of complex matrices in the outer layer and germ, and rich in minerals, oils, proteins, carbohydrates, vitamins, mono and polyunsaturated fatty acids, and antioxidants that protect the plant's DNA from oxidative stress, thus facilitating the perpetuation of the species. Some edible seeds are: flaxseed (linseed), sesame seed, chia seed, quinoa seed, pumpkin seed, sunflower seed, and hemp seed. Sunflower seed, rapeseed, and cottonseed are used commercially in the production of oils. However, some seeds, such as castor seed of the plant *Ricinus communis*, seed of the strychnine tree, and seeds of bitter almond, peach, and apricot, are toxic. Ricin, a water-soluble lectin present in castor seed, is highly toxic and can cause death if consumed (154). In contrast, castor oil extracted from castor seed is not toxic and can be used in food additives or in pharmacy as a laxative because ricin is not soluble in castor oil. Seed of the strychnine (*Strychnos nux-vomica*) tree can cause deadly convulsion. Seeds of bitter almond, apricot, and peach, containing amygdalin, may cause cyanide poisoning with high intake. Except for some particular cases cited above, most seeds frequently consumed such as flaxseed, sesame seed, chia seed, and quinoa seed, are good for health.

2.3.13.1 Flaxseed or Linseed

Flaxseed or linseed is seed of a flax plant or Lin plant of the genus Linus in the family Linaceae. Flaxseed is a rich source of fiber and omega-3 fatty acids, particularly alpha-linolenic acid (ALA), the precursor of active eicosapentaenoic acid (EPA) and docosahexaenoic acid (DHA) (, 155). It also contains linoleic acid (an omega-6 fatty acid), oleic acid (an omega-9 fatty acid), proteins, manganese, magnesium, and vitamin B1 in moderate levels. In addition, linseeds contain different polyphenol antioxidants, especially lignan, a type of phytoestrogen, which may help relieve menopausal symptoms such as hot flashes. These compounds provide health benefits to humans through their anti-inflammatory action, antioxidative capacity, and lipid modulating properties (155). However, the conversion of ALA into EPA and DHA is limited in the biological media, especially in seniors. Therefore, high consumption of flaxseed is not beneficial for the health of elderly people. The presence of phytoestrogens with adverse health effects and toxic compounds in flaxseed cannot be neglected (155). Flaxseed oil does not contain fibers. So, the health benefits related to flaxseed depend on the type of product. The effects of flaxseeds in the reduction of cholesterol levels and cardiovascular diseases are still controversial, mostly in the elderly.

2.3.13.2 Sesame Seed

Sesame seed is the seed of the plant *Sesamum indicum*, family Pedaliaceae. Similar to flaxseed, sesame seed is rich in oil, omega-3 alpha-linolenic acid, omega-6 fatty acids, vitamin E, fibers, phytic acid, proteins, and minerals. Sesame seeds and oil also contain a lot of lignans (non-flavonoid polyphenols), particularly sesamin and sesamolin, substances that may help lower blood cholesterol levels, and may have antihypertensive, immunoregulatory, anticarcinogenic, and anti-aging activities (156–157). Sesame seeds and oils might prevent some cardiac diseases and inflammation such as atherosclerosis and arthritis (156–157). However, sesame seed and oil can cause allergy, including anaphylaxis. Sesame seed and oil are used as ingredients in various cuisines in the world (Mexico, Eastern Asia, Middle Eastern, etc.).

2.3.13.3 Chia Seed

Chia (*Salvia hispanica*) is an annual herbaceous plant belonging to the family Lamiaceae. Chia fruits are round, and contain many tiny, oval seeds of two mm in length and one mm in width. Colors of chia seeds may vary from black and brown to off-white. Chia plants are grown particularly in Mexico and South America (158–159). Chia seeds are ascribed high nutritive value particularly thanks to their high contents of dietary fiber (23–41%) and fat (20–34%). Chia seeds are an excellent source of fat (20– 34%), particularly polyunsaturated fatty acids such as α-linolenic (60%) and linoleic (20%) acids (158–159). Moreover, chia seeds have high levels of protein such as prolamins, amino acids (16% to 26%), vitamins B complex, vitamins E, and minerals (phosphorus, magnesium, potassium, calcium). Due to the absence of gluten, these seeds are appropriate for celiac patients. Additionally, chia seeds are also a source of polyphenol antioxidants, such as gallic, chlorogenic, ferulic, caffeic acids, quercetin, epicatechin, and kaempferol (158–159). Chia seeds have different medicinal effects, particularly anti-inflammatory and antidiabetic activities, and positive effects on blood lipid profile, cardiovascular disease, and hypertension. Chia seeds also have antimicrobial and immunostimulatory effects (158–159).

2.3.13.4 Quinoa Seed

Quinoa (*Chenopodium quinoa*) is an herbaceous plant of the Chenopodiaceae or Amaranthaceae family for its edible seeds. Quinoa originated in the South American Andes region (Peru, Bolivia, Chile) and was first cultivated by the Incas as staple food for 7,000 years (160–162). There are hundreds of quinoa varieties, but the most consumed are white, red, and black quinoas. Quinoa has an outer seed coat containing bitter saponin that acts as an insecticide and is removed by simple rinsing with water before cooking. Quinoa seeds are high in proteins, amino acids, starch, fibers, minerals (iron, zinc, copper, magnesium, manganese), B vitamins (B1, B2, B6, folate), and some antioxidants (160–162). Moreover, due to the absence of gluten, quinoa is suitable for celiac patients or gluten related disorders. Fats are rich in unsaturated fatty acids like oleic acid and alpha-linolenic acid. Quinoa gives energy to the body. It helps regulate the digestive system and may prevent hypercholesterolemia and cardiovascular diseases (160–162).

2.3.14 Nuts

In botany and in general language, a nut is a dry fruit comprising an inedible hard shell and a dry edible seed. Nuts are used mostly in cuisine or roasted as snack foods. The nuts most commonly eaten are: walnut, pistachio, pecan, almond, cashew nut, peanut, macadamia, Brazil nut, chestnut, ginkgo nut, and more (163–165). Nuts are an important source of nutrients and energy for humans because nuts have high oil contents – mostly essential monounsaturated and polyunsaturated fatty acids. The main monounsaturated fats are oleic acid and palmitoleic acid, while polyunsaturated fatty acids include linoleic acid (LA) and alpha linolenic acid (ALA), which are omega-6 fatty acid and omega-3 fatty acid, respectively (163–165). They are an excellent source of protein and essential amino acids, especially L-arginine (164). As this amino acid is the precursor of the endogenous vasodilator nitric oxide (NO), nut intake might help improve the vascular system. Nuts also are a good source of dietary fiber (4 to 11 g per 100 g), and some essential minerals like magnesium, phosphorus, potassium, copper, and selenium (163–165). Many nuts are rich in vitamins such as vitamin E, vitamin B_2, folate, phytosterols, and polyphenolic antioxidants like carotenoids (163–164). Thanks to their rich nutrient composition, nuts have a beneficial impact on human health. Many epidemiological studies have associated nut consumption with a reduced incidence of cardio vascular diseases in both sexes and of diabetes in women, but not in men (163–165). Feeding trials have clearly demonstrated that consumption of all kinds of nuts has a cholesterol-lowering effect (165). Nuts may aid in weight loss and hypertension, as well as prevent oxidative stress and inflammation (163–165). However, prevention or treatment of cancer and other pathologies by nuts are still not evident (163). Another aspect that should be taken into consideration is the allergenic potential of nuts, especially walnuts and peanuts (163–164). Allergy of nuts affects principally young children and may be particularly severe, even life-threatening (163–164). Processed foods such as snacks and juices containing nuts, can also cause allergic reactions. Thus, do not eat nuts and their processed foods if you are allergic to nuts. In addition, bitter almonds are rich in cyanides which are very toxic and fatal. In contrast, sweet almonds are not toxic. Heating like boiling, drying, or grilling can destroy toxic cyanide in nuts and other vegetables like manioc.

2.3.14.1 Roles of Four Main Nuts: Almond, Walnut, Pistachio and Peanut

The four most consumed nuts are: almond, walnut, pistachio, and peanut.

The benefits of almond intake to human health include reduction of cardiovascular risk, with evident benefits for diabetic, hyperlipidemic, and obese individuals. Another benefit is the improvement in diet quality and gut microbiota, especially in children, because almond is rich in dietary fibers (163).

The consumption of walnuts (Figure 5.4) may be related to the reduction of cardiovascular risk both by improvement in lipid profile and reduction of inflammatory and atherogenic processes which are due to the high concentration of antioxidants present in walnuts, such as α-linolenic acid and alpha-tocopherol (163).

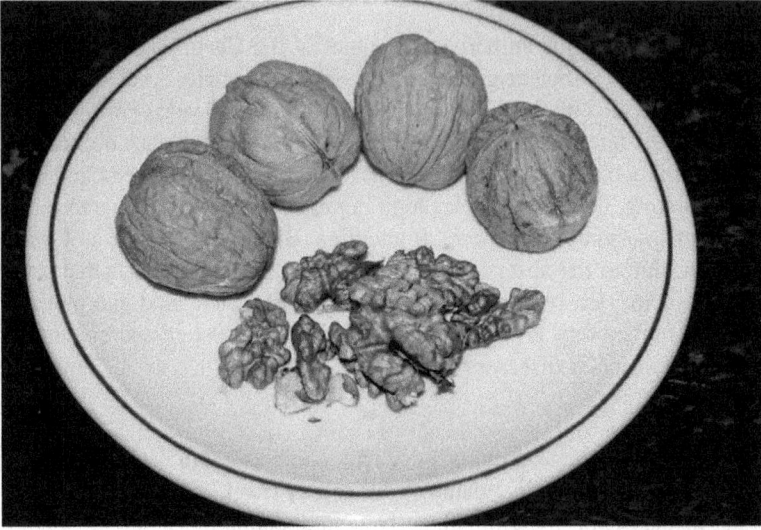

FIGURE 5.4   Walnut.

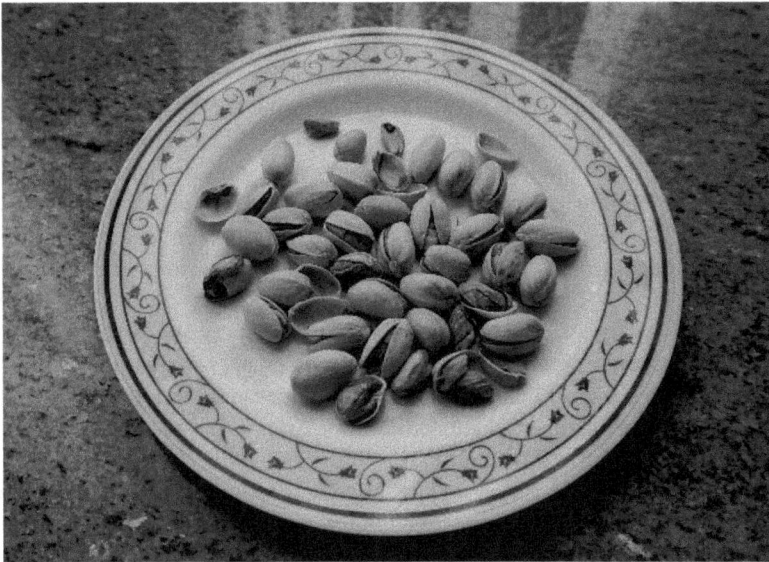

FIGURE 5.5   Pistachio.

Pistachio (Figure 5.5) consumption (range 25–84 g/day) may be beneficial to ameliorate lipid profile and attenuate inflammatory markers and blood pressure in obese individuals. Moreover, pistachio consumption may improve glucose metabolism, vascular function, and systemic hemodynamics (163).

Peanuts have a higher content of protein and fiber when compared to tree nuts. Therefore, peanut consumption (42.5–75 g/day) in a period of three weeks, independent of body composition alteration, improves glycemic control, induces satiety, and attenuates non-esterified fatty acid (NEFA) concentration. Therefore, the inclusion of peanuts in the diet not only improves the quality of the diet, but also stimulates satiety, increases fat oxidation and thermogenesis, and reduces glycemic response. Moreover, the consumption of peanuts in large portions (70 g) does not result in body weight gain (163). In addition, Brazil nut, hazelnut, cashew nut, macadamia, and ginkgo nut are also good sources of nutrients and antioxidants. They are often consumed as dessert, or snack. In conclusion, nuts have nutritional characteristics that can benefit human health, in particular, regarding the prevention and treatment of diseases.

2.3.15 Tubers

Some main tubers or roots used as vegetables are: carrot, onion, garlic, bunching or Welsh onion, leek, shallot, beetroot, chive, scallion, radish, and turnip. Other tubers rich in carbohydrates such as beets, potatoes, cassava, yam, are not considered vegetables and are generally classified as staple foods. Only carrot, onion, garlic, Welsh onion, leek, shallot, and beetroot will be examined below, due to their high health benefits.

2.3.15.1 Carrot

Carrot (*Daucus carota* L.), among the most important root vegetables in the Apiaceae family, is a multi-nutritional food source. It is rich in natural bioactive compounds like carotenoids, flavonoids, polyacetylenes, vitamins (vitamin C, B1, B2, B3 or niacin), minerals (Ca, Fe, Mg, Na, K, Cu, Zn), and fibers, all of which possess numerous nutraceutical effects and health benefits (166–169). These chemicals may reduce cancer and cardiovascular diseases due to their antioxidant, anti-inflammatory, antitumor, and immune-enhancing properties (166–169). Carrot root is a good protector of eye health thanks to its high levels of α and β -carotenes and lutein, which are well-known nutrients for the eyes (168). Anti-diabetic, anti-hypertensive, hepatoprotective properties, hypercholesterolemia and nephropathy prevention, have also been reported in many studies concerning the roles of carrots in human health (166–169). Numerous factors influence the amount and type of phytochemicals present in carrots. Genotype (color differences) plays an important role; high contents of α and β -carotene are present in orange carrots, lutein in yellow carrots, lycopene in red carrots, anthocyanins in the root of purple carrots, and phenolic compounds abound in black carrots (168). The consumption of carrot and its products is increasing steadily due to it being recognized as an important source of natural antioxidants with anticancer activity (167). Carrot root is eaten raw, cooked or processed as juice, dried powder, canned, preserves, candy, or pickle. Carrot pomace containing about 50% of β-carotene could be utilized for the supplementation of products like cake, bread, biscuits, and preparation of several types of functional products (167).

2.3.15.2 Onion and Welsh Onion

Onion (*Allium cepa* L.) is the most widely cultivated species of the Liliaceae or Amaryllidaceae family, which has over 700 members such as garlic, leek, shallot, scallion, chive, and so on (170–173). The plant part commonly used is the bulb, which is utilized as a food ingredient to give flavor and aroma to a great variety of dishes, and also as medicines. Flavors can be sweet and juicy to sharp, spicy, and pungent. The most common type consumed is white onion; some other varieties like yellow and red onions are also eaten. All onion types are an important source of several phytonutrients such as flavonoids (quercetin, kaempferol, anthocyanin, flavonol), fructo-oligosaccharides, homocysteine, folate, calcium, thiosulfinates, and other sulfur compounds (170–172). Anthocyanins belonging to flavonoids are mainly present in red onions, while yellow onions are rich in flavonols. Onions as well as all *Allium* vegetables, are characterized by their rich content of thiosulfinates and other volatile organosulfur compounds which are responsible for their particular odor and flavor and are also their lachrymatory or tear factor (171–172). The thiosulfinates or alkane(ene) thial-S-oxide are formed by the action of the enzyme alliinase from their respective S-alk(en)yl cysteine sulfoxides, which are mainly responsible for onion flavor, producing the eye-irritating compounds that induce lacrimation (172). To avoid this disagreeable sensation (lacrimation) while cutting onion, cut onion under a running tap water or in a receptacle filled with water.

These volatile lachrymatory compounds are also active antimicrobial agents; hence, onions may be used as natural food preservatives to inhibit microbial growth (170–172). Eating raw onion will maximize sulfur compounds, while boiling onions for five minutes will decrease them, except at a low heat. Therefore, avoid 'ready-to-eat onion' because these onions do not contain the volatile sulfur compounds which are active antimicrobial agents (173). Consuming onions freshly cut is the best way to preserve thiosulfinates and other antioxidants. In onions, sulfur compounds are responsible for typical odor and flavor and are also active antimicrobial agents; hence, onions may be used as natural preservatives to control microbial growth (170). Numerous studies have shown that a high consumption of onion and garlic may play a role in the prevention of cancer and cardiovascular disorders. Furthermore, onion and garlic extracts have strong antioxidant, hypocholesterolemic, hypolipidemic, anti-hypertensive, anti-diabetic, antithrombotic, anti-inflammatory, antiallergic, anti-viral, anti-protozoa, anti-parasitic, and neuroprotective properties (170–171). They also stimulate immune and kidney function, prevent atherosclerosis, and have anti-bacterial/ fungal activity, as well as prebiotic effect (171). The therapeutic properties of onion and garlic are caused by the combination and biological activity of pungent organo-sulfur compounds such as S-allyl-l-cysteine, diallyl disulfide, diallyl trisulfide, ajoene, and allicin. Studies suggest that the biological and therapeutic properties of garlic and onions are mainly due to their highly smelly organo-sulfur compounds (171).

In brief, eating raw onion or slightly cooked onion may prevent cancers, CVDs and neurological diseases, and may treat some benign infections, inflammation, and osteoporosis. However, excessive intake of fresh or semi-cooked onion and garlic may cause indigestion and flatulence.

2.3.15.3   Garlic

Garlic (*Allium sativum*, family Liliaceae) has been used both as a food flavoring and as a prophylactic as well as a therapeutic medicinal plant for several thousand years (171, 174–176). The bulb of the garlic plant is the most commonly used part, and each bulb contains many white fleshy cloves. Garlic cloves have a pungent and spicy flavor when cut or chewed, and are eaten raw or cooked as a seasoning or condiment. They are also processed in the form of garlic extracts, garlic oil and garlic powder with differences in chemical composition and bioactive compound content between the various forms (174). Garlic is important due to its use in therapeutic and preventive purposes in both traditional and modern medicine. The chemical composition of garlic is similar to that of onion (171). Like onion, garlic is considered one of the richest vegetable sources of total phenolic compounds, but its bioactive properties are attributed to its organosulfur compounds. The two main classes of organosulfur compounds found in whole garlic cloves are L-cysteine sulfoxides and γ-glutamyl-L-cysteine peptides. About 80% of cysteine sulfoxide in fresh garlic is alliin or S-allyl-L-cysteine sulfoxide. Alliin is a strong antioxidant and immunostimulant (175). Crushing or chopping garlic releases an enzyme called alliinase that catalyzes the formation of allicin from alliin. Therefore, allicin is not present in fresh and intact garlic cloves. It is instantaneously formed when garlic clove is broken in the mouth or cut by a knife. Allicin (diallyl-thiosulfinate) is one of the major organosulfur compounds in garlic considered to be biologically active. Allicin is a powerful anti-infective, and is also responsible for the heady, pungent garlic smell. Making garlic odorless by different processing treatments can also diminish its health benefits (174–176). However, allicin is very unstable. It is rapidly broken down in the body in about one hour, forming different active and inactive organosulfur compounds. Apart from its sulfur compounds, garlic is also rich in vitamins (vitamin B complex and vitamin C), antioxidants, flavonoids, minerals (phosphorous, potassium, selenium), saponins, and allixin (175). Numerous preclinical and clinical studies have reported that organosulfur compounds from garlic could exert antioxidant, antimicrobial, anticancer, anti-inflammatory, and cardio-protective activities (174–176). Research suggests that eating garlic can reduce the risk of developing colon or rectal cancer and can reduce high blood glucose levels. However, the mechanisms of all phytochemicals of garlic and their long-term effects are still ambiguous (175).

Recently, Korean researchers found that sprouted garlic formed from old garlic bulbs with bright green shoots sprouting from their cloves has higher antioxidant activity than fresher, younger bulbs (177). They observed that garlic sprouted for 5 days had the highest antioxidant activity. Therefore, sprouting may be a useful way to improve the antioxidant potential of garlic (177). Contrary to some sprouted plant foods like potatoes, which are harmful, sprouted garlic makes many new beneficial compounds that may present more health benefits than fresh intact garlic.

Black garlic, another artificial form of white garlic, is also developed in Korea, Japan, and Thailand. Black garlic is a functional food produced from fresh garlic (*Allium sativum* L.) via fermentation with the whole bulbs or peeled cloves in a chamber in which temperature (60–90°C) and humidity (70–90%) are regulated for a period of time (30–90 days) (178). Only the enzymes in the fresh garlic will transform white garlic into its black color. There are no addition of yeasts, bacteria or chemicals in this fermentation. Black garlic has an abundant amount of antioxidant compounds such as polyphenols, flavonoids, tetrahydro-β-carboline derivatives, and organosulfur compounds, including S-allyl-mercaptocysteine and S-allyl-cysteine, as compared with fresh garlic (178). A growing body of evidence in the past few decades demonstrates therapeutic effects of black garlic, including antioxidant, anticancer, anti-obesity, hypolipidemic, immunomodulatory, hepatoprotective, and neuroprotective effects.

Further studies are needed to elucidate the pathophysiological mechanisms of garlic and its derivatives (sprouted garlic, black garlic) as well as its efficacy and safety in the treatment of various diseases.

2.3.15.4   Other Allium Species: Welch Onion, Shallot and Leek

Beside the two main Allium species cited previously – onion and garlic – three other Allium species frequently consumed are Welsh onion, shallot, and leek.

In Asia, there is a species of onion called Welsh or bunching onion (*Allium fistusolum*, family Liliaceae) which is very similar in taste and odor to the related common onion but possesses hollow leaves and does not develop a bulb. The Welsh onion, raw or cooked, is a common ingredient in Asian cuisine and is also used in traditional Asian medicine as a bactericide, diuretic, and digestive due to its high content in sulfur compounds. In addition, it is used as an ethno-medicinal herb for the treatment of common colds, headaches, eyesight problems, heart problems, wounds, and festering sores (179).

Shallot (*Allium ascalonicum*) and leek (*Allium ampeloprasum*) are two close relatives of onion and belong to the same family, Liliaceae (171, 180). Shallot and leek are also both food and medicine. The main chemicals in shallot are mannose-specific lectin, furostanol saponins, selenium, sulfur compounds, antifungal peptide, and flavonol glucosides (171). Leek is a rich source of flavonoids (kaempferol), flavonoid polymers (proanthocyanidins or condensed tannins), and sulfur compounds, and therefore has significant health benefits (180). Components of shallot and leek have antioxidant, antibacterial, anti-fungal, anti-inflammatory, anti-angiogenic, hepatoprotective, hypolipidemic, and hypocholesterolemic properties (171, 180). Regular intake of shallot and leek is beneficial for health and may prevent cancer and cardiovascular diseases.

2.3.15.5   Beetroot

Beetroot – also known as beet, red beet, and table beet – is a tuber or root vegetable of the plant *Beta vulgaris* in the Chenopodiaceae family (classical classification) or Amaranthaceae family (phylogenetic classification). There are several cultivated varieties of beetroot: sugar beet, red beetroot, and yellow or golden beetroot. Sugar beet with white flesh is used for cuisine and sugar production as cited previously in this chapter. Red beetroot and golden beetroot with violet red and yellow flesh, respectively, are mostly used for cuisine and medicine, but they cannot produce sugar (181–183). Beetroot can be eaten raw, used for juice extraction, baked, or boiled. Beets have been used in traditional medicine to treat constipation, gut, and joint pain. Modern pharmacology shows that red beet extracts exhibit antihypertensive and hypoglycemic activity as well as excellent antioxidant property (181). The past decade is characterized by an explosive growth of interest in the impact of red beetroot on human health (181–185).

Red beetroot or *Beta vulgaris rubra* is a rich source of several biologically active phytochemicals such as betalains, betaine, nitrate (NO_3^-), ascorbic acid, carotenoids, phenolic acids, and flavonoids. Beetroot also contains several highly bioactive phenolics, such as rutin, epicatechin, and caffeic acid, which are also known to be excellent antioxidants. Nevertheless, the most important red beetroot phytochemicals are secondary metabolites: betalains, betaine, and nitrates (181–185).

Betalains are water-soluble bioactive pigments classified into betacyanin pigment, which is red-violet in color, and betaxanthin pigment, which is yellow-orange in color. The major betalain in red beetroot is betanin, which belongs to red betacyanin pigment. Betalains have high antioxidant and anti-inflammatory properties and are used to fight oxidative stress and chronic inflammation such as liver disease, arthritis, and even cancer (181–185). Red beetroot or *Beta vulgaris rubra* is richer in antioxidants than other *Beta vulgaris* varieties.

Betaine (trimethylglycine) is a derived form of amino acid. The principal physiological role of betaine is as an osmolyte and methyl donor (transmethylation). Inadequate dietary intake of betaine often leads to hypo-methylation in many important pathways, including disturbed hepatic protein (methionine) metabolism, and inadequate hepatic fat metabolism, which leads to steatosis and plasma dyslipidemia. Betaine has a principal role in lowering the blood level of homocysteine, which is the key element in cascading development of atherosclerosis (181).

Beetroot contains about 250mg/kg of nitrate (183). Nitrate itself is not considered to mediate any specific physiological function; rather, nitrate's beneficial effects are attributed to its *in vivo* reduction to nitrite (NO_2^-), then to nitric oxide (NO), through bacterial nitrate reductases in the digestive tract from the tongue to the stomach. Nitric oxide is a multifarious messenger molecule with important vascular and metabolic functions (183).

Many observations showed that fresh red beetroot and its supplements such as juice might reduce blood pressure in different populations, probably through the nitrate/nitrite/nitric oxide ($NO_3^-/NO_2^-/NO$) pathway and other compounds found in *Beta vulgaris* (181–184). In addition, some recent studies have reported that beetroot ingestion or supplementation as beetroot juice may improve clinical outcomes for some diseases such as atherosclerosis, vascular dysfunction, cardiorespiratory disorders, Type 2 diabetes, cancer, and senile cognitive decline (181–185). Nitric oxide (NO) is also a good neurotransmitter, and immunostimulant, but excessive production of NO is harmful to the body. NO is also produced in the body by the amino acid L-arginine.

Nitrate was long considered to be a harmful substance contaminating vegetables. Nitrate was thought to be harmful due to the potential production of carcinogenic nitrosamines under certain conditions, such as an acidic stomach (181, 186). Nitrosamines were reported to be related to esophageal cancer, gastric cancer, colon cancer, and other endocrinological diseases, or fetus defection (181, 186). However, recent epidemiological investigations of nitrates and tumors have shown that no clear evidence has verified that dietary nitrate could increase the occurrence of tumors (186). Therefore, exogenous dietary nitrate plays an important role in various physiological activities as an effective supplement of nitrogen oxide (NO) in human body. In contrast, beetroot contains oxalic acid, an anti-nutrient. Therefore, regular consumption of red beet and other *Beta vulgaris*, as well as other vegetables like lettuce, is contraindicated for people with urolithiasis (kidney stone disease) (181).

2.3.16 Asparagus Sprouts or Shoots

Garden asparagus is the species *Asparagus officinalis L.* in the family Asparagaceae. It is an herbaceous, perennial plant. Garden asparagus is cultivated for its sprout or shoot, called its spear, which has many specific flavors and nutrients used in cuisine and medicinal purposes (187–191).

There are three varieties of *Asparagus officinalis*: white, green, and purple asparagus. Green and white asparagus are the most consumed worldwide. Agronomically, the key difference is whether the shoots are harvested above ground (green and purple varieties) or underground before they reach the surface or sunlight (white asparagus) (188). When the shoots are above ground, photosynthesis in the shoot turns is green or green-purple due to the formation of chlorophyll. In contrast, when the shoots are underground, the shoots remain white.

Garden asparagus has a wide range of bioactive components with great health benefits (187–191). Its bioactive components include flavonoids (i.e., tannin, anthocyanin, quercetin, kaempferol, rutin), steroidal saponins, other phenolics, dietary fibers (lignins), and essential oils, which can potentially be used to develop novel cosmetic or health food ingredients (187–191). Pharmacological activities of garden asparagus include anticancer, antioxidant, antifungal, antibacterial, anti-dysenteric, anti-inflammatory, anti-abortifacient, antiulcer, anti-hypertensive, and anticoagulant effects. Moreover, it may reduce the risk of constipation, colon cancer, diarrhea, osteoporosis, cardiovascular disease, obesity, rheumatism, and diabetes, as well as improve fertility and vitality in women and men (187–191).

Asparagus sprouts can be eaten raw or cooked; however, the longer the cooking times, the more health benefits decrease. It should also be noted that consuming asparagus can cause the urine to smell very badly if eaten excessively.

2.4 SPICES

A spice is generally a root, bark, dried seed, or fruit and used to give flavor or color to a food. Many spices have medicinal properties like antiseptic, digestive, stimulant, and so on. They are often used in traditional medicine and recently in modern medicine and cosmetology.

The spices most commonly used as medicine, food colorant, and flavor are turmeric, galangal, ginger, pepper, chili, and cinnamon.

2.4.1 Turmeric

Turmeric is a rhizomatous herbaceous perennial plant (*Curcuma longa*) of the Zingiberaceae family. Turmeric is a spice that has received much interest from both the medical areas as well as from the culinary world since antiquity through today (192–210). Turmeric is a tropical plant mostly cultivated in India and Southeast Asia (Myanmar, Thailand, Cambodia, Vietnam, Indonesia, etc.) and recently in Taiwan, Jamaica, Haiti, and Hawaii. About 133 species of Curcuma and approximately 70 varieties of *Curcuma longa* are found around the world (192, 193). Turmeric rhizome has a tough brown skin and bright orange flesh, and measures 2.5–7.0 cm (1–3 inches) in length and 1–2.5 cm (0.4–1 inch) in diameter, with smaller tubers branching off (192, 197) (Figure 5.6). The rhizome can

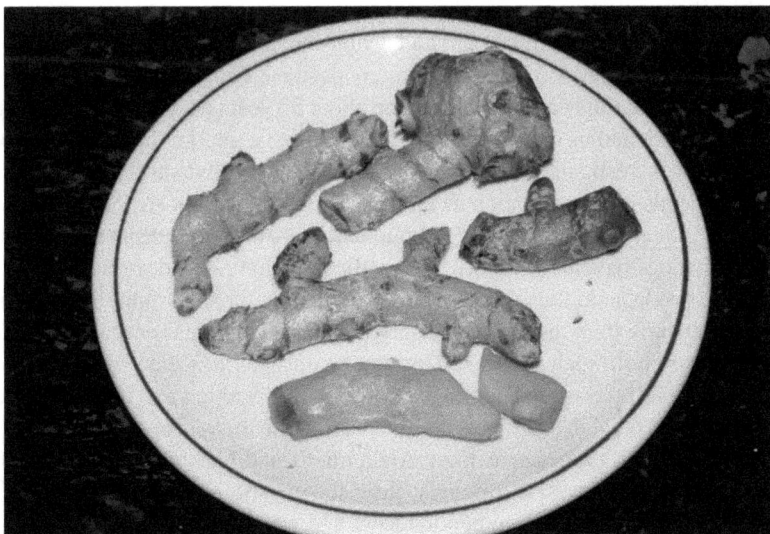

FIGURE 5.6   Turmeric.

be eaten fresh or cooked after peeling for culinary or medicinal uses. When the rhizome is dried, it can be ground to a yellow powder with a bitter, slightly acrid, yet sweet, taste. In general, fresh turmeric rhizome is better than its dried powder because all nutritional benefits are preserved in fresh product. Moreover, turmeric contains a number of polyphenol antioxidants which are easily oxidized by air, heat, and sunlight. To preserve all nutrients, fresh rhizome must be kept in sealed plastic bag at freezer temperature for no more than two weeks. Dried turmeric powder is used as colorant or flavor for cuisine. For turmeric supplements, the quality of turmeric obtained depends on the processing mode of each producer.

More than 200 chemical compounds, primarily the volatile oils and the orange-yellow coloring pigments named curcuminoids, have been isolated from turmeric rhizome (192–197). The volatile oils are mainly constituted of terpenoids, while the curcuminoids (diarylheptanoids) are phenolic compounds. They are the major bioactive ingredients of turmeric rhizomes. The essential oils from leaves and flowers are usually dominated by monoterpenes while those from roots and rhizomes contain primarily sesquiterpenes. Different volatile oils include turmerone, arturmerone, atlantone, zingiberene, cineole, d-α-phellandrene, d-sabinene, borneol, aneole, dehydroturmerone, mono-terpenes, and a variety of sesquiterpenes (192–197). The orange-yellow curcuminoids are strong phenolic antioxidants including curcumin, mono-desmethoxycurcumin, di-desmethoxycurcumin, p-coumaroylferuloyl-methane, and di-p-coumaroylmethane (192–195). Curcumin or diferuloyl-methane is a yellow polyphenol pigment with a 77% level of of total curcuminoids; it is also the main therapeutic agent of turmeric. Each 100 g of turmeric contains about 5–6.6% curcumin and 3.5% volatile oils (192–195). However, the amounts of curcumin and volatile oils in the *Curcuma longa* rhizome vary with its varieties. Turmeric grown in India and Southeast Asian areas are con-sidered the best varieties found in the world. Besides the two main nutrient groups cited above, tur-meric also contains sugars, protein, polysaccharides (starch, ukonanes), minerals (iron, potassium, etc.), niacin, vitamins A, C, omega-3 fatty acid, α-linolenic acid, alkaloid, and sterols, and more (192–195).

In Asian cooking, turmeric is used as a coloring and flavoring for various dishes and bever-ages like curries, rice, meat, tea, soup, and so on. In Western countries, turmeric powder is a safe coloring for foods and referred to as E-100 in food industry. The consumption of fresh turmeric in Asian countries in humans is in the range of 200–1000 mg/day or 160–440 g/person/year (192). In traditional medicine, turmeric has been used for thousands of years in India, China and other Asian countries for different ailments such as rheumatoid arthritis, wound healing, chronic anterior uve-itis, conjunctivitis, skin cancer, small pox, chicken pox, insect bites, urinary tract infections, asthma, and digestive ailments (colic, abdominal pain and distension, appetite stimulant, digestive disorders, constipation, jaundice, etc.) (192–202). Concerning modern medicine, turmeric has drawn the atten-tion of scientists to its potential health benefits since about 30 years ago. Many in vitro, in vivo, clin-ical, and epidemiological studies on turmeric and its bioactive compound curcumin as well as other constituents have been investigated in different laboratories and industries worldwide for finding their different therapeutic effects and their exact mechanisms of action. According to the Curcumin Resource Database edited in 2015, over 9,000 publications and 500 patents concerning turmeric, curcumin, and its analogs have been recorded over the past three decades (200). This explains the importance of these products in the prevention and treatment of a large number of human diseases. Most of these studies have demonstrated a variety of pharmacological properties of turmeric and its main compound curcumin such as anti-inflammatory, anti-carcinogenic, anti-neurodegenerative, antioxidant, antimicrobial, and wound healing actions, in vitro and in vivo. In humans, turmeric and its curcumin may be beneficial in a number of ailments like rheumatoid arthritis, osteoarthritis, can-cer, cardiovascular diseases, diabetes, asthma, Alzheimer's and Parkinson's diseases, autoimmune disease, gastro-intestinal diseases, pulmonary disease, metabolic disease, infection, and more. Turmeric is also found useful in healing peptic ulcers and wounded skin in patients (192–208).

Despite the important evidence of these tests in vitro and in animals of curcumin against differ-ent forms of cancer and neurological diseases, the clinical application of curcumin remains limited due to its low bioavailability and rapid metabolism in human body (192, 197, 199, 205–209). To overcome the problem of the poor pharmacokinetic characteristics of curcumin, several associated compounds have been tested to improve curcumin's bioavailability by using different mechanisms. Most of them have been developed to block the metabolic pathway of curcumin in order to increase its bioavailability. For example, piperine, a known bioavailability enhancer, is the major active component of black pepper and is associated with an increase of 2,000% in the bioavailability of curcumin (199). As curcumin is water-insoluble and oil-soluble (lipophilic), the association of curcumin or curcuminoids with phospholipids or lecithin has been proposed to increase their absorption in the human intestinal tract. Therefore, eating turmeric or curcumin supplement with foods rich in phospholipids or lecithin like egg yolks, milk, fishes, fish oil, omega-3, soybeans, and olive oil, may increase its bioavailability. Recently, it has been hypothesized that curcumin could exert direct regulative effects primarily in the gastrointestinal tract, where high concentrations of curcumin have been detected after oral administration. Consequently, it might be hypothesized that curcumin directly exerts its regulatory effects on the gut microbiota, thus explaining the paradox between its low systemic bioavailability and its wide pharmacological activities (209). Another way to overcome the problem of the poor pharmacokinetic of curcumin is the use of nanotechnology (see Chapter 5, monograph Nano food). Different nanoparticles such as liposomes, micelles, carbon nanotubes, and superparamagnetic ferric oxide (Fe_3O_4) have been proposed as nanocarriers of curcumin for enhancing its absorption in therapy (210–212).

Several studies comparing the incidences of cancer and cancer related deaths in India and the United States have revealed lower risk of different forms of cancer in India than in the United States, from five to ten times (208). It is proposed that one of the major reasons for the drastic difference in cancer occurrences in these regions is the increased intake of dietary agents such as turmeric, and other herbs like galangal, cumin, black pepper, chili, and coriander, which are important ingredients for curries, the favorite dish of India. Therefore, the association of turmeric or curcumin with these herbs may enhance the absorption of curcumin and curcuminoids. However, tea may reduce the absorption of turmeric; therefore, it is to avoid taking tea and turmeric at the same time.

Curcuminoids have been approved by the US Food and Drug Administration (FDA) as 'Generally Recognized As Safe' (GRAS), and good tolerability and safety profiles have been shown by clinical trials, even at doses between 4,000 and 8,000 mg/day and of doses up to 12,000 mg/day of 95% concentration of three curcuminoids: curcumin, bisdemethoxycurcumin, and demethoxycurcumin (192, 199). In general, three to six g of fresh peeled turmeric rhizome per day mixed with milk, egg, olive oil, black pepper, galangal or soybeans, is considered safe to use. No evident toxicity or grave side effects were found when used for a long term. However, taking large amounts of turmeric by mouth for long periods of time may cause some digestive problems like stomach upset, flatulence, nausea and, in extreme cases, gastric ulcers. Allergic reactions like skin rash are possible for some people. Moreover, consult a doctor if you have gall bladder disease, gallstones, bile duct obstruction, stomach ulcers, jaundice, toxic liver disorders, or congestive heart disease before eating turmeric rhizome or curcumin supplement. In brief, fresh turmeric is considered safe when taken at the recommended doses. The doses of turmeric or curcumin supplements depend on the manufacture method of each producer. It is important to highlight that whole fresh turmeric tuber could have different dietary and therapeutic effects in the body greater than curcumin alone because of the synergistic effects of numerous compounds like terpenoids, polyphenols, vitamins, and so on, present in whole fresh turmeric. More research about whole turmeric, curcumin alone, and combined with different spices or herbs, in clinical applications are needed because this spice has various biological and pharmacological activities which have been demonstrated in numerous *in vitro* and *in vivo* studies.

2.4.2 Galangal

Galangal is a perennial herb in the Zingiberaceae family. Galangal includes more than 200 species distributed in tropical and subtropical Asia, Australia, and the Pacific Islands. However, only

Lesser Galangal and Greater Galangal are the two species most used as both spice and medicinal herb (213–226). Lesser galangal has the taxonomic name *Alpinia officinarum* and is originated in Southeast China (Yunnan, Hainan isle), Vietnam, Laos, and Japan (Okinawa). Greater galangal, named *Alpinia galanga*, is native to Indonesia, and now cultivated in Southeast Asia (Thailand, Malaysia, Cambodia, India), and in Australia and Hawaii (213–218). Different galangal species vary in their hotness and flavor. Flavor ranges from flowery to ginger-like to peppery-cinnamon. Greater Galangal rhizome has an orange-brown skin with pale yellow or white interior and is milder in flavor but larger in size (Figure 5.7). Lesser Galangal rhizome has a red-brown interior and fibrous texture. Both species can be eaten as fresh rhizome, sliced or powdered (213). Both the Greater and Lesser Galangal species have similar effects in cookery and medicine. Besides the two previous galangals, Kaempferia Galangal, another galangal species with red skin and white flesh in interior, is also sometimes used as a condiment and medicinal herb (213).

Galangal contains several important chemical compounds that give it its different medicinal properties. In total, 544 compounds were isolated from 35 Alpinia species (218). Different compounds in galangal are: 210 terpenoids, 143 diarylheptanoids, 71 flavonoids, 66 phenolics (including 2 abundant phenol derivatives named acetoxychavicol acetate and acetoxyeugenol acetate), 24 lignans, 6 stilbenes, 4 steroids, 3 fatty acids, 2 alkaloids, 2 glycosides, 1 ester, and some vitamins and minerals (215–222). Previous phytochemical investigations have shown that both *A. galanga* and *A. officinarum* have some similar chemical constituents, such as diarylheptanoids, flavonoids, volatile oil, terpenes, phenylpropanoids, and glycosides, though the main chemical components are different. *A. galanga* is rich in a variety of phenolic compounds and essential oils, whereas *A. officinarum* is rich in flavonoids and diarylheptanoids (222). Investigations have shown *A. galanga* and *A. officinarum* to have many biological activities, including effectiveness as anti-inflammatory, antiviral, antimicrobial, antioxidant, antitumor, anti-allergic, and gastro-protective agents (222).

The two main compounds in *Alpinia galanga* and *Alpinia officinarum* are volatile oil known as galangol, and non-volatile polyphenol antioxidants. The major compounds identified in the oils of *A. galanga* and *A. officinarum* are primarily constituted of different terpenoids such as 1,8-cineole (63.4 and 44.2%), α-terpineol (2.8 and 6.3%), α-pinene (1.9 and 2.0%), β-pinene (0.8 and 5.7%), and terpinen-4-ol (2.8 and 4.5%), respectively. Some additional compounds identified in

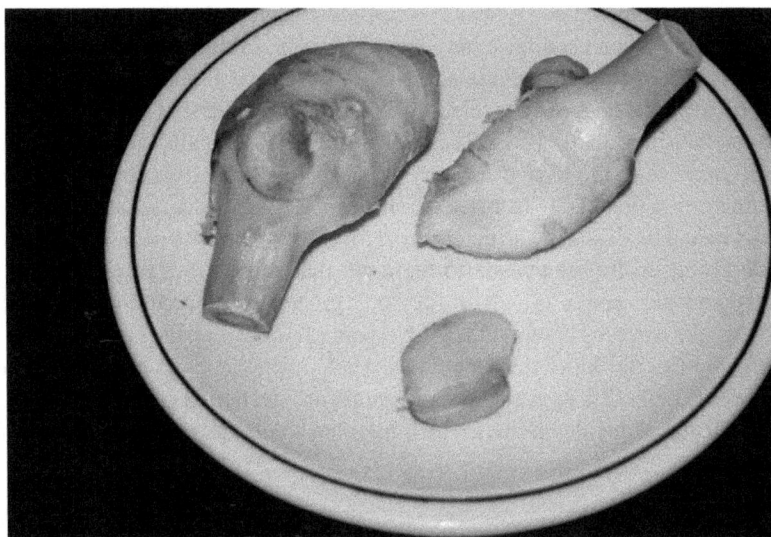

FIGURE 5.7   Greater galangal (*Alpinia galanga*).

A. officinarum oil are camphor (4.0%) and α-fenchyl acetate (8.9%), while chavicol (0.9%), (*E*)-β-farnesene (8.4%), β-sesquiphellandrene (2.6%), β-bisabolene (0.3%), and eugenol acetate (3.3%) are present in *A. galanga* oil. (219, 220). Many terpenoids in volatile oil, especially 1,8-cineole or eucalyptol, a monoterpenoid, are reported to possess expectorant, antiseptic, and analgesic properties and are used widely in pharmaceutical preparations for the treatment of cold, bronchitis, and cough, based on traditional Chinese and Indian medicine (213–220). Diarylheptanoids, characterized by a 1,7-diphenylheptane skeleton, are natural phenols and constitute a group of 400 natural products often present in different plants such as galangal, ginger, turmeric, alder (alnus), maple (acer), bayberry (myrica), and walnut (juglans) (223, 224). They are divided into linear-diarylheptanoids and cyclic-diarylheptanoids (223, 224). Different bioactivities of diarylheptanoids in galangal are: antioxidant, antibacterial, anticancer, anti-inflammatory, anti-emetic, hepato-protective, and antiosteoporotic properties, which have been discovered recently by many scientists (220, 224).

The two main phenolic compounds, acetoxychavicol acetate and acetoxyeugenol acetate, present in galangal were recently reported to have anti-ulcer, anti-leishmanial, and antitumor bioactivities (218). Furthermore, acetoxychavicol acetate isolated from *Alpinia galanga* also showed antiallergic, anti-asthmatic, anti-HIV (human immunodeficiency virus), antiviral (especially herpes simplex virus), antibacterial, anti-cancer, gastro-protective, efflux pump inhibitory, NO production inhibitory, xanthine oxidase inhibitory, plant growth-inhibitory, and fungal growth inhibitory activities by different tests in vitro and in animals over the past two decades (218, 223, 225–226). The association of galangal and turmeric might enhance the antiviral and antibacterial effects of these two herbs.

Galangin, kaempferol, and kaempferide are the major flavonoids in galangal and have strong antioxidant activities. A recent study reported that galangin may be a promising candidate for cancer prevention (218).

In both Chinese and Ayurvedic (Indian) traditional medicine since ancient times, *Alpinia galanga* and *Alpinia officinarum* were and still are used as aphrodisiacs for both sexes, especially promoting sexual appetite in women (221). Other traditional medicinal properties of galangal include: stomachic, carminative, antiseptic, antifungal, anti-itching, anti-emetic, and expectorant (213–221). The rhizome of *Alpinia officinarum*, due to its warming effect on the body, or yang property according to Chinese medicine, has been used in China for treating colds, diabetes, relieving stomach ache, reducing swelling, invigorating the circulatory system, and has antiulcer, anti-diarrhea, analgesic, anti-inflammatory, and anticoagulation effects (213, 220). *Alpinia galanga* has been used in traditional medicine for the treatment of cough, coryza, bronchitis, halitosis (bad breath), throat infections, voice roughness, measles, pityriasis versicolor (a yeast dermatitis), eczema, otitis, gastritis, mouth ulcers, gum inflammation, and rheumatoid arthritis (213, 221). The choice between the two main Alpinia species for medical use depends on the type of ailment and must be consulted with an herbalist. Consult your physician to avoid eventual incompatibility or interaction between galangal and your pathology or your drug. However, for culinary use, galangal is likely safe at small doses of about one to three g/day. The smaller rhizomes are usually preferred instead of larger and harder roots that are more difficult to slice. Before used, the rhizomes must be washed and the outer skin removed, and then can be cut into small pieces for culinary uses (217). Do not heat galangal for a long time because it contains volatile compounds. Large amounts of fresh galangal root, dried sliced root, and prolonged usage can irritate the mouth, the stomach, and the guts and can cause gastric ulcers or other ailments like flatulence and nausea.

Although a large spectrum of therapeutic properties of diverse galangals has been reported in traditional medicine as well as in recent research, more efforts are needed to standardize their therapeutic uses and to explain their mechanisms. Moreover, it is interesting to discover the synergistic effects of galangal with other natural herbs such as turmeric and ginger in the treatment and prevention of many dreadful ailments such as rheumatoid arthritis, osteoarthritis, asthma, cardiovascular diseases, infectious diseases (AIDS, candidiasis), and cancer – which are almost all still not cured through today.

2.4.3 Ginger

Ginger, the rhizome of *Zingiber officinale*, a member of the Zingiberaceae family, is a popular spice used for cooking, snack foods, and traditional medicine, especially in Asia and the Middle East (195, 227–234). Its rhizomes are aromatic, thick lobed, and pale yellowish (Figure 5.8) (227). Several dozen hybrid varieties of ginger are grown in the South Asian region. The cultivars depend upon climate, soil, and local conditions (227). In the past, ginger has been widely used in Chinese, Ayurvedic (Indian), and Unani-Tibb (Greco-Arab) medicines to cure a variety of diseases like arthritis, rheumatism, nausea, vomiting, asthma, cough, inflammation, pain, hypertension, constipation, indigestion, and infection (195, 227–234). Recently, ginger has attracted the attention of Western countries not only on its culinary properties, but also for its therapeutic benefits. Several scientific research concerning the constituents and the pharmacology of ginger have been intensively investigated in the last three decades.

The constituents of ginger are numerous and vary depending on its origin and the appearance of the rhizomes – for example, fresh or dry. They may be due to several dozen chemicals and several hundred compounds (230, 232). *Zingiber officinale* is reported to possess essential oils, phenolic compounds, flavonoids, terpenoids, steroids, tannin, alkaloids, glycosides, saponins, carbohydrates, and proteins, as the major phytochemical groups (227–232). Terpenoids of ginger include terpineol, borneol, zingiberene, β-sesquiphellandrene, β-bisabolene, α-farnesene, and α-curcumene, while phenolic compounds include gingerol, paradols, shogaol, and diarylheptanoids. Gingerols and shogaol are the major phenolic compounds in ginger. Terpenoids, flavonoids, and phenolic compounds are strong antioxidants. Besides these, amino acids, raw fiber, phytosterols, vitamins (nicotinic acid and vitamin A), protein, and minerals are also present (227–232).

Ginger contains two classes of active constituents: volatile essential oils and non-steam volatile components. The aroma and flavor of ginger are due to its steam volatile oil, while the pungency is produced by non-steam volatile components (227–228). The steam volatile oils are comprised mainly of sesquiterpenes, monoterpenes, and oxygenated monoterpenes. The monoterpenes are the most important contributors to the aroma of ginger and more abundant in the fresh rhizome than in dried ginger. Zingiberol is the principal volatile aroma of fresh ginger rhizome (227–228). The non-volatile pungent constituents include gingerols, shogaols, paradols, gingerdiols, and zingerone,

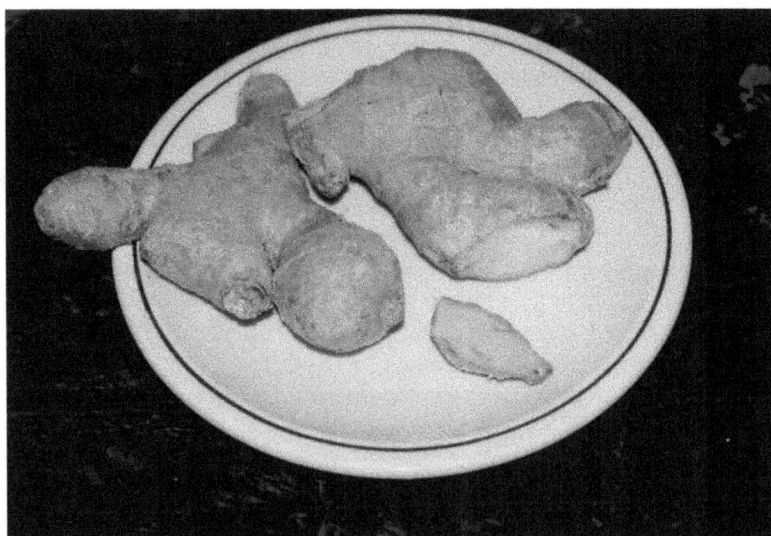

FIGURE 5.8   Ginger (In: Chapter 5: 'Plant source foods', page: XX).

that produce a 'hot' sensation in the mouth (227, 231). The main pungent compounds in fresh ginger are gingerols, whereas the pungency of dry ginger is mainly due to shogaols, which are dehydrated forms of gingerols. Because gingerols are thermally labile, the concentrations of gingerols in dry ginger are reduced slightly in comparison to fresh ginger, whereas the concentrations of shogaols increase (228, 231). Zingerone is produced during drying, cooking or roasting of ginger directly and also by thermal degradation of gingerols or shogaols, possessing potent pharmacological activities (231). Different main biological and pharmacological properties of ginger are: antioxidant, anti-microbial, anti-inflammatory, analgesic, anti-pyretic, anti-osteoarthritis, anti-rheumatoid arthritis, antidiabetic, anti-cancer (especially anti-gastrointestinal cancer), anti-vomiting, anti-nausea, anti-diarrheic, anti-gastric ulcer, anti-hypertensive, anti-hypercholesterolemia, anti-obesity, cardio-protective, liver-protective, and neuro-protective activities (195, 227–234). However, these findings are still not officially recognized by different healthcare organizations. More studies are needed in animals and humans on the pharmacokinetics of ginger and its constituents and on the eventual synergistic effects with other herbs or drugs for the treatment of different chronic ailments. Ginger is classified as a 'Generally Recognized As Safe' (GRAS) product by the Food Drug Administration in the United States and has few side effects (228–230). However, gastric irritation could occur if ginger is taken over six g/day (228).

2.4.4   Chili Pepper and Bell Pepper

Pepper is the fruit of plants belonging to the genus *Capsicum* which is a member of the Solanaceae family. The genus *Capsicum* consists of approximately 31 species of which the five domesticated species are *Capsicum annuum*, *Capsicum baccatum*, *Capsicum chinense*, *Capsicum frutescens*, and *Capsicum pubescens* (235–241). Several universal English names of the genus *Capsicum* include chili pepper, chili, hot pepper, tabasco pepper, cayenne pepper, paprika, African chili, bell pepper, and sweet pepper. All these species are native to Central and South America since antiquity. In the sixteenth century, *Capsicum annuum* and *Capsicum frutescens* were widely distributed from America to other continents. Different varieties of the genus Capsicum are widely grown for their fruits, which may be eaten fresh, cooked, as a dried powder, in a sauce, or processed into oleoresin. Three major products traded on the world market for use in food processing are paprika, oleoresin, and dried chili (both whole and in powdered form). Oleoresin is a viscous liquid derived by polar solvent extraction from ground powder of any Capsicum species (240). The tabasco pepper is a variety of the chili pepper species *Capsicum frutescens* for the preparation of Tabasco sauce in Mexico. Paprika is the ground dried fruits of the red chili pepper species *Capsicum annuum* in Hungarian cuisine, and is also used to make hot sauce for Latin-American dishes. Nowadays, *Capsicum annuum* is cultivated worldwide and used not only as spice but also as traditional medicine due to the presence of many healthy nutrients in its fruits (235–241). Chili peppers have a hot and burning flavor and are sold in two forms: red fruits and green fruits. Red chili peppers are mature fruits which are more spicy and richer in nutrients than green immature fruits, and are eaten fresh, dried or ground. All varieties of peppers contain high amount of vitamin C and other vitamins such as A, E, K, B5, B6, and minerals like calcium, magnesium, folate, potassium, thiamin, iron, and copper (235–241). The red color of ripe pepper fruit is due to several carotenoid pigments, including capsanthin, capsorubin, zeaxanthin and cryptoxanthin, while lutein is high in green peppers. They are all antioxidants (235–239). The hotness (pungency) in Chili pepper fruit is due to the alkaloid compounds called capsaicinoids which are pungent phenol compounds (235–239). Capsaicin is their major compound and constitutes about 70% of their total levels (236). Capsaicin and capsaicinoids in pepper have different medicinal properties such as anti-microbial, anti-carcinogenic, anti-inflammatory, anti-arthritic, anti-rhinitis, anti-coagulant, analgesic, and immunomodulatory effects. Chili pepper and capsaicin are also used for the prevention of cardiovascular diseases, Type 2 diabetes, hypercholesterolemia, and obesity, and might stop the spread of prostate cancer (235–239). The consumption of hot red chili pepper is reported to be associated with reduced mortality in human beings (237). Green chili shows promise as a memory enhancer (239). Capsaicin and capsaicinoids are absent in bell peppers, therefore, bell peppers do not have a hot, burning taste.

Besides some beneficial effects of chili peppers cited above, they possess some main adverse reactions due to their hot, burning flavor on digestive tube, mouth, throat, and eyes. The substance responsible is capsaicin. In high amounts, the hot *Capsicum annuum* variety can be harmful for the digestive system as it can cause irritation and inflammation to mucous membrane of the mouth, stomach, throat, and intestines. It should not be used on open wounds or abrasions, or near the eyes (236, 239). It has antagonistic effects on α-adrenergic blockers, clonidine, and methyldopa (239). The hot varieties are generally not recommended for young children because they do not yet have well-developed digestive systems (236). High chili pepper consumption can increase risk of cancer, especially in the mouth, throat, gallbladder, and stomach. To avoid these dangerous effects of fresh red chili peppers, replace them by their sauce, their powder paprika, or another variety such as bell pepper.

Bell pepper or sweet pepper is the fruit of plants belonging to a cultivar group of the species *Capsicum annuum*. Bell pepper contains all vitamins, minerals, and antioxidants cited previously for hot chili pepper, except capsaicin and capsaicinoids (240–241). It is the only member of the *Capsicum* genus that does not contain capsaicin and capsaicinoids, the main chemicals responsible for hot, burning sensations; therefore, it does not have the adverse effects cited above. It has a cubic or bell-shaped form with different colors like green, red, yellow, and orange. Red and green bell peppers are the most consumed and can be eaten raw or cooked.

2.4.5 Black Pepper and White Pepper

Black pepper and white pepper are both the same fruit of the *Piper nigrum* plant, a species belonging to the Piperaceae family. The pepper berries have a green color. They become different in color and flavor due to their method of processing. Their well-known black color, is due to the enzymatic oxidation of polyphenolic substrates present in the skin of green pepper under sun exposure. White pepper is produced from black pepper by removal of the black outer skin, leaving only the white inner seed. This decortication is conducted either by fermentation, by lowering them in bags in streams, or by mechanical methods that grind off the outer layer (242). Consequently, the color and taste of black and white pepper differ. White pepper is hotter than black pepper, but black pepper has more nutrients and antioxidants than white pepper because the outer skin is preserved. The oil fraction of the pepper is extracted from dry powdered peppercorns (242). Black pepper and white pepper are used as separate dry whole grain, mixed whole grain, or dry powder for culinary or medicinal purposes. In general, black pepper is more consumed than white pepper, especially for therapeutic use. Pepper oil and spirit are used in many medicinal and cosmetic products.

Pepper berry (*Piper nigrum*) contains a variety of phytochemicals including: phenolics, flavonoids, amides, alkaloids, steroids, terpenes, chalcones, fibers, essential oils, piperine, eugenol, the enzyme lipase, and minerals (243–245). Piperine is the major alkaloid present in both black and white peppers, and has numerous pharmacological actions. Essential oil components of black pepper include α- and β-pinene, limonene, β-caryophyllene, and α-terpinene (243–245). Black pepper is richer in phytochemicals than white pepper.

The scientific literature provides evidence that black pepper and piperine may have health benefits, particularly for the function of the digestive tract in enhancing digestion, stimulating appetite and digestive enzymes, and reducing stomach gas (243–245). Piperine exhibits diverse pharmacological activities like antihypertensive, antiplatelets, antioxidant, antitumor, antipyretic, analgesic, anti-inflammatory, anti-diarrheal, antibacterial, antifungal, anti-reproductive, and insecticidal activities. *Piper nigrum* also has been found to decrease lipid peroxidation *in vivo*. It has been reported to possess antioxidant activity that may be due to the presence of flavonoids and phenolic contents (245). Black pepper and piperine have been observed to inhibit cytochrome P450 enzymes. Black pepper enhances absorption of curcumin in turmeric, and other nutrients like β-carotene, coenzyme Q10, and flavonoids (244). For example, coadministration of black pepper and curcumin or curcuma to rats or humans enhances the levels of curcumin in blood because piperine inhibits the cytochrome P450 enzymes that metabolize all xenobiotics (phytochemicals and drugs). In healthy human volunteers, piperine administration increased blood levels of the antiepileptic drug phenytoin, the antihypertensive drug propranolol, and the anti-asthmatic drug theophylline (244). Therefore, notify your doctor if you consume high amounts of black pepper. Based on the current scientific evidence, more information and research are needed on the health benefits of black pepper in cancer, stroke, obesity, and other diseases, particularly in human subjects.

2.4.6 Cinnamon

Cinnamon is a spice obtained from the inner bark of several *Cinnamomum* trees belonging to the family Lauraceae. There are four main types of cinnamon: True cinnamon or Ceylon cinnamon (*Cinnamomum veranicum*), Vietnamese cinnamon (*Cinnamomum loureiroi*), Chinese cinnamon or Cassia cinnamon (*Cinnamomum aromaticum*), and Indonesian cinnamon (*Cinnamomum burmanni*) (246–247). In the market, pure cinnamon is sold as brown sticks (rolls), brown powder, or oil extract.

A wide range of phytochemical compounds including cinnamaldehyde, eugenol, terpinenes, flavonoids, alkaloids, anthraquinones, coumarins, phenols, saponins, tannins, carboxylic acid, camphene, fatty acids, actinodaphnine, butanolides, lignans, steroids, propenoids, and kaempferol glycosides are found in various parts of the plant such as bark, oil extract, and leaves (247). Cinnamon is rich in aromatic oils like cinnamaldehyde (in the bark oil), eugenol (in the leaf oil), and camphor (in the root-bark oil) (246).

Due to its exotic flavor and hot taste, cinnamon is used as a culinary spice and also a traditional medicine since antiquity. In traditional medicine, cinnamon is used in the treatment of respiratory and digestive ailments, as a stimulant, and as an anointment since antiquity (246). Recently, many experimental and clinical trials have explored its antimicrobial, anti-inflammatory, antidiabetic, antioxidant, antilipemic, and cognition enhancer effects for the treatment of infection, diabetes, depression, hypercholesterolemia, and Parkinson's disease (246–248). However, Cassia cinnamon (Chinese cinnamon) contains high levels of coumarins, about ten times more than Ceylon cinnamon. Coumarin is toxic to the liver in high doses. Therefore, its addition into food products is prohibited. Due to a lack of awareness regarding the standard limits of cinnamon in these products, it is advisable for patients of hepatic disorders to avoid cinnamon (246). In addition, a daily intake of coumarin more than 0.1 mg/kg body weight can lead to conspicuous effect on the blood coagulation profile if the patient is simultaneously on drugs such as warfarin. However, these results are still contradictory (246). So, it is recommended not to take a lot of pure cinnamon product or supplement. High intake of cinnamon can cause liver damage, mouth sore, cancer, hemorrhage, and breathing problems.

2.5 ALGAE AND SEAWEEDS

Algae are aquatic plants and can live in seawater and freshwater. Algae living in seawater only are called seaweeds. Some algae can live in both kinds of water, like chlorella, spirulina, and dunaliella. Algae are divided into two groups based on their size: microalgae and macroalgae. Microalgae are unicellular forms such as spirulina, chlorella, and the diatoms, while macroalgae are multicellular structures like giant kelp, a large brown alga. Seaweeds are seawater macroalgae including green algae, brown algae, and red algae, and are widely eaten as seafood around the world, especially in East Asia (249–255).

Macroalgae are abundant plant species commonly found in coastal areas and belong to seaweed. They are classified into brown seaweed (Phaeophyta), green seaweed (Chlorophyta), and red seaweed (Rhodophyta) based on their pigmentation. They are multicellular forms and vary greatly in size. Some brown algae such as kelps may reach 70m long (251–253). Red algae are considered the most important source of many biologically active metabolites in comparison to other algal classes.

Seaweeds are used for a great number of applications by man. The principal uses of seaweeds are as a source of human food and as a source of gums (phycocollides). Phycocolloides like agar agar, alginic acid, and carrageenan are primarily constituents of brown and red algal cell walls and are widely used in industry (251).

Microalgae are microscopic single cells (from some ten µm to some hundreds µm), and comprise more than 50,000 different types of microalgal species (254–255). Some wild green microalgae like spirulina, chlorella, and dunaliella can easily grow in either seawater (oceans) or freshwater (lakes, ponds, and rivers); among these species, only 30,000 have been studied (254–255). Other microalgae include blue green algae, dinoflagellates, and bacillariophyta (diatoms) (251). The microalgae phyla have been recognized to provide chemical and pharmacological novelty and diversity. Moreover, microalgae produce many highly bioactive compounds found in marine resources (251).

Like plants, micro- and macroalgae can transform carbon dioxide (CO_2) in the atmosphere by photosynthesis into organic molecules like glucose in their cells with the aid of sunlight and water, and then release oxygen in the air. Algae produce approximately half of the atmospheric oxygen and use gas carbon dioxide to grow and constitute the basic foodstuff for numerous aquaculture species such as fishes, mollusks, crustaceans, and so on (249–255).

Algae synthesize a number of nutrients like vitamins, omega-3 fatty acids, minerals, and antioxidants that are consumed by aquatic animals and humans. Macro- and microalgae are especially rich in iodine, calcium, magnesium, iron, zinc, copper, selenium, sulfur, and phosphorous. They are also high in vitamins and antioxidants such as vitamins C, E, K, carotenoids (β-carotene, astaxanthin, fucoxanthin, canthaxanthin, lutein), and many of the B-complex vitamins, in particular vitamin B12. Contrary to other vegetables, macro- and microalgae are the unique plants containing vitamin B12 in the high quantity (249–260). Fruits and vegetables cannot produce vitamin B12. Moreover, they also contain different omega-3 fatty acids including alpha-linoleic acid (ALA), eicosapentaenoic acid (EPA) and docosahexaenoic acid (DHA), proteins, amino acids, and polysaccharides (dietary fibers, alginates, fucoidans, carrageenan, beta-glucans, ulvans, agar) (249–260). It is noteworthy that only algae can synthesize the two active forms omega-3 EPA and DHA, contrary to other vegetables and fruits that only contain ALA, an inactive form of omega-3 unsaturated fatty acids. As other animals, fishes and crustaceans cannot synthesize omega-3 fatty acids, they get them by consuming algae. ALA, EPA, and DHA are essential fatty acids for humans. Concerning vitamin D, some microalgae contain cholesterol and some provitamin D3 sterols like sitosterol, desmosterol, and fucosterol (261). However, it is difficult to make any conclusions about algae's production of vitamin D3 in fish (261).

Brown algae like kelp, rockweed, mozuku, kombu, wakame, limu moui, and bladderwrack contain high levels of fucoidan, fucoxanthin, iodine, alginic acid, and omega-3 fatty acids. The brown seaweeds containing fucoidan are widely consumed as part of the normal diet in East Asia, mostly Japan, Korea, China, and Philippines (250–253, 257–259). The Japanese, in particular the Okinawans, enjoy the longest life expectancies in the world, thanks to their dietary intake of fish, seaweed (mozuku, kombu, wakame), and soy (253). Green microalgae like chlorella and green macroalgae like sea lettuce are abundant in omega-3 unsaturated fatty acids (ALA, EPA and DHA), chlorophylls, and minerals. Red macro-algae like Irish moss or carrageen moss (*Chondrus crispus*) and freshwater green microalgae like *Haematococcus pluvialis* are considered the highest sources of astaxanthin (249–250, 254, 255, 260). *Spirulina*, especially the variety *Spirulina platensis* is a blue-green filamentous microalga that became famous after it was successfully used by NASA (National Aeronautics and Space Administration) as a dietary supplement for astronauts on space missions (256). It is high in protein (up to 70%), and also contains vitamins, especially B12, vitamin D3, and provitamin A (β-carotenes), as well as minerals, especially iron. It is also rich in phenolic acids, tocopherols, and γ-linolenic acid. This alga represents an important staple diet in humans and has been used as a source of protein and vitamin supplement in humans without any significant side effects. *Spirulina* may improve several symptoms of hypercholesterolemia and allergic rhinitis, and may even have anticancer, antiatherogenic, antiviral, and immunomodulator properties (254, 256).

Nowadays, among different phytochemicals present in macro and microalgae, the three compounds most cited in scientific literature as well as in industrial investigation include fucoidan, astaxanthin, and iodine.

2.5.1 Fucoidan

Fucoidan or fucoidans cover a family of sulfated fucose-rich polysaccharides, and are found in brown seaweeds and echinoderms (marine animals like starfish, sea urchin) (257–260). Despite their phylogenetic proximity to brown algae, red and green algae do not have fucoidan in their cell walls (262).

Fucoidan has potential therapeutic properties, including anti-proliferative effects on cancer cells, antioxidant, immunoregulatory, hepatoprotective, anti-inflammatory, anti-viral, as well as anti-thrombotic and anti-coagulant activities (257–260, 262–263). It has anti-cancer activity against various cancer types by targeting key apoptotic molecules. It also has beneficial effects as it can protect against toxicity associated with radiation and chemotherapeutic agents. Thus, the synergistic effect of fucoidan with current anti-cancer agents is of great interest (257, 258, 262). Fucoidan also has nutraceutical and cosmeceutical applications.

Currently, fucoidans are available for use in cosmetics, functional foods, dietary supplements, and for inclusion in pet, livestock, and aquaculture feed supplements. To date there are no approved uses for fucoidan fractions in biomedical applications, either within biomaterials, or via direct administration (intravenous, intraperitoneal, intramuscular, or subcutaneous) (260). However, research on the use of fucoidan in the delivery of drugs and biomaterials as a topical agent and as an orally administered agent for a variety of pathologies appears promising. There is also a wealth of evidence to support an anticancer function of fucoidan, but the majority of evidence comes from in vitro or animal studies. The exact mechanism of action of fucoidan in cancer treatment remains unknown (262–263). As fucoidan is not a drug approved by the FDA, it is still a dietary supplement; therefore, its quality and purity in the market vary enormously and leave much to be desired. So, consult a doctor before use of fucoidan for any treatment.

2.5.2 Astaxanthin

Astaxanthin is a red xanthophyll carotenoid which is mainly found in green microalgae (264–267). It is considered a 'super antioxidant' among different natural antioxidants. Green microalgae include more than 7,000 species growing in a variety of habitats (264). The main microalgae containing astaxanthin include: *Haematococcus pluvialis*, *Chlorella zofingiensis*, *Chlorococcum*, and *Phaffia rhodozyma* (265). Among them, *Haematococcus pluvialis* (Chlorophyceae, Volvocales) is considered the richest source of natural astaxanthin with the best quality. It is a unicellular freshwater microalga distributed in many habitats worldwide. *H. pluvialis* is harvested for the production of pure natural astaxanthin (266–267). Astaxanthin is also present in many seafood including salmon, trout, red sea bream, shrimp, lobster, and fish eggs. These animals consume algae, therefore they accumulate astaxanthin, a red pigment, in their body, giving them the reddish color which brightens the flesh, skin, or exoskeleton. Wild caught salmon and large trout are good sources of astaxanthin (265).

Recently, astaxanthin from artificial sources has entered the marketplace. The primary alternative source in the human nutritional supplement market has been a synthetic form of astaxanthin produced from petrochemicals (266). Additionally, a very small amount of astaxanthin from a genetically-manipulated yeast *Xanthophyllomyces dendrorhous* is also available in some supplement products (266). The three forms: natural astaxanthin, synthetic astaxanthin, and semi-synthetic astaxanthin have substantial chemical differences. In addition to the chemical differences between sources of astaxanthin, *in vitro* research has demonstrated profound differences in antioxidant strength, and animal research has revealed fundamental differences in health benefits. In all cases, only natural astaxanthin obtained by direct extraction of astaxanthin from *H. pluvialis* has proven more biologically active than the other sources (266). Currently, over 95% of the astaxanthin available in the market is produced synthetically; while *H. pluvialis* derived natural astaxanthin corresponds to <1% of the commercialized quantity (264). Synthetic astaxanthin has 20 times lower antioxidant capacity than its natural counterpart and to date has not been approved for human consumption (264). Therefore, be careful when you buy astaxanthin supplement in the market because supplement is not a controlled product, contrary to drug. Synthetic astaxanthin is used as a colorant for foodstuffs and for aquaculture.

In terms of antioxidant activity, natural astaxanthin is 65 times more powerful than vitamin C, 54 times stronger than β-carotene, ten times more potent than canthaxantin, zeaxanthin, and lutein, and 100 times more effective than α-tocopherol (vitamin E) (264). Therefore, astaxanthin is named a 'super antioxidant'. Many studies have shown that astaxanthin has protective effects against diseases, such as cancers, eye diseases, inflammatory diseases, metabolic syndrome, diabetes, diabetic nephropathy, and neurodegenerative diseases. In addition, astaxanthin enhances the immune system and inhibits cancer proliferation in animal as well as in vitro studies (255, 264–267). Regular consumption of red seafood such as salmon, trout, crustaceans, and some comestible algae is the best way to provide astaxanthin and other antioxidants to the body.

2.5.3 Iodine

Marine algae or seaweeds are a good nutritional source for iodine (250, 253, 263, 268–272). Seaweeds have the unique ability to concentrate iodine from the ocean, with certain types of brown seaweed accumulating over 30,000 times the iodine concentration of seawater (272). The genus Laminaria of brown algae is the strongest accumulator of iodine currently known and is a major emitter of both molecular iodine (I_2) and iodinated organics (CH_3I and CH_2I_2) into the atmosphere (268). These compounds (I_2, CH_3I and CH_2I_2) are thus considered a major carrier of gas phase iodine from the ocean to atmosphere, which in turn supplies iodine in precipitation to marine and terrestrial environments (271). The emission of these gasses from seaweeds also contributes to the destruction of the tropospheric ozone layer; an important link between ocean biology, atmospheric composition, and climate (268, 271–272).

However, not all brown algae accumulate high levels of iodine; for example, the kelps Undaria (wakame) and Alaria (Atlantic wakame) have lower iodine levels that are comparable to Palmaria palmata (dulse, a red sea vegetable) (250). The knowledge of iodine levels in algae, mostly in seaweeds is important to maintain good iodine concentrations in the human body and to avoid toxicity. Nevertheless, there is clear evidence that algal food consumption leads to elevated iodine levels in humans. In the Laminariales, iodine is mostly stored as inorganic iodine (I_2, I^-, IO_3^-) which amounts to 80–90% of the total iodine content, the remainder consisting of the iodinated amino acids, mono- and diiodotyrosine (271). In seaweeds, iodine (I_2) can be bound to organic compounds like proteins and fatty acids to form an unstable complex. Iodine (I_2) and organic iodine (CH_3I and CH_2I_2) become volatile when cooking. Therefore, the levels of iodine before and after cooking of seaweeds are largely different and depend on cooking modes. It is noteworthy that the levels of iodine in table salt or iodized salt used as supplement remain invariable before and after cooking because iodine is in iodide (I^-) form only.

Iodine is an essential micromineral (metalloid) required for the synthesis and function of triiodothyronine (T3) and thyroxine (T4), thyroid hormones of the thyroid gland (263, 269). In humans, these hormones are required for growth and development of the brain and the central nervous system. They also control the carbohydrate, fat, protein, vitamin, and mineral metabolism (269). An insufficient or excessive supply of iodine from foods is harmful to the body (see the description in Chapter 2 of this book). The current recommended daily iodine intake (RDI) level, as suggested by WHO and UNICEF, depend on age, gender, and health status. General guidelines propose 90–120 μg/day for infants and children, 150 μg/day for adults, and 200 μg/day for pregnant and lactating women (269). An iodine deficient diet may lead to major health concerns such as the dysfunction and/or an enlargement of the thyroid gland. On the other hand, ingestion of iodine at levels above the RDI can also negatively affect human health (269). Currently in Japan, iodine intake ranges from one to three mg/day, and is largely due to the daily consumption of edible seaweeds; iodine intake by the Japanese is among the highest in the world (269, 272). The epidemiological evidence detailing the risks and benefits of iodine intake from seaweeds remains inconclusive (263). Seaweed consumption was associated with increased risk of papillary carcinoma of the thyroid in Japanese postmenopausal women but not premenopausal women. However, another study found no association between seaweed consumption and total thyroid cancer risk or papillary carcinoma in premenopausal or postmenopausal women (263). In most cases, avoid consumption of iodine supplement (iodized salts) over the RDA (recommended daily allowance). The quantity of iodine ingested from seaweeds depends on their species, their cooking modes, and their quantity consumed. In Japan, over 20 species of red, green, and brown seaweeds are included in meals (272). The three most popular seaweed products in Japan are nori (Porphyra), wakame (Undaria), and kombu (Laminaria). Dried iodine contents range from 16 μg/g in nori to over 8,000 μg/g in kelp flakes; Japanese kombu and wakame contain an estimated 2,353 μg/g and 42 μg/g, respectively (272). When kombu is boiled in water for 15 minutes it can lose up to 99% of its iodine content, while iodine in sargassum, a similar brown seaweed, loses around 40% (272). The myriad variations in iodine concentration between seaweed species, season, and harvest location present challenges to the food industry (263). Algae also contain some contaminants such as mercury, arsenic, and industrial wastes. Therefore, do not consume wild seaweeds. The best way is to consume cultivated or Japanese seaweeds. In conclusion, algae are a rich and sustainable source of many essential macronutrients and micronutrients that are not found in other plant and animal foods. More studies in humans are necessary on fucoidan, astaxanthin, and iodine in algae.

2.6 PLANT-BASED FOOD PRODUCTS

Plant-based food products are products obtained from plants for food purposes via various modes of processing. They mainly include vegetable oils, cocoa and chocolate, and plant-based beverages.

2.6.1 Vegetable Oils

Vegetable oils are lipid liquid extracted from different parts of plants such as seeds (rapeseed, sunflower seed), legumes (peanut, soybean), nuts (walnut, almond), or the flesh of some fruits (olives) (273–276). Vegetable oils are pressed from the plants and are then processed and refined to produce high-quality oils suitable for use as an ingredient in recipes, for frying, in salad dressings, and in the production of margarines and spreads (273). Culinary oils are liquid at room temperature. Major edible vegetable oils in terms of production include soybean, sunflower, palm oil, and rapeseed, which together account for approximately 79% of the total production in the world (273–275). Other oils such as olive oil, sesame oil, peanut oil, corn oil, canola oil, flaxseed oil, and coconut oil are also used for frying, salad dressing, and snack food processing. Some oils extracted from nuts like almond oil, walnut oil, cashew oil, and pine nut oil are very expensive and mainly used as flavoring agents or in traditional medicine. Oils obtained by distillation are called essences, which are mainly destined for medicinal or cosmetic uses.

Vegetable oils contain different triacylglycerols (triglycerides) and fatty acids (saturated and unsaturated). Their composition and concentration vary according to each type of oil. Most culinary oils tend to be predominantly unsaturated and high in either monounsaturated fatty acid (e.g., rapeseed oil, olive oil, peanut oil) or polyunsaturated fatty acid (e.g., corn oil, sunflower oil, walnut oil) (273–275). However, there are some vegetable oils that are high in saturated fatty acid, particularly coconut oil (86%) and palm kernel oil (82%) (273). In addition, vegetable oils also contain vitamin E (tocopherols and tocotrienols) in appreciable amounts, as well as some minor components like phospholipids, sphingolipids, and squalene, all of which may provide a range of health benefits such as antioxidant, anti-inflammatory, antidiabetic, and cardio-protective effects (273–275). Contrary to animal fats, pure vegetables oils are safe and cannot cause cancer. However, some culinary oils such as peanut oil, sesame oil, and soybean oil can cause allergy for some people who are sensitive to the corresponding nuts and seeds. Remember that used oils must be discarded because they can contain acrolein and other toxic products formed during frying foods. High consumption of fried foods might increase the risk of obesity, cardiovascular disease (CVD), and diabetes (276). Some recent studies did not support the myth that frying foods is generally associated with a higher risk of CVD. They also observed that frying foods with virgin olive oil significantly reduces the risk of CVD clinical events (276). However, heating any type of unsaturated oil at high temperatures will result in the breakdown of double bonds present in the fat, which leads to the formation of compounds such as short-chain aldehydes (273). Therefore, do not fry meat or foods to the point of carbonization or dark color because of the formation of acrolein and other carcinogenic compounds. In addition, high intake of fried foods such as French fries may cause overweightness and obesity (276).

In recent years there has been an increasing use of plant oils for production of biofuels and chemical feedstocks. Biodiesel is already a major fuel derived from plant oils such as rapeseed, sunflower, or palm (274–275). There are also numerous uses and applications of plant oils for plant-derived industrial feedstocks such as the fabrication of detergent, soap, cosmetic, toothpaste, pharmaceutical, food, lubricant, and so on (274–275).

The chemical composition and health benefits of some common plant oils such as olive oil, soybean oil, sunflower oil, peanut oil, flaxseed oil, rapeseed oil, palm oil, and microalgae oil, are described below.

2.6.1.1   Olive Oil

Olive oil is mainly produced and consumed in the Mediterranean area and is a major component of the Mediterranean diet (273). In recent years, it has become more popular in Northern Europe, the United States and Canada. This increase in popularity is attributable to studies showing that the consumption of a Mediterranean-style diet, including olive oil, is beneficial in the prevention of cardiovascular diseases and the promotion of longevity (273, 276). The beneficial properties of olive oil are mainly attributable to the high content of oleic acid, vitamin E, and phenolic compounds. The fatty acid composition of the olive oil is around 14% saturates, 73% monounsaturates (oleic acid, an omega-9), and 8% polyunsaturates (mainly in the form of linoleic acid, an omega-6) (273). Eating about two tablespoons of uncooked olive oil a day may reduce the risk of heart disease due to hypercholesterolemia (273). Food fried with olive oil does not lead to overweightness or obesity, unlike other vegetable oils (276). Olive oil is used as a dressing for salads and for frying foods. It is thermo-stable and gives a pleasant taste.

2.6.1.2   Soybean Oil

Soybean oil is the most widely used oil in the world because soybeans are a commonly produced agricultural crop. Soybean oil comprises approximately 60% polyunsaturates (primarily linoleic acid, an omega-6, and also relatively high amounts of alpha-linolenic acid, an omega-3 fatty acid), 20% monounsaturates, and 15% saturates. It also contains some minor components, such as gamma-tocopherol (vitamin E) and phytosterols (273). About 95% of the soybean oil produced worldwide is used in food applications such as the production of margarine and cooking oils and the preparation of salad. Health benefits of soybean oil are still not evident. A clinical study found that soybean germ oil reduced serum total cholesterol and low-density lipoprotein (LDL), or bad cholesterol, compared with a control group using safflower oil (273). Soybean, soybean oil, fish, and seaweed are the main components of the Japanese diet.

2.6.1.3   Sunflower Oil

Sunflower seeds have a high oil content. They are very high in polyunsaturates and low in saturates. The oil is used in cooking and for dressing salads. The seeds can also be eaten as a snack. Sunflower oil has a high polyunsaturated content (typically 65–70% linoleic acid, an *n*-6 fatty acid) and a minor monounsaturated acid (oleic acid). Sunflower oil also contains a number of other compounds including tocopherols, plant sterol and stanol esters, and phospholipids. The high proportion of linoleic acid in sunflower oil may improve blood lipid profile and thus reduce risk of cardiovascular diseases (CVDs) (273).

2.6.1.4   Peanut Oil

Peanut oil is extracted from peanuts. It is most commonly used for frying and cooking, as well as in salad dressings. It is suitable for deep-fat frying as it has a high smoke point (229.4°C), which allows the food to cook quickly and develop a crisp coating without absorbing too much oil. Peanut oil is particularly popular in Chinese cookery because of its subtle flavor. The fatty acid composition of peanut oil is around 20% saturates, 50% monounsaturates (oleic acid), and 30% polyunsaturates (linoleic acid). Contrary to whole peanuts, the beneficial effects of peanut oil in the prevention of CVDs are not evident (273). As whole peanuts, unrefined peanut oils can cause allergy in sensitive individuals. In refined peanut oil, all allergens are removed, so this oil is not allergenic. Peanut oil must be labelled as an allergen, whether it is fully refined or not. One of the problems with peanuts and peanut oil production is the potential for contamination with aflatoxin. This is a potentially carcinogenic compound produced by *Aspergillus* and *Aspergillus parasiticus*, which can contaminate peanuts as well as corn and other food commodities (273).

2.6.1.5   Flaxseed Oil

The oil extracted from flaxseed is often called linseed oil and has been widely used for non-culinary purposes. Flaxseed oil has become a popular dietary supplement because of its reputed health-promoting properties. Flaxseed is a cultivar of *Linum usitatissimum* (family Linaceae). The fatty acid profile of flaxseed oil is largely comprised of polyunsaturates (66%), primarily the omega-3 fatty acid alpha-linolenic acid (ALA) (over 50%), and it is this that makes the oil oxidize rapidly (273). The oil also contains 440–588 mg/100 g of tocopherols. Flaxseed oil may reduce platelet aggregation for the prevention of blood clots and may improve autoimmune disorders. However, excessive intake of flaxseed supplement may cause hemorrhage. Due to its low oxidative stability, it has little use in food preparation.

2.6.1.6   Rapeseed Oil

Rapeseed oil is the oil extracted from the seed of rape or colza or canola that is the *Brassica* genus of the Cruciferae family (broccoli, cabbage, and cauliflower). Rapeseed is intended for the production of culinary oils and biodiesel. The byproduct of oil production is rich in protein and is used as animal feeds. Rapeseed oil is lower in saturates (6.6 g/100 g) than all other vegetable oils, high in mono-unsaturated fatty acids (59.3 g/100 g), and has a high ALA (9.6 g/100 g) and lower LA (19.7 g/100 g) content compared to other vegetable oils (273). It therefore provides a good balance of omega-3 to omega-6 polyunsaturated fatty acids. However, rapeseed oils produced from the cultivars of *Brassica napus* or *Crambe abyssinica* are rich in erucic acid (55–60%) which is toxic to cardiac muscles (273–275). In addition, rapeseed oils contain glucosinolates, which interfere with the uptake of iodine by the thyroid gland in animals (273). Rapeseed is cheap; therefore, it is used to produce biodiesel. Rapeseed oil is commonly used as a cooking oil, in pan frying and salad dressings.

2.6.1.7   Palm Oil

Palm oil is the cheapest of all the major edible oils and fats. There are two types of oil obtained from the fruit: oil from the flesh of the fruit and oil from the kernel inside the nut (palm kernel oil). The latter is primarily used for the oleochemical industry, although it does have some food applications. The oil from the flesh of the fruit can be separated into liquid and solid fractions (olein and stearin, respectively). From these, the refining industry produces various types of palm oil for different applications. Palm oil and palm oil products are commonly used in the food manufacturing industry (273). Palm oil has equal proportions of saturated and unsaturated fatty acids. Saturated fatty acids are represented by palmitic acid (44%) and stearic acid (5%). Unsaturated fatty acids are represented by oleic acid (37%), a monounsaturated fatty acid, and linoleic acid (9%), a poly-unsaturated omega-6 fatty acid. The minor components of palm oil also vary depending on the conditions of refining. Crude palm oil is rich in carotenes, tocopherols, tocotrienols, sterols, and squalene (273). Concerning palm oil and health, some studies gave contradictory results on CVDs. Some authors concluded that palm oil had no adverse health consequences. However, studies that have compared the effects of palm oil with other oils have reported adverse effects on heart health of both palm oil and hydrogenated oils (273). Therefore, it is prudent not to consume palm oil too often or in large quantity.

2.6.1.8 Algae Oil

Algae is the unique plant that produces active omega-3 fatty acids: eicosapentaenoic acid (EPA) and docosahexaenoic acid (DHA). Microalgae is a potential source for the production of algae oil. Some microalgae such as *Mortierella alpina, Fistulifera, Phaedodactylum tricornutum* species and diatoms have been used to produce oil for commercial use (274). However, many of these microalgae are not suitable for large scale production, and the technology needs further optimization, as obtainment of oils is costly and still not profitable (274). Therefore, fish oils are still a good source for dietary supplements of omega-3 EPA and DHA in the market.

In conclusion, vegetable oils are better than animal fats because most vegetable oils are richer in unsaturated fatty acids than animal fats, except seafoods. The choice of different types of vegetable oils depends on the availability of this vegetable oil in the market, its price, its flavor, its cooking mode, and the scientific knowledge of the consumer. Vegetable oils are also used in different industries for the production of biofuel, pharmaceuticals, soaps, candles, cosmetic products, and so on.

2.6.2   Cocoa and Chocolate

Cocoa is the dried and fully fermented fatty seed (bean) of the fruit of the cacao tree, *Theobroma cacao,* belonging to the family Sterculiaceae (277–279). Chocolate is the food prepared from roasted cacao seeds. Foods, beverages, and medicines made from beans of the fruit cacao have been consumed by Mayas and Aztecs in Mesoamerica (from Mexico to Costa Rica) since antiquity, maybe more than 3,000 years ago (277–279). Cacao was diffused to Europe in the mid-1500s and now cultivated in Indonesia and Brazil, as well as some countries in Africa. Cocoa liquor is the paste made from ground, roasted, shelled, and fermented cocoa beans, called nibs, which have a dark brown color. Cocoa liquor is not a liquid, as its name implies. It contains both nonfat cocoa solids and cocoa butter. Cocoa butter is the viscous oil made from pressing fresh cocoa seeds and has a white color. Cocoa powder is made by removing some of the cocoa butter from the liquor. Most chocolate recipes are made by combining dark brown cocoa liquor with white cocoa butter and sugar. The proportion of cocoa liquor in the final product determines how dark the chocolate is (277–278). White chocolate contains only pure cocoa butter mixed with sugar and eventually milk solids. Milk chocolate is a mixture of milk powder and brown chocolate. The seeds of cacao fruit contain an enormous quantity of beneficial components. However, many bioactive compounds have been altered by the processing and manufacturing of dark chocolate, especially during the roasting, fermentation, and drying of cacao seeds (278–279). Therefore, white chocolate is considered healthier than dark chocolate because it contains only untreated cocoa butter, though its flavor is not the same.

Cocoa liquor is a complex food and contains many bioactive compounds. Cocoa butter contains significant amounts of fatty acids, whereas the nonfat cocoa solids contain vitamins, minerals, fiber, and polyphenols (277–279). The oil in cocoa butter is a mixture of monounsaturated and saturated fatty acids. In the monounsaturated fraction, oleic acid, predominates, with a concentration of about 33%. The majority of the saturated fatty acids are palmitic acid (25%) and stearic acid (33%). Oleic acid has a positive effect by decreasing lipid and cholesterol levels, while saturated fats like stearic acid and palmitic acid adversely increase them. However, in the case of cocoa butter, stearic acid may not have any effect on lipid levels; it does not elevate serum lipid levels to the same degree that other saturated fatty acids do (277, 279). Therefore, obesity has not been observed due to moderate consummation of dark chocolate.

Cocoa is a rich source of polyphenolic antioxidants with high amounts of flavonoids such as epicatechin, catechin, and procyanidins (277–279). Dark chocolate contains considerably higher amounts of flavonoids than milk chocolate. Moreover, the milk may slow down the intestinal absorption of flavonoids (277, 279). Due to their high amounts of polyphenol antioxidants, cocoa and chocolate increase the production or bioavailability of endothelial nitric oxide (NO). Nitric oxide regulates vasodilation and the environment of the blood vessel wall. Therefore, cocoa and chocolate may be useful for the prevention of hypertension and atherosclerosis. In addition, cocoa contains theobromine (2–3%) and caffeine (0.2%) (277). Theobromine is a purine alkaloid. It stimulates heart muscle and relaxes bronchial smooth muscles for the treatment of asthma. In addition, theobromine has antioxidant activity and may be used for depression therapy (278). Chocolate and cacao bean are rich in essential minerals like magnesium, copper, potassium, and iron – mostly magnesium (277–279). These minerals may enhance the activities of some polyphenol antioxidants.

Briefly, moderate consumption of cocoa and chocolate is safe and healthful. They might prevent some diseases like hypertension, atherosclerosis, asthenia, asthma, stress, aging, and dry skin. However, excess intake of chocolate tablets and drinks may cause obesity, constipation, palpitation, insomnia, migraine, and acne due to the presence of theobromine, caffeine, tannins, saturated fatty acids, and sugar in cocoa products.

2.6.3 Plant-Based Beverages: Tea, Coffee, Juice Fruits, Alcohols

Beverages obtained from plants via different industrial processing or individual preparation such as tea, coffee, juice fruits, and alcohols, have been described in Chapter 4, paragraph 'Beverage types' of this book.

Tea is the most widely consumed beverage in the world, aside from water. Green tea contains strong antioxidants mainly due to catechins belonging to the polyphenolic flavonoids which may prevent many ailments such as cancer, cardiovascular diseases, and inflammatory diseases (280).

2.7 MEDICINAL PLANTS AND THEIR ACTIVE COMPOUNDS

The list of plants used in traditional medicine as well as in modern medicine is extensive. They are used either as supplements or as drugs prescribed by a doctor. Medicinal plants can have side effects or interferences with other drugs. Only a few of them that are considered nontoxic and legal to sell over the counter as supplements are listed below. Most medicinal plants are not used as foods or for culinary purposes.

2.7.1 Ginkgo Biloba Leaves

Ginkgo biloba (family Ginkgoceae) is a unique tree, known to be among the oldest living species on this planet, and has flourished in forests for over 150 million years. A single tree can live as long as 1,000 years, even 2,000 years, and can have a large trunk with a girth of about 7 m (23 feet) and a height of about 30 m (110 feet) (281–283). It can resist weather changes, bad environment, parasite, or insect invasion, and even radiation from a nuclear bomb. The leaves of Ginkgo are deciduous and have two lobes, hence the name biloba. *Ginkgo biloba* leaves and seeds have been used as a traditional herbal remedy for thousands of years in China, Japan, Korea, and its leaf extract has been consumed as a botanical dietary supplement in capsule form for therapeutic use in modern medicine in Western countries for half a century (281–283). *Ginkgo biloba* leaf extract is one of the best-selling botanical dietary supplements in the United States (282). Cooked or roasted nuts from ginkgo fruits are used as food and traditional medicine in many Asian countries. However, these nuts are not authorized to commercialize as supplement in Western countries because they become toxic in case of excessive intake. Moreover, the healthy compounds of ginkgo nuts are much lower than those of ginkgo leaves.

There are numerous chemical compounds present in *Ginkgo biloba* leaf. The two main pharmacologically active groups of compounds contained in Ginkgo leaf extract are the flavonoids and the terpenoids (281–283). Only two types of terpenoids are found in Ginkgo leaf: ginkgolides and bilobalide. Ginkgolides are diterpene trilactones with five types (A, B, C, J, and M), while bilobalide is a unique sesquiterpene trilactone (281, 283). Flavonoids frequently present in Ginkgo leaf extract are: flavones, biflavones (bilobetol, amentoflavone, 5 methoxybilobetol, ginkgetin, isoginkgetin and sciadopitysin), flavonols, tannins, and glycosides of quercetin and kaempferol (283). The standardized preparation of Ginkgo leaf extract made from the dried green leaves is named EGb 761 and contains two main bioactive constituents, flavonoid glycosides (about 24%) and terpene lactones (ginkgolides and bilobalide about 6%), along with less than five ppm of the allergenic component, ginkgolic acid (281, 283). Terpenoids such as ginkgolides and bilobalide help vasodilation, blood circulation, platelet anti-aggregation, and more.

The main pharmacological and therapeutic properties of ginkgo leaf extract include (281–283):

- Neuroprotection for the treatment of some neurological disorders and neural damage such as cerebral vascular disease, dementia, Alzheimer's disease, shaking hand, memory and learning loss, cognitive function disorder, anxiety, depression, schizophrenia, vertigo, attention deficit hyperactivity disorder, etc.
- Antioxidant and anti-inflammatory activities for the treatment of asthma, chronic bronchitis, aging, tinnitus (ringing in the ears), glaucoma, macular degeneration, intermittent claudication, etc.
- Vasodilatation and platelet anti-aggregation for the prevention and treatment of some diseases like hypertension, ischemia, leg pain, premenstrual syndrome by improvement of coronary blood flow.

However, the results found in a recent clinical study of ginkgo extract supplements make them controversial for many reasons. The main reason is due to its extraction. The commercial extracts of ginkgo leaves could be 'full extracts', 'crude extracts', or 'simple extracts' that are complex mixtures consisting of active principles, inert plant constituents, and in some cases, constituents that may cause adverse side effects (281). The standardized extract named EGb761 is now prepared by many manufacturers in the world. In addition, herbal remedies are not held to the same standards of purity and efficacy. As such, tremendous variability of the same product can occur between manufacturers and from batch to batch because herbal dietary supplement products are not submitted to the FDA (281). That may explain some contradictory results and side effects found in the recent literature. Therefore, the choice of ginkgo biloba supplements in the market is a great problem for consumers. In general, ginkgo leaf extract has some side effects. Adverse effects of high ginkgo intake include excessive bleeding, gastrointestinal upset, headache, dizziness, and hives (282). However, recently *Ginkgo biloba* leaf extract has been classified as a possible human carcinogen (Group 2B) by the International Agency for Research on Cancer (IARC) (282). Consult a doctor before using ginkgo supplement alone or in combination with other drugs. More research regarding ginkgo is needed.

2.7.2 Ginseng

Ginseng is the root of plants belonging to the genus Panax of the Araliaceae family. Ginseng is both food and medicine, mostly used as ginseng-infused tea or liquor since antiquity in Asian traditional medicine and now as powder or extract in capsule for dietary supplement (284–290). There are 12 species of the genus Panax. The most well-known are *Panax ginseng* or Korean ginseng, *Panax japonicas* or Japanese ginseng, *Panax notoginseng* or Chinese ginseng, *Panax quinquefolius* or American ginseng, and *Panax vietnamensis* or Vietnamese ginseng (284). Ginseng is native in Northeast Asia (Korea, China, Japan, Far East Siberia of Russia), and now also cultivated in North America (Canada, USA) and Vietnam. Ginseng roots are available in the market in wild and cultivated form. Wild ginseng grows naturally mainly in forest and is rare and very expensive because it is more appreciated than cultivated ginseng. Cultivated species can be classified by its processing methods and include fresh ginseng (raw ginseng), white ginseng (air-dried), and red ginseng (steamed, then sun-dried) (286, 287). As fresh ginseng tends to be easily degraded at room temperature, it has traditionally been processed into white ginseng through air drying of the root or into red ginseng through root steaming without peeling the root, followed by sun drying (284, 286–287, 289). White ginseng is cited as a monograph in different international pharmacopeias. But until now, international ginseng monographs including those of the World Health Organization have been based on data on white ginseng and have mentioned red ginseng only partly (286). Red ginseng is mainly produced in Korea. Red ginseng was originally developed for the purpose of improving the preservation of ginseng for long-term storage. Both white and red ginsengs have similar chemical properties and pharmacological activities (285). They both have potential anti-inflammatory activities that relate to immunomodulation. Results suggest that both white ginseng and red ginseng may have an anticancer effect, though their mechanisms or pathways may differ (285). However, white ginseng has an anti-inflammatory effect that is stronger than that of beclomethasone, while red ginseng shows no significant effect (285). Red ginseng occupies an important position as a healthy functional food.

Ginseng roots contain various functional constituents, including mainly ginseng saponins called ginsenosides, and secondary non-saponin compounds such as polysaccharides, polyacetylenes, phenolic compounds, sesquiterpenes, alkaloids, and oligopeptides (284–290). Ginsenosides have anti-inflammatory and antioxidant properties. The amounts of ginsenosides vary according to harvest time, storage condition, and processing methods. Concerning ginsenoside levels and their biological benefits, red Korean ginseng is considered better than fresh and white Korean ginseng, and also better than other varieties throughout the world (285–287).

In Asian traditional medicine, ginseng has been used for its tonic and aphrodisiac effects since antiquity. In Korea, China, and Japan, ginseng is used not only as a nourishing and tonifying agent but also as a therapeutic agent for a variety of diseases including immune diseases, liver diseases, and cancer. Many researchers have scientifically proven its diverse effects through in vitro studies, animal experiment models, and clinical research (286). Recently, ginseng is known to possess various biological activities including boosting the immune system, improving blood circulation, enhancing spermatogenesis, stimulating sexual rapport, treatment of erectile dysfunction, stimulating memory, anti-fatigue effects, and positive effects on menopausal disorder (284–290). In moderate intake, ginseng is considered safe. It has a clear efficacy and no major side effects (287–288). However, insomnia is a common side effect reported. Headache, dizziness, and gastric disturbance have also been observed in long-term intake of ginseng (288). Several studies have warned about adverse effects of red ginseng, including allergies and toxicity to the heart, kidney, liver, and reproductive organs (287). Ask a doctor before taking ginseng supplement with other drugs.

2.7.3   Angelica

Angelica or Radix Angelicae Sinensis (also named Dong Quai or Danggui in Chinese) is the dried root of *Angelica sinensis* (Apiaceae) which is a fragrant and perennial herb native to China, Japan, and Korea. It has been used in Chinese traditional medicine since antiquity (291–293). The chemical constituents of the Angelica extract are classified into essential oil and water-soluble parts. The volatile oil is constituted of many alkyl phthalides (ligustilides) and some terpenes. The water-soluble part or non-volatile fraction includes phenylpropanoids (ferulic acid, coniferyl ferulate), phenolic compounds, carbohydrates, organic acids, benzenoids, and coumarins. Polysaccharide fractions of low relative molecular mass are also present (291–293). In traditional Chinese medicine, Angelica root replenishes blood, promotes blood circulation, relieves pain, and moistens the intestines. It is used to treat chronic constipation and menstrual disorders (291–293). Research has found that Angelica and its active components have anti-hypertensive, antioxidant, anti-arthrosclerotic, and anti-inflammatory properties (293). However, the therapeutic properties of Angelica are still not approved by the Food and Drug Administration or the World Health Organization. Angelica should not be administered to children or patients with diarrhea, hemorrhage or hypermenorrhea, and should not be used during pregnancy or lactation (291–292). Some side effects such as headaches have been observed. Dried crude powder and fluid extracts of Angelica root are the two forms orally used (291–292).

2.7.4 Oregano

Oregano (*Origanum vulgare*), belonging to family Lamiaceae, is a perennial herb native to temperate regions like Mediterranean and Eurasian countries. The leaf is used as medicine, culinary spice and food preservative. The major components associated with antimicrobial activities in oregano include carvacrol and thymol which are terpenoid phenols (248, 294). In ancient Greek and Roman empires, applications of the leaves on the skin were used as an antiseptic and to treat skin sores and aching muscles (cramping) (294). Nowadays, in Western traditional medicine, oregano oil is used to treat cold and troubles of the respiratory and digestive tracts (248, 294). Based on the current scientific literature, oregano extracts have demonstrated antimicrobial effects in vitro, especially on Salmonella serotypes, although the capacity to counter human infections was not well-studied (248, 294). Some preliminary studies showed that oregano exhibited benefits toward the cardiovascular and nervous systems, relieved symptoms of inflammation, and modulated blood sugar and lipids. Well-controlled human studies substantiating these health effects were lacking (294). More research are needed for oregano leaf extracts.

2.7.5 Artemisia

Artemisia is a genus of small herbs and shrubs found in northern temperate regions and belongs to the family Asteraceae (295). Many species of Artemisia are known for their essential oils, mainly in the leaves which have strong aromas and bitter tastes. These volatile oils are constituted of diverse terpenoids and sesquiterpene lactones which have strong pharmacological activities (295). Artemisia is used as flavoring for food and as antiseptic, antiparasitic, antibacterial, antifungal, and more in the treatment of various infections. Here, only two Artemisia species: *Artemisia annua* and *Artemisia herba-alba* are examined as follows.

2.7.5.1 Artemisia Annua

Artemisia annua or sweet wormwood, an herb used in Chinese traditional medicine, has been successfully applied to treat malaria in patients resistant to quinine and its derivatives (296). Malaria is a disease caused by a parasite named Plasmodium which is transmitted from an infected female *Anopheles* mosquito. The discovery of artemisinin, a sesquiterpenoid, isolated from *Artemisia annua* (leaves and stems) and its derivative, dihydro-artemisinin, has saved millions of lives suffering from dreadful malaria around the world. This discovery is due to a Chinese botanist and professor in pharmacy, Mrs. Tu Youyou, born 1930 in China, who received the 2015 Nobel Prize of Medicine and the 2011 Lasker Award in clinical medicine (297). Additionally, research related to artemisinin has been a hot topic in malaria and other fields such as antiviral and anticancer treatment in the past 15 years (297).

2.7.5.2 Artemisia Herba-Alba

This plant is known also as desert wormwood and is mainly found in North African countries. *Artemisia herba-alba* is rich in cineole (eucalyptol) and oxygenated monoterpenes (camphor, borneol). Herbal tea from this species has been used as analgesic, antibacterial, antispasmodic, and hemostatic agents (298). Recently, a study has demonstrated the powerful antimicrobial activity of *Artemisia herba-alba* against different germs in periodontal disease, a dental infection (299).

2.7.6 Ursolic Acid

Ursolic acid (UA) is a natural pentacyclic triterpene compound found in various fruits and vegetables such as the leaves of various plants (rosemary, marjoram, lavender, thyme, oregano, sage, eucalyptus, loquat, and hawthorn), fruits (apple fruit peel), flowers, and berries (300–301). Ursolic acid exhibits excellent anticancer, antimicrobial, antiviral, antiarrhythmic, anti-hyperlipidemic, anti-hypercholesterolemic, cardioprotective, anti-obesity, antidiabetic, neuroprotective, hepatoprotective, and antioxidant properties (300–301). Ursolic acid can be used to prevent or treat various forms of cancer, inflammatory diseases, diabetes, neurodegenerative diseases, muscle atrophy (sarcopenia) in the elderly, and so on (300–301). Ursolic acid also exhibits anti-microbial features against numerous bacteria (Bacillus subtilis, Escherichia coli, Streptococcus pneumoniae, Staphylococcus aureus, Klebsiella pneumoniae), viruses like Hepatitis B virus, Hepatitis C virus, human immunodeficiency virus (HIV), influenza virus, and parasite Plasmodium protozoa causing malaria (301). Recently, a preliminary research showed that ursolic acid and its derivatives (oleanolic acid, carvacrol), might be potential inhibitors against the main protease of Covid-19 by controlling viral replication (302). Ursolic acid is more potent than oleanolic acid and carvacrol in the *in vitro* inhibition of protease of Covid-19. Oleanolic acid is a pentacyclic triterpenoid compound and is found in the same plants as ursolic acid. Carvacrol is a monoterpenoid phenol, possessing a wide range of strong antimicrobial and antiviral activity such as herpes simplex virus, retrovirus, and human respiratory syncytial virus. It is present in essential oil of oregano and thyme plants (302). More researches concerning the interesting phytochemicals ursolic acid and its derivatives are needed in the future for the sake of human health.

2.7.7 Sallow Plant and its Product: Salicylic Acid, Acetylsalicylic Acid or Aspirin

The story of the discovery of aspirin stretches back more than 3,500 years ago when bark from the willow tree was used as a pain reliever and antipyretic (303). Salicylic acid is a secondary metabolite synthetized in the barks and leaves from the willow or sallow tree, a medicinal and ornamental plant. Salicylic acid was first isolated from willow bark in 1828 by Buchner, then refined by Leroux in 1829 and crystallized by Piria in 1838. In 1852, the French chemist Charles Gerhardt (1816–1856) was the first to modify salicylic acid with the introduction of an acetyl group in place of a hydroxyl group, to produce acetylsalicylic acid or aspirin for the first time (303). Rapidly absorbed from the intestine, the pro-drug Aspirin is broken down by hydrolysis in the body to liberate its active compound, salicylic acid. Aspirin is now used as an antipyretic, analgesic, antiplatelet, and anti-inflammatory agent, and has recently been used to prevent stroke and heart attack.

2.7.8 Other Plant-Based Medicines

The list of chemicals obtained from plants and used as medicines is extensive. They are often secondary metabolites of plants including different chemical groups such as flavonoids, terpenoids, alkaloids, glycosides, phenolics, and so on. They are used in modern therapy as well as in traditional medicine (304–306). For example, quinine, an anti-malaria alkaloid, is extracted from the cinchona barks. Digoxin and digitoxin, two cardio-tonic glycosides, are isolated from the plants *Digitalis lanata* and *purpurea*, respectively. Morphine and codeine, two alkaloids used as strong analgesic and antitussive drugs, respectively, are obtained from the opium poppy latex. Cocaine, an alkaloid used as local anesthetic, is isolated from *Erythroxylum coca* leaves. Atropine, an alkaloid used as anticholinergic, is obtained from *Atropa belladonna* leaves. Paclitaxel or Taxol[R], a diterpenoid with strong anticancer activity found in recent years, is isolated from *Taxus brevifolia* and *bacata*, a Pacific yew. Despite their toxicity, these drugs are still used today because of their high therapeutic efficacy (304). Other compounds often present in our habitual foods such as menthol from mint leaves, theobromine and theophylline from cocoa and tea, beta-glucan from oat and yeast, and so on, also have therapeutic activity. They are both food and medicine.

3 DISCUSSION

Cereals (wheat, rice, corn, oats, barley, millets, etc.), potato, sweet potato, and cassava (manioc) are rich in carbohydrates and are used as staple food by many countries in the world. However, people in many areas in the world lack staple food due to drought and heat. Famine still exists through today. Fruits, vegetables whole grains, and other plant foods are universally promoted as healthy.

Regular consumption of fruits and vegetables has been observed with the decrease of chronic ailments such as cardiovascular diseases, cancer, obesity, and diabetes (307). Additionally, they supply dietary fiber, and fiber intake is linked to lower incidence of cardiovascular disease and obesity (307). Fruits and vegetables also supply energy, vitamins, and minerals to the diet and are sources of phytochemicals that function as antioxidants, phytoestrogens, bactericides, and anti-inflammatory agents, as well as through other protective mechanisms (307–308). Fruits and vegetables contain not only vitamins, antioxidants, essential minerals, but also other compounds such as coenzymes and cofactors which enable the bioavailability of vitamins, antioxidants, and minerals in our body. So, consumers should obtain their nutrients, antioxidants, and bioactive compounds from a balanced diet with a wide variety of fruits, vegetables, whole grains, and other plant foods for optimal nutrition, health, and well-being – not from dietary supplements (308). In the United States, fruit and vegetables have been a cornerstone of healthy dietary recommendations; as demonstrated by the 2015–2020 U.S. Dietary Guidelines for Americans which recommend that fruit and vegetables constitute one-half of the plate at each meal (309).

Because vegetables, fruits, tubers, grains, and stems contain most of the essential components of human nutrition (aside from vitamin B12, which exists only in seaweed), vegetarian humans can live as normally, healthfully, and long as their omnivore counterparts. Moreover, products synthetized by plants are very pure and easily absorbable and better than the same products obtained by artificial synthesis.

Thanks to the genes that Nature has assigned to each plant, the number of natural chemical compounds synthesized by plants can be estimated in the millions all over the world. In addition, plants are not only a good source of nutrients, but also an immense treasure of drugs which are still not well-exploited for therapeutic uses.

Moreover, plants furnish not only foods and medicines for humans – they produce oxygen to the atmosphere and protect the environment. Plants have been used since antiquity for the well-being of humans such as in the construction of houses, manufacture of furniture, paper, textile, perfume, rubber, the production of 'green energy' fuel for machinery, and so on.

Protecting forests and cultivating plants are two of the most important missions for all people in the world for the sake of human health.

4   REFERENCES

1. Levetin E., McMahon K. (2011). Chapter 9. Diversity of Plant Life. In: *Plants and Society*. 6th edition. McGraw-Hill Education, New York, 544 pages.
2. National Council of Educational Research and Training (NCERT). (2006). Chapter 3. Plant Kingdom, pp. 29–32. In: *Biology Textbook for Class 11*. https://ncert.nic.in/textbook.php?kebo1 = 3-22.
3. Christenhusz M.J.M, Byng J.W. (2016). The Number of Known Plants Species in the World and Its Annual Increase. *Phytotaxa*, **261**(3): 201–217.
4. Wheeler G.L., Carstens B.C. (2018). Evaluating the Adaptive Evolutionary Convergence of Carnivorous Plant Taxa Through Functional Genomics. *PeerJ.*, **6**: e4322, 1–28.
5. Bentham A.R., De la Concepcion J.C., Mukhi N., Zdrzałek R., Draeger M., Gorenkin D., Hughes R.K., Banfield M.J. (2020). A Molecular Roadmap to the Plant Immune System. *J. Biol. Chem.*, **295**(44): 14916–14935.
6. Heldt H-W., Piechulla B., Heldt F. (2011). *Plant Biochemistry*. 4th Edition. Academic Press, Elsevier, Cambridge, USA, 618 pages.
7. Levetin E., McMahon K. (2011). Chapter 4. Plant Physiology. In: *Plants and Society*. 6th edition. McGraw-Hill Education, New York, 544 pages. http://highered.mheducation.com/sites/0072909498/index.html.
8. Wurtzel E.T., Kutchan T.M. (2016). Plant Metabolism, the Diverse Chemistry Set of the Future. *Science*, **353**(6305): 1232–1236.
9. Keegstra K. (2010). Plant Cell Walls. *Plant Physiol.*, **154**: 483–486.
10. Anderson J., Baird P., Davis R., Ferreri S., Knudtson M., Koraym A., Waters V., Williams C. (2009). Health Benefits of Dietary Fiber. *Nutr. Rev.*, **67**(4): 188–205.

11. Tungland B.C., Meyer D. (2002). Nondigestible Oligo- and Polysaccharides (Dietary Fiber): Their Physiology and Role in Human Health and Food. *Compr. Rev. Food Sci. Food Saf.*, **3**: 90–109.

12. Mudgil D., Barak S. (2013). Composition, Properties and Health Benefits of Indigestible Carbohydrate Polymers as Dietary Fiber: A Review. *Int. J. Biol. Macromol.*, **61**: 1–6.

13. Sabater B. (2018). Evolution and Function of the Chloroplast. Current Investigations and Perspectives. *Int. J. Mol. Sci.*, **19**(10): 3095, 1–5 pages.

14. Fristedt R. (2017). Chloroplast Function Revealed Through Analysis of GreenCut2 Genes. *J. Exp. Bot.*, **68**(9): 2111–2120.

15. Pareek S., Sagar N.A., Sharma S., Vinay K., Agarwal T., Gonzalez-Aguilar G.A., Yahia E.M. (2018). Chapter 14. Chlorophylls: Chemistry and Biological Functions, pp. 269–284. In: *Fruit and Vegetable Phytochemicals: Chemistry and Human Health*, Volume I. 2nd edition. Editor: Elhadi M. Yahia. John Wiley & Sons Ltd, Hoboken, New Jersey, USA.

16. Johnson M.P. (2016). Photosynthesis. *Essays Biochem.*, **60**(3): 255–273.

17. Haryasz J. (2021). Different Types of Evergreen Trees (with Pictures). Identification Guide, April 18. www.gardeningchores.com/types-of-evergreen-trees/.

18. Wyka T.P., Oleksyn J. (2014). Photosynthetic Ecophysiology of Evergreen Leaves in the Woody Angiosperms – A Review. *Dendrobiology*, **72**: 3–27.

19. Verhoeven A. (2014). Sustained Energy Dissipation in Winter Evergreens. Review. *New Phytol.*, **201**: 57–65.

20. Barrett D.M., Beaulieu J.C., Shewfelt R. (2010). Color, Flavor, Texture, and Nutritional Quality of Fresh-Cut Fruits and Vegetables: Desirable Levels, Instrumental and Sensory Measurement, and the Effects of Processing. *Crit. Rev. Food Sci. Nutr.*, **50**: 369–389.

21. Schwab W., Davidovich-Rikanati R., Lewinsohn E. (2008). Biosynthesis of Plant-Derived Flavor Compounds. *Plant J.*, **54**: 712–732.

22. Tanaka Y., Sasaki N., Ohmiya A. (2008). Biosynthesis of Plant Pigments: Anthocyanins, Betalains and Carotenoids. *Plant J.*, **54**: 733–749.

23. Hsu C-Y., Chao P-Y., Hu S-P., Yang C-M. (2013). The Antioxidant and Free Radical Scavenging Activities of Chlorophylls and Pheophytins. *Food Nutr. Sci.*, **4**: 1–8.

24. Fernández-García E., Carvajal-Lérida I., Jarén-Galán M., Garrido-Fernández J., Pérez-Gálvez A., Hornero-Méndez D. (2012). Carotenoids Bioavailability from Foods: From Plant Pigments to Efficient Biological Activities. *Food Res. Int.*, **46**: 438–450.

25. Shi J., Le Maguer M. (2000). Lycopene in Tomatoes: Chemical and Physical Properties Affected by Food Processing. *Crit. Rev. Food Sci. Nutr.* **40**(1): 1–42.

26. Khoo H.E., Azlan A., Tang S.T., Lim S.M. (2017). Anthocyanidins and Anthocyanins: Colored Pigments as Food, Pharmaceutical Ingredients, and the Potential Health Benefits. *Food Nutr. Res.*, **61**(1): 1361779, 1–21.

27. Miguel M.G. (2018). Betalains in Some Species of the Amaranthaceae Family: A Review. *Antioxidants*, **7**(53): 1–33.

28. Rahimi P., Abedimanesh S., Mesbah-Namin S.A., Ostadrahimi A. (2019). Betalains, the Nature-Inspired Pigments, in Health and Diseases. *Crit. Rev. Food Sci. Nutr.*, **59**(18): 2949–2978.

29. Riley P.A. (1997). Melanin. *Int. J. Biochem. Cell Biol.*, **29**(11): 1235–1239.

30. Varga M., Berkesi O., Darula Z., May N.V., Palágyi A. (2016). Structural Characterization of Allomelanin from Black Oat. *Phytochemistry*, **130**: 313–320.

31. ElObeid A.S., Kamal-Eldin A., Abdelhalim M.A.K., Hasee A.M. (2017). Pharmacological Properties of Melanin and Its Function in Health. *Basic Clin. Pharmacol. Toxicol.*, **120**: 515–522.

32. Peter K.V. (2006). *Handbook of Herbs and Spices*, Volume 3. Editor: K.V. Peter. Woodhead Publishing Limited, Cambridge, England, and CRC Press LLC, FL, 559 pages.

33. Hounsome N., Hounsome B., Tomos D., Edwards-Jones G. (2008). Plant Metabolites and Nutritional Quality of Vegetables. *J. Food Sci. J.*, **73**(4): R48–R65.

34. Hussein R.A., El-Anssary A.A. (2018). Chapter 2. Plants Secondary Metabolites: The Key Drivers of the Pharmacological Actions of Medicinal Plants. In: *Herbal Medicine*. Editor: Philip F. Builders. IntechOpen. doi:10.5772/intechopen.76139.

35. Pagare S., Bhatia M., Tripathi N., Pagare S., Bansal Y.K. (2015). Secondary Metabolites of Plants and Their Role: Overview. *Curr. Trends Biotechnol. Pharm.*, **9**(3): 293–304.

36. Wang G., Tang W., Bidigare R.R. (2005). Chapter 9. Terpenoids As Therapeutic Drugs and Pharmaceutical Agents, pp. 197–227. In: *Natural Products: Drug Discovery and Therapeutic Medicine*. Editors: Lixin Zhang, Arnold Demain. Humana Press, Totowa, NJ, 382 pages.

37. Hossain M.T., Asadujjaman Md., Manik Md I.R., Matin Md A., Chowdhury R.Z., Rashid Md H. (2019). A Study on the Pharmacological Effects and Mechanism of Action of Alkaloids, Glycosides and Saponins. *Pharm. Chem. J.*, **6**(2): 112–122.

38. Poudel R., Bhatta M. (2017). Review of Nutraceuticals and Functional Properties of Whole Wheat. *J. Nutr. Food Sci.*, **7**(1): 1–6.

39. Sramkova Z., Gregova E., Sturdík E. (2009). Chemical Composition and Nutritional Quality of Wheat Grain. *Acta Chimica Slovaca*, **2**(1): 115–138.

40. Zilic S. (2013). Chapter IV. Wheat Gluten: Composition and Health Effects, pp. 71–86. In: *Gluten.* Editor: Dane B. Walter. Nova Science Publishers, Inc., New York.

41. Henrion M., Francey C., Lê K.A., Lamothe L. (2019). Cereal B-Glucans: The Impact of Processing and How It Affects Physiological Responses. *Nutrients*, **11**(1729): 1–14.

42. Chaudhari P.R., Tamrakar N., Singh L., Tandon A., Sharma D. (2018). Rice Nutritional and Medicinal Properties: A Review Article. *J. Pharmacogn. Phytochem.*, **7**(2): 150–156.

43. Kang M-Y., Rico C., Lee S-C. (2010). Physicochemical Properties of Eight Popular Glutinous Rice Varieties in Korea. *Plant Prod. Sci.*, **13**(2): 177–184.

44. Ravichanthiran K., Ma Z.F., Zhang H., Cao Y., Wang C.W., Muhammad S., Aglago E.K., Zhang Y., Jin Y., Pan B. (2018). Phytochemical Profile of Brown Rice and Its Nutrigenomic Implications. *Antioxidants (Basel)*, **7**(71), 16 pages.

45. Shah T.R., Prasad K., Kuma P. (2016). Maize – A Potential Source of Human Nutrition and Health: A Review. *Cogent Food Agric.*, **2**: 1166995, 9 pages.

46. Ghete A.B., Duda M.M., Varban D.I., Varban R., Moldovan C., Muntean S. (2018). Maize (Zea Mays), a Prospective Medicinal Plant in Romania. *Hop Med. Plants*, **26**(1–2): 44–51.

47. Kumar A., Tomer V., Kaur A., Kumar V., Gupta K. (2018). Millets: A Solution to Agrarian and Nutritional Challenges. *Agric. Food Sec.*, **7**(31), 15 pages.

48. Ezekiel R., Singh N., Sharma S., Kaur A. (2013). Beneficial Phytochemicals in Potato. A Review. *Food Res. Int.*, **50**: 487–496.

49. Navarre D.A., Goyer A., Shakya R. (2009). Chapter 14. Nutritional Value of Potatoes: Vitamin, Phytonutrient, and Mineral Content, pp. 395–424. In: *Advances in Potato Chemistry and Technology.* Editors: J. Singh, L. Kaur. Elsevier, New York, USA, 528 pages.

50. Camire M.E., Kubow S., Donnelly D.J. (2009). Potatoes and Human Health. *Crit. Rev. Food Sci. Nutr.*, **49**(10): 823–840.

51. Organization for Economic Co-operation and Development. (2002). Consensus Document on Compositional Considerations for New Varieties of Potatoes: Key Food and Feed Nutrients, Anti-Nutrients and Toxicants. In: Series on the Safety of Novel Foods and Feeds, No. 4, Published in Paris, January 9, 26 pages. www.oecd.org/env/ehs/biotrack/46815167.pdf.

52. Matthäus B., Haase N.U. (2014). Acrylamide – Still a Matter of Concern for Fried Potato Food? *Eur. J. Lipid Sci. Technol.*, **116**: 675–687.

53. Bovell-Benjamin A.C. (2007). Sweet Potato: A Review of Its Past, Present, and Future Role in Human Nutrition. *Adv. Food Nutr. Res.*, **52**: 1–59.

54. Motsa N.M., Modi A.T., Mabhaudhi T. (2015). Sweet Potato (Ipomoea Batatas L.) as a Drought Tolerant and Food Security Crop. *S. Afr. J. Sci.*, **111**(11, 12): 1–8.

55. Ayeleso T.B., Ramachela K., Mukwevho E. (2016). A Review of Therapeutic Potentials of Sweet Potato: Pharmacological Activities and Influence of the Cultivar. *Trop. J. Pharm. Res.*, **15**(12): 2751–2761.

56. Neela S., Fanta S.W. (2019). Review on Nutritional Composition of Orange-Fleshed Sweet Potato and Its Role in Management of Vitamin A Deficiency. *Food Sci. Nutr.*, **7**: 1920–1945.

57. Amoanimaa-Dede H., Hongbo Z., Kyereko W.T., Yeboah A., Agyenim-Boateng K.A. (2019). Structure, Functions and Biosynthetic Pathway of Naturally Occurring Anthocyanin in Sweet Potato – A Review. *J. Plant Biochem. Physiol.*, **7**(234), 9 pages.

58. Chandrasekara A., Kumar T.J. (2016). Roots and Tuber Crops as Functional Foods: A Review on Phytochemical Constituents and Their Potential Health Benefits. *Int. J. Food Sci.*, **2016**, Article ID 3631647, 15 pages.

59. Burns A.E., Gleadow R.M., Zacarias A.M., Cuambe C.E., Miller R.E., Cavagnaro T.R. (2012). Variations in the Chemical Composition of Cassava (Manihot Esculenta Crantz) Leaves and Roots as Affected by Genotypic and Environmental Variation. *J. Agric. Food Chem.*, **60**: 4946–4956.

60. Montagnac J.A., Davis C.R., Tanumihardjo S.A. (2009). Nutritional Value of Cassava for Use as a Staple Food and Recent Advances for Improvement. *Compr. Rev. Food Sci. Food Saf.*, **8**: 181–194.

61. Salvador E.M., Steenkamp V., McCrindle C.M.E. (2014). Production, Consumption and Nutritional Value of Cassava (Manihot esculenta, Crantz) in Mozambique: An Overview. *J. Agric. Biotech. Sustain. Dev.*, **6**(3): 29–38.

62. O'Sullivan J.N. (2010). Yam Nutrition: Nutrient Disorders and Soil Fertility Management. ACIAR Monograph No. 144. Australian Centre for International Agricultural Research: Canberra, 112 pages.

63. Singh A., Lal U.M., Mukhtar H.M., Singh P.S., Shah G., Dhawan R.K. (2015). Phytochemical Profile of Sugarcane and Its Potential Health Aspects. *Pharmacogn. Rev.*, **9**(17): 45–54.

64. Organization for Economic Co-operation and Development (OECD). (2011). Consensus Document on Compositional Considerations for New Varieties of Sugarcane (*Saccharum* ssp. Hybrids): Key Food and Feed Nutrients, Anti-Nutrients and Toxicants. Environment, Health and Safety Publications. Series on the Safety of Novel Foods and Feeds. No. 23., October 25, 43 pages. www.panelamonitor.org/documents/582/consensus-document-compositional-considerations/.

65. Janikula M. (2002). Polycosanol: A New Treatment for Cardiovascular Disease? *Altern. Med. Rev.*, **7**(3): 203–217.

66. Kassis A.N., Jones Peter J.H. (2006). Lack of Cholesterol-Lowering Efficacy of Cuban Sugar Cane Policosanols in Hypercholesterolemic Persons. *Am. J. Clin. Nutr.*, **84**: 1003–1008.

67. Biancardi E., McGrath J.M., Panella L.W., Lewellen R.T., Piergiorgio S. (2010). Chapter 6. Sugar Beet, pp. 173–219. In: *Root and Tuber Crops, Handbook of Plant Breeding 7.* Editor: J.E. Bradshaw. Springer Science + Business Media, LLC 2010. doi:10.1007/978-0-387-92765-7_6.

68. Finkenstadt V.L. (2013). A Review on the Complete Utilization of the Sugar Beet. *Sugar Tech.*, **16**(4): 339–346.

69. Organization for Economic Co-operation and Development (OECD). (2002). Consensus Document on Compositional Considerations for New Varieties of Sugar Beet: Key Food and Feed Nutrients and Anti-Nutrients. Environment, Health and Safety Publications. Series on the Safety of Novel Foods and Feeds. No. 3, February 01, 26 pages. www.oecd.org/env/ehs/biotrack/46815157.pdf.

70. International Agency for Research on Cancer of World Health Organization (IARC). (2003). *Handbooks of Cancer Prevention. Fruit and Vegetables*, Volume 8. IARC Press, Lyon, France, 384 pages.

71. Zhao C-N., Meng X., Li Y., Li S., Liu Q., Tang G-Y., Li H-B. (2017). Fruits for Prevention and Treatment of Cardiovascular Diseases. *Nutrients*, **9**(598), 29 pages.

72. Hyson D.A. (2011). A Comprehensive Review of Apples and Apple Components and Their Relationship to Human Health. *Adv. Nutr.*, **2**(5): 408–420.

73. Boyer J., Liu R.H. (2004). Apple Phytochemicals and Their Health Benefits. *Nutr. J.*, **3**(5): 15 pages.

74. Wassermann B., Müller H., Berg G. (2019). An Apple a Day: Which Bacteria Do We Eat with Organic and Conventional Apples? *Front. Microbiol.*, **10**: 1629, 1–13.

75. Singh B., Singh J.P., Kaur A., Singh N. (2016). Bioactive Compounds in Banana and Their Associated Health Benefits – A Review. *Food Chem.*, **206**: 1–11.

76. Netshiheni R.K., Omolola A.O., Anyasi T.A., Jideani A.I.O. (2019). Banana Bioactives: Absorption, Utilisation and Health Benefits. In: *Banana Nutrition – Function and Processing Kinetics*. Editors: Afam I.O. Jideani, Tonna A. Anyasi. IntechOpen, October 9. www.intechopen.com/books/banana-nutrition-function-and-processing-kinetics/banana-bioactives-absorption-utilisation-and-health-benefits.

77. Ollat N., Carde J-P., Gaudillère J-P., Barrieu F., Diakou-Verdin P., Moing A. (2002). Grape Berry Development: A Review. *OENO One*, **36**(3): 109–131.

78. Conde C., Silva P., Fontes N., Dias A.C.P., Tavares R.M., Sousa M.J., Agasse A., Delrot S., Gerós H. (2007). Biochemical Changes Throughout Grape Berry Development and Fruit and Wine Quality. *Food*, **1**(1): 1–22.

79. Skrovankova S., Sumczynski D., Mlcek J., Jurikova T., Sochor J. (2015). Bioactive Compounds and Antioxidant Activity in Different Types of Berries. *Int. J. Mol. Sci.*, **16**(10): 24673–24706.

80. Nile S.H., Park S.W. (2014). Edible Berries: Bioactive Components and Their Effect on Human Health. *Nutrition*, **30**: 134–144.

81. Kaume L., Howard L.R., Devareddy L. (2012). The Blackberry Fruit: A Review on Its Composition and Chemistry, Metabolism and Bioavailability, and Health Benefits. *J. Agric. Food Chem.*, **60**: 5716–5727.

82. Kresty L.A., Mallery S.R., Stoner G.D. (2016). Black Raspberries in Cancer Clinical Trials: Past, Present and Future. *J. Berry Res.*, **6**(2): 251–261.

83. Miller K., Feucht W., Schmid M. (2019). Bioactive Compounds of Strawberry and Blueberry and Their Potential Health Effects Based on Human Intervention Studies: A Brief Overview. *Nutrients*, **11**(7): 1510, 12 pages.

84. Neto C.C., Vinson J.A. (2011). Chapter 6. Cranberry. In: *Herbal Medicine: Biomolecular and Clinical Aspects*. 2nd edition. Editors: I.F.F Benzie, S. Wachtel-Galor. CRC Press/Taylor & Francis, Boca Raton, FL. www.ncbi.nlm.nih.gov/books/NBK92762/.

85. Bucheli P., Gao Q., Redgwell R., Vidal K., Wang J., Zhang W. (2011). Chapter 14. Biomolecular and Clinical Aspects of Chinese Wolfberry. In: *Herbal Medicine: Biomolecular and Clinical Aspects*. 2nd edition. Editors: I.F.F Benzie, S. Wachtel-Galor. CRC Press/Taylor & Francis, Boca Raton, FL. www.ncbi.nlm.nih.gov/books/NBK92756/.

86. Zibaee E., Kamalian S., Tajvar M., Amiri M.S., Ramezani M., Moghadam A.T., Emami S.A., Sahebkar A. (2020). Citrus Species: A Review of Traditional Uses, Phytochemistry and Pharmacology. *Curr. Pharm. Des.*, **26**(1): 44–97.

87. Peterson J.J., Dwyer J.T., Beecher G.R., Bhagwat S.A., Gebhardt S.E., Haytowitz D.B., Holden J.M. (2006). Flavanones in Oranges, Tangerines (Mandarins), Tangors, and Tangelos: A Compilation and Review of the Data from the Analytical Literature. *J. Food Comp. Anal.*, **19** (Suppl.): S66–S73.

88. Rafiq S., Kaul R., Sofi S.A., Bashir N., Nazir F., Nayik G.A. (2018). Citrus Peel as a Source of Functional Ingredient: A Review. *J. Saudi Soc. Agric. Sci.*, **17**: 351–358.

89. Etebu E., Nwauzoma A.B. (2014). A Review on Sweet Orange (Citrus Sinensis Osbeck): Health, Diseases, and Management. *Am. J. Res. Commun.*, **2**(2): 33–70. www.usa-journals.com, ISSN: 2325–4076.

90. Karthikeyan V., Karthikeyan J. (2014). *Citrus Aurantium* (Bitter Orange): A Review of Its Traditional Uses, Phytochemistry and Pharmacology. *Int. J. Drug Discov. Herb. Res. (IJDDHR)*, **4**(4): 766–772.

91. Sarker S.K., Tun K.D., Eva E.O., Paul R. (2015). Grapefruit Juice: Nutritional Values and Drug Interactions. *Int. J. Integr. Med. Sci.*, **2**(10): 186–189.

92. Wong R.W.K. (2008). The Pharmacological Actions of Grapefruit Extracts: Naringin and Naringinin. *Tree For. Sci. Biotech.*, **3** (Special Issue 1): 127–138.

93. Kiani J., Imam S.Z. (2007). Medicinal Importance of Grapefruit Juice and Its Interaction with Various Drugs. *Nutr. J.*, **6**(33): 9 pages.

94. Deng W., Liu K., Cao S., Sun J., Zhong B., Chun J. (2020). Chemical Composition, Antimicrobial, Antioxidant, and Antiproliferative Properties of Grapefruit Essential Oil Prepared by Molecular Distillation. *Molecules*, **25**(217): 12 pages.

95. Peterson J.J., Beecher G.R., Bhagwat S.A., Dwyer J.T., Gebhardt S.E., Haytowitz D.B., Holden J.M. (2006). Flavanones in Grapefruit, Lemons, and Limes: A Compilation and Review of the Data from the Analytical Literature. *J. Food Comp. Anal.*, **19** (Suppl.): S74–S80.

96. Vicente A.R., Manganaris G.A., Cinseros-Zevallos L., Crisosto C.H. (2011). Chapter 13. Prunus, pp. 238–259. In: *health Promoting Properties of Fruits and Vegetables*. Editor: Leon Terry. CABI, Wallingford, UK.

97. Poonam V., Raunak K.G., Reddy L.C.S., Jain R., Sharma S.K., Prasad A.K., Parmar V.S. (2011). Chemical Constituents of the Genus Prunus and Their Medicinal Properties. *Curr. Med. Chem.*, **18**(25): 3758–3824.

98. Kant R., Shukla R., Shukla A. (2018). A Review on Peach (Prunus persica): An Asset of Medicinal Phytochemicals. *Int. J. Res. Appl. Sci. Eng. Tech. (IJRASET)*, **6**(I): 2186–2199.

99. Bozhkova V. (2014). Chemical Composition and Sensory Evaluation of Plum Fruits. *Trak. Univ. J. Nat. Sci.*, **15**(1): 31–35.

100. Walkowiak-Tomczak D. (2008). Characteristic *of* Plums as a Raw Material with Valuable Nutritive and Dietary Properties – A Review. *Pol. J. Food Nutr. Sci.*, **58**(4): 401–405.

101. Stacewicz-Sapuntzakis M., Bowen P.E., Hussain E.A., Damayanti-Wood B.I., Farnsworth N.R. (2001). Chemical Composition and Potential Health Effects of Prunes: A Functional Food? *Crit. Rev. Food Sci. Nutr.*, **41**(4): 251–286.

102. Fatima T., Bashir O., Gani G., Bhat T., Jan N. (2018). Nutritional and Health Benefits of Apricots. *Int. J. Unani Integr. Med.*, **2**(2): 05–09.

103. Ferretti G., Bacchetti T., Belleggia A., Neri D. (2010). Cherry Antioxidants: From Farm to Table. *Molecules*, **15**(10): 6993–7005.

104. Kelley D.S., Adkins Y., Laugero K.D. (2018). A Review of the Health Benefits of Cherries. *Nutrients*, **10**(3): 368, 22 pages.

105. Reiland H., Slavin J. (2015). Systematic Review of Pears and Health. *Nutr. Today*, **50**(6): 301–305.

106. Dreher M.L., Davenport A.J. (2013). Hass Avocado Composition and Potential Health Effects. *Crit. Rev. Food Sci. Nutr.*, **53**(7): 738–750.

107. Pavan R., Jain S., Kumar S., Kumar A. (2012). Properties and Therapeutic Application of Bromelain: A Review. *Biotechnol. Res. Int.*, **2012**, Article ID 976203, 6 pages.

108. Ahmed J., Aljasass F., Siddiq M. (2014). Chapter 11: Date Fruit Composition and Nutrition, pp. 261–284. In: *Dates: Postharvest Science, Processing Technology and Health Benefits*. 1st edition. Editors: Muhammad Siddiq, Salah M. Aleid, Adel A. Kader. John Wiley & Sons, Ltd., Hoboken, New Jersey.

109. Vella F.M., Cautela D., Laratta B. (2019). Characterization of Polyphenolic Compounds in Cantaloupe Melon By-Products. *Foods*, **8**(6): 196, 10 pages.

110. Erhirhie E.O., Ekene N.E. (2013). Medicinal Values on Citrullus Lanatus (Watermelon): Pharmacological Review. *Int. J. Res. Pharmac. Biomed. Sci.*, **4**(4): 1305–1312.

111. Richardson D.P., Ansell J., Drummond L.N. (2018). The Nutritional and Health Attributes of Kiwifruit: A Review. *Eur. J. Nutr.*, **57**(8): 2659–2676.

112. Yaqub S., Farooq U., Shafi A., Akram K., Murtaza M.A., Kausar T., Siddique F. (2016). Chemistry and Functionality of Bioactive Compounds Present in Persimmon. *J. Chem.*, **2016**, Article ID 3424025, 13 pages.

113. Gao Q.H., Wu C.S., Wang M. (2013). The Jujube (Ziziphus Jujuba Mill.) Fruit: A Review of Current Knowledge of Fruit Composition and Health Benefits. *J. Agric. Food Chem.*, **61**(14): 3351–3363.

114. Chen J., Liu X., Li Z., Qi A., Yao P., Zhou Z., Dong T.T.X., Tsim K.W.K. (2017). A Review of Dietary *Ziziphus Jujuba* Fruit (Jujube): Developing Health Food Supplements for Brain Protection. *Evid. Based Complement. Alternat. Med.*, **2017**, Article ID 3019568, 10 pages.

115. Lauricella M., Emanuele S., Calvaruso G., Giuliano M., D'Anneo A. (2017). Multifaceted Healthy Benefits of *Mangifera Indica* L. (Mango): The Inestimable Value of an Orchard Recently Rooted in Sicilian Rural Areas. *Nutrients*, **9**(525): 14 pages.

116. Gutierrez-Orozco F., Failla M.L. (2013). Biological Activities and Bioavailability of Mangosteen Xanthones: A Critical Review of the Current Evidence. *Nutrients*, **5**(8): 3163–3183.

117. Aizat W.M., Ahmad-Hashim F.H., Jaafar S.N.S. (2019). Valorization of Mangosteen, "The Queen of Fruits," and New Advances in Postharvest and in Food and Engineering Applications: A Review. *J. Adv. Res.*, **20**: 61–70.

118. Aizat W.M., Jamil I.N., Ahmad-Hashim F.H., Noor N.M. (2019). Recent Updates on Metabolite Composition and Medicinal Benefits of Mangosteen Plant. *PeerJ*, **7**: e6324, 25 pages.

119. Kaliyaperumal K., Kim H-M., Jegajeevanram K., Xavier J., Vijayalakshmi J. (2014). Papaya: A Gifted Nutraceutical Plant – A Critical Review of Recent Human Health Research. *Int. J. Genuine Tradit. Med.*, **4**: 1–17.

120. Osuki N., Dang N.H., Kumagai E., Kondo A., Iwata S., Morimoto C. (2010). Aqueous Extract of Carica Papaya Leaves Exhibits Anti-Tumor Activity and Immunomodulatory Effects. *J. Ethnopharmacol.*, **127**(3): 760–767.

121. Emanuele S., Lauricella M., Calvaruso G., D'Anneo A., Giuliano M. (2017). Litchi Chinensis as a Functional Food and a Source of Antitumor Compounds: An Overview and a Description of Biochemical Pathways. *Nutrients*, **9**(9): 992, 15 pages.

122. Omar S.H. (2008). Olive: Native of Mediterranean Region and Health Benefits. *Pharmacogn. Rev.*, **2**(3): 135–142.

123. Lima E.B., Sousa C.N., Meneses L.N., Ximenes N.C., Santos Júnior M.A., Vasconcelos G.S., Lima N.B., Patrocínio M.C., Macedo D., Vasconcelos S.M. (2015). Cocos Nucifera (L.) (Arecaceae): A Phytochemical and Pharmacological Review. *Braz. J. Med. Biol. Res.*, **48**(11): 953–964.

124. DebMandal M., Mandal S. (2011). Coconut (Cocos Nucifera L.: Arecaceae): In Health Promotion and Disease Prevention. *Asian Pac. J. Trop. Med.*: 241–247.

125. Suryakumar G., Gupta A. (2011). Medicinal and Therapeutic Potential of Sea Buckthorn (Hippophae Rhamnoides L.). *J. Ethnopharmacol.*, **138**: 268–278.

126. Singh I.P., Ahmad F., Gore D.D., Tikoo K., Bansal A., Jachak S.M., Jena G. (2019). Therapeutic Potential of Sea Buckthorn: A Patent Review (2000–2018). *Expert Opin. Ther. Pat.*, **29**: 9, 733–744.

127. Olas B., Skalski B., Ulanowska K. (2018). The Anticancer Activity of Sea Buckthorn [Elaeagnus Rhamnoides (L.) A. Nelson]. *Front. Pharmacol.*, **9**: 232, 8 pages.

128. Ordás A., Cartea M.E. (2008). Cabbage and Kale. In: *Vegetables I. Handbook of Plant Breeding*. Editors: J. Prohens, F. Nuez, Volume 1. Springer, New York. https://doi.org/10.1007/978-0-387-30443-4_4.

129. Di Gioia F., Petropoulos S.A. (2021). Chapter 2. Glucosinolates. In: *Food Bioactives and Health*. Editor: C.M. Galanakis. Springer Cham, Switzerland. https://doi.org/10.1007/978-3-030-57469-7_5.

130. Podsedek A. (2007). Natural Antioxidants and Antioxidant Capacity of Brassica Vegetables: A Review. *LWT*, **40**: 1–11.

131. Higdon J.V., Delage B., Williams D.E., Dashwood R.H. (2007). Cruciferous Vegetables and Human Cancer Risk: Epidemiologic Evidence and Mechanistic Basis. *Pharmacol. Res.*, **55**(3): 224–236.

132. Ahmed F.A., Ali R.F.M. (2013). Bioactive Compounds and Antioxidant Activity of Fresh and Processed White Cauliflower. *BioMed Res. Int.*, **2013**, Article ID 367819, 9 pages.

133. Sachin C., Hazar H., Doha M. (2018). A Review on Phytochemical and Pharmacological Potential of Watercress Plant. *Asian J. Pharmac. Clin. Res.*, **11**(12): 102–107.

134. Al-Snafi A. (2014). The Pharmacology of Apium Graveolens. -A Review. *Int. J. Pharm. Res. Scholars (IJPRS)*, **3**: 671–677.

135. Khalil A., Nawaz H., Ghania J., Rehman R., Nadeem F. (2015). Value Added Products, Chemical Constituents and Medicinal Uses of Celery (Apium Graveolens L.) -A Review. *Int. J. Chem. Biochem. Sci. (IJCBS)*, **8**: 40–48.

136. Al-Asmari A.K., Athar M.T., Kadasah S.G. (2017). An Updated Phytopharmacological Review on Medicinal Plant of Arab Region: *Apium Graveolens* Linn. *Pharmacogn. Rev.*, **11**(21): 13–18.

137. Kim M.J., Moon Y., Tou J.C., Mou B., Waterland N.L. (2016). Nutritional Value, Bioactive Compounds and Health Benefits of Lettuce (Lactuca Sativa L.). *J. Food Compos. Anal.*, **49**: 19–34.

138. Kim M.J., Moon Y., Kopsell D., Park S., Tou J.C., Waterland N.L. (2016). Nutritional Value of Crisphead 'Iceberg' and Romaine Lettuces (Lactuca Sativa L.). *J. Agr. Sci.*, **8**(11): 1–10.

139. Mampholo B.M., Maboko M.M., Soundy P., Sivakumar D. (2016). Phytochemicals and Overall Quality of Leafy Lettuce (*Lactuca Sativa* L.) Varieties Grown in Closed Hydroponic System. *J. Food Qual.*, **39**: 805–815.

140. Gutierrez R.M.P., Velazquez E.G., Carrera S.P.P. (2019). Spinacia Oleracea Linn Considered as One of the Most Perfect Foods: A Pharmacological and Phytochemical Review. *Mini. Rev. Med. Chem.*, **19**(20): 1666–1680.

141. Roberts J.L., Moreau R. (2016). Functional Properties of Spinach (Spinacia Oleracea L.) Phytochemicals and Bioactives. *Food Funct.*, **7**(8): 3337–3353.

142. Amarathunga A.A.M.D.D.N., Kankanamge S.U. (2017). A Review on Pharmacognostic, Phytochemical and Ethnopharmacological Findings of Peperomia Pellucida (L.) Kunth: Pepper Elder. *Int. Res. J. Pharm.*, **8**(11): 16–23.

143. Perveen R., Suleria H.A.R., Anjum F.M., Butt M.S., Pasha I., Ahmad S. (2015). Tomato (Solanum Lycopersicum), Carotenoids and Lycopenes Chemistry; Metabolism, Absorption, Nutrition, and Allied Health Claims-A Comprehensive Review. *Crit. Rev. Food Sci. Nutr.*, **55**(7): 919–929.

144. Nasir M.U., Hussain S., Jabba S. (2015). Tomato Processing, Lycopene and Health Benefits: A Review. *Sci. Lett.*, **3**(1): 1–5.

145. Story E.N., Kopec R.E., Schwartz S.J., Harris G.K. (2010). An Update on the Health Effects of Tomato Lycopene. *Annu. Rev. Food Sci. Technol.*, **1**: 1–24.

146. Khatib S.E., Muhieddine M. (2019). Nutritional Profile and Medicinal Properties of Pumpkin Fruit Pulp. In: *The Health Benefits of Foods – Current Knowledge and Further Development*. Editor: Liana Claudia Salanţă. IntechOpen, London.

147. Abdulqader A., Ali F., Ismail A., Norhaizan M.E. (2018). Gac (Momordica Cochinchinensis Spreng.) Fruit and Its Potentiality and Superiority in-Health Benefits. *J. Contemp. Med. Sci.*, **4**(4): 179–186.

148. Polak R., Phillips E.M., Campbell A. (2015). Legumes: Health Benefits and Culinary Approaches to Increase Intake. *Clin. Diabetes*, **33**(4): 198–205.

149. Winham D.M., Webb D., Barr A. (2008). Beans and Good Health. *Nutr. Today*, **43**(5): 201–209.

150. Messina V. (2014). Nutritional and Health Benefits of Dried Beans. *Am. J. Clin. Nutr.*, **100** (Suppl.): 437S–442S.

151. Rizzo G., Baroni L. (2018). Soy, Soy Foods and Their Role in Vegetarian Diets. *Nutrients*, **10**(1): 43, 51 pages.

152. Hassan S.H. (2013). Soybean, Nutrition and Health. In: *Soybean – Bio-Active Compounds*. Editor: Hany A. El-Shemy. IntechOpen. www.intechopen.com/books/soybean-bio-active-compounds/soybean-nutrition-and-health.

153. Ros E., Hu F.B. (2013). Consumption of Plant Seeds and Cardiovascular Health: Epidemiological and Clinical Trial Evidence. *Circulation*, **128**(5): 553–565.

154. Franke H., Scholl R., Aigner A. (2019). Ricin and *Ricinus Communis* in Pharmacology and Toxicology-from Ancient Use and "Papyrus Ebers" to Modern Perspectives and "Poisonous Plant of the Year 2018". *Naunyn-Schmiedeberg's Arch. Pharmacol.*, **392**: 1181–1208.

155. Carraro J., Dantas M., Espeschit C., Martino H., Ribeiro S. (2012). Flaxseed and Human Health: Reviewing Benefits and Adverse Effects. *Food Rev. Int.*, **28**(2): 203–230.

156. Namiki M. (2007). Nutraceutical Functions of Sesame: A Review. *Crit. Rev. Food Sci. Nutr.*, **47**(7): 651–673.

157. Hsu E., Parthasarathy S. (2017). Anti-Inflammatory and Antioxidant Effects of Sesame Oil on Atherosclerosis: A Descriptive Literature Review. *Cureus*, **9**(7): e1438, 16 pages.

158. Kulczyński B., Kobus-Cisowska J., Taczanowski M., Kmiecik D., Gramza-Michałowska A. (2019). The Chemical Composition and Nutritional Value of Chia Seeds-Current State of Knowledge. *Nutrients*, **11**(6): 1242, 16 pages.

159. Melo D., Machado T.B., Oliveira M.B.P.P. (2019). Chia Seeds: An Ancient Grain Trending in Modern Human Diets. *Food Funct.*, **10**: 3068–3089.

160. Angeli V., Miguel Silva P., Crispim Massuela D., Khan M.W., Hamar A., Khajehei F., Graeff-Hönninger S., Piatti C. (2020). Quinoa (*Chenopodium Quinoa* Willd.): An Overview of the Potentials of the "Golden Grain" and Socio-Economic and Environmental Aspects of Its Cultivation and Marketization. *Foods*, **9**(2): 216, 31 pages.

161. Pereira E., Encina-Zelada C., Barros L., Gonzales-Barron U., Cadavez V., Ferreira I. (2019). Chemical and Nutritional Characterization of Chenopodium Quinoa Willd (Quinoa) Grains: A Good Alternative to Nutritious Food. *Food Chem.*, **280**: 110–114.

162. Vega-Galvez A., Miranda M., Vergara J., Uribe E., Puente L., Martinez E.A. (2010). Nutrition Facts and Functional Potential of Quinoa (Chenopodium Quinoa Willd.), an Ancient Andean Grain: A Review. *J. Sci. Food Agric.*, **90**(15): 2541–2547.

163. de Souza R.G.M., Schincaglia R.M., Pimentel G.D., Mota J.F. (2017). Nuts and Human Health Outcomes: A Systematic Review. *Nutrients*, **9**(12): 1311, 23 pages.

164. Ros E. (2010). Health Benefits of Nut Consumption. *Nutrients*, **2**(7): 652–682.

165. Ros E. (2015). Nuts and CVD. *Br. J. Nutr.*, **113**: S111–S120.

166. Silva Dias J.C. (2014). Nutritional and Health Benefits of Carrots and Their Seed Extracts. *Food Nutr. Sci.*, **5**: 2147–2156.

167. Sharma K.D., Karki S., Thakur N.S., Attri S. (2012). Chemical Composition, Functional Properties and Processing of Carrot-a Review. *J. Food Sci. Technol.*, **49**(1): 22–32.

168. Ahmad T., Cawood M., Iqbal Q., Ariño A., Batool A., Tariq R.M.S., Azam M., Akhtar S. (2019). Phytochemicals in *Daucus Carota* and Their Health Benefits-Review Article. *Foods*, **8**(9): 424, 22 pages.

169. Que F., Hou X., Wang G., Xu Z-S., Tan G-F., Li T., Wang Y-H., Khadr A., Xion A-S. (2019). Advances in Research on the Carrot, an Important Root Vegetable in the Apiaceae Family. *Hortic. Res.*, **6**(69), 15 pages.

170. Liguori L., Califano R., Albanese D., Raimo F., Crescitelli A., Di Matteo M. (2017). Chemical Composition and Antioxidant Properties of Five White Onion (*Allium Cepa* L.) Landraces. *J. Food Quality*, **2017**, Article ID 6873651, 9 pages.

171. Bisen P.S., Emerald M. (2016). Nutritional and Therapeutic Potential of Garlic and Onion (*Allium* sp.). *Curr. Nutr. Food Sci.*, **12**: 190–199.

172. Benkeblia N., Lanzotti V. (2007). *Allium* Thiosulfinates: Chemistry, Biological Properties and Their Potential Utilization in Food Preservation. *Food*, **1**(2): 193–201.

173. Bahram-Parvar M., Lim L-T. (2018). Fresh-Cut Onion: A Review on Processing, Health Benefits, and Shelf-Life. *Compr. Rev. Food Sci. Food Saf.*, **17**: 290–308.

174. Bayan L., Koulivand P.H., Gorji A. (2014). Garlic: A Review of Potential Therapeutic Effects. *Avicenna J. Phytomed.*, **4**(1): 1–14.

175. Martins N., Petropoulos S., Ferreira I.C.F.R. (2016). Chemical Composition and Bioactive Compounds of Garlic (*Allium Sativum* L.) as Affected by Pre- and Post-Harvest Conditions: A Review. *Food Chem.*, **211**: 41–50.

176. Micova M., Bystricka J., Kovarovic J., Harangozo L., Lidikova A. (2018). Content of Bioactive Compounds and Antioxidant Activity in Garlic (*Allium Sativum* L.). *Acta Agric. Slov.*, **111**: 581–595.

177. Zakarova A., Seo J.Y., Kim H.Y., Kim J.H., Shin J-H., Cho K.M., Lee C.H., Kim J-S. (2014). Garlic Sprouting Is Associated with Increased Antioxidant Activity and Concomitant Changes in the Metabolite Profile. *J. Agric. Food Chem.*, **62**(8): 1875–1880.

178. Tran G-B., Pham T-V., Trinh N-N. (2019). Black Garlic and Its Therapeutic Benefits. In: *Medicinal Plants – Use in Prevention and Treatment of Diseases*. Editor: Bassam Abdul Rasool Hassan. IntechOpen, March 29. doi:10.5772/intechopen.85042.

179. Singh B., Ramakrishna Y. (2017). Welsh Onion (Allium Fistulosum L.): A Promising Spicing-Culinary Herb of Mizoram. *Indian J. Hill Farming*, **30**(2): 201–208.

180. Strati I.F., Kostomitsopoulos G., Lytras F., Zoumpoulakis P., Proestos C., Sinanoglou V.J. (2018). Optimization of Polyphenol Extraction from *Allium Ampeloprasum* var. *Porrum* Through Response Surface Methodology. *Foods*, **7**(10): 162, 10 pages.

181. Babarykin D., Smirnova G., Pundinsh I., Vasiljeva S., Krumina G., Agejchenko V. (2019). Red Beet (Beta Vulgaris) Impact on Human Health. *J. BioSci. Med.*, **7**(3): 61–79.

182. Masih D., Singh N., Singh A. (2019). Red Beetroot: A Source of Natural Colourant and Antioxidants: A Review. *J. Pharmacogn. Phytochem.*, **8**(4): 162–166.

183. Clifford T., Howatson G., West D.J., Stevenson E.J. (2015). The Potential Benefits of Red Beetroot Supplementation in Health and Disease. *Nutrients*, **7**(4): 2801–2822.

184. Bonilla Ocampo D.A., Paipilla A.F., Marín E., Vargas-Molina S., Petro J.L., Pérez-Idárraga A. (2018). Dietary Nitrate from Beetroot Juice for Hypertension: A Systematic Review. *Biomolecules*, **8**(4): 134, 12 pages.

185. Lechner J.F., Stoner G.D. (2019). Red Beetroot and Betalains as Cancer Chemopreventative Agents. *Molecules*, **24**(8): 1602, 12 pages.

186. Ma L., Hu L., Feng X., Wang S. (2018). Nitrate and Nitrite in Health and Disease. *Aging Dis.*, **9**(5): 938–945.

187. Guo Q., Wanga N., Liua H., Lia Z., Lua L., Wang C. (2020). The Bioactive Compounds and Biological Functions of Asparagus Officinalis L. – A Review. *J. Funct. Foods*, **65**: 103727, 1–12.

188. Pegiou E., Mumm R., Acharya P., de Vos R.C.H., Hall R.D. (2020). Green and White Asparagus (Asparagus officinalis): A Source of Developmental, Chemical and Urinary Intrigue. *Metabolites*, **10**: 17, 23 pages.

189. Iqbal M., Bibi Y., Raja N.I., Ejaz M., Hussain M., Yasmeen F., Saira H., Imranet M. (2017). Review on Therapeutic and Pharmaceutically Important Medicinal Plant Asparagus Officinalis L. *J. Plant Biochem. Physiol.*, **5**: 180, 6 pages.

190. Mfengwana P-M-A.H., Mashele S.S. (2019). Medicinal Properties of Selected Asparagus Species: A Review. In: *Phytochemicals in Human Health*. Editors: Venketeshwer Rao, Dennis Mans, Leticia Rao. IntechOpen, August 9. doi:10.5772/intechopen.87048. www.intechopen.com/books/phytochemicals-in-human-health/medicinal-properties-of-selected-asparagus-species-a-review.

191. Al-Snafi A.E. (2015). The Pharmacological Importance of Asparagus Officinalis – A Review. *J. Pharm. Biol.*, **5**: 93–98.

192. Prasad S., Aggarwal B.B. (2011). Chapter 13. Turmeric, the Golden Spice: From Traditional Medicine to Modern Medicine. In: *Herbal Medicine: Biomolecular and Clinical Aspects*. 2nd edition. Editors: I.F.F. Benzie, S. Wachtel-Galor. CRC Press/Taylor & Francis, Boca Raton, FL. www.ncbi.nlm.nih.gov/books/NBK92752/.

193. Li S., Yuan W., Deng G., Wang P., Yang P., Aggarwal B. (2011). Chemical Composition and Product Quality Control of Turmeric (Curcuma Longa L.). *Pharmaceutical Crops*, **2**: 28–54.

194. Aggarwal B.B., Bhatt I.D., Ichikawa H., Ahn K.S., Sethi G., Sandur S.K., Sundaram C., Seeram N., Shishodia S. (2007). Chapter 10: Curcumin – Biological and Medicinal Properties, pp. 297–368. In: *Turmeric: The Genus Curcuma*. Editors: P.N. Ravindran, K. Nirmal Babu, K. Sivaraman. CRC Press, Taylor & Francis Group, Boca Raton, FL, 504 pages.

195. Prabhakaran Nair K.P. (2013). *The Agronomy and Economy of Turmeric and Ginger. The Invaluable Medicinal Spice Crops*. 27 Chapters. Elsevier, 544 pages. https://doi.org/10.1016/C2011-0-07514-2.

196. Amalraj A., Pius A., Gopi S., Gopi S. (2017). Biological Activities of Curcuminoids, Other Biomolecules from Turmeric and Their Derivatives – A Review. *J. Tradit. Complement Med.*, **7**(2): 205–233.

197. Alsamydai A., Jaber N. (2018). Pharmacological Aspects of Curcumin: Review Article. *Int. J. Pharmacogn.*, **5**(6): 313–326.

198. Aggarwal B.B., Harikumar K.B. (2009). Potential Therapeutic Effects of Curcumin, the Anti-Inflammatory Agent, Against Neurodegenerative, Cardiovascular, Pulmonary, Metabolic, Autoimmune and Neoplastic Diseases. *Int. J. Biochem. Cell Biol.*, **41**(1): 40–59.

199. Hewlings S.J., Kalman D.S. (2017). Curcumin: A Review of Its' Effects on Human Health. *Foods*, **6**(92), 11 pages.

200. Nelson K.M., Dahlin J.L., Bisson J., Graham J., Pauli G.F., Walters M.A. (2017). The Essential Medicinal Chemistry of Curcumin. *Miniperspective. J. Med. Chem.*, **60**(5): 1620–1637.

201. Pulido-Moran M., Moreno-Fernandez J., Ramirez-Tortosa C., Ramirez-Tortosa M.C. (2016). Curcumin and Health. *Molecules*, **21**: 264–285.

202. Priyadarsini K.I. (2014). The Chemistry of Curcumin: From Extraction to Therapeutic Agent. *Molecules*, **19**: 20091–20112.

203. Jana S., Swarnakar S. (2013). Chapter: 26: Curcumin and Cardiovascular Diseases, pp. 487–500. In: *Cardiovascular Diseases: Nutritional and Therapeutic Interventions*. 1st edition. Editor: Nilanjana Maulik. CRC Press; Taylor & Francis Group, Boca Raton, FL, April 9, 614 pages.

204. He Y., Yue Y., Zheng X., Zhang K., Chen S., Du Z. (2015). Curcumin, Inflammation, and Chronic Diseases: How Are They Linked? *Molecules*, **20**: 9183–9213.

205. Heger M., van Golen R.F., Broekgaarden M., Michel M.C. (2014). The Molecular Basis for the Pharmacokinetics and Pharmacodynamics of Curcumin and Its Metabolites in Relation to Cancer. *Pharmacol. Rev.*, **66**: 222–307.

206. Lopresti A.L. (2018). The Problem of Curcumin and Its Bioavailability: Could Its Gastrointestinal Influence Contribute to Its Overall Health-Enhancing Effects? *Adv. Nutr.*, **9**(1): 41–50.

207. Teiten M-H., Dicato M., Diederich M. (2014). Hybrid Curcumin Compounds: A New Strategy for Cancer Treatment. *Molecules*, **19**: 20839–20863.

208. Salem M., Rohani S., Gillies E.R. (2014). Curcumin, a Promising Anti-Cancer Therapeutic: A Review of Its Chemical Properties, Bioactivity and Approaches to Cancer Cell Delivery. *R.S.C. Adv. (Royal Society of Chemistry Advances)*, **4**: 10815–10829.

209. Scazzocchio B., Minghetti L., D'Archivio M. (2020). Interaction Between Gut Microbiota and Curcumin: A New Key of Understanding for the Health Effects of Curcumin. *Nutrients*, **12**(9): 2499, 18 page.

210. Qi M., Zhang K., Li S., Wu J., Pham-Huy C., Diao X., Xiao D-L., He H. (2016). Superparamagnetic Fe3O4 Nanoparticles: Synthesis by a Solvothermal Process and Functionalization for a Magnetic Targeted Curcumin Delivery System. *New J. Chem.*, **40**: 4480–4491.

211. Yallapu M.M., Ebeling M.C., Khan S., Sundram V., Chauhan N., Gupta B.K., Puumala S.E., Jaggi M., Chauhan S.C. (2013). Novel Curcumin Loaded Magnetic Nanoparticles for Pancreatic Cancer Treatment. *Mol. Cancer Ther.*, **12**: 1471–1480.

212. He H., Xiao D-L., Pham-Huy A.L., Dramou P., Pham-Huy C. (2017). Chapter 6. Carbon Nanotubes Used as Nanocarriers in Drug and Biomolecule Delivery, pp. 163–212. In: *Drug Delivery Approaches and Nanosystems, Volume 1. Novel Drug Carriers.* Editors: R.K. Keservani, A.K. Sharma, R.K. Kesharwani. Apple Academic Press Inc., Palm Bay, Florida

213. Ghosh S., Rangan L. (2013). Alpinia: The Gold Mine of Future Therapeutics. *3 Biotech.*, **3**(3): 173–185.

214. Pillai M.K., Young D.J., Bin Hj Abdul Majid H.M. (2018). Therapeutic Potential of Alpinia Officinarum. *Mini Rev. Med. Chem.*, **18**(14): 1220–1232.

215. Abubakar I.B., Malami I., Yahaya Y., Sule S.M. (2018). A Review on the Ethnomedicinal Uses, Phytochemistry and Pharmacology of Alpinia Officinarum Hance. *J. Ethnopharmacol.*, **5**(224): 45–62.

216. Chouni A., Paul S. (2018). A Review on Phytochemical and Pharmacological Potential of Alpinia Galanga. *Pharmacog. J.*, **10**(1): 9–15.

217. Das G., Patra J.K., Gonçalves S., Romano A., Gutiérrez-Grijalva, E.P., Heredia J.B., Talukdar A.D., Shome S., Shin H-S. (2020). Galangal, the Multipotent Super Spices: A Comprehensive Review. *Trends Food Sci. Technol.*, **101**: 50–62.

218. Ma X-N., Xie C-L., Miao Z., Yang Q., Yang X-W. (2017). An Overview of Chemical Constituents from Alpinia Species in the Last Six Decades. *RSC Adv.*, **7**: 14114–14144.

219. Raina A.P., Verma S.K., Abraham Z. (2014). Volatile Constituents of Essential Oils Isolated from *Alpinia Galanga* Willd. (L.) and *A. Officinarum* Hance Rhizomes from North East India. *J. Essent Oil Res.*, **26**(1): 24–28.

220. Basri A.M., Taha H., Ahmad N. (2017). A Review on the Pharmacological Activities and Phytochemicals of *Alpinia Officinarum* (Galangal) Extracts Derived from Bioassay-Guided Fractionation and Isolation. *Pharmacogn. Rev.*, **11**(21): 43–56.

221. Raviraja Shetty G., Monisha S. (2015). Pharmacology of an Endangered Medicinal Plant *Alpinia Galanga* – A Review. *Res. J. Pharm. Biol. Chem. Sci. (RJPBCS)*, **6**(1): 499–511.

222. Zhou Y-Q., Liu H., He M-X., Wang R., Zeng Q-Q., Wang Y., Ye W-C., Zhang Q-W. (2018). Chapter 11: A Review of the Botany, Phytochemical, and Pharmacological Properties of Galangal, pp. 351–396. In: *Natural and Artificial Flavoring Agents and Food Dyes.* Elsevier, Amsterdam, the Netherlands, 542 pages.

223. Alberti Á., Riethmüller E., Béni S. (2018). Characterization of Diarylheptanoids: An Emerging Class of Bioactive Natural Products. *J. Pharm. Biomed. Anal.*, **147**: 13–34.

224. Ly H., She G. (2012). Naturally Occurring Diarylheptanoids – A Supplementary Version. *Rec. Nat. Prod.*, **6**(4): 321–333.

225. Ye Y., Li B. (2006). 1'S-1'-Acetoxychavicol Acetate Isolated from Alpinia Galanga Inhibits Human Immunodeficiency Virus Type 1 Replication by Blocking Rev Transport. *J. Gen. Virol.*, **87**: 2047–2053.

226. Seo J-W., Cho S-C., Park S-J., Lee E-J., Lee J-H., Han S-S., Pyo B.S., Park D-H., Kim B-H. (2013). 1'-Acetoxychavicol Acetate Isolated from Alpinia Galanga Ameliorates Ovalbumin-Induced Asthma in Mice. *PLoS One*, **8**(2): e56447–e56455.

227. Dhanik J., Arya N., Nand V. (2017). A Review on *Zingiber officinale*. *J. Pharmacogn. Phytochem.*, **6**(3): 174–184.

228. Gunathilake K.D.P.P., Vasantha Rupasinghe H.P. (2015). Recent Perspectives on the Medicinal Potential of Ginger. *Botanics: Targets and Therapy*, **5**: 55–63.

229. Rahmani A.H., Al Shabrmi F.M., Aly S.M. (2014). Active Ingredients of Ginger as Potential Candidates in the Prevention and Treatment of Diseases Via Modulation of Biological Activities. *Int. J. Physiol. Pathophysiol. Pharmacol.*, **6**(2): 125–136.

230. Ali B.H., Blunden G., Tanira M.O., Nemmar A. (2008). Some Phytochemical, Pharmacological and Toxicological Properties of Ginger (Zingiber Officinale Roscoe): A Review of Recent Research. *Food Chem. Toxicol.*, **46**: 409–420.

231. Ahmad B., Rehman M.U., Amin I., Arif A., Rasool S., Bhat S.A., Afzal I., Hussain I., Bilal S., Mir M.R. (2015). A Review on Pharmacological Properties of Zingerone (4-(4-Hydroxy-3-methoxyphenyl)-2-but anone). *Sci. World J.*, **2015**, Article ID 816364, 6 pages.

232. Prasad S., Tyagi A.K. (2015). Ginger and Its Constituents: Role in Prevention and Treatment of Gastrointestinal Cancer. *Gastroent. Res. Pract.*, **2015**, Article ID 142979, 11 pages.

233. Choi J.G., Kim S.Y., Jeong M., Oh M.S. (2018). Pharmacotherapeutic Potential of Ginger and Its Compounds in Age-Related Neurological Disorders. *Pharmacol. Ther.*, **182**: 56–69.

234. Selga G., Sauka M., Aboltina L., Davidova A., Kaipainen P., Kheder D., Westermarck T., Atroshi F. (2014). Chapter 10. Pharmacological and Clinical Effectiveness of *Zingiber Officinale* and *Alpinia Galanga* in Patients with Osteoarthritis, pp. 255–264. In: *Pharmacology and Nutritional Intervention in the Treatment of Disease*. Editor: Faik Atroshi. InTech, London, 426 pages.

235. Saleh B.K., Omer A., Teweldemedhin B. (2018). Medicinal Uses and Health Benefits of Chili Pepper (Capsicum Spp.): A Review. *MOJ Food Process Technol.*, **6**(4): 325–328.

236. Olatunji T.L., Afolayan A.J. (2018). The Suitability of Chili Pepper (Capsicum Annuum L.) for Alleviating Human Micronutrient Dietary Deficiencies: A Review. *Food Sci. Nutr.*, **6**: 2239–2251.

237. Chakrabarty S., Mominul Islam A.K.M., Aminul Islam A.K.M. (2017). Nutritional Benefits and Pharmaceutical Potentialities of Chili: A Review. *Fundam. Appl. Agric.*, **2**: 2518–2021.

238. Srinivasan K. (2016). Biological Activities of Red Pepper (Capsicum annuum) and Its Pungent Principle Capsaicin: A Review. *Crit. Rev. Food Sci. Nutr.*, **56**(9): 1488–1500.

239. Parvez G.M.M. (2017). Current Advances in Pharmacological Activity and Toxic Effects of Various Capsicum Species. *Int. J. Pharm. Sci. Res.*, **8**(5): 1900–1912.

240. Nadeem M., Anjum F.M., Khan M.R., Saeed M., Riaz A. (2011). Antioxidant Potential of Bell Pepper (Capsicum Annum L.) – A Review. *Pak. J. Food Sci.*, **21**(1–4): 45–51.

241. Blanco-Ríos A.K., Medina-Juarez L.A., González-Aguilar G.A., Gamez-Meza N. (2013). Antioxidant Activity of the Phenolic and Oily Fractions of Different Sweet Bell Peppers. *J. Mex. Chem. Soc.*, **57**: 137–143.

242. van Ruth S.M., Silvis I.C.J., Ramos M.E., Luning P.A., Jansen M., Elliott C.T., Alewijn M. (2019). A Cool Comparison of Black and White Pepper Grades. *LWT – Food Sci. Technol.*, **106**: 122–127.

243. Damanhouri Z.A., Ahmad A. (2014). A Review on Therapeutic Potential of Piper Nigrum L. (Black Pepper): The King of Spices. *Med. Aromat. Plants*, **3**: 161, 6 pages. doi:10.4172/2167-0412.1000161.

244. Singletary K. (2010). Black Pepper. Overview of Health Benefits. *Nutr. Today*, **45**(1): 43–47.

245. Srivastava A., Singh V. (2017). Biological Action of Piper Nigrum – the King of Spices. *Eur. J. Biol. Res.*, **7**: 223–233.

246. Kawatra P., Rajagopalan R. (2015). Cinnamon: Mystic Powers of a Minute Ingredient. *Pharmacognosy Res.*, **7** (Suppl. 1): S1–S6.

247. Kumar S., Kumari R., Mishra S. (2019). Pharmacological Properties and Their Medicinal Uses of Cinnamomum: A Review. *J. Pharm. Pharmacol.*, **71**: 1735–1761.

248. Liu Q., Meng X., Li Y., Zhao C.N., Tang G.Y., Li H.B. (2017). Antibacterial and Antifungal Activities of Spices. *Int. J. Mol. Sci.*, **18**(6): 1283, 62 pages.

249. Graham L.E., Graham J.M., Wilcox L.W. (2009). *Algae*. 2nd edition. Benjamin Cummings, San Francisco, 720 pages.

250. Wells M.L., Potin P., Craigie J.S., Raven J.A., Merchant S.S., Helliwell K.E., Smith A.G., Camire M.E., Brawley S.H. (2017). Algae as Nutritional and Functional Food Sources: Revisiting Our Understanding. *J. Appl. Phycol.*, **29**: 949–982.

251. El-Gamal A. (2010). Biological Importance of Marine Algae. *Saudi Pharm. J.*, **18**: 1–25.

252. Smit A.J. (2004). Medicinal and Pharmaceutical Uses of Seaweed Natural Products: A Review. *J. Appl. Phycol.*, **16**: 245–262.

253. Brown E.M., Allsopp P.J., Magee P.J., Gill C.I.R., Nitecki S., Strain C.R., McSorley E.M. (2014). Seaweed and Human Health. *Nutr. Rev.*, **72**(3): 205–216.

254. Barkia I., Saari N., Manning S.R. (2019). Microalgae for High-Value Products Towards Human Health and Nutrition. *Mar. Drugs*, **17**(5): 304, 29 pages.

255. Sathasivam R., Radhakrishnan R., Hashem A., Abd-Allah E.F. (2019). Microalgae Metabolites: A Rich Source for Food and Medicine. *Saudi J. Biol. Sci.*, **26**(4): 709–722.

256. Tang G., Suter P.M. (2011). Vitamin A, Nutrition, and Health Values of Algae: Spirulina, Chlorella, and Dunaliella. *J. Pharm. Nutr. Sci.*, **1**: 111–118.

257. Ale M.T., Meyer A.S. (2013). Fucoidans from Brown Seaweeds: An Update on Structures, Extraction Techniques and Use of Enzymes as Tools for Structural Elucidation. *RSC Adv.*, **3**: 8131–8141.

258. Atashrazm F., Lowenthal R.M., Woods G.M., Holloway A.F., Dickinson J.L. (2015). Fucoidan and Cancer: A Multifunctional Molecule with Anti-Tumor Potential. *Mar. Drugs*, **13**: 2327–2346.

259. Zayed A., Ulber R. (2020). Fucoidans: Downstream Processes and Recent Applications. *Mar. Drugs*, **18**(3): 170, 22 pages.

260. Fitton J.H., Stringer D.N., Karpiniec S.S. (2015). Therapies from Fucoidan: An Update. *Mar. Drugs*, **13**(9): 5920–5946.

261. Japelt R.B., Jakobsen J. (2013). Vitamin D in Plants: A Review of Occurrence, Analysis, and Biosynthesis. *Front Plant Sci.*, **4**: 136, 1–20.

262. van Weelden G., Bobiński M., Okła K., van Weelden W.J., Romano A., Pijnenborg J.M.A. (2019). Fucoidan Structure and Activity in Relation to Anti-Cancer Mechanisms. *Mar. Drugs*, **17**(1): 32, 30 pages.

263. Cherry P., O'Hara C., Magee P.J., McSorley E.M., Allsopp P.J. (2019). Risks and Benefits of Consuming Edible Seaweeds. *Nutr. Rev.*, **77**(5): 307–329.

264. Shah M.M.R., Liang Y., Cheng J.J., Daroch M. (2016). Astaxanthin-Producing Green Microalga Haematococcus pluvialis: From Single Cell to High Value Commercial Products. *Front. Plant Sci.*, **7**(531): 1–28.

265. Ambati R.R., Phang S.M., Ravi S., Aswathanarayana R.G. (2014). Astaxanthin: Sources, Extraction, Stability, Biological Activities and Its Commercial Applications – A Review. *Mar. Drugs*, **12**(1): 128–152.

266. Capelli B., Talbott S., Ding L. (2019). Astaxanthin Sources: Suitability for Human Health and Nutrition. *Funct. Foods Health Dis.*, **9**(6): 430–445.

267. Shah M.M., Liang Y., Cheng J.J., Daroch M. (2016). Astaxanthin-Producing Green Microalga Haematococcus pluvialis: From Single Cell to High Value Commercial Products. *Front Plant Sci.*, **7**, Art. 531, 1–28.

268. Küpper F.C., Carrano C.J. (2019). Key Aspects of the Iodine Metabolism in Brown Algae: A Brief Critical Review. *Metallomics*, **11**: 756–764.

269. Roleda M.Y., Skjermo J., Marfaing H., Jónsdóttir R., Rebours C., Gietl A., Stengel D.B., Nitschke U. (2018). Iodine Content in Bulk Biomass of Wild-Harvested and Cultivated Edible Seaweeds: Inherent Variations Determine Species-Specific Daily Allowable Consumption. *Food Chem.*, **254**: 333–339.

270. La Barre S., Potin P., Leblanc C., Delage L. (2010). The Halogenated Metabolism of Brown Algae (Phaeophyta), Its Biological Importance and Its Environmental Significance. *Mar. Drugs*, **8**(4): 988–1010.

271. Leblanc C., Colin C., Cosse A., Delage L., La Barre S., Morin P., Fievet B., Voiseux C., Ambroise Y., Verhaeghe E., Amouroux D., Donard O., Tessier E., Potin P. (2006). Iodine Transfers in the Coastal Marine Environment: The Key Role of Brown Algae and of Their Vanadium-Dependent Haloperoxidases. *Biochimie*, **88**: 1773–1785.

272. Zava T.T., Zava D.T. (2011). Assessment of Japanese Iodine Intake Based on Seaweed Consumption in Japan: A Literature-Based Analysis. *Thyroid Res.*, **4**: 14, 7 pages.

273. Foster R., Williamson C.S., Lunn J. (2009). Culinary Oils and Their Health Effects. *Nutr. Bull.*, **34**(1): 4–47.

274. Kumar A., Sharma A., Upadhyaya K.C. (2016). Vegetable Oil: Nutritional and Industrial Perspective. *Curr. Genomics*, **17**(3): 230–240.

275. Dyer J.M., Stymne S., Green A.G., Carlsson A.S. (2008). High-Value Oils from Plants. *Plant J.*, **54**(4): 640–655.

276. Sayon-Orea C., Carlos S., Martinez-Gonzalez M.A. (2015). Does Cooking with Vegetable Oils Increase the Risk of Chronic Diseases? A Systematic Review. *Br. J. Nutr.*, **113**: S36–S48.

277. Katz D.L., Doughty K., Ali A. (2011). Cocoa and Chocolate in Human Health and Disease. *Antioxid. Redox Signal.*, **15**(10): 2779–2811.

278. Scapagnini G., Davinelli S., Di Renzo L., De Lorenzo A., Olarte H.H., Micali G., Cicero A.F., Gonzalez S. (2014). Cocoa Bioactive Compounds: Significance and Potential for the Maintenance of Skin Health. *Nutrients*, **6**(8): 3202–3213.

279. Latif R. (2013). Chocolate/Cocoa and Human Health: A Review. *Neth. J. Med.*, **71**(2): 63–68.

280. Pham-Huy N.L.A., He H., Pham-Huy C. (2008). Green Tea and Health. An Overview. *J. Food Agric. Environ. (JFAE)*, **6**: 6–13.

281. Chan P.-C., Xia Q., Fu P.P. (2007). *Ginkgo Biloba* Leave Extract: Biological, Medicinal, and Toxicological Effects. *J. Environ. Sci. Health Part C*, **25**: 211–244.

282. Mei N., Guo X., Ren Z., Kobayashi D., Wada K., Guo L. (2017). Review of Ginkgo Biloba-Induced Toxicity, from Experimental Studies to Human Case Reports. *J. Environ. Sci. Health C Environ. Carcinog. Ecotoxicol. Rev.*, **35**(1): 1–28.

283. Mahadevan S., Park Y. (2008). Multifaceted Therapeutic Benefit of Ginkgo Biloba L.: Chemistry, Efficacy, Safety, and Uses. *J. Food Sci.*, **73**(1): R14–R19.

284. Shin B.-K., Kwon S.W., Park J.H. (2015). Chemical Diversity of Ginseng Saponins from Panax Ginseng. *J. Ginseng Res.*, **39**: 287–298.

285. He M., Huang X., Liu S., Guo C., Xie Y., Meijer A.H., Wang M. (2018). The Difference Between White and Red Ginseng: Variations in Ginsenosides and Immunomodulation. *Planta Med.*, **84**: 845–854.

286. So S-H., Lee J.W., Kim Y-S., Hyun S.H., Han C-K. (2018). Red Ginseng Monograph. *J. Ginseng Res.*, **42**(4): 549–561.

287. Lee Y-M., Yoon H., Park H-M., Song B.C., Yeum K-J. (2017). Implications of Red Panax Ginseng in Oxidative Stress Associated Chronic Diseases. *J. Ginseng Res.*, **41**(2): 113–119.

288. Kim Y-S., Woo J-Y., Han C-K., Chang I-M. (2015). Safety Analysis of *Panax Ginseng* in Randomized Clinical Trials: A Systematic Review. *Medicines*, **2**: 106–126.

289. Kim K.H., Lee D., Lee H.L., Kim C-E., Jung K., Kang K.S. (2018). Beneficial Effects of Panax Ginseng for the Treatment and Prevention of Neurodegenerative Diseases: Past Findings and Future Directions. *J. Ginseng Res.*, **42**(3): 239–247.

290. Leung K.W., Wong A.S.T. (2013). Ginseng and Male Reproductive Function. *Spermatogenesis*, **3**(3): e26391–1–e26391–6.

291. World Health Organization (WHO). (2004). Radix Angelicae Sinensis, pp. 25–34. In: *Monographs on Selected Medicinal Plants*, Volume 2. Editor: Dr Xiaorui Zhang. Acting Coordinator of Traditional Medicine of WHO, 358 pages. https://apps.who.int/iris/bitstream/handle/10665/42052/9241545372.pdf?sequence=2.

292. Fang L., Xiao X-F., Liu C-X., He X. (2012). Recent Advance in Studies on Angelica Sinensis. *Chin. Herb. Med.*, **4**(1): 12–25.

293. Wu Y.C., Hsieh C.L. (2011). Pharmacological Effects of Radix Angelica Sinensis (Danggui) on Cerebral Infarction. *Chin. Med.*, **6**: 32, 5 pages.

294. Singletary K.W. (2010). Oregano: Overview of the Literature on Health Benefits. *Nutr. Today*, **45**: 129–138.

295. Abad M.J., Bedoya L.M., Apaza L., Bermejo P. (2012). The *Artemisia* L. Genus: A Review of Bioactive Essential Oils. *Molecules*, **17**: 2542–2566.

296. Tu Y. (2011). The Discovery of Artemisinin (qinghaosu) and Gifts from Chinese Medicine. *Nat. Med.*, **17**(10): 1217–1220.

297. Su X.Z., Miller L.H. (2015). The Discovery of Artemisinin and the Nobel Prize in Physiology or Medicine. *Sci. China Life Sci.*, **58**(11): 1175–1179.

298. Mohamed A.E-H.H., El-Sayed M.A., Hegazy M.E., Helaly S.E., Esmail A.M., Mohamed N.S. (2010). Constituents and Biological Activities of *Artemisia herba-alba*. *Rec. Nat. Prod.*, **4**(1): 1–25.

299. Arbia L., Chikhi-Chorfi N., Betatache I., Pham-Huy C., Zenia S., Mameri N., Drouiche N., Lounici H. (2017). Antimicrobial Activity of Aqueous Extracts from Four Plants on Bacterial Isolates from Periodontitis Patients. *Environ. Sci. Pollut. Res.*, **24**(15): 13394–13404.

300. Seo D.Y., Lee S.R., Heo J.W., No M.H., Rhee B.D., Ko K.S., Kwak H.B., Han J. (2018). Ursolic Acid in Health and Disease. *Korean J. Physiol. Pharmacol.*, **22**(3): 235–248.

301. Woźniak L., Skąpska S., Marszalek K. (2015). Ursolic Acid. A Pentacyclic Triterpenoid with a Wide Spectrum of Pharmacological Activities. *Molecules*, **20**(11): 20614–20641.

302. Kumar A., Choudhir G., Shukla S.K., Sharma M., Tyagi P., Bhushan A., Rathore M. (2020). Identification of Phytochemical Inhibitors Against Main Protease of COVID-19 Using Molecular Modeling Approaches. *J. Biomol. Struct. Dyn.*: 1–11. https://doi.org/10.1080/07391102.2020.1772112.

303. Desborough M.J.R., Keeling D.M. (2017). The Aspirin Story – From Willow to Wonder Drug. *Br. J. Haematol.*, **177**(5): 674–683.

304. Fabricant D.S., Farnsworth N.R. (2001). The Value of Plants Used in Traditional Medicine for Drug Discovery. *Environ. Health Perspect.*, **109** (Suppl. 1): 69–75.

305. World Health Organization (WHO). (2009). WHO Monographs on Selected Medicinal Plants, Volume 4. Geneva, Switzerland, 28 Monographs, 456 pages. www.who.int/medicines/areas/traditional/SelectMono Vol4.pdf.

306. Rates S.M.K. (2001). Plants as Source of Drugs. *Toxicon*, **39**: 603–613.

307. Slavin J.L., Lloyd B. (2012). Health Benefits of Fruits and Vegetables. *Adv. Nutr.*, **3**: 506–516.

308. Liu R.H. (2013). Health-Promoting Components of Fruits and Vegetables in the Diet. *Adv. Nutr.*, **4**: 384S–392S.

309. Wallace T.C., Bailey R.L., Blumberg J.B., Burton-Freeman B., Chen C-Y.O., Crowe-White K.M., Drewnowski A., Hooshmand S., Johnson E., Lewis R., Murray R., Shapses S.A., Wang D.D. (2020). Fruits, Vegetables, and Health: A Comprehensive Narrative, Umbrella Review of the Science and Recommendations for Enhanced Public Policy to Improve Intake. *Crit. Rev. Food Sci. Nutr.*, **60**(13): 2174–2211.

6 Animal Source Foods

1 INTRODUCTION

Food products of animal origin occupy the second place after plant foods within the human diet domain. Animals including humans are classified under the Kingdom Animalia, also called Metazoa (1–4). Over a million to 1.5 million species of animal have been described until now on this planet (1, 3).

In spite of differences in structure and form of different animals, there are fundamental features common to various individuals in relation to the arrangement of cells, body symmetry, nature of coelom, patterns of digestive, circulatory, and reproductive systems. These features are used as the basis of animal classification (1). Animals are divided into various sub-groups called phyla. Biologists have identified about 36 phyla within the animal kingdom including humans, mammals, birds, reptiles, fish, amphibians, insects, and so on (1–2). Animals can be divided into vertebrates and invertebrates. Vertebrates have a backbone or spine, and comprise about 5% of all animal species. They include fish, amphibians, reptiles, birds, and mammals, including humans. The remaining animals are invertebrates, which lack a backbone. These include mollusks (oysters, clams, squid, cuttlefish, snails, octopuses), arthropods (shrimp, crabs, lobsters, insects, spiders, scorpions, millipedes), annelids (earthworms, leeches), nematodes (filarial worms, hookworms), flatworms (liver flukes, tapeworms), cnidarians (jellyfish, sea anemones, sea pens, corals), ctenophores (comb jellies), echinoderms (starfish, sea urchins, sea cucumbers, sand dollars, sea lilies or crinoids), and sponges (1–2). Most animals live on land (80%), the rest inhabit oceans (15%) or freshwater (5%) (3).

2 ANIMAL BIOLOGY AND PHYSIOLOGY

All members of Animalia are multicellular, eukaryotic, mobile, and heterotrophic organisms (1–2, 4). That means that animals have many cells with nucleus inside (eukaryote) and can move independently and spontaneously to search food from other organisms – plants and animals. All animals are heterotrophs, meaning that they feed directly or indirectly on other living things, contrary to plants that are autotrophs. They are often further subdivided into groups such as carnivores, herbivores, omnivores, and parasites. When an animal eats plants or other animals, the food becomes a source of energy and building materials for the animal. Digestion takes place in the internal cavity called the digestive system for advanced animals like mammals, birds, and fish, and in vacuoles for primitive animals such as amoeba and paramecium (1, 2, 4). Animals follow a definite growth pattern; the adults have a definite shape and size. Animals can be categorized on the basis of their symmetry. Most of the animals (mammals, birds, fishes, insects, etc.) are bilaterally symmetrical, while primitive animals (sponges) are asymmetrical. Ctenophores (comb jellies), cnidarians (corals, sea anemones, sea pens, jellyfish), and echinoderms (starfish, sand dollar, sea urchin, sea cucumber) have radial symmetry (1, 2, 4). Most animals can move, due to their locomotive organs like legs, wings, fits, and body muscle, according to each species. Sexual reproduction is achieved by the copulation of male and female which is followed by the development of an embryo. Respiration is a gaseous exchange of oxygen and carbon dioxide and takes place in lungs, gills, book gills, book lungs, or skin. In animals the nervous system consists of the brain, spinal cords and nerves (1, 2, 4).

Coloration or pigmentation in animals mediates the relationship between an organism and its environment in important ways, including camouflage, mimicry, social signaling, antipredator defenses, parasitic exploitation, thermoregulation, and protection from ultraviolet light, microbes, and abrasion (5–6). Some aquatic animals such as fish, amphibians and cephalopods use pigmented

DOI: 10.1201/9781003220817-6

chromatophores to provide camouflage. Pigmentation is used in signalization between animals, such as in courtship and sexual relation. For example, some cephalopods use their chromatophores to communicate. Across animals, coloration serves as a dynamic form of information (5–6).

In humans, the main pigment is black melanin which is found in skin, hair, eye iris, inner ear (stria vascularis), brain (substantia nigra), and adrenal gland (zona reticularis) (5–7). Black melanin in humans is able to dissipate over 99.9% of absorbed UVB radiation of sunlight, therefore it is thought to protect skin cells from solar radiation damage, reducing the risk of skin cancer or melanoma (5–7). However, UVB of sunlight is also necessary for the production of vitamin D3 that is formed from cholesterol in the skin under the action of sunlight. Too much melanin in the skin will stop the production of vitamin D3 due to the absence of UVB of sunlight. The black color of melanin is predominant; melanin hides other colors. When this black pigment is absent, other colors like white, blue or yellow will appear and, therefore skin, eyes, hair becomes white, blue, or blonde, respectively. Melanin is produced by a melanocyte which is located in the skin, hair, and eyes. It is noteworthy that the colors of the skin and hair are not related to the intelligence of an individual or a human race. A person's intelligence comes from their genes and brain. In brief, the color of human skin plays important roles in the protection of excess UVB from sunlight and the synthesis of vitamin D3 in the skin. This means that the absence of melanin in the skin may engender skin cancer and its excess can cause vitamin D3 deficiency.

3 ORIGIN OF ANIMAL SOURCE FOODS

Animal source foods have always been a constituent of human diets since antiquity. Before two million years ago, meat in particular was acquired via hunting of small animals (8). Animal source foods can provide a variety of micronutrients that are difficult to obtain in adequate quantities from plant source foods alone (8). Animal source foods supply not only high-quality, easily digested protein and energy, but are also an efficient source of available micronutrients such as iron, zinc, calcium, vitamin A, and vitamin B12 (8–10). Vitamin B12 and omega-3 fatty acids DHA and EPA are not found in common vegetables and fruits.

Edible animals used for food have two origins: wild animals and farmed animals. Wild animals used for food are mainly found in fresh and salt water such as fishes, crustaceans, and mollusks. Wild terrestrial animals like deer, wild birds, wild boar, insects, and kangaroo are not considered important food sources for humans, though they are often consumed by people living in forests or tropical areas, such as some autochthonous people. In contrast, farmed land animals such as pig, cow, lamb, and poultry are the most consumed by humans and marketed worldwide. In recent years, fish cultivated via aquaculture have begun to appear more in the market. The byproducts of farmed animals such as milk, egg, honey, and roes are also favorite foods for adults and children. Processed foods such as ham, sausage, and pâté are frequently consumed in Western countries. However, excessive intake of animal foods is harmful to health.

3.1 FOOD FROM WILD FISH

Among wild animals, fish and shellfish living in sea water and fresh water are an important source of food for humans, especially for people in coastal countries such as Japan, the Mediterranean region, Australia, and Indonesia, as well as Arctic regions like Alaska, Iceland, Scandinavia, and Siberia. More than 3.5 billion people depend on the ocean for their primary source of food, while wild land animals like birds, frogs, insects, wild boar, tortoise, turtle, and some terrestrial crustaceans, are less hunted for food (11–12).

3.1.1 Food from Wild Saltwater Fish and Shellfish or Seafood

Wild animals living in water and used for food mainly comprise fish and shellfish. They are divided into two groups: wild seawater fish and wild freshwater fish (13–15). Seafood is food obtained from the sea and mainly includes fish, shellfish (crustaceans, mollusks, echinoderms), and seaweed. Fish are the most consumed worldwide. Over 32,000 fish species have been described; about 60% of them are marine (14).

Fish play an important role in global food provision, accounting for about 20% of animal protein and 6.7% of all protein consumed by humans (13). Over 3 billion people worldwide now obtain approximately 17–20% of their animal protein from fish (15). In addition to protein, food from the sea provides essential vitamins (especially vitamin B12), minerals, long chain omega-3 fatty acids, and other nutrients not found in plant-source foods or other animal proteins (13–15). Fish has been shown to have positive effects in relation to heart disease, some cancers, inflammatory disease, high blood pressure, stroke, and muscular degeneration (15). However, most humans commonly eat only small amounts of marine fishes.

Marine fishes are divided in three categories: big-size, medium-size, and small-size (14). Big-sized fishes such as whales and dolphins belonging to sea mammals have been captured for food-stuffs and cosmetic industry, but their fishing is now banned because they are endangered species. Sharks are harvested primarily for their meat, fins, skin, cartilage, and liver (16). Shark fins are the most valuable of shark products and are used to make traditional shark fin soup, a delicacy and luxurious meal, in many Asian countries, especially in China (16). Shark meat is a preferred food in Japan, Australia, India, and some European countries. Shark cartilage is used for food and medicine in China and Japan. It is high in chondroitin and glucosamine sulfate, compounds used effectively in treating arthritis (16). However, shark as well as swordfish, tilefish, and king mackerel are high in mercury content and are now banned for children and pregnant women (12, 16–17). The most consumed medium- and small-sized fishes are: salmon, tuna, sardine, anchovy, pollock, trout, mackerel, sturgeon, cod, herring, eel, halibut, turbot, flying fish, cuttlefish, squid, sea bass, bonito, and so on. These wild fishes, especially salmon, sardine, pollock, anchovy, and mackerel, are generally safe and low in mercury content (17–18).

Shellfish include various species of crustaceans (krill, shrimp, prawn, lobster, crayfish, crab, copepod), mollusks (oyster, mussels, snails, cockle, abalone, clam as geoduck, scallop, octopus), and echinoderms (sea star, sea urchin, sea cucumber, sea horse). Krill, shrimp, and prawn are all crustaceans, but shrimp and prawn are about twice the size of krill. Krill has three segments: the head, thorax, and abdomen, while shrimp has two parts: a cephalothorax and the abdomen. Krill is vegetarian (algae) and lives in the Antarctic, while shrimp and prawn are omnivorous. Shrimp is found near the sea floor, while prawn prefers fresh water (river) (12–14, 19). Shellfish, in general, contain appreciable quantities of digestible proteins, essential amino acids, bioactive peptides, omega-3 fatty acids (DHA, EPA), astaxanthin and other carotenoids, vitamin B12 and other vitamins, and minerals (iodine, selenium), which offer a variety of health benefits to the consumer (19). Although shellfish are generally safe for consumption, some shellfish such as oysters, clams, and mussels may occasionally present health risks because of possible presence of various hazards including microbes, parasites, biotoxins, environmental pollutants, heavy metals, and also presence of allergy-causing compounds in their bodies (18). However, shrimp is rich in omega-3 fatty acids (EPA, DHA) and has low levels of mercury (14, 19). Sea cucumbers belonging to the class *Holothuroidea* are marine invertebrate echinoderm, habitually found in the benthic areas and deep seas across the world (20). They have a soft and cylindrical body like cucumber fruit; worm-like organisms with a leathery skin. Sea cucumbers, informally named as bêche-de-mer, or gamat, have long been used for food and folk medicine in the communities of Asia and Middle East. They are rich in vitamins (A, B1, B2, B3, B12) and minerals (calcium, magnesium, iron, zinc). Scientific studies have found that sea cucumbers have different biological and pharmacological activities including antioxidant, anticancer, anticoagulant, anti-hypertension, anti-inflammatory, antimicrobial, antithrombotic, anti-angiogenic, and wound healing (20–21). Therapeutic properties of sea cucumbers are due to a wide array of bioactive compounds like triterpene glycosides (saponins), glycosaminoglycan, chondroitin sulfates, polysaccharides, sterols, phenolics, cerebrosides (*cardiac glycosides*), peptides, glycoprotein, glycosphingolipids, lectins, and essential fatty acids (20–21). Small fish species, such as sardines and anchovies are often eaten whole, meaning the skin, head, bones, and viscera of these fishes are all consumed, while these organs in larger fish species are usually discarded. Therefore, a meal with whole small fish (sardine, anchovy) gives more minerals, especially calcium and phosphorous, than a meal with a fillet of large fish. Fish liver deteriorates very rapidly in air and therefore must be preserved as soon as possible after being extracted. Fish eggs of salmon, trout, mackerel, sturgeon, and so on are yellow-red and rich in astaxanthin.

3.1.2   Food from Wild Freshwater Fish

A freshwater fish is any species of fish that spends some or all of its life in freshwater. Freshwater fish is divided into three categories: (1) exclusively freshwater, (2) occurring in fresh and brackish waters, (3) or occurring in fresh, brackish, and marine waters (22). By nomenclature, a 'potamodromous' fish migrates wholly within freshwater, whereas a 'diadromous' fish can move between fresh and saltwater (22). Diadromous fishes are divided into 'anadromous', 'catadromous', or 'amphidromous' fishes (22). 'Anadromous' fish is fish spending most of its life in marine waters and only migrating to fresh water to breed, while 'catadromous' fish is fish spending most of its life in fresh water and only migrating to the sea to breed (22). Fish regularly migrating from fresh water to the seas, or vice versa, but not for breeding, is called 'amphidromous' (22). Except some anadromous fish and catadromous fish, the great majority of fish have a specific environment where they live.

Freshwater fish include catfish, charr, cisco, mooneye, gar, shiner, trout (apache, blueback, brook, brown and cutthroat), sunfish, pike, salmon (pink, coho, chum, Chinook and altantic), and whitefish (23). Saltwater fish includes albacore, certain types of bass, bluefish, common dolphin, butterfish, eels, flounder, cod, marlin, mackerel, herring, shark, snapper, tuna, and yellowtail (23). Wild fish living in river, lake, and pond are called freshwater fishes or potamodromous fishes, and are usually classified by the water temperature in which they survive, and thus named cold-water, cool-water, and warm-water species (23).

Anadromous fish such as salmon, sturgeon, trout, shad, herring, sawfish, sea lamprey, and striped bass spend most of their adult life in the sea, but when they reproduce, they migrate into freshwater to spawn (deposit eggs). In contrast, catadromous fish, like anguillid eels, are born in a marine habitat, but migrate into freshwater area to grow and mature. When they become adults they return to the sea to spawn (23–24). Some wild freshwater fish mostly commonly consumed are: carp, catfish, charr, bluegill, pike, brown trout, perch, charr, crappie, and mooneye (23). Some common edible wild freshwater crustaceans are: crawfish (crayfish or freshwater lobster), shrimp (prawn), and freshwater crab. The main freshwater mollusks include around 1,200 species of freshwater bivalves (mussels, clams), and around 4,000 species of freshwater gastropods (snails) (25). Mussels have historically not only been eaten, but also used for tempering pottery and for making utensils, tools, and jewelry. Freshwater snails also serve as a food source for humans in many parts of the world.

3.1.3   Difference in Physiology between Saltwater and Freshwater Fish

Anatomically, there is no difference between saltwater fish and freshwater fish. Both saltwater and freshwater fish breathe through specialized gills, which are openings located on their skin (23). The main difference resides in the regulation of salt and water contents in their tissues by osmosis in order to maintain the ratio of salt and water levels constant with their water environment – saltwater or freshwater. Freshwater fish have gills that function to diffuse water while ensuring bodily fluids remain inside the fish (23). Freshwater fish have large, well-developed kidneys that are able to process large amounts of urine in order to avoid an excess of water in their body tissues (23). Saltwater fish lose large quantities of internal body fluids through their gills because of osmosis. Since saline water is less diluted than the internal fluids of the fish, the saline water rushes in to replace the internal fluids in an effort to form an equilibrium. They replace lost water by consuming large quantities of saltwater (23).

3.1.4   Difference in Nutrient Content between Saltwater and Freshwater Fish

Concerning the nutrient contents, the difference between saltwater fish and freshwater fish is difficult to evaluate. In general, both kinds of fish are rich in proteins, amino acids, fats, unsaturated fatty acids, fat-soluble vitamins, and antioxidants, and low in carbohydrates. However, the main difference resides in the quantity of each nutrient. Recent data revealed that marine water fish is a better source of omega-3 essential fatty acids (ranged from 4.54% to 25.61%), while freshwater fish is a good source of omega-6 essential fatty acids (ranged from 5.66% to 12.15%) (26). Generally, the results showed that global fatty acid compositions of marine water fish species are comparable to those of freshwater fish species as sources of polyunsaturated fatty acids (PUFA) (26–27). It is noteworthy that omega-3 fatty acids, including docosahexaenoic acid (DHA) and eicosapentaenoic acid (EPA), are responsible for the prevention and treatment of inflammatory diseases (arthritis, asthma), cardiovascular diseases, and more, while omega-6 fatty acids do not. Moreover, the fatty acid composition of fishes depends on their species, diet, and environmental factors such as salinity, temperature, season, and geographical location, as well as whether the fish are farmed or wild (26–27). Fish cannot synthesize omega-3 and omega-6 fatty acids. They obtain them by eating algae and plankton present in their environment. It is noteworthy that freshwater microalgae contain plenty of omega-6 fatty acid and alpha-linolenic acid (ALA), an inactive form of omega-3 fatty acid. Therefore, freshwater fish are richer in these unsaturated fatty acids (omega-6 and ALA) than seawater fish, which mainly contain DHA and EPA, the two active forms of omega-3 fatty acids in the human body (27). As marine algae and plankton are rich in DHA and EPA, seawater fish are therefore rich in these two active forms of omega-3 fatty acids. Some fish can convert ALA to DHA and EPA, and many fish are carnivorous. Therefore, some freshwater fish also contain DHA and EPA in comparable levels to seawater fish.

3.1.5   Fish Feeding Habits

Fish are classified as carnivorous (meat eating), herbivorous (plant eating), omnivorous (meat and plant eating), and detritivorous (detritus feeder) based on their usual food source preferences in their natural habitats (27). Carnivorous fish include salmon, perch, basses, breams, halibut, flounders, groupers, shark, dolphin, whale, and cod; while carp, tilapia, milkfish, surgeonfish, parrotfish, and manatees are herbivorous. Omnivorous fish such as carp, catfish, grey mullet, eels, brown trout, buffalo fish, sunfish, minnows, and shrimp are the most abundant in sea as well as in rivers, lakes, and ponds. In aquatic environments, common detritivorous or detritivores are crustaceans (lobsters, fiddler crabs), echinoderms (sea cucumbers, sea stars), and mud carp (*Cirrhinus molitorella*). Carnivorous, herbivorous, and omnivorous fish are rich in nutrients and popular among consumers (27).

3.1.6   Fish Meat

Fish meat is classified as white meat which also includes poultry meat. Fish and poultry meats are called white meats because they contain lower myoglobin and heme iron levels than red meats from mammals. Fish meat is an important source of energy, high-quality proteins, good fats, vitamins, antioxidants, and minerals (13, 17, 28–32). It is the main food source for populations living near ocean, sea, lake, or river. In several African and Asian countries, fish provide more than half of the animal protein supply and are a food staple (28). Fish meat has been recently discovered to prevent some chronic ailments, in particular cardiovascular diseases. Studies have reported the absence of CVDs among Inuit in Greenland and the Arctic region, who eat most fatty fish and shellfish daily (31–32).

3.1.6.1   *Constituents and Benefits of Fish Meat*

The benefits of seafood as well as of freshwater fish for health maintenance and disease prevention are well-known through valuable studies worldwide. Regular intake of seawater fish and freshwater fish is good for health because fish is not only high in protein and amino acids but also rich in vitamins A and D, as well as strong essential antioxidants, and mostly omega-3 polyunsaturated fatty acids (n-3 PUFAs) (13–14, 17, 27–34).

Thus, the levels of the two active forms docosahexaenoic acid (DHA) and eicosapentaenoic acid (EPA) of omega-3 fatty acids in fish and shellfish are strongly dependent on the species consumed. Fish species that provide the highest levels of n-3 PUFAs are sockeye salmon, farmed trout, farmed salmon, Copper River salmon, Coho salmon, brozini, fresh bluefin tuna, albacore tuna canned in water, and toothfish (17). Species providing less than 150 mg of n-3 PUFAs per 100 g fish meals include mahi-mahi, skate, triggerfish, monkfish, red snapper, wahoo, grouper, corvina, and tuna canned in oil (17). Species intermediate in n-3 PUFAs are haddock, cod, halibut, sole, flounder, crustacea, perch, black bass, tilapia, and swordfish (17). Shrimp and krill are also good sources of n-3 PUFAs. DHA and EPA play an important role in health promotion and chronic disease prevention like cardiovascular diseases, neurodegenerative disease, and cancer (30–34). DHA has a major role in the development of brain and retina during fetal development and the first two years of life, and positively influences neurodevelopment, mainly visual acuity and cognitive functions (17, 29–30, 33). Meta-analyses of cohort studies concerning fish intake also suggest a strong protective effect of stroke. This effect cannot be exclusively attributed to EPA and DHA, but also to other fish components such as taurine, an abundant sulfur amino acid in fish and shellfish (29–30). This amino acid is known for its role in the formation and excretion of bile salts, which are the breakdown cholesterol products. It also plays a role in the function of the neonatal retina and in cognitive function (29).

In fish and shellfish, omega-3 unsaturated fatty acids are mainly esterified either in phospholipids (PLs) or triglycerides (TGs) or, due to a partial hydrolysis, are present in the free form (35). TGs are highly hydrophobic, whereas PLs are hydrophilic due to the polar headgroup. Hence, the physical-chemical properties of these two groups of lipid structures (PLs and TGs) are different, and only PLs are able to form micelles and liposomes, and are thereby more absorbable in the body. Marine sources such as salmon, tuna, rainbow trout, mackerel, fish roe, and krill oil contain high amounts of EPA and DHA under PLs (35).

Fish and shellfish are considered a good source of minerals such as calcium (Ca) (about 10–100 mg/100 g), magnesium (Mg) (10–170 mg/100 g), and phosphorus (P) (200–300 mg/100 g), as well as fluorine (F) (300–400mg/100 g), iodine (I) (10–300 mg/100 g), selenium (Se) (35–45mg/100 g), iron (Fe) (0.3–2.8 mg/100 g), zinc (Zn) (0.3–1.3 mg/100 g), and copper (Cu) (0.1–0.2 mg/100 g) (30, 33). However, fish is a poor source of sodium (Na) (20–140 mg/100 g) but rich in potassium (K) (200–400 mg/100 g). Seafood products are one of the few natural sources of I and Se and omega-3 phospholipids (13, 29, 30, 33). The highest Se levels are usually present in tuna, swordfish, and scad (30). Mussels, scad, and sardines are the fresh species with the highest Zn levels. Mollusks and crustaceans have high levels of Cu and Fe; their remarkable level of Cu could be accounted for by the presence of hemocyanin, a Cu-containing respiratory protein found in the blood of those species (30).

Fish is rich in vitamins, namely thiamin (vitamin B1) (40–210mg/100 g), riboflavin (vitamin B2) (50–360 mg/100 g), niacin (vitamin B3) (2–10 mg/100 g), pyridoxine (200–980mg/100 g), and specially cobalamin (vitamin B12) (1–9mg/100 g). Herrings, shads, sardines, hilsa, and menhadens of the fish family Clupeidae. Anchovies of the family Engraulidae exhibit the highest content of vitamin B12 (30). Liposoluble vitamins, mainly vitamins A and D, are mostly accumulated in the liver of codfish species, therefore cod liver oil is a good supplement for people with deficiencies of vitamins A and D. Vitamin A in fish fillet ranges 3–180 mcg (micrograms)/100 g. The vitamin D content of fish may vary enormously and it is not well correlated with the fat content, with values ranging from 3–20 mg/100 g (30). Fish is also a good source of co-enzyme Q10 which is a strong antioxidant at the sub-cellular level (29). Additionally, astaxanthin, a xanthophyll carotenoid red-orange pigment, is a powerful biological antioxidant present naturally in a wide variety of marine organisms such as microalgae, salmon, trout, crayfish, krill, shrimp, lobster, crustaceans, fish eggs and crab eggs. Astaxanthin is 65 times more powerful than vitamin C and 54 times stronger than beta-carotene and plays an important role in the prevention of many ocular diseases such as glaucoma, cataract, and macular degeneration (36). Among small crustaceans, *Calanus finmarchicus* living in the North Sea, the Norwegian Sea and the North Atlantic, is rich in protein and contains high amounts of omega-3 fatty acids and diverse antioxidants such as astaxanthin (30).

Seafood consumption may protect the heart and vessels as well as reduce inflammatory diseases like asthma and rheumatoid arthritis, and prevent stroke and diabetes. It is also shown to reduce blood pressure and decrease triglyceride levels in blood (30–33). For example, Japanese people are high consumers of seafood (fish, shellfish, seaweed), therefore, they have very low cardiovascular disease death rates (e.g., 87% lower than comparable Western populations) (32). For the neurodevelopmental benefits of seafood intake during pregnancy, one observational cohort study reported beneficial effects to children with improved neuro-behavioral development when maternal seafood intake exceeded 340 g per week compared to mothers not consuming seafood (17, 31, 33). Because the brain is made mainly of fat, and omega-3 fatty acids, seafood is also a good food for supporting brain activity and for the prevention of neurodegenerative diseases and depression. Although some cohort studies show that fish intake is not associated with either increase or decrease in the risk of cancer overall, there is significant evidence of protection for colorectal cancer and some evidence in relation to prostate cancer in people who frequently consume seafood or freshwater fish (30).

3.1.6.2   Risks of Fish Meat

In contrast to the potential health benefits of dietary fish consumption, concern has arisen over potential risks from certain chemical and organic pollutants, namely mercury, arsenic, dioxins, polychlorinated biphenyls (PCBs), and plastics present in some seawater and freshwater fish species (11, 30–33).

Mercury is a heavy, liquid metal emitted from natural sources (volcanoes and some ores) and human sources from industrial wastes. From the atmosphere, mercury cycles from rainwater into lakes and oceans, where it is converted by microbial activity into organic methylmercury (32). Mercury in fish exists in the form of methylmercury $(CH_3\text{-}Hg)^+$ which is a fat-soluble organic compound and highly toxic for the human central nervous system. Inorganic mercury liquid (for example, from ancient thermometers) is poorly absorbed following ingestion, and elemental mercury does not readily cross tissue barriers (32). In contrast, methylmercury is readily absorbed and actively transported into tissues, then accumulated in the brain and nerves. Methylmercury causes neuropathy (ataxia, numbness, paralysis, coma, death) in humans and mammals like cats, but is not toxic in fish and shellfish except for in very high doses (32). Methylmercury can cross the placenta, and fetal exposure correlates with maternal exposure. The famous poisoning of methylmercury by eating fish contaminated from industrial wastes is called Minamata disease or syndrome (11, 31–32).

Methylmercury was first recognized as a hazard in seafood as a result of large-scale industrial poisonings during the 1950s in Minamata Bay, Japan, where recorded mercury levels in local seafood reached 36 ppm (31). It was caused by the release of methylmercury in industrial wastewater from a chemical factory located near Minamata Bay. This toxic compound accumulated in all fish and shellfish in this sea caused mercury poisoning for the population of Minamata Bay for many years. Concentrations of methylmercury in aquatic species depend on levels of environmental contamination and on the predatory nature and lifespan of the species. Larger, longer-living predators (swordfish, shark) have higher tissue concentrations of mercury than smaller or shorter-lived species (shellfish, salmon, sardine) (32–33). For example, mercury levels are found inferior to 0.05ppm (μg/g) in anchovy, catfish (farmed), Atlantic herring, Atlantic mackerel, Alaskan pollock, salmon wild and farmed, sardines, clams, oysters, scallops, shrimp, fish fat food, and frozen fish (32–33). They vary from 0.10 ppm to 0.20 ppm in Atlantic cod, Atlantic tilefish, mahi-mahi, trout, tuna light, and crab. Mercury levels are found very high – about 1ppm (μg/g) – in both shark and swordfish, 0.73ppm in king mackerel, and 1.45ppm in tilefish in the Gulf of Mexico (32–33). It is noteworthy that mercury level for tilefish in Atlantic (0.14ppm) is 10 times lower than for the same tilefish in the Gulf of Mexico (1.45ppm) (18, 32). This great difference in mercury levels in the same species found in two different regions may be explained by the presence of many submarine volcanoes in the Gulf of Mexico.

Besides mercury, arsenic is also found in seafood, in particular crustaceans like lobsters and crabs, and bivalves like clams, oysters, scallops, and mussels. Arsenic is a metalloid that occurs in different inorganic and organic forms, which are found in the environment both from natural occurrence and from anthropogenic activity. The mineral forms of arsenic are more toxic than the organic arsenic (37). In fish and crustaceans, the toxic mineral arsenic is transformed into soluble organic form named arsenobetaine, which becomes nontoxic and easily excreted via human urine (37). Other organic arsenic forms found in fish, shellfish, and marine algae are arsenocholine, arsenosugars, and arsenolipids, which are considered nontoxic (37).

Dioxins and polychlorinated biphenyls (PCBs) are produced by industrial wastes and household garbage discharged into the environment, often contaminating fish. PCBs are synthetic organochlorine compounds previously used in industrial and commercial processes (18, 32). Dioxins, commonly referring to as dibenzodioxins and dibenzofurans, are organochlorine byproducts of waste incineration, pesticide production, paper bleaching, and production of polyvinyl chloride plastics. Manufacture and processing of PCBs was prohibited in 1977 and regulatory and industry efforts have reduced dioxin emissions by more than 90% since 1987 (32). Nevertheless, these contaminants persist for long periods in the environment, and thus remain in the environment, while levels are steadily declining. Dioxins and PCBs are both carcinogenic (see Chapter 8 of this book).

3.1.7 Choice of Fish

Selection of fish depends on three factors: the mode of fish living, in other words, wild fish or farmed fish; the area where fish live, whether marine or freshwater; and the quality of fish meat including nutrients, contaminants, and taste.

3.1.7.1 Mode of Fish Obtention

Obtaining wild fish and shellfish by capture in ocean, sea, sea coast, river, lake, or pond, is called fishing, hunting, or capture fisheries; while cultivating wild seawater, freshwater fish, and shellfish via industry or individuals is classified as aquaculture, mariculture, or fish farming, in the case of fish only (13, 28). A fishery or mariculture is an area where marine or freshwater animals and plants are farmed and harvested for commercial benefits. The fish species that are widely farmed are: salmon, basses, breams, halibut, catfish, eels, carp, tilapia, eels, flounders and groupers (27). In general, wild fish captured in open ocean may be healthier and safer than farmed fish because they are far from pollution zone and their nutrients are naturally formed (13, 29). However, nowadays, some farmed fish have the same quality as fish captured in ocean. In general, farmed fish are often cheaper than wild-caught fish.

3.1.7.2 Choice of Seawater Fish and Freshwater Fish

As cited above, both seawater and freshwater fish have similar nutrient contents, but the difference between them resides in the levels of these nutrients. In general, seawater fish is higher in omega-3 essential fatty acids (EPA and DHA) than freshwater fish, while freshwater fish is a good source of omega-6 essential fatty acids like linoleic acid (LA) and alpha-linolenic acid (ALA), an inactive form of omega-3 fatty acids (26). However, some freshwater fish can convert ALA into DHA and EPA and many fish are carnivorous. Therefore, some freshwater fish like carp, rainbow trout, have amounts of DHA and EPA as high as seawater fish (38). Capture fisheries in oceans need large boats with elaborate equipment, while those in freshwater like river, pond, only need some banal tools like nets, fishing rods, or small boats. Therefore, freshwater fish are cheaper than seawater fish and are often consumed by people living in developing countries or in areas with many rivers, lakes, and ponds, such as in Southeast Asia. The levels of proteins and other nutrients in seawater fish and freshwater fish are generally the same (26–27). So, people in industrial countries prefer seafoods because of their abundance in active omega-3 fatty acids, while people in developing areas choose freshwater fish due to their low cost and their availability.

3.1.7.3 Choice of Fish Based on Nutrients and Contaminants

As cited above, fish is a choice meat because fish is not only high in protein, amino acids, vitamins, and antioxidants, but also rich in active omega-3 polyunsaturated fatty acids (EPA and DHA), which are not found in other animal meat. EPA and DHA are two important nutrients necessary for brain and heart activities. However, fish meat also contains mercury in the form of methylmercury, a neurotoxin for adults and children. In addition, fish are also contaminated by some other organic toxic compounds such as dioxins and polychlorinated biphenyls (PCBs) which are industrial wastes discharged into the environment. The levels of these toxins (mercury, dioxins) vary with the environment, thereby with fish species. So, the choice of fish and shellfish depends not only on their nutrient levels, but also on their contaminated toxic contents. Fish rich in healthy nutrients and very low in mercury and industrial contaminants include small fish living in large oceans and far from volcanoes and industrial areas. Salmon, sardine, Alaskan pollock, anchovy, herring, Atlantic mackerel, Atlantic cod, Atlantic tilefish, mahi-mahi, trout, tuna, shrimp, scallop, and crab – all harvested in large oceans – are good seafood because they contain very low levels of mercury, dioxins, and PCBs. In contrast, big fish like shark, swordfish, and tilefish, must be avoided because of their high mercury content (30–32). Freshwater fish like carp, rainbow trout, and catfish, living in 'green areas' are also good for health. In general, all fish of small or medium sizes living far from volcanoes and industrial areas are considered safe to eat.

3.1.8 Recommendations Concerning Fish Intake

Overall, concerning the risk/benefit assessments of fish consumption, most studies and international organizations such as the World Health Organization (WHO), the Food and Agriculture Organization (FAO) of the United Nations, the International Agency for Research on Cancer (IARC), and the American Heart Association (AHA) have found that the benefits far outweigh the risks among the general population (30–32, 39). According to the AHA, it is recommended to eat fatty fish at least two times a week for the prevention of cardiovascular diseases. The FAO/WHO Expert Committee stated that the fish species, the frequency of consumption, and the meal size are essential issues for an adequate balance of the health benefits and risks of regular fish intake (30).

Briefly, for major health outcomes among adults, the vast majority of epidemiological studies have proven that the benefits of fish intake exceed the potential risks, excepting a few cases in sensitive populations such as pregnant women. Many people in the world such as Inuit, Japanese, and Mediterranean populations have less incidence of cardiovascular diseases than others because their favorite foods are seafood. The use of fish oil or omega-3 supplements cannot replace the intake of fish meat because these supplements do not contain other necessary nutrients present in fish meat. However, excessive intake of fish and shellfish, especially fish oil supplement, can increase bleeding risks like epistaxis and cerebral hemorrhage, or cause hypoglycemia or hypotension, as observed in Inuit peoples who only eat seafood.

3.2 FOOD FROM WILD LAND ANIMALS

Some wild terrestrial animals such as wild boar, deer, kangaroo, bison, jackrabbit, frog, wild duck, goose, birds, pigeon, insects, and tortoise are still hunted for foods by humans today, mostly in tropical regions and developing countries. Some big animals, like kangaroos, wild boars, and deer are killed or caught in their natural environments, mostly in forests or meadows. For catching these wild animals, a hunting permit is required in many countries. The hunting of some wild animals such as elephant, polar bear, African lion, Siberia tiger, Indian rhinoceros, hippopotamus, Vietnamese pheasant, and lesser white-fronted goose is now banned because they are endangered species.

In some tropical countries, wild insects are also consumed, such as grasshopper, cricket, silkworm pupa, bee, beetle, wasp, dragonfly, caterpillar, cockroach, and earthworms because they are rich in proteins and easy to obtain (40). Some advantages of wild animals in comparison with farmed animals are the absence of pesticides, insecticides, or other artificial chemicals (hormones, antibiotics, etc.) in their meat or organs. Moreover, their meat is better; for example, pigeon, wild duck, or wild boar is richer in proteins and lesser in fats than farmed duck or pig. However, wild land animal meats are rarely found in the markets of industrialized countries, but are still present in developing communities.

3.3   FOOD FROM FARM LAND ANIMALS

Animals raised by farmers are called farmed or farm animals. Common farm land animals include: cattle, pigs, goats, sheep, horses, poultry and sometimes bees. They produce meat, fat, milk, eggs, or honey for human consumption. Eggs, milk, and honey are called animal byproducts and are produced by animals during their lifetimes. To produce animal meat, farm animals are bred until they reach a target weight, then are killed, processed, and sold to consumers.

3.3.1   Types of Land Animal Feed

Animal feed is food given to farm animals. Animal feeds are either classified as fodder, forage, or mixed or compound feeds (41). Each type of these feeds has its own uses and benefits (41). Animal feed plays an important part in the food chain and the composition and quality of the livestock products (milk, meat, and eggs) that people consume (41).

Fodders could be classified as roughages (fresh cut forage, hay or dry forage, straw, root crops, stover, and silage) and concentrates such as grains, legumes and byproducts of processing (41). The most common feed grains include corn, soybeans, sorghum, oats, and barley (41–42). Other grains like rice, wheat, and oat are often given to poultry. Dry bean and other crop residue are of lesser importance (42). Fodders are the most used by farmers in industrialized countries because they are practical, cheap and give a high meat yield.

Fresh plants that are grown in pasture land or meadow and are consumed by various farmed animals (livestock) are known as forage (41). Pasture can be composed of herbaceous legumes (alfalfa), native and improved grasses, crop residues, agro-industrial byproducts, non-conventional feed resources such as cereals, and other edible plants (41–42). During winter, dried gras (hay) is given to animals raised by forage. Animals raised by forage give superior food to consumers because they eat fresh plants in nature and they have space to move. Forage-raised animals have better meat than fodder-raised animals, because grass-fed beef contains less saturated fat and cholesterol than grain-fed beef. In addition, it is richer in vitamins A and E and antioxidants than grain-fed beef (43). Other studies have found that compared to eggs of the caged hens, pastured hens' eggs had twice as much vitamin E and long-chain omega-3 fatty acids, and less than half the ratio of omega-6/omega-3 fatty acids (44). Moreover, forage-raised animals are exempt of artificial chemicals like hormones and antibiotics. However, the production of animal food obtained from forage-raised animals diminishes today, mostly in industrialized countries, and is replaced by animals grown with grains in feedlots, due to the low cost of farming by grains.

Mixed feeds are produced from several feed ingredients combined in different proportions to achieve a particular nutritional quality. Feed ingredients, including additives, may or may not add any nutritional value to the mixed feed. They comprise of components originating from plant, animal, or aquatic sources, organic and inorganic in nature (41). Like vitamin supplements for humans, mixed feeds are often complemented with extra vitamins and minerals. Mixed feeds are usually produced in the form of pellets or mash (41). It is important to consider that livestock feed affects not only animal health, but also consumer health.

3.3.2   Problems of Land Animal Feed

In some industrialized countries, animal feeds contain mixtures of plant-based products, as well as other ingredients ranging from rendered animals and animal waste to pharmaceutical and industrial sources such as antibiotics and organo-arsenicals (45). The inclusion of these ingredients in animal feeds can result in the presence of a range of biological, chemical, and other etiologic agents in feed that can affect the quality and safety of animal-based food products and pose potential risks to human health. Specific feed ingredients vary depending upon the animal (i.e., poultry, swine, cattle) (45). Currently, the use of animal feed ingredients, including rendered animal products, animal waste, antibiotics, metals, and fats, could result in higher levels of bacteria, antibiotic resistant bacteria, prions, arsenic, and dioxin-like compounds in animals and resulting animal-based food products intended for human consumption. Subsequent human health effects among consumers could include increases in bacterial infections (antibiotic resistant and nonresistant) and increases in the risk of developing fatal chronic diseases such as variant Creutzfeldt-Jakob disease (vCJD) (45). Recently, three problems found in the literature concerning farm animals raised by fodder are 'mad cow' disease, antibiotic resistance, and beef hormones (hormone-treated beef).

3.3.2.1 Mad Cow Disease

Bovine spongiform encephalopathy (BSE) is a progressive neurological disorder of cattle first recognized in 1986 in the United Kingdom which results from infection by an unusual transmissible agent called a prion (46). The nature of the transmissible agent is not well understood. Currently, the most accepted theory is that the agent is a modified form of a normal protein known as prion protein. This prion changes into a pathogenic (harmful) form that then damages the central nervous system of cattle (46). BSE possibly originated as a result of feeding cattle meat-and-bone meal that contained BSE-infected products (46).

The BSE epizootic in the United Kingdom peaked in January 1993 at almost 1,000 new bovine deaths per week. Since then, the annual numbers of BSE death cases in the United Kingdom have dropped sharply from about 14,560 cases in 1995 to 1,443 cows in 2000 (46). Over 150 human deaths from bovine spongiform encephalopathy (BSE)-contaminated food products were counted in the UK population in this period (47). Nowadays, mad cow disease is not observed due to the ban of this mode of cattle feeding.

3.3.2.2 Antibiotic Use and Antibiotic Resistance

The use of antibiotics for animal feeds began in the 1950s after farmers observed that livestock eating antibiotic supplements gained meaty weight more rapidly (48). The mechanism of this weight gain due to antibiotic use for farmed animals is not known. Some ten years later, many scientists published their landmark study demonstrating a direct link between antibiotic use on farms and the spread of antibiotic resistance to human populations (49). Recently, many scientific studies have recognized some evidence of links between antimicrobial use in the food chain and antimicrobial resistance in humans (50). Therefore, the European Union banned the use of antibiotic growth promoters in animal feed in 2006 and the United States FDA curtailed antibiotic use in livestock since 2017 after years of debate (48).

3.3.2.3 Beef Hormones

The polemic about selling beef containing hormones or meat hormones was a commercial dispute between the United States, Canada, and the European Union (EU) since 1989 until recently. This 'beef war' was due to the use of many growth hormones such as recombinant bovine growth hormone (rBGH), or recombinant bovine somatotropin (rBST), which are authorized for beef farming in the United States and Canada, while the EU considers this addition to be harmful for human health and have banned the importation of beef meat made in these two countries (51). In June 2019, the European Union and the United States have reached an agreement on imports of hormone-free beef (52).

4 BENEFITS AND RISKS OF LAND ANIMAL SOURCE FOOD

Foods obtained from land animals may be helpful or harmful to health, depending on the different types of meat, animal species, cooking types, livestock farming, and so on.

4.1   Benefits of Land Animal Source Food

In general, land animal source foods (ASF) are excellent sources of energy because they are rich in both macronutrients and micronutrients. Macronutrients include proteins, fats, amino acids, and micronutrients are essential minerals (calcium, iron, zinc) and vitamins (A, B_{12}, B_2 or riboflavin) (8–11, 53–54). Vitamin B_{12} levels (µg/100g) are highest in rabbit meat (6.5 µg), then beef meat (2.4 µg), goat meat (1.2 µg), eggs (1.0 µg), fish (0.6 µg), cow's milk (0.3 µg), and are not found in vegetables (0.0 µg), like maize, wheat, bean, soy, and spinach, except for algae (9, 11). Therefore, vegetarians must take Vitamin B_{12} supplement to avoid anemia. In contrast, vitamins C, B1, B2, and calcium are present in different animal and vegetable source foods. For example, calcium levels (mg/100g) found in some animal and vegetable foods are the following: cow's milk (76 mg), goat's milk (90 mg), beef (7 mg), chicken (13 mg), fish (37 mg), eggs (50 mg), maize (47 mg), wheat (0 mg), beans (35 mg), soy (zero mg), and spinach (122 mg) (11). However, for the same concentration, calcium absorption in humans from land animal source foods such as milk is better than that of plant source foods because it is in organic form (11). It is important to note that the proteins in animal source foods are considered the highest quality available, as they contain a full complement of essential amino acids and most resemble the proteins of the human body in their amino acid composition. Animal source foods also provide high biological value protein and energy owing to hemoprotein, a complex of porphyrin with iron (Fe^{2+}), present only in meat, fish, and fowl.

4.2   Red Meat and White Meat

Among land animal foods, meat is the food most consumed by humans. There are two kinds of meat: red meat and white meat. Red meats originate from the flesh of farm mammals like beef, veal, pork, lamb, sheep, and horse, and of wild mammals such as kangaroo, deer, wild boar; while white meats are obtained from chicken, duck, turkey, fish and shellfish (55). Some internal organs and offal like heart, liver, kidneys, intestines, and brains of different mammals and poultry are also used. In general, meat can be classified as 'red' or 'white' based on their myoglobin concentration in muscle fiber (55). Myoglobin is a complex of protein-like hemoglobin in red blood cells. It is combined with iron and oxygen found in the muscle tissue of all mammals. When myoglobin makes contact with oxygen, a reddish pigment called oxymyoglobin develops, making meat appear red. Myoglobin levels in mammal meat are higher than those in poultry and fish. This classification is arbitrary and varies with country and organism. For example, in Australia, the term 'red meat' is used by the meat industry to refer to meat from cattle, sheep, and goat (i.e., beef, veal, lamb, mutton, and goat meat). It does not include meat from pigs (e.g., pork, bacon, ham) or kangaroo, buffalo, and camel (56). Purchased red meat usually consists of both lean tissue (muscle) and fat tissue, which can be either distributed throughout the muscle as marbling (internal fat) or surrounding the muscle meat as selvage or external fat (56).

4.3   Benefits of Red Meat for Health

Red meat contains high biological value protein and important micronutrients that are needed for good health throughout life (56). In general, lean red meat is a particularly good source of protein, amino acids, niacin, vitamin B6, vitamin B12, phosphorus, zinc, and iron, with 100 g providing more than 25% RDI (recommended daily intake) of these nutrients (56–58). It also provides more than 10% RDI of riboflavin, pantothenic acid, and selenium. These compounds play an important role in the growth of children and adolescents and give strength to people who do physical work (56–58). Red meat is an excellent source of vitamin B12 and iron. Vitamin B12 and iron are two essential micronutrients for hematopoiesis that is necessary for the formation of red blood cells. Vegetables do not contain vitamin B12, except algae. Iron in vegetables is not more or less digestible because it is in inorganic form. In contrast, 50–60% of iron in red meat is in heme form, an easily absorbed organic form (57). Anemia is often observed in vegans or people who do not eat red meat due to poverty or another reason like religion. In general, lean red meat has a relatively low-fat content, and is moderate in cholesterol (56). In contrast, fat red meat is high in saturated fatty acids and cholesterol. Of the four meats (beef, veal, lamb, and mutton), mutton is particularly nutrient-dense, and the richest source of thiamin, vitamins B6 and B12, phosphorus, iron, and copper (56). Lean pork meat and lean beef meat have the same nutrients, but beef meat in general contains more saturated fatty acids, iron, and flavor than pork meat. Ground beef and ground pork are rich in fats of different amounts. Western people prefer beef meat, while Asian people and people in developing countries like pork meat.

4.4 Risks of Red Meat and Processed Red Meat for Health

Concerning human health, red meats and their processed foods (ham, sausage, bacon, corned beef, beef jerky, hot dogs etc.) are now the subjects of many debates between academic researchers and industrial furnishers about their effects on the development of many chronic diseases.

Recently, a 2017 literature review reported that for 100g or more per day of unprocessed red meat consumed, the risk increased 11% for breast cancer, 17% for colon cancer, 19% for prostate cancer, 11% for stroke, and 15% for cardiovascular mortality (59). For each additional 50g per day of processed red meat (ham, sausage, bacon, etc.) consumed, the risks still increased for most studied diseases from cancer to CVDs, stroke, and diabetes. The evidence-based conclusion is that high consumption of red meat, and especially processed meat, is associated with an increased risk of several major chronic diseases and preterm mortality (59). Many scientific publications about health problems with red meat and processed meat consumption are also reported in the literature (58–76). While more evidence regarding the health effects of red and processed meats is needed, the body of epidemiologic data showing their associations with Type 2 diabetes, CVD, and cancer is large and consistent (62). Nevertheless, some studies do not support the association between red meat or processed meat and cancer or other chronic diseases such as CVD and diabetes (67–68).

4.4.1 Consumption of Red Meat and Processed Red Meat and Cancer

In October 2015, 22 scientists from ten countries met at the International Agency for Research on Cancer (IARC), the cancer agency of the World Health Organization, in Lyon, France, to evaluate the carcinogenicity of the consumption of red meat and processed meat. They classified the consumption of red meat as probably carcinogenic to humans (Group 2A), based on limited evidence that the consumption of red meat causes cancer in humans and strong mechanistic evidence supporting a carcinogenic effect of processed meat (Group 1) (60–61). According to IARC, red meat refers to all types of mammalian muscle meat, such as beef, veal, pork, lamb, mutton, horse, and goat; while processed meat refers to meat that has been transformed through salting, curing, fermentation, smoking, or other processes to enhance flavor or improve preservation such as ham, saucisson, sausages, corned beef, beef jerky, and canned meat (60). Other studies in men and women confirmed the carcinogenic properties of processed meat and the probable carcinogenic effects of red meat with frequent consumption over a long period (62–66).

Nevertheless, other publications do not support significant links between red meat consumption and cancers. In a review article, McAffee et al. (67) concluded that moderate intake of lean red meat as part of a balanced diet is unlikely to increase risk for colon cancer or CVD, but may positively influence nutrient intakes and fatty acid profiles, thereby impacting positively on long-term health. After reviewing numerous studies, Truswell concluded that the relationship of colorectal cancer with meat consumption appeared weaker than the 'probable' status given by the World Cancer Research Foundation in 1997 (68).

Meat cooking also plays an important role in cancer development (see Chapter 4, paragraph: Cooking). For example, eating rare steak or medium-rare beefsteak has less of an association with stomach cancer than eating medium-well or well-done steak because the former contains less carcinogenic compounds formed by meat heating than the latter.

4.4.2   Consumption of Red Meat and Processed Red Meat and Cardiovascular Diseases

There are still controversies in different studies found in the literature about the link between red meat and processed meat consumption and cardiovascular diseases (CVDs) (69–71). However, many scientists observed that processed meats are more harmful to the heart and vessels than unprocessed meats because processed meats contain salt and preservatives which are harmful to the cardiovascular system and can cause hypertension. Fats in red meat play a minor role in CVDs. McAfee et al suggested that future studies investigate lean red meat trimmed of excess fat to find the exact cause of CVD in relation to red and processed meat consumption (67).

4.4.3   Consumption of Red Meat and Processed Red Meat and Diabetes

The relation between consumption of different types of red meats and risk of Type 2 diabetes (T2D) remains uncertain. Based on 3 cohorts in 1986–2006 with 37,083 men participants, 1980–2008 with 79,570 women participants, and 1991–2005 with about 87,504 women participants, and an updated meta-analysis, a group of American researchers found that red meat consumption, particularly processed red meat, is associated with an increased risk of T2D (72). Other groups found that only processed meat intake was associated with 19% higher risk of diabetes mellitus (69).

4.4.4   Consumption of Red Meat and Processed Red Meat and Obesity

In 2010, a study entitled the European Prospective Investigation into Cancer and Nutrition – Physical Activity, Nutrition, Alcohol, Cessation of Smoking, Eating Out of Home and Obesity (EPIC-PANACEA) published that meat consumption is positively associated with weight gain in men and women, after tracking 373,803 people over a period of 8 years and across 10 countries (73). In contrast, the National Cattlemen's Beef Association opposed by stating that meat consumption is not associated with fat gain (74). Another publication in 2014 revealed that red and processed meat intake is directly associated with risk of obesity, and positively linked with greater weight gain (75).

4.4.5   Consumption of Red Meat and Processed Red Meat and Mortality

A 1999 meta-study combined data from five prospective studies to compare the death rates from common diseases of vegetarians with those of non-vegetarians with similar lifestyles (76). Mortality from ischemic heart disease was 24% lower in vegetarians than in non-vegetarians. Further categorization of diets showed that, in comparison with regular meat eaters, mortality from ischemic heart disease was 20% lower in occasional meat eaters, 34% lower in people who ate fish but not meat, 34% lower in lacto-ovo-vegetarians, and 26% lower in vegans (76). According to these authors (76) there were no significant differences between vegetarians and non-vegetarians in mortality from all forms of cancer (colon, stomach, lung, breast, prostate cancers), or all other causes combined. However, some other scientists recently found that greater consumption of unprocessed and processed red meats is associated with higher mortality risk of all forms of diseases, cancer included (58–63). Compared to red meat, other dietary components, such as fish, poultry, nuts, legumes, low-fat dairy products, and whole grains, were associated with lower risks. These results indicate that replacement of red meat with alternative healthy dietary components may lower the mortality risk of all disease causes (62–63).

4.4.6   Consumption of Red Meat and Processed Red Meat and Pathology Mechanisms

Several mechanisms have been proposed to explain the adverse effects of unprocessed and processed red meat intake on disease development and mortality risk. Unprocessed red meats like beef and pork contain more saturated fats, cholesterol, arachidonic acid, heme iron, and homocysteine compared to white meats such as poultry and fish (59, 63, 77–78). One of the components of red meat, heme iron (an iron porphyrin pigment present at ten-fold higher concentrations in red meat compared to white meat), has been ascribed a role in cancer development (59). Free ferrous iron is released from heme and iron itself plays a role in the increased production of free radicals (ROS), especially H_2O_2, which may further induce lipid peroxidation, inflammation, cytotoxic effects, and genetic mutations (changes in DNA) (59). Heme iron in red meat under certain conditions may act as a nitrosating agent, responsible for cancer development (59). Saturated fatty acids and cholesterol found in red meat have been reported to be associated with significantly raised risks of colorectal cancer and cardiovascular diseases such as myocardial infarction, coronary heart disease, and stroke. They may also increase insulin resistance causing Type 2 diabetes (59, 63). Furthermore, dietary iron, particularly heme iron, rich in red meat, has been positively associated with myocardial infarction and fatal coronary heart disease (59, 63).

Processed meats like ham, sausage, summer sausage, and saucisson (dried sausage) contain on average about 50% more nitrates and 400% more salt (sodium chloride) than unprocessed red meat. Nitrites and nitrates used in processed meat for preservation are converted to nitrosamines by binding to amino compounds within food or in the stomach (59). Nitrosamines are toxic to pancreatic tissue, decrease insulin secretion, and increase the risk of diabetes. Nitrosamines can cause DNA damage and produce free radicals that generate protein adduct formation, lipid peroxidation, and pro-inflammatory cytokine activation (59). High salt contents are the cause of high blood pressure, chronic kidney disease, edema, stroke, CVD, and more.

Briefly, it is important to note that unprocessed red meats like beef and pork are rich in absorbable proteins, vitamin B12, antioxidants, and essential micronutrients which play an important role in human health maintenance. Therefore, it is likely that maintaining intakes of unprocessed red meat at or below the current advised level (70 g/day), whilst reducing intakes of processed meat such as ham, sausage, and saucisson, may reduce the risks of chronic disease development (67). Moreover, some nutrients, vitamins, and antioxidants in processed meat, can be partially or totally destroyed during processing and storage.

In summary, red meat is a food rich in protein and minerals such as iron and zinc as well as a variety of vitamins, in particular vitamin B12. However, red meat is higher in cholesterol and saturated fat than some other food groups such as white meat (fish, poultry) and vegetables (77–78). Processed meats are usually made of red meat that are cured, salted, or smoked in order to improve the durability of the food and/or to improve color and taste. Hence, high consumption of processed foods may lead to an increased intake of saturated fats, cholesterol, salt, nitrite, hem iron, colorants, flavors, and preservatives (78). Several large cohort studies have shown that a high consumption of processed red meat increased risk of chronic diseases (CVD, diabetes mellitus, or some types of cancer) and overall mortality (77–78). To avoid these side effects of red meat, it is important to limit its consumption to 70 g/day and to avoid processed meat in case of chronic diseases (67).

For these reasons, some scientists observed that to improve human health, dietary guidelines should continue to emphasize dietary patterns low in red and processed meats and high in sea foods, plant foods such as fruits, vegetables, grains, and nuts, and spices (77).

4.5   BENEFITS AND RISKS OF WHITE MEATS

Meats obtained from poultry and fish are called white meats because they contain lower myoglobin and heme iron levels than red meats from mammals. In general, white meats are safer than red meats.

4.5.1   Poultry Meat

Poultry meat including chicken, duck, turkey, goose, pigeon, and quail, is a valuable food because it contains variable but moderate quantities of energy with highly digestible proteins of good nutritional quality and low saturated fats (except its skin which is easily removed) (79–83). Moreover, poultry meat is rich in B-group vitamins (mainly thiamin, vitamin B6, and pantothenic acid), and minerals (like iron, zinc, copper). Chicken meat is also an excellent source of selenium, an essential mineral and antioxidant for the activity of many enzymes (79–82). Moreover, chicken meat contains low collagen levels, which is another positive characteristic. Collagen is a structural protein that reduces meat digestibility, so chicken meat is easier to digest than other types of meat (81). Chicken and turkey meat are slightly higher in protein and slightly lower in fat than beef and other red meats. Chicken meat is known by its nutritional quality, as it contains significant amount of high-quality and easily digestible protein and a low portion of saturated fat (80–81). In addition, it is a rich source of all essential amino acids. For example, a 100 g serving of baked chicken breast contains 4 g of fat and 31 g of protein, compared to 10 g of fat and 27 g of protein for the same portion of broiled, lean beefsteak (81–82). Therefore, chicken meat is recommended for consumption by all age groups. However, lipid intake associated with poultry meat is variable and dependent on the cut (79). For example, chicken skin contains high amounts of fat and bad saturated fat. It is important to mention that chicken with skin contains two to three times more fat than chicken without skin, so it should be eaten without skin to ensure the intake of high-quality protein without extra calories and fat (81). For this reason, do not consume chicken or poultry skin. Poultry skin (chicken, dusk, turkey, etc.) should be removed before or after cooking. The skin of duck and goose is particularly high in fat content. The total fat level in duck meat is 8% of the edible portion, and in the meat plus skin, the total fat content is 28% of the edible portion (80). The total lipid content of goose meat is 7% of the edible portion, but in goose meat plus skin, the fat content rises to 34% of the edible portion (80). In chicken meat, the dark meat is higher in fat than the light meat or white meat. Chicken breast muscle is an important component of a modern healthy diet (80).

The composition of poultry fat is favorable. Only a third of total fat is made up of saturated fatty acids (bad fats) such as palmitic acid (21–24%), stearic acid (15–17%) and myristic acid (0.4–1%). The rest (two-thirds) includes significant amounts of monounsaturated fatty acids (good fats), in comparison with bovine, ovine, or pig meat (79–80). The main monounsaturated fatty acids are oleic acid and palmitoleic acid. Substantial amounts of polyunsaturated fats are the omega-6 fatty acids such as linoleic acid or LA, (16.1%), and arachidonic acid or AA (1.5–5.6%) (79–80). The dominant omega-3 fatty acid is α-linolenic ALA, with a range of 1.15 to 2.51%. The least abundant omega-3 fatty acid is eicosapentaenoic acid (EPA), comprising 0.24 to 0.96%. The other omega-3 fatty acid is docosahexanoic acid (DHA), comprising 0.67 to 3.35%. The n-6/n-3 ratios vary from 3.37 to 11.35 (80). Keep in mind that the omega-3 ALA is an inactive form; it must be hydrolyzed in the body into the two active forms, EPA and DHA. Hydrolysis decreases with age to almost none in the elderly. As poultry eat grains and cereals, their levels of alpha-linoleic acid (ALA) are much higher than its two active forms, EPA and DHA (79–83). Therefore, chicken meat cannot replace fish meat and fish oil. Chicken meat quality depends on various factors such as keeping conditions, feeding treatment, feed composition, and more (81). When compared to red meat, the main advantage of white chicken meat is in its low caloric value and low level of saturated fat; so, consumption of white chicken meat is recommended to people who want to reduce fat intake, as well as to people suffering from cardiovascular diseases (81). When compared to cholesterol content, white chicken meat does not differ much from other types of meat (81). From a nutritional point of view, the composition of poultry fat is favorable because only a third of total fat is made up of 'bad' saturated fatty acids; the rest includes significant amounts of 'good' monounsaturated fatty acids (79–81).

4.5.1.1 Benefits of Poultry Meat

High protein content makes chicken meat an ideal foodstuff for all consumers who need high-quality, easily degradable protein (athletes, children, pregnant women, the elderly). Poultry meat consumption also contributes to the overall quality of the diet in specific ages and conditions (prior to conception, during pregnancy up to the end of breastfeeding, during growth, and in the geriatric age) and is suitable for those who have an increased need for calorie and protein compared to the general population (79). Because of all stated above, chicken meat is recommended as a rich source of high-quality protein in human nutrition (81). In addition, consumption of poultry meat is associated with a reduction of developing overweight and obesity, cardiovascular diseases, and Type 2 diabetes mellitus. Also, white meat (and poultry in particular) is considered moderately protective or neutral on cancer risk (79). The relationship between meat intake and lung cancer risk appears to depend on the types of meat consumed (84–85). A high intake of red meat may increase the risk of lung cancer by about 35%, while a high intake of poultry decreases the risk by about 10% (84). More cohort studies about the association between meat and lung cancer are needed to observe meat mutagens based on meat cooking preferences (84). Additionally, no association with intake of poultry, seafood, and colorectal cancer has been observed in almost all of the cohort studies that have examined this relationship (85). The European Prospective Investigation into Cancer and Nutrition (EPIC) supports the hypothesis that colorectal cancer risk is positively associated with high consumption of red and processed meat and inversely associated with the intake of fish and poultry (85). Fish and poultry intakes were not associated with colorectal cancer risk in the most recently published prospective and cohort studies (85).

4.5.1.2   Risks of Poultry Meat

Three main types of food risk, namely, microbiological risk, chemical risk, and technological risk related to chicken have been identified (86).

Some microbiological risks for consumers of poultry, meat, and eggs are due to bacterial infections caused by *Staphylococcus aureus*, Salmonella, Campylobacter, and avian influenza virus (86). Poultry products may become contaminated by these bacteria during handling, processing, marketing, or storage, resulting in food-borne disease if the product is improperly cooked or handled. Thorough cooking of the product would kill these bacteria, but there is always a risk of cross-contamination due to improper handling of the raw product (86). This contamination is also observed with red meat and seafood.

Chemical risk includes residues in food due to antibiotics fed to chickens as well as the remnants of agricultural chemicals (pesticides, fertilizers, etc.) in animal feed. Exposure to chemical residues in food may cause cancer, chronic fatigue syndrome, immune deficiencies, and lung and nerve damage (86).

Technological risk refers to the possible negative consequences of technological advancements in food products, such as genetic modification (GM) of food (86). Technology has contributed multiple benefits in terms of food safety and increased food availability in general. There may also be public health risks associated with potential toxic or allergic effects of GM organisms or environmental effects resulting from the accidental release of GM organisms (86). People tend to be suspicious of new technologies, often perceiving that the risks will outweigh the potential benefits, especially when the relative advantage of the technology is untested or unclear (86).

In summary, poultry meat is healthy and rich in necessary nutrients such as proteins, 'good fats', vitamins, and minerals. However, poultry skin is rich in saturated fats ('bad' fats) and must be removed when eating. It may be superior to red meat in certain aspects because the cancer risks due to poultry meat are lower than those caused by red meat and processed meats, and obesity is rarely observed. The levels of active omega-3 fatty acids DHA and EPA in poultry meat are lower than those in seafood. The ease of farming chicken meat and its resulting low cost make it an appealing choice.

4.6   Meat Cooking

Other problems of meat consumption have to do with cooking and preparation. The mode of cooking meat plays an important role in health and disease of the consumer. In general, grilled meat, fumed meat, fried meat, and so on can contain toxic compounds due to direct contact of meat with a high heat source; hence, it may be advisable to consume them in moderation, about two to three times a week, because frequent intake of barbecued or fried foods may lead to obesity, CVDs, and cancer formation (87–89). Cooking with moderate heat, like boiling, steaming, braising, and stewing, is the best choice for meat cooking (see Chapter 4). However, it is advised to avoid eating raw meat due to bacterial and/or parasitic contamination.

5 ANIMAL BYPRODUCTS

Animal byproducts are products directly obtained from animals and are used as foods and in some cases as medicines. The most consumed whole animal byproducts are milk, egg, and honey which are mainly produced by farmed animals. Fish oil, cod liver oil, and krill oil are byproducts of seawater fish and shellfish, and are destined for the preparation of omega-3 unsaturated fatty acid dietary supplements. Velvet antler is a cartilaginous byproduct of deer, elk, moose, and caribou. In addition, edible bird's nest and fish fins are byproducts of wild swiftlet birds and shark, respectively, and are employed as luxurious food for festivities in many Asian countries, and also for their tonic effects. Silk, skin, and fur are also animal byproducts used for clothing manufacture.

5.1 MILK AND DAIRY PRODUCTS

Milk is a complex nourishing liquid directly produced by different female mammals and humans, and is used as primary food for their baby. Dairy products are foods derived from animal milk and are processed by farmers or industrial companies. The main dairy products are yogurt, cheese, butter, cream, and kefir.

5.1.1 Milk

Milk from human and animal origins provides essential nutrients and is an important source of dietary energy, high-quality proteins, and fats. For babies, milk is the primary source of nutrition and comes from maternal milk (breast feeding) or from animal milk, especially cow's milk. It is considered a complete liquid food for the growth of babies of all mammals. Milk contains not only all nutrients but also all defensive materials such as antibodies, immune cells for the protection of babies against microbes during the first months of their life (90–99). Therefore, breastfeeding is the best nourishment for babies. Sources of animal milk and milk products include cows, sheep, camels, goats, yaks, horses, donkeys, and buffaloes.

In India, Western, and Middle Eastern countries, humans continue to consume milk and its byproducts beyond infancy, using the milk of other animals as a beverage, or as processed milk products like cheese, yogurt, and butter, as foods. However, many people in East Asia never consume milk and dairy products throughout their adult life. The consumption of milk and milk products varies from about 180 kg yearly per capita in Iceland and Finland to less than 50 kg in Japan and China (93).

5.1.1.1 Composition of Cow's and Other Animal Milks

Bovine milk is the most consumed because of its high nutritional quality, its extensive production, and its easy farming. In general, the gross composition of cow's milk is 87.7% water, 4.9% lactose (carbohydrate), 3.4% fats, 3.3% protein, 0.8% minerals and 0.1% vitamins (90, 92–99). Cow's milk contains several vitamins (A, E, D, and B group) and minerals (calcium, magnesium, selenium, phosphate, iodine, etc.) easily consumable in significant quantity (90, 92–95). Milk composition varies depending on the species (cow, goat, sheep, horse, yak, camel, buffalo), breed, the animal's feed (forage or fodder), and the stage of lactation (92). Sheep milk has higher fat and protein contents than cow and goat milk (90, 92, 94–95, 99). Fats in sheep milk are about 6.4 g/100g, while those in cow and goat are about 3.3–3.6 g/100g and 3.6–3.9 g/100g, respectively (92, 94–95). Sheep milk also generally has a higher lactose content than milk from cows, buffaloes, and goats (90). The high protein and overall solid contents of sheep milk make it particularly appropriate for cheese and yogurt making. Milk from sheep is important in the Mediterranean region, where most of it is processed into cheeses such as pecorino and feta (90, 92).

Carbohydrates. Lactose is the main sugar of all milks, and its levels vary between 2–8% depending on the species. It is a disaccharide composed of galactose and glucose and its flavor is less sweet than sucrose. It is hydrolyzed by a β-galactosidase known as lactase (92, 94–95).

This enzyme is located in small intestine mucosa membrane and after lactose is hydrolyzed, the two monosaccharides glucose and galactose are absorbed and transported to the liver through the portal vein where galactose is converted to glucose. Lactose is responsible of milk intolerances in some people who lack an enzyme named lactase that hydrolyzes lactose into galactose and glucose. Lactose non-hydrolyzed – intact – moves to the large intestine where it is fermented by bacteria and can cause intestinal troubles (92, 94–96). Interestingly, intake of lactose, as opposed to glucose and fructose, does not appear to be associated with diabetes incidence (96). Even though the evidence in favor or against lactose use by diabetic patients is scant, the American Diabetes Association recommends the use of milk and dairy products (96). This is partly because milk has a relatively low glycemic index due to dairy proteins, in particular casein, which exhibit insulinogenic properties and facilitates glycemic regulation through a mechanism involving elevation of certain plasma amino acids and stimulation of incretins, a group of metabolic hormones used to decrease blood glucose levels (96).

Proteins. Milk is generally considered an important protein source in the human diet, supplying approximately 32 g protein/L (92–99). Its protein fraction can be divided into soluble and insoluble proteins. Soluble proteins, named whey proteins, represent approximatively 20% of milk protein fraction, whereas the insoluble proteins, namely caseins, represent about 80% and may vary slightly depending on the species (92–96). The casein family contains phosphorus and will coagulate at pH 4.6.

The soluble whey protein family is globular protein and consists of approximately 50% ß-lactoglobulin, 20% α-lactalbumin, blood serum albumin, immunoglobulins (Ig) or antibodies, lactoferrin, transferrin, lactoperoxidase, lysozyme, and many minor proteins and enzymes (92–96). Lactoferrin, lactoperoxidase, and lysozyme are important antimicrobial agents, whereas lactoferrin together with β-lactoglobulin and α-lactalbumin has shown suppressing action in tumor development (93–94). Whey is the liquid remaining after milk has been curdled to produce cheese, and it is used in many products for human consumption, such as ricotta and brown cheese, and concentrated whey is an additive to several products such as bread, crackers, pastries, and animal feed (93).

The main role attributed to insoluble caseins is mineral binding and their capacity as carriers, mainly for calcium and phosphorus (90–95). Total caseins can be divided in α-, β-, and κ-caseins. They transport calcium and phosphorus, forming a coagulum and improving their digestibility in the stomach. In addition, caseins give several bioactive peptides that have antioxidant, immuno-modulatory, cyto-modulatory, antihypertensive, and antithrombotic actions in the cardiovascular, nervous, immune, and digestive systems (90–94). Milk protein is especially rich in amino acids that stimulates muscle synthesis, and some proteins and peptides in milk have positive health effects on blood pressure, inflammation, oxidation, and tissue development. The amino acid profile is quite different between the two fractions. Whey is especially rich in branched chain amino acids such as leucine, isoleucine, and valine as well as lysine; whereas casein has a higher proportion of histidine, methionine, and phenylalanine (90–94). The benefits of drinking whey have been known for centuries. An ancient proverb from the Italian city of Florence says: 'If everyone was raised on whey, doctors would be bankrupt' (93).

Fats. Most milks consumed now contain a standardized fat content of around 3.4 g/100 g (92–94). Milk fat contains approximately 65% saturated, 30% monounsaturated, and 5% polyunsaturated fatty acids. Triacylglycerol (TAG) forms 95–98% of milk fat fraction, whereas other lipids like diacylglycerol (2%), cholesterol (< 0.5%), phospholipids (about 1%), and free fatty acids (0.1%) also can be found (92–94). Milk fat is the most complex of all natural fats considering that more than 400 different fatty acids make up its triacylglycerol (93). Within saturated fatty acids (SFAs), the most important are palmitic acid (30%), myristic acid (11%), and stearic acid (12%). Short-chain fatty acids can also be found and make up 11% of SFAs, mainly butyric (4.4%), and caproic acids (2.4%) (93). A moderate intake of milk fat has no negative health effects; on the contrary, many milk fat components may be harmful to the body (92). In the market, bovine milk is prepared by ultra-high temperature (UHT) and is classified in three categories according to its fat content: whole milk, semi-skimmed milk or low-fat milk, and skimmed milk. For example, UHT whole milk contains 3.5 g fats/100 g, UHT semi-skimmed milk 1.6% fats, and UHT skimmed milk 0.2% fats (92, 94). Cholesterol levels also vary with the concentration of fats. They are 13 mg/100 g in whole bovine milk UHT, 8 mg/100 g in semi-skimmed cow milk UHT and 1 mg/100 g in skimmed bovine milk UHT (94). Whole bovine milk and whole sheep milk have the highest cholesterol concentrations (99). Cheese had the weakest effect on increasing LDL cholesterol, but whole milk increased concentrations of LDL cholesterol (bad cholesterol), similar to butter (96). Therefore, the intake of whole milk products might theoretically have detrimental effects on cholesterol concentrations. However, it is noteworthy that the contribution of dietary cholesterol to cardiovascular risk is being debated and might likely depend on individual predisposition to synthesizing versus absorbing cholesterol (96).

Vitamins, Minerals and Antioxidants. Milk contains the water-soluble vitamins: thiamin (vitamin B1), riboflavin (vitamin B2), niacin (vitamin B3), pantothenic acid (vitamin B5), vitamin B6 (pyridoxine), vitamin B12 (cobalamin), vitamin C, and folate. Milk is a good source of thiamin, riboflavin, and vitamin B12, but is not considered a major source of niacin, pantothenic acid, vitamins B6, C, E and K, or folate (92–95). Milk is a great source of calcium, magnesium, phosphorus, potassium, selenium, and zinc. The calcium concentration in bovine milk is about one g/l (93). Calcium in milk is in organic form such as calcium lactate; it is more assimilable in the human body than calcium in mineral form such as calcium carbonate and phosphate. Calcium, magnesium, phosphate, and fluoride present in milk are necessary for the skeletal growth of the baby. Milk contains small amounts of iron, manganese, copper, fluoride, and sodium and is not considered a major source of these minerals in the diet (92, 97). Dairy products contain antioxidant compounds in varying proportions depending on the matrix type (i.e., milks, yogurts, fermented milks, and cheeses) and processing (i.e., mechanical, thermal, and fermentative) (100). These compounds include both lipophilic and hydrophilic antioxidants: proteins (especially casein), peptides, antioxidant enzymes (i.e., superoxide dismutase, catalase, and glutathione peroxidase), coenzyme Q10, lactoferrin, vitamins (C, E, A, and D3), carotenoids, and some minerals (selenium, iron) (100). In brief, cow milk and other animal milks can make a significant contribution to the required nutrient intakes for calcium, magnesium, selenium, riboflavin, vitamin B12, and pantothenic acid (94). The species of dairy animal, its breed, age, and diet, along with the stage of lactation, parity (number of parturitions), farming system, physical environment and season, influence the composition of milk and allow the production of a variety of milk products. Animal milk can play an important role in the diets of children in populations with very low fat intakes and limited access to other animal source foods. For adults, consumption of 0.5 L animal milk daily supplies a significant amount of many of the nutrients that are required daily (93).

5.1.1.2 Composition and Role of Human Milk

The composition of human milk is the biologic norm for infant nutrition (91). Human milk also contains many hundreds to thousands of distinct bioactive molecules including antibodies and immune cells that protect against infection and inflammation and contribute to immune maturation, organ development, and healthy microbial colonization for the baby. Human milk is a dynamic, bioactive fluid that changes in composition from colostrum to late lactation, and varies within feeds, diurnally, and between mothers (91).

The colostrum or early breast milk is the first form of milk produced by the mammary glands of all mammals immediately following delivery of the newborn (91). Colostrum, produced in low quantities in the first few days postpartum, is rich in immunologic components such as secretory immunoglobulin A (IgA) or antibody A, lactoferrin, and leukocytes, as well as developmental factors such as epidermal growth factor (91). These immunologic products in colostrum absorbed by the baby are to ensure immunity defense against microbes. It is important to note that antibodies are transferred from placenta to the fetus, which justifies the low concentrations after birth. Colostrum has 100 times more antibodies than milk (94). Colostrum only lasts a few days and is then replaced by milk. It is reported that the antibodies in cow colostrum have no effect on the human body because the antibodies are generally specific to each species; they will be destroyed as other proteins in the human digestive tract. Therefore, giving the mother's colostrum to the baby is very necessary for the sake of the newborn's health. Exclusive human milk feeding for the first six months of a baby's life, with continued breastfeeding for one to two years or longer, is recognized as the normative standard for infant feeding that promotes survival and healthy development (91).

While cow milk and human milk contain a similar percentage of water, the relative amounts of protein, carbohydrate, fat, vitamins and minerals vary widely (91–93). For example, cow's milk contains 120 mg/100g calcium, 11 mg/100g magnesium, 94 mg/100g phosphorous, 156 mg/100g potassium, and 43 mg/100g sodium. Human milk has 34 mg/100g calcium, 3 mg/100g magnesium, 15 mg/100g phosphorous, 15 mg/100g sodium, 58 mg/100g potassium (90–91). Although human milk contains less calcium, it is more easily absorbed than that found in cow milk. The fat content of women's milk (2.1–4.0%) was greater than that of non-ruminants, but less than that of ruminants (99).

Human milk and cow's milk differ in the amounts of various proteins they contain. The most abundant proteins of human milk are casein, α-lactalbumin, lactoferrin, secretory immunoglobulin IgA, lysozyme, and serum albumin (91). Cow's milk contains more protein (3.2%) than does human milk (1.2%), but human milk contains more lactose (6.7 to 7.8%) than does cow milk (4.7%), resulting in comparable energy contents (92, 94). In cow's milk, levels of casein are 26 g/L – about ten folds greater than those in human milk (2.7 g/L) (94). Caseins can form leathery curds in the stomach and be difficult to digest for human babies. In addition, the type of caseins that predominate in the two milks also differs; human milk contains more β-casein, which is more susceptible to peptic hydrolysis than αS-casein, particularly αs1-casein, which predominates in cow milk (92). Human milk does not contain β-lactoglobulin, one of the main proteins associated with cow milk allergy. A review of 20 studies of cognitive function of breast-fed infants compared to infants fed on formula concluded that the nutrients in breast milk may have a significant effect on neurological development in infants. More recent work indicates that compared to formula milk, nutrients in breast milk may confer better cognitive and motor development in infants (91).

Fat is the most highly variable macronutrient of milk. The percentage of saturated fatty acids (bad fats) reported in cow milk were higher (65.6%) than in human milk (48.2%). On the other hand, the mono- and polyunsaturated fatty acids (good fats) were higher in human milk than in cow milk (39.8% and 10.8% vs. 30.3% and 4.5%) (99). Breast milk contains both long-chain polyunsaturated fatty acids and essential fatty acids. Colostrum contains high levels of arachidonic acid (omega-6 unsaturated fatty acids) (more than 1% of total fatty acids) and docosahexaenoic acid (omega-3 unsaturated fatty acids) (above 0.50%) (99).

Indeed, the popular consensus among health care professionals is that ordinary cow's milk, goat's milk, condensed milk, dried milk, evaporated milk, or any other type of milk should not be given to a child under the age of one (92). Breastfeeding is the exclusive food for babies under 6 months old.

5.1.1.3   Roles of Milk and Dairy Products in Human Health and Disease

Milk is widely consumed in Western countries from childhood to old age because it is an important source of macro- and micronutrients. It is considered a complete nutrient-dense food for everybody. Milk is recognized as being useful during childhood and adolescence because milk is rich in calcium, vitamins, proteins, and so on that are the main compounds necessary for the growth of children. However, there exist some minor negative effects of milk on human health, such as the presence of some saturated fats in milk that may increase high cholesterol in blood, as well as lactose intolerance in some individuals (94, 96, 101).

5.1.1.3.1   Obesity   Recent evidence suggested that intake of milk and dairy product was associated with reduced risk of childhood obesity. In adults, intake of dairy products was shown to improve body form and facilitate weight loss during energy restriction (101). Of all the bioactive milk components, calcium and vitamin D have been chiefly studied for their effects on body weight and adipose tissue. Studies have been performed on these compounds as either isolated molecules or as components of milk and dairy products (96). Proposed mechanisms include thermogenesis and lipid oxidation (which are enhanced by calcium and vitamin D) and increased lipid fecal excretion (96). In addition, dairy proteins are being suggested as reducers of adipose mass (namely, visceral fat) and body weight. While whey protein appears to be particularly effective and their actions seem to be mediated by several mechanisms that include increased satiety and decreased appetite (96).

5.1.1.3.2   Bone Diseases and Growth   Milk and dairy products are high in calcium, phosphate, vitamin D2, lactose, and proteins that are required for building strong bones in children and for their maintenance during adulthood with the aim to reduce osteoporosis and bone fractures in elderly people (94, 96, 98, 101). Cow milk has good bioavailability of calcium; its calcium absorption is good in humans because it contains not only high quantities of calcium but also other compounds that aid in its absorption, namely lactose, vitamin D2, casein phospho-peptides. These components act synergistically to promote calcium absorption, playing an important role in bone density (94, 96, 98). In addition, calcium (Ca) in milk and dairy foods are more soluble and absorbed in intestinal transit than calcium in plant foods because milk contains lactose that helps calcium absorption and transportation in the body. Among dairy products, hard cheeses such as parmesan, gouda, cheddar, gruyere, Emmental, and pecorino are the richest sources of calcium and can provide 1 g of Ca per 100 g, whereas milk and yogurt can furnish between 100 mg to 180 mg of Ca per 100 g (102). Some plant foods can be a source of calcium. However, plant foods can contain many inhibitory compounds, such as oxalates and phytates that inhibit the absorption of calcium and iron. Oxalates and phytates bind to calcium and form insoluble salt complexes, thus decreasing calcium absorption. In adults, interactions between calcium, phosphorus, protein, and vitamin D reduce bone resorption and increase bone formation, thereby attenuating age-related bone loss (101, 103). A recent systematic review concluded that calcium and dairy products are important contributors to bone health in adults (101). Low bone mass is the main risk factor for osteoporosis and bone fractures (94). As milk and dairy products should still be considered the superior sources of calcium, their regular intake is necessary for growth of children, for protection against tooth decay, and for the prevention of osteoporosis and bone fracture in the elderly (94, 103). East Asian people are often small because they do not consume milk and dairy products from infancy to adulthood. For all these reasons, hard cheese and skimmed milk or semi-skimmed milk intake is globally recommended as a promoter of good bone health (94, 103).

5.1.1.3.3   Type 2 Diabetes   Few epidemiologic studies have addressed the possible effect of milk intake in risk for Type 2 diabetes (94, 96). However, many results from long cohort studies have shown that higher milk and dairy product intake was associated with a reduced relative risk, which was confirmed by the most recent meta-analysis (94, 96). This protective effect may be due to milk's richness in calcium and magnesium, two minerals that have been found crucial in insulin sensitivity and glucose tolerance as reported in experimental and cohort studies, as well as in a recent meta-analysis (94, 96). Finally, data from the EPIC (European Prospective Investigation into Cancer and Nutrition) study relative to 16,835 healthy and 12,403 diabetic participants of 8 European nations confirmed the inverse association between cheese and fermented dairy consumption and incidence of diabetes (96). In particular, 55 g/day of cheese and yogurt were associated with a 12% reduction in incidence of Type 2 diabetes (96, 101). Therefore, regular consumption of fermented dairy products (cheese, yogurt) might reduce the risk of Type 2 diabetes.

5.1.1.3.4   Cancer   It is not completely clear if milk consumption increases or decreases the risk for cancer (94, 96–97, 101, 103–104). Cancer has a complex and multifactorial etiology, thus there is no available evidence to prove the effect of a single food and/or nutrient on its origin and development. Moderate dairy product consumption has been recommended as a healthy food habit suggested as part of a protective dietary pattern involved in the prevention of several chronic diseases, including cancer (94). In population studies, dairy has been associated positively and negatively with various cancers, but most have been based on limited evidence, and very few findings remain robust (96, 97, 101). Dairy products contain a variety of bioactive compounds that could exert both positive and negative effects on carcinogenesis. The positive effects may be related to the content of whey proteins, calcium, lactoferrin, and fermentation products, whereas the negative effects could be linked to the content of insulin-like growth factor I (IGF-1) (101, 104). Whey proteins are Sulfur containing Amino Acids, (SAA)-rich proteins, and have been reported to possess anticarcinogenic properties. Indeed, through provision of methionine and cysteine, they have a positive influence on cellular methylation, and, by stabilizing DNA, they retard the development of colon tumors and tumor precursors (104). The anticarcinogenic activity of whey proteins and their individual components is well-documented, and these proteins offer protection against colon and mammary cancers (104). In addition, other studies have shown that the minor milk protein lactoferrin has anticancer properties (103). In research on mice containing a human gene that induces lung tumors, lactoferrin significantly decreased the proliferation of cancer cells and lung cell inflammation (103). Considering these data, it is possible to suggest that the complex etiology of cancer does not allow a clear and evident conclusion about a positive or negative role of milk consumption in risk for cancer; however, some assumptions can be made (94). Excessive milk intake can increase prostate and ovarian cancers due to calcium and lactose consumption, respectively. Concerning calcium, the suggested hypothesis is that excessive calcium intake impairs the synthesis of vitamin D and possibly promotes vitamin D receptor gene polymorphisms, which suppress its modulating role in prostate cell tumor growth and development (94). Whole-milk consumption also can increase risk for breast and prostate cancers due to the influence of fat in androgens and estrogens, as well as to the increased energy availability, which would facilitate carcinogenesis process (94). However, moderate milk consumption, regardless of fat content, has a protective effect in colorectal cancer (94, 96). According to the World Cancer Research Fund reports and the latest meta-analyses, consumption of milk and dairy products probably protects against colorectal cancer, bladder cancer, gastric cancer, and breast cancer (101). Dairy intake does not seem to be associated with risk of pancreatic cancer, ovarian cancer, or lung cancer, whereas the evidence for prostate cancer risk is inconsistent (101). In women, dairy offers robust and significant health benefits in reducing the risk of common and serious colorectal cancer and, possibly, also the risk of breast cancer. In men, the benefit of the protective effect of milk and dairy on common and serious colorectal cancer is judged to outweigh a potentially increased risk of prostate cancer (101).

5.1.1.3.5 Cardiovascular Diseases Milk and dairy products (cheese, butter) contain cholesterol and saturated fats, namely palmitic, myristic and lauric acids; therefore, the intake of these products might theoretically have detrimental effects on cholesterol and lipid levels in blood. However, the effects of these products on cholesterol production in humans are different depending on the dairy products used. Many scientists reported that whole milk increased LDL-cholesterol (bad cholesterol) in blood similar to butter; while cheese decreased it (96, 103). This contrasting phenomenon is due to the presence of bacteria used for the processing of cheese and the higher amounts of calcium in cheese than in butter and whole milk (103). Several potential explanations have been proposed to elucidate the different effects of cheese and butter on cholesterolemia. One hypothesis is that calcium, the concentrations of which are higher in cheese than in butter, combines with fatty acids in the intestine and forms insoluble detergents as suggested by the observation of a higher-fat fecal excretion in the cheese compared with the butter groups (96, 103). The higher protein and probiotic content of cheese could also speculatively contribute to its almost neutral effect on plasma cholesterol. One of the original studies investigating the link between CVDs and milk intake was the Honolulu Heart Program, where over 8,000 men of Japanese ancestry were followed up for 22 years to study the relationship between milk intake, calcium intake, and risk of stroke (97). The study found that risk of stroke decreased as the men increased their milk intake, where men who were non-drinkers of milk had twice the risk of stroke compared to men who did. It was hypothesized that high levels of calcium in milk were responsible for the decrease; however, the study found that calcium intake from non-dairy sources like vegetables did not decrease risk of stroke (97). Additionally, some limited evidence suggests that calcium, albeit non-dairy calcium, may in fact lead to higher incidences of myocardial infarction (97). Another study reported that high-fat dairy products like butter and whole milk are known to increase high density lipoprotein (HDL) and low-density lipoprotein (LDL)-cholesterol concentrations (101). The latter, called 'bad cholesterol', normally predicts risk of cardiovascular disease, but this may depend on the size of the LDL-cholesterol particles. Small, dense LDL particles are more atherogenic (causing fatty deposits in the arteries) than their larger counterparts due to their lower affinity for the LDL-receptor and higher susceptibility to oxidation (101). Among dairy products, cheese does not seem to increase LDL cholesterol because cheese is high in minerals, especially high in calcium (101). The association Dietary Approaches to Stop Hypertension (DASH) recommends a daily consumption of low-fat milk and other dairy products for the prevention of cardiovascular diseases (94). Accordingly, a meta-analysis on dairy and cardiovascular disease found that intake of cheese and milk as well as yogurt was inversely associated with cardiovascular disease risk (96, 101). Another study found that dairy intake was associated with a 12% lower risk of cardiovascular disease and 13% lower risk of stroke as compared to individuals with no or a low dairy consumption (101). Indeed, low-fat milk, yogurt, and cheese might be helpful for the prevention of some CVDs such as hypercholesterolemia, hypertension, and stroke. In contrast, whole milk and butter may be avoided due to their high saturated fat content. Briefly, to avoid accumulation of high cholesterol and lipids in blood, the best way is to replace whole milk by skimmed milk, low-fat milk, or cheese, and to avoid butter – especially people with CVDs. The available evidence of an effect (whether beneficial or detrimental) of milk and dairy products on CVDs is mixed and does not allow for drawing firm conclusions.

5.1.1.3.6   Milk and Blood Pressure   Evidence from epidemiological studies suggests that an increase in milk consumption may reduce blood pressure in hypertensive individuals (93, 94, 96–97, 101, 103). Whey proteins in milk and yogurt have long been studied for their potentially positive effects on blood pressure (96). In fact, dairy products are frequently pointed out as important diet components in hypertension treatment and prevention. One of the main lines of evidence for this comes from the Dietary Approaches to Stop Hypertension (DASH) study. The DASH study indicates that the intake of low-fat dairy products can improve high blood pressure in hypertensive patients (94, 97). Several studies have suggested that there is an association between milk consumption and blood pressure, as hypertension is inversely related to milk consumption in some epidemiological- and intervention studies (93). It has been suggested that some milk peptides have antihypertensive effects by inhibiting angiotensin-converting enzyme (ACE) (93–94, 96–97, 101, 103). The caseins in milk facilitate absorption of calcium and phosphate in the small intestine and are the main substrates for production of bioactive peptides (103). These small dairy peptides are the product of either fermentation of milk by Lactobacilli or by digestion of milk protein in the small intestine. These lactotripeptides inhibit angiotensin-converting enzyme (ACE), thereby lowering blood pressure (103). It is noteworthy that ACE converts angiotensin I to angiotensin II, a hormone that restricts blood vessels and leads to hypertension (103). Briefly, dairy products are frequently pointed out as important dietary components in a cardioprotective food pattern for the treatment and prevention of hypertension. DASH and many scientists recommend a daily consumption of low-fat milk (about 200 ml/day) and other dairy products like cheese and yogurt for health maintenance and disease prevention (94, 101).

5.1.1.4   Side Effects of Milk

For some people, milk can engender two main adverse reactions, namely lactose intolerance and cow milk protein allergy (93–94). These two phenomena, caused by two different origins, do not occur in all people.

5.1.1.4.1   Lactose Intolerance   Lactose, a disaccharide, is the main carbohydrate (sugar) present in milk. Lactose must be hydrolyzed into glucose and galactose by an enzyme named lactase, or more precisely, β-galactosidase, present in the small intestine (93–94). In mammals, lactase activity decreases significantly after weaning; this apparently does not happen at the same rate in humans. Lactose intolerance is common in many adults throughout the world and is caused by deficiency of intestinal lactase (hypolactasia) (93). Its activity continues through adulthood, and intolerance symptoms occur when, for some reason, there is an enzymatic deficiency (94). Lactose intolerance itself causes several gastro-intestinal symptoms provoked by lactose and sugar fermentation in the colon. Abdominal cramps and bloating, flatulence, diarrhea, nausea, and vomiting are frequent adverse events observed in lactose intolerance. During fermentation several compounds are formed such as short-chain fatty acids, methane, and carbon dioxide, which also can affect intestinal motility, causing increased bowel internal pressure and increased bowel transit time due to non-absorbed lactose (94). The amount of lactose that can cause these symptoms can vary within individuals, as well as with the consumption of other foods and the degree of β-galactosidase deficiency (93–94). If a lactose-intolerant individual continues to ingest elevated doses of lactose, high levels of galactitol formed by reductase NADPH can cause blindness and be fatal, because this conversion can occur in eye lenses or in neural tissue (94). The only treatment possibility for lactose intolerance is to avoid lactose products or to use lactose-free milk. Colon bacteria also can adapt their metabolic activity to improve lactose tolerance, bolstered by the consumption of lactic bacteria or specific probiotics (94). As hard cheese and yogurt contain less amounts of lactose, eating these dairy products may not cause side effects in some people who have milk intolerance (93–94).

5.1.1.4.2   Cow's Milk Protein Allergy   Cow's milk protein allergy is generally the first food allergy observed in children, mostly in small children (0–3 years), and its prevalence varies around 2–7.5% (93–94). After the age of three, there is no longer a problem for most children (93). Milk allergy is an immunologic-mediated adverse reaction to cow's milk protein and it can be developed in the neonatal period or during the first years of life. Cow's milk protein allergy can be caused by the antibody IgE, named immediate hypersensitivity, or IgE-mediated allergy or delayed (non-IgE-mediated) hypersensitivity. The immediate reaction symptoms include anaphylaxis, cutaneous reactions with urticaria and edema, respiratory episodes, and gastro-intestinal distress including vomiting, diarrhea, and bloody stools (94). Similarly, the delayed allergy is also characterized by cutaneous, respiratory, and gastro-intestinal symptoms, including disorders like atopic dermatitis, milk-induced pulmonary disease, chronic diarrhea, and gastroesophageal reflux disease (94). These aftereffects can happen one hour to several days after ingestion of cow milk. Most frequently, these allergies are due to whey proteins, mainly β-lactoglobulin, but also can be promoted by caseins (93). In breast-fed infants, mothers are commonly advised to avoid all cow milk-derived products; whereas in formula-fed children, the alternative is to replace cow's milk products with hydrolyzed or amino acid options or eventually soy milk (94).

Despite being rare, some cow's milk allergy cases in adulthood can been found and clinical research has shown that symptoms are quite severe, even when compared with children, including respiratory and cardiovascular impairments, as well as some frequency of anaphylactic shock (94). This allergy type requires immediate medical attention. In adults, it has been shown that respiratory symptoms were not associated with milk intake, and concluded that consumption of milk does not seem to exacerbate the symptoms of asthma, but in a few cases, people with cow's milk allergy may have asthma-like symptoms after milk consumption (93).

In summary, the totality of available scientific evidence supports that intake of milk and dairy products contribute to meeting nutrient recommendations, and may protect against the most prevalent chronic diseases, whereas very few adverse effects have been reported (101).

5.1.2 Different Forms of Milk

In the market, milk exists in different forms such as liquid milk, condensed milk, evaporated milk, dried milk, and milk powder.

5.1.2.1 Liquid Milk

Liquid milk is the form of milk most consumed worldwide and is considered a beverage. It is directly obtained from mammals like cow, goat, and sheep. It can also be classified according to the processing procedures it has undergone, such as pasteurized milk, sterilized milk, extended shelf-life (ESL) milk, and fortified milk with vitamins and ultra-high-temperature (UHT)-treated milk, among others (90, 92). Worldwide, less and less liquid milk is consumed in its raw form, except in some developing countries and rural regions.

5.1.2.2 Condensed Milk

The aspect of condensed milk is viscus or syrupy. Condensed milk is whole or skimmed cow milk from which water has been removed. Processing includes heat-treating and concentration. Condensed milk is generally sweetened by adding sugar. In Latin America, for example, condensed milk is often used in cooking and baking instead of jam (90, 92).

5.1.2.3 Evaporated Milk

The processing is the same as condensed milk without the concentration step. Processing includes heat-treating to make the milk bacteriologically safe and stable. Evaporated milks are generally mixed with other foods, such as in milky tea (90, 92).

5.1.2.4 Dry Milk or Milk Powder

It is obtained from the dehydration of milk and is usually in the form of powder or granules. The advantage of milk powder is its long preservation and its easy transportation because it does not need to be refrigerated due to the absence of water (90, 92). It is used by people in areas far from market and in some countries such as some Eastern Asian countries where liquid milk is not marketed.

5.1.3 Dairy Products

They include yogurt, cheese, cream, butter, whey, and casein.

5.1.3.1 Yogurts

Yogurt is a fermented dairy product derived from the fermentation of milk by two species of bacterial cultures, *Streptococcus thermophilus* and *Lactobacillus bulgaricus*, to reach a desired level of acidity (90, 105–106). Milk is often first pasteurized, then fermented with various live bacteria cultures, and incubated at a specific temperature to encourage bacteria growth. The lactose in milk is transformed into lactic acid by the action of bacteria. The fermented yogurt base is then cooled to 4°C to arrest further growth of the culture and further acid development (106). Other probiotic organisms are permitted as additional cultures. Probiotic bacteria, such as *L. acidophilus* and *Bifidobacterium* spp., are commonly included in probiotic yogurt to enhance the health benefits of yogurt (106). Yogurts contain protein, calcium, magnesium, potassium, vitamin B12, and other vitamins of the B group. Yogurts enhance healthy gut bacteria and can restore the intestinal flora destroyed after an oral antibiotic treatment. Health benefits range from protecting against osteoporosis to relieving irritable bowel disease and aiding digestion, but these depend on the type of yogurt consumed. Yogurt bacteria, in particular, have been scientifically demonstrated to assist in lactose digestion, reduce or prevent diarrhea episodes, and strengthen immune defenses of the host (106).

Several hundred bacterial species inhabit the human digestive tract. Their population in the colon is about 100 trillion. Their functions include modulation of cell growth and differentiation, antagonistic activity against pathogens and other infections, immune stimulation of gut-associated lymphoid tissue, reduction of blood lipids, and biosynthesis of vitamins (106). In healthy individuals, the colonies of diverse gut bacteria exist in equilibrium. Factors such as gastrointestinal disturbances, stress, age, or antibiotic therapy are known to upset the balance of gut microflora and the resultant malfunctioning of their digestive and metabolic effects. Probiotics in yogurt help in restoring balance (106). Therefore, regular consumption of natural yogurt or yogurt fortified with probiotics is better for the health than regular intake of yogurt mixed with diverse sugar ingredients. In general, one pot of natural yogurt a day may help keep the gut working properly. Some varieties of yogurt are kefir (a fermented milk drink), skyr (an Icelandic yogurt), and koumiss (a fermented product obtained from goat or mare milk), among others. (90, 92, 105–106). Kefir is made from milk in the presence of yeast and bacteria.

5.1.3.2 Cheeses

Cheeses are produced through the coagulation of milk protein (casein), which is separated from milk's whey. Most cheeses are fermented by bacteria, which turn milk lactose into lactic acid; then, the addition of the rennet, a complex of enzymes, completes the curdling. Diverse characteristics of cheese depend on the compositions and types of milk, processes applied and bacteria used (90, 92, 107–109). Cheese can be obtained from whole milk or skimmed milk. Besides cheese from cow's milk, cheeses are also obtained from goat milk and sheep milk (90, 92). Over a thousand varieties of cheese are produced, many of them being characteristic to a particular region of the globe. Cheese can be soft, semi-hard, hard, hard ripened, or unripened. Some soft cheeses in the market are cream cheeses, camembert, brie, Roquefort, Neufchâtel, and feta. Semi-hard cheeses frequently consumed include Mozzarella, Edam, Cantal, Emmental, and Gruyere. Hard cheeses frequently consumed are Cheddar, Pecorino, Parmesan, Brick, Gouda, Grana Padano, and more.

From a nutritional point of view, cheese is a rich source of essential nutrients such as proteins, bioactive peptides, amino acids, fat, fatty acids, vitamins, and minerals (calcium, phosphate) that are important for a healthy diet (92, 107–108). Cheese can enhance health benefits by the production of certain peptides and free amino acids which have various bioactive properties, such as antimicrobial, anti-carcinogenic, anti-thrombotic, and so on (107). Certain biologically active lipids, such as conjugated fatty acid (CLA) and milk fat globule membrane (MFGM), present in cheeses are also found to be beneficial to health. Thus, cheese plays a very important role in the diet of humans; however, it suffers from an adverse nutritional image due to the presence of saturated fatty acid, cholesterol, and salt content. These can be overcome by the production of cheese with low fat or cholesterol removal and by the addition of certain functional living materials, such as probiotic bacteria (107). Despite the presence of a notable amount of saturated and trans-fatty acids, there is no clear evidence relating the consumption of cheese to any disease (108). Ripened cheese is free of lactose and therefore suitable for the nutrition of lactose-intolerant individuals. Conjugated linoleic acid and sphingolipids present in cheese may have anti-carcinogenic properties. The high concentration of essential amino acids in cheese contributes to growth and development of the human body (108). The high concentration of calcium in cheese is well known to contribute to the formation and maintenance of strong bones and teeth, but also shows a positive effect on blood pressure and helps in losing weight in combination with low-energy diets (108). Calcium in cheese and milk is more absorbable than calcium in vegetable food. Calcium levels of hard cheese are the highest among different dairy products and about ten times more abundant than those of milk and yogurt.

5.1.3.3 Cream

Cream is a fluid milk product comparatively rich in fat, in the form of an emulsion of fat-in-skimmed milk, obtained by physical separation (centrifugation or skimming) from milk (90, 92).

Cream products include recombined cream, reconstituted cream, prepared cream, pre-packaged liquid cream, cream packed under pressure, whipped cream, fermented cream, and acidified cream (90, 92).

5.1.3.4   Butter and Ghee

Are fatty milk products. Butter is produced by churning milk or cream; in many developing countries, traditional butter is obtained by churning sour whole milk. Ghee is obtained by removing the water from butter and is especially popular in India and South Asia. Ghee has a very long shelf-life of up to two years. Butter and ghee are rich in saturated fatty acids that can cause hypercholesterolemia and other cardiovascular diseases (90, 92).

5.1.3.5   Whey Products

Whey is a byproduct of the dairy industry. Whey is the liquid part of the milk that remains after the separation of curd in cheese making. Its main food use is in the preparation of whey cheese, whey drinks, and fermented whey drinks. The main industrial uses are in the manufacture of lactose, whey paste, and dried whey. Whey can be sweet or acidic depending on the method of cheese-making (90, 92, 109). Recent studies found that whey proteins have antimicrobial, antiviral, and antioxidant effects (109). Other whey properties are cited above. Whey products are the favorite food of Italians.

5.1.3.6   Casein

Casein is the principal protein in milk and is used as an ingredient in several products, including cheese, bakery products, paints, and glues (90). Casein is extracted from skimmed milk by precipitation with rennet or by harmless lactic acid-producing bacteria (90, 92).

In summary, liquid milk, cheese, and yogurt are the three dietary products the most consumed worldwide and are considered complete, safe, and healthy foods. They are indispensable for the growth and the corporal development of children and adolescents. They also may help maintain good health and prevent diseases in adults and the elderly. Breast feeding is necessary for the life of the baby because only maternal milk can furnish all essential nutrients and materials not only for the development of baby but also for the defense against microbes and infection. However, some dietary products rich in saturated fats like whole cow milk, butter, and cream may cause some cardiovascular diseases like hypercholesterolemia and hyperlipidemia, hence they may be avoided or consumed with moderation. These fatty dietary products can be replaced by their equivalents like skimmed milk, low fat milk, cheese, and yogurt.

5.2   Egg

The eggs of most animals are giant single cells. An egg is an animal reproductive body and contains stockpiles of all the materials needed for initial development of the embryo through the stage at which the new individual can begin feeding (110). Before the feeding stage, the giant cell cleaves into many smaller cells, but no net growth occurs. The mammalian embryo is an exception. It can start to grow early by taking up nutrients from the mother via the placenta (110). For poultry, birds, turtles, fish, snakes, and insects, the egg is released outside of the animal body. In general, eggs are typically spherical or ovoid, with a diameter of about 0.1 mm in humans and sea urchins, 1 mm to 2 mm in frogs and fishes, and many cm in birds and reptiles (110–114). Eggs sold in the market are not fertilized and cannot have the potential to be a chick. Eggs used as foods include those of chicken, duck, goose, quail, turkey, pigeon, and fish. The most commonly consumed eggs are chicken egg and duck egg. One duck egg weighs 70 g, while one chicken egg weighs about 50 g. Fish eggs called roes like caviar, lumpfish roe, and salmon roe, are also eaten.

The different parts of a poultry egg include: shell, thin proteinaceous membranes, air cell, albumen, chalazae, vitelline membrane, yolk, and germinal disk (111–114). Albumen, or egg white, is rich in albumin and accounts for about 63% of the whole egg. Yolk is the yellow part in the middle of an egg and comprises the second most content of the egg (27.5%) (114). It is surrounded by the white and is rich in protein and fat, and is used to nourish the developing embryo. The chalazae are two spiral bands in the white of a poultry egg that hold the yolk in the center of the albumen. The vitelli membrane is the membrane surrounding the yolk. The germinal disk is a disk of cells lying on the yolk from which the embryo develops after fertilization occurs. Albumen and yolk are two important parts of eggs used in nutrition (111–112).

5.2.1 Composition of an Egg

All eggs are particularly rich in proteins, fats, and many essential vitamins, minerals, and antioxidants. They are low in energy. In general, for 100 g whole raw egg, there are about: 140 kcal energy, 12 g protein, 10 g total fats, and 1.1 g carbohydrates, as well as different vitamins such as vitamins: A, D, E, B2, B12, B9 (folate), and different minerals like iodine, selenium, calcium, iron, and so on (111–115).

Protein is distributed in both egg white and yolk. Egg white is mainly composed of protein (11%), with ovalbumin being the most abundant (54%), followed by ovotransferrin (12%), ovomucoid (11%), lysozyme (3.5%), and ovomucin (3.5%) (111–115). Other minor proteins such as ovoglycoprotein, ovoflavoprotein, ovomacroglobulin, avidin, cystatin, and ovoinhibitor have also been identified (112, 114–115). The main components of the yolk are lipids (31–35%), although it also has 15–17% of proteins including lipovitellins (36%), livetins (38%), phosvitin (8%), and low-density lipoproteins (17%) (115). Egg yolk is covered with the vitelline membrane which separates it from the egg white. It is also a good source of proteins, being composed mostly of protein fibers (115).

Fats in eggs include saturated fatty acids, monounsaturated fatty acids, and polyunsaturated fatty acids (omega-3 and omega-6 fatty acids), and are only concentrated in the egg yolk (112–115). Eggs are also the principal source of dietary cholesterol of which the mean levels are about 400 mg per 100g of whole egg or about 200 mg of a medium egg (55 g). All cholesterols are found in the yolk (111–115). In addition, eggs are a rich source of phospholipids (PL) and choline (111–112, 116–117). The average large egg contains about 1.3 g of phospholipids, also known as egg yolk lecithin, which are almost exclusively found in the yolk (117). Eggs are also an excellent source of choline which is an amino alcohol. Choline is an essential nutrient and is mainly found in the yolk (680 mg/100 g in the egg yolk versus 1 mg/100 g in the egg white) (112, 116). In foods, choline is found in both water-soluble (free choline, phosphocholine, and glycerophosphocholine) and lipid-soluble forms (phosphatidylcholine and sphingomyelin), and has important and diverse functions in both cellular maintenance and growth through all life stages (112). Hard-boiled egg represents the second major source of choline after beef liver and the first source of choline in the US diet (112).

In addition, eggs contain different antioxidants. Numerous compounds in both egg white and yolk exhibit antioxidant properties. Many egg proteins such as ovalbumin, ovotransferrin, phosvitin, egg lipids such as phospholipids, as well as certain micronutrients such as vitamin E, vitamin A, selenium, and carotenoids, are reported to have antioxidant properties (114). Some of these proteins have antioxidant properties by themselves, but it has been demonstrated that peptides derived from them, usual fragments of 2–20 amino acid residues, have the higher bioactive potential (115).

Amino acids in eggs like glutamine, asparagine, and the hydrophobic proline, alanine, cysteine, valine, methionine, isoleucine, leucine, phenylalanine, tyrosine, and tryptophan amino acids have strong positive effects on antioxidant activity (115).

In addition, eggs can be naturally fortified by feeding hens with grains and seeds rich in antioxidants (i.e., carotenoids, vitamin E, selenium, and iodine) and/or in omega-3 fatty acids such as alpha linoleic acid (ALA) (114–115). Consequently, the eggs obtained are high in these nutrients. This type of egg is called a fortified egg. Therefore, the levels of these macro- and micronutrients in eggs can vary according to the species, the poultry farming, the animal feed type, and the life mode of the poultry.

5.2.2 Egg Benefits

Eggs are of particular interest from a nutritional point of view, containing essential proteins, lipids, amino acids, vitamins, antioxidants, minerals, and trace elements, while offering a moderate calorie source (about 140 kcal/100 g), great culinary potential, and low economic cost. Indeed, eggs have been identified to represent the lowest-cost animal source for proteins, vitamin A, iron, vitamin B12, riboflavin, and choline, and the second lowest-cost source for zinc and calcium (112). The amino acid profile of egg protein (approximately 6.5 g/egg) is similar to that of beef steak, but has greater bioavailability (113). Thanks to these nutrients, eggs lead to strong muscles and help hematopoiesis, immune functioning, and enzyme activity.

Vitamin A, lutein, and zeaxanthin are abundant in eggs and help to prevent macular degeneration, the leading cause of age-related blindness, and also to promote good vision. Lutein and zeaxanthin in eggs may fight some types of cancer and carotid artery atherosclerosis (116).

Antioxidant peptides from eggs can inhibit oxidative stress, which plays an important role in human health, and in food systems, and increase the quality and the shelf life of products (114–115). Antioxidants play important roles in the prevention of chronic diseases such as inflammatory diseases (arthritis, asthma, arthrosis), CVDs, cancer, and so on.

Dietary phospholipids or lecithin in egg yolk have emerged as a potential source of bioactive lipids that may have widespread effects on pathways related to inflammation, cholesterol metabolism, and HDL function (117). Lecithin is also necessary for the functioning of a number of tissues and organs such as brain, lungs, blood, bile, and more. Large intakes of dietary lecithin have long been known to influence serum cholesterol levels in humans by inhibiting cholesterol absorption when cholesterol is in significant amounts in the diet (117).

Eggs are also an excellent source of choline, which plays an important role in fetal and neonatal brain development (116). Inadequate choline intake during pregnancy increases the risk for neural tube defects such as spina bifida (116). Choline intake is also associated with decreased plasma levels of homocysteine and inflammatory factors. Recent studies have also shown that high intake of choline is associated with reduced breast cancer incidence and mortality (116). However, studies also show that a majority of the population, including a majority of pregnant and lactating women, do not have adequate choline intakes and that adding an egg a day to the diet could alleviate this inadequacy (116). The importance of choline in fetal and neonatal brain development has been shown in numerous studies, and inadequate choline intakes during these critical periods can have very negative effects (116). Choline plays roles in neurotransmission, brain development, and bone integrity (112). For example, acetylcholine is a well-known neurotransmitter of the central nervous system. Moreover, dietary choline is considered especially important for maintaining a healthy liver (117). Dietary sources of choline include egg yolk, organ meat such as liver, and wheat germ. Eggs have also been shown to promote weight loss in overweight and obese subjects by increasing feelings of satiety and reducing short-term energy intake (113). Briefly, thanks to myriad biologically active components, egg provides well-balanced nutrients for infants and adults.

5.2.3 Egg Risks

Since eggs are high in cholesterol and saturated fatty acids, their consumption may lead to risks of hypercholesterolemia and cardiovascular diseases. Other concerns of egg consumption are diabetes, bacterial contamination, and allergy (112–113, 116–122).

5.2.3.1 *Egg Consumption and Risks of Hypercholesterolemia and Cardiovascular Diseases*

Eggs represent the principal source of dietary cholesterol, which has been a major barrier to the popularity of egg intake, primarily because of the outdated, but widespread misconception that egg cholesterol converts directly into serum cholesterol, and thus increases risk of CVD (113). Recently, a growing body of evidence from prospective cohort studies, systematic reviews, and meta-analyses has culminated in a consensus that eggs exert a relatively small and clinically insignificant effect on serum LDL-cholesterol (bad cholesterol) in comparison with other lifestyle factors (111–113, 116–117, 119–122).

In 1968, based on some publications concerning the relationship between egg consumption and population health risks, the American Heart Association (AHA) recommended to consume no more than three egg yolks per week because eggs are rich in cholesterol, and frequent consumption of egg yolks may lead to cardiovascular disease (CVD) risks (112, 116). However, in the early twenty-first century, several publications and cohort studies to date have indicated very little association between a high egg intake (i.e., seven eggs per week) and cardiovascular disease or cardiac mortality in the general population (112–113, 116–117, 119–122). Most studies show no association between egg consumption and CVD risk in a healthy population, while others suggest an increased risk of CVD with higher egg consumption (greater than seven eggs per week), especially in people with diabetes mellitus (120). In 2019, the Hellenic National Nutrition and Health Survey published that eggs do not increase the risk of dyslipidemia and can be consumed as part of a healthy diet that is high in fiber and low in saturated fat, without excessive energy intake, by all individuals (119). Another study regarding egg consumption in adolescent girls followed for ten years suggested that eggs may be included as part of a healthy adolescent diet without adverse effects on glucose, lipid levels, or insulin resistance (121). A meta-analysis suggests that egg consumption is not associated with the risk of CVD and cardiac mortality in the general population (122). However, egg consumption may be associated with an increased incidence of Type 2 diabetes among the general population and CVD comorbidity among diabetic patients (122).

Indeed, the effect of egg consumption on blood cholesterol is minimal when compared with the effect of trans-fats and saturated fats often present in fast foods and processed foods. The risk of heart disease may be more closely tied to processed foods such as bacon, sausages, ham, butter, and margarine that accompany the eggs. Therefore, do not cook egg with butter or margarine, and consume eggs with vegetable foods to avoid hypercholesterolemia and hyperlipidemia. Because eggs contain both good nutrients and cholesterol, healthy people should not consume more than seven chicken eggs per week; while people with diabetes, hypercholesterolemia, or heart disease, should limit this consumption to three chicken eggs per week. It is noteworthy that duck egg contains more cholesterol than chicken egg.

5.2.3.2 Egg Consumption and Risks of Diabetes

Evidence for associations between egg intake and increased incidence of diabetes in meta-analyses of prospective cohort studies has been inconsistent, some of which support associations, while others do not (113, 120). Of the eight studies evaluating incidence of Type 2 diabetes mellitus (T2DM) associated with egg consumption, four prospective studies found a statistically significant association (123). In contrast, studies among healthy subjects found that egg intake may reduce the risk of T2DM and metabolic syndrome (123). In conclusion, there was no consistency in the findings for an association between egg intake and incidence of Type 2 diabetes mellitus.

5.2.3.3 Bacterial Contamination

Another risk of egg consumption is potential for bacterial contamination (112, 118). Eggs may become contaminated by a number of different types of bacteria during production such as *Salmonella typhimurium*, *Salmonella enterica*, mycoplasma, infectious bronchitis virus, and avian influenza virus (112, 118). The egg shell is a hermetic seal, but this seal can be broken by improper handling, or if the egg is laid by unhealthy chickens. So, consumers are advised to avoid eating raw or undercooked eggs and to wash eggs with tap water before breaking them.

5.2.3.4 Egg Allergy

Egg is one of the most important allergens in childhood feeding, and egg allergy can pose quality of life concerns (124). Most of the allergenic egg proteins are found in egg white, including ovomucoid, ovalbumin, ovotransferrin, and lysozyme. Although ovalbumin is the most abundant protein comprising hen's egg white, ovomucoid has been shown to be the dominant allergen in egg. Egg allergy is closely associated with atopic dermatitis and was found to be present in about two-thirds of children (124). Processed foods containing egg such as cookies must signal its presence to consumers on the labels.

5.2.4 Comparison between Chicken Egg and Other Poultry Eggs

Having undergone divergent evolution processes, poultry eggs from different species (chicken, duck, goose, turkey, quail, and pigeon) vary significantly in egg size and nutritional composition (125). According to the study of Sun et al., egg weights of chicken, duck, goose, turkey, quail, and pigeon were about 58 g, 74 g, 139 g, 90 g, 11 g, and 23 g, respectively (125). Yolk and albumen weights were respectively 16 g and 36 g for chicken, 24 g and 43 g for duck, 53 g and 73 g for goose, 27 g and 55 g for turkey, 3.3 g and 6.7 g for quail, and 4.3 g and 16.6 g for pigeon (125). Due to its large size, goose egg also had the heaviest yolk, albumen, and eggshell. Eggs of the six bird species had a similar conical shape, however goose and turkey eggs had a much sharper shape than others. The proportion of yolk to egg weight was highest in goose (37.91%), followed by duck (32.40%), quail (30.19%), turkey (29.83%), chicken (27.52%), and pigeon (19.33%) (124). Similarly, significant differences were observed in albumen percentage among different species. Pigeon eggs had the highest (73%) egg albumen percentage. Goose egg had the highest yolk to albumen ration (73%), and the lowest was pigeon egg (26%) (125).

Chicken eggs are the most widely consumed in Western countries, while duck eggs are preferred by Eastern Asian people. In Eastern Asia, duck eggs are used to prepare salted egg for long conservation by immersing duck eggs in a concentrated solution of salt, or coating them with a paste of salt and mud. They are also used to prepare a specialty called bahut which is a fertilized developing egg embryo after an incubation period of two to three weeks.

Quail eggs are the eggs laid by various species of quail, which are mid-sized birds found in Eastern Asia, Europe, the United States, North Africa, and more. Quail eggs are a favorite food of the Japanese. Quail eggs are smaller than chicken and duck eggs. The mean quail egg weight is about 11g (125–126). Chemical composition of quail egg is similar to chicken egg (126). Quail eggs have lower fat content as compared to chicken eggs; however, the cholesterol levels are similar. It is worth emphasizing that quail eggs are richer than chicken eggs in essential amino acids and minerals such as calcium, phosphate, and iron (126). According to traditional medicine, quail eggs have some tonic effects, but these properties are not proven scientifically.

5.2.5 Fish Eggs

Fish eggs are also called roes. The most consumed fish roes are caviar, lumpfish roes, and salmon roes. Roes are also the preferred marine foods for many people in the world. Roes can be obtained from wild fishes or cultivated fishes (127). They are occasionally consumed and often more expensive than chicken or duck eggs.

Caviars are the salted, cured, and preserved eggs obtained from sturgeons. Caviar or sturgeon roe is delicious, but very costly and often reserved for festivities. The most famous are the black caviars produced from the wild Russian and Iranian Beluga and Osetra sturgeons which are harvested in the Caspian Sea (127). Caviars are now obtained from sturgeons elevated in aquaculture from different countries in Europe, North America, and Central Asia. Roes of other fishes and crustaceans such as lumpfish, salmon, steelhead, trout, whitefish, crab roe, sea urchin, and so on are cheaper than caviar and also tasty.

Lumpfish roe is obtained from the marine lumpfish *Cyclopterus lumpus* and is generally red or black in color. It is cheaper than caviar and is also delicious. Lumpfish roe is also consumed for popular festivities (127). Salmon roe is red in color and is also called red caviar or Ikura in Japan. It is mainly produced in North Pacific countries from Alaska to Japan and Siberia (127).

Sizes of sturgeon roe (caviar), salmon roe, and lumpfish roe are about 2.5 mm, 4–5 mm, and 2–5 mm in diameter, respectively (127). Roe from Chinook salmon has the largest diameter of about

7 mm (127). The nutrient contents of caviar, lumpfish roe, salmon roe, and poultry egg are about the same with a slight decrease in cholesterol for caviar and fish roes. Moreover, fish roes and crustacean roes like crab roes contain astaxanthin (a carotenoid) and more omega-3 polyunsaturated fatty acids such as docosahexaenoic acid (DHA) and eicosapentaenoic acid (EPA) than poultry eggs (127).

In summary, an egg is equipped to support life, with a profile of essential nutrients that is unparalleled by any other food. However, eggs are also high in cholesterol; their consumption is limited for certain individuals who have hypercholesterolemia, atherosclerosis, or diabetes. For normal people, egg intake in moderation is good for the health and the prevention of some chronic diseases.

5.3   Honey, Royal Jelly, Propolis

Honey, royal jelly, and propolis are three main byproducts of honeybees. These compounds are mainly produced by honeybees belonging to the species *Apis mellifera* of the family Apidae. In Sri Lanka, the predominant honey-making bee is *Apis cerana* (128–130). Honeybees are social insects, often regarded as superorganisms. In a hive or colony, there are three types of bees: one fertile female called queen, many fertile males or drones, and many sterile females or worker bees (131). Among them, only worker bees collect and regurgitate the nectar from various floral sources and store it as honey which serves as food for bees during winter. The honeybees' nutrition is divided into two categories: nectar and pollen collected from flowers. Floral nectar is the primary source of carbohydrates, while pollen provides the proteins, lipids, vitamins, essential sterols, and other micronutrients they need to survive (128). Honeybees make a journey of nearly 55,000 miles to gather nectar from approximately 2 million flowers for accumulating 1 pound of honey (131). Honeybees pollinate three-quarters of the world's angiosperm plants and increase the yields of crops by one-third (130). Queens can mate with many fertile males or drones a day and may lay up to 3,000 eggs a day and survive as long as five years compared with infertile female workers that live up to 45 days only (132).

5.3.1   Honey

Honeybees produce honey by collecting sugar-rich nectar from flowers, which is a clear liquid consisting of nearly 80% water and complex sugars. In the hive, the bees use their 'honey stomachs' to ingest and regurgitate the nectar many times until it is partially digested. They continue this process until the product reaches the desired quality (129). After the final regurgitation, the honeycomb is left unsealed. Raw honey is then stored in honeycomb cells to dry. Honeybees use their wings to fan the honey comb, to evaporate about 80% of the water from the raw honey, thereby preventing fermentation of the honey (129, 131). Once dried, the cells of the honeycomb are sealed with wax to preserve the honey. Ripe honey, as removed from the hive by a beekeeper, has a long shelf life and will not ferment if properly sealed (129).

Honey has been used both as food and medicine since the ancient times, nearly 5,500 years ago (133). Most ancient populations, including the Greeks, Chinese, Egyptians, Romans, Mayans, and Babylonians consumed honey for both its nutritional purposes and medicinal properties (133).

Honey is a viscous liquid and has a very complex chemical composition that varies depending on the botanical source. Today, there are approximately 300 types of honey in the world (133). These varieties are related to the different types of nectar collected by the honeybees. Depending on its origin, honey can be classified in different categories among which monofloral honey seems to be the most promising and interesting as a natural remedy. Manuka honey, a monofloral honey obtained from the manuka tree (*Leptospermum scoparium*) of the Myrtaceae family, which grows as a shrub or a small tree throughout New Zealand and eastern Australia, has greatly attracted the attention of researchers for its biological properties, especially its antimicrobial and antioxidant capacities (134).

Honey is a natural source of interesting macro- and micronutrients. Honey is a saturated solution of soluble carbohydrates (sugars) with a content of 95–97% of its dry weight. Furthermore, honey includes important compounds such as proteins, enzymes, vitamins, amino acids, minerals, antioxidants, and organic acids. Pure honey also consists of flavonoids, polyphenols, reducing compounds, alkaloids, glycosides, cardiac glycosides, anthraquinone, and volatile compounds (133–138). About 95% of honey's dry matter is composed of soluble sugars including fructose (32–38%) and glucose (28–31%). Other sugars include disaccharides such as maltose, sucrose, isomaltose turanose, nigerose, melibiose, panose, maltotriose, and melezitose. Honey contains 4 to 5% fructooligosaccharides, which serve as probiotic agents (133–138). Furthermore, natural honey contains about 200 minor constituents, especially phenolic compounds (flavonoids), antioxidants, enzymes, amino acids, minerals, vitamins, aromatic compounds, and small amounts of proteins (133–138). Organic acids constitute 0.6% of honey and include gluconic acid which is a byproduct of the enzymatic digestion of glucose. The concentration of mineral compounds ranges from 0.1% to 1.0%. Potassium is the major mineral present, followed by calcium, magnesium, sodium, phosphorus, sulfur, and more. Trace elements include iron, copper, zinc, and manganese (133–138). Vitamins of B group like B1, B2, B3 (niacin), B5 (pantothenic acid), and B6, as well as ascorbic acid (vitamin C) and tocopherols (vitamin E), are also found. However, protein content is very low – about 0.1–0.5%. Fats, cholesterol, and polyunsaturated fatty acids such as omega-3 and omega-6 are absent in honey (133–138). A variety of enzymes such as oxidase, invertase, amylase, and catalase are also present in honey. The main enzymes invertase (saccharase), diastase (amylase), and glucose oxidase play an important role in the formation of honey (133–138). The enzyme glucose oxidase produces hydrogen peroxide (which provides antimicrobial properties) along with gluconic acid from glucose which helps in calcium absorption. Invertase converts sucrose to fructose and glucose. Other antioxidants and specific antioxidant enzymes are also present including catalase, superoxide dismutase, reduced glutathione, peptides, and Maillard reaction products such as methylglyoxal, glyoxal, 3-deoxyglucosulose (133–138). Moreover, most natural honey contains flavonoid antioxidants such as apigenin, kaempferol, quercetin, galangin, pinocembrin, catechin, luteolin, naringenin, myricetin, chrysin, and hesperetin, as well as phenolic acids such as gallic, benzoic, ellagic, syringic, caffeic, p-coumaric, and ferulic acids (133–138). Most of those products works together to provide a synergistic antioxidant effect. There are approximately 600 volatile compounds in honey that contribute to its potential biomedical effects. The volatile compounds of honey include aldehydes, alcohols, ketones, hydrocarbons, acid esters, pyran, terpene, norisoprenoids, sulfur, furan, and cyclic compounds (134). The composition of honey is rather variable and depends primarily on its floral source; seasonal and environmental factors can also influence its composition and its biological effects. Several studies have shown that the antioxidant potential of honey is strongly correlated not only with the concentration of total phenolic compounds present, but also with the color, with dark colored honeys being reported to have higher total phenolic contents and, consequently, higher antioxidant capacities (134, 136). This is explained by the fact that colors are often due to the presence of double bonds in the chemical structure of antioxidants, especially phenolic compounds.

Honey has been shown to possess antimicrobial, antiviral, anti-parasite, anti-inflammatory, antioxidant, antimutagenic, and antitumor effects (138–139). It also has immunomodulatory and healing properties. The antimicrobial activity in most honeys is due to the enzymatic production of hydrogen peroxide (H_2O_2) and methylglyoxal (138). Recently, an antimicrobial peptide named bee defensin-1, discovered by Kwakman et al., was shown to have strong bactericidal activity (139). Bee defensin-1, also called 'royalisin', is isolated from royal jelly, the major food source for queen bee larvae, and is found in the hypopharyngeal gland of young worker bees that produce royal jelly (139). Briefly, the factors contributing to antimicrobial activity of honeys are due to the presence of hydrogen peroxide, methylglyoxal, and defensin-1 in honey, and their high sugar concentration and their low pH level (3.2–4.5).

Thanks to high levels of different antioxidants, honey can fight oxidative stress and may prevent or treat some dreadful ailments such as inflammatory diseases (asthma, arthritis, arthrosis), cardiovascular diseases, gastrointestinal disorders, leukemia, and some other cancer forms (129, 131, 133, 135, 137, 140). Honey is highly cytotoxic against cancer cells while it is non-cytotoxic to normal cells.

However, some precautions regarding the use of honey and its side effects should be reported to the users.

As honey is rich in sugars, excessive consumption of honey may cause diabetes and obesity. Therefore, limit the consumption of honey to one to two spoons a day. In addition, the key to honey preservation is limiting its exposure to humidity. In its cured state, honey has a sufficiently high sugar content to inhibit fermentation. However, raw honey can contain bacterial spores, mainly those of Bacillus spp., and spores of the notorious pathogen *Clostridium botulinum*, which can cause wound botulism or gangrene, are incidentally detected (139). Medical-grade honey intended for clinical application therefore must be sterilized to destroy potentially present bacterial spores. This is generally achieved by gamma irradiation or pasteurization (139). Honey is prohibited in children under one year old because their immune system is still immature to fight against the *Clostridium botulinum* spores potentially present.

As the global honeybee population decreases each year due to degraded ecosystems, it is necessary to protect honeybees by banning the use of insecticides (neonicotinoids) and pesticides for floral gardens, as well as floral fields such as sunflower and lavender fields. Protect them not only for the survival of bees, but also for the survival of apiculturists and the health of honey consumers. Moreover, honeybees contribute to the pollination of angiosperm plants and the yields of crops (130).

In brief, honey is not a complete food like milk and egg, due to the absence of proteins and fats and the high presence of soluble sugars. High intake of honey might lead to obesity or diabetes. But it is a special animal byproduct because it contains a variety of antibacterial and antiviral compounds and is very rich in various antioxidants which are not found in other foods. Honey is good for convalescents and the elderly.

5.3.2 Royal Jelly

Royal jelly is a white or yellowish creamy substance secreted from the mandibular and hypopharyngeal glands of the worker honeybee *Apis mellifera*. It is the food of the bee queen throughout her life and also the food of all bee larvae during their first three days of life (132, 141–144). The consumption of this magical liquid by the queen bee generates many advantages such as their size, which is double in comparison to worker bees, a longer lifespan, and a better function of their reproductive system. It is suggested that royal jelly is a potent promoter of healthy aging and longevity, because it enhances overall health and fertility of queen bees (132, 141–142). Royal jelly prevents senescence of human tissues in cell cultures. However, clinical studies of the effect royal jelly on longevity in humans are scarce and are still not confirmed (132).

Unlike honey, royal jelly is a rich source of proteins, peptides, amino acids, and fatty acids (132, 141–144). Fresh royal jelly is a solution containing 60–70% of water with pH ranging between 3.6 and 4.2 (132, 142). Proteins are the dominant ingredient of royal jelly (50% of its dry matter). More than 80% of royal jelly proteins are soluble proteins. Carbohydrates, vitamins, lipids, minerals, flavonoids, polyphenols, as well as several biologically active substances are also present (132, 161–162) Sugars mainly constituted of glucose and fructose comprise 7.5–15% of royal jelly content. Lipids constitute 7–18% of royal jelly content. The most prominent royal jelly fatty acids in order are 10-hydroxydecanoic acid, 10-hydroxy-2-decenoic acid, and sebacic acid (132). In addition, royal jelly contains different amino acids, organic acids, steroids, esters, phenols, sugars, minerals, trace elements, and other constituents (132, 141). The composition of royal jelly varies with seasonal and regional conditions. Royalisin and jelleines are two royal jelly antimicrobial peptides that enhance efficiency of the immune response of bee larvae to various infections (132). Its antioxidant potency is due to the presence of some polyphenolic compounds and flavonoids. Royal jelly is rich in pantothenic acid (vitamin B5), niacin, and nucleotides such as adenosine triphosphate (ATP), adenosine monophosphate (AMP), and adenosine diphosphate (ADP), and contains small amounts of various B group vitamins (132).

Royal jelly may possess numerous functional properties such as antibacterial activity, anti-inflammatory activity, vasodilative and hypotensive activities, disinfectant action, antioxidant activity, anti-hypercholesterolemic activity, and antitumor activity and might enhance longevity in humans by promoting general health (132, 141–142). In addition, this product has demonstrated its efficiency in the alleviation of postmenopausal complaints (142). However, the exact mechanism through which royal jelly may extend lifespan is not well-understood (132). The biological activities of royal jelly are mainly attributed to its bioactive fatty acids, proteins, and phenolic compounds (141). Royal jelly may cause allergy such as asthma in some hypersensitive people.

A handful of studies concerning the possible contamination of royal jelly have been published. However, the extent of this contamination was relatively low (141). In contrast, royal jelly adultera-tion is the most important quality problem. Adulteration with honey is more probable, causing an increase of the sugar values. Royal jelly may spoil or deteriorate and lose its commercial value eventually when it is stored improperly, hence it should be stored at 4–8° C or less to guarantee its good quality (141). Royal jelly is sold as a dietary supplement (capsule, oral solution).

5.3.2 Propolis

Propolis, generally known as the 'bee glue', is a resinous mixture produced by honeybees from dif-ferent leaf and flower buds, stems, and bark cracks of numerous species of plants (143–144). Bees use it mainly as a sealant and a disinfecting material for the reconstruction of the beehive. It is also used for smoothing the inner surface of the beehive, retaining the hive's internal temperature (35°C), and preventing weathering and invasion by predators. Furthermore, propolis hardens the cell wall and contributes to an aseptic internal environment. Propolis generally becomes soft and sticky upon heating (143–144). Raw propolis contains 50–60% resins and balms (including phenolic compounds), 30–40% waxes and fatty acids, 5–10% essential oils, 5% pollen, and about 5% other substances including amino acids, micronutrients, and vitamins (B1, B2, B6, C, and E) (143–144). In addition, more than 300 compounds belonging to polyphenols, terpenoids, steroids, sugars, amino acids, and others have been identified in propolis. Propolis and its extracts have numerous applications in treating various diseases due to its antiseptic, anti-inflammatory, antioxidant, anti-bacterial, antimycotic, antifungal, antiulcer, anticancer, and immunomodulatory properties as well as neuroprotective effects (143–144).

In conclusion, many in vitro and animal studies seem to confirm the usefulness of using bee products (honey, royal jelly, propolis) as natural agents capable of counteracting the effects of oxida-tive stress underlying the pathogenesis of numerous diseases, such as inflammatory diseases, neu-rodegenerative disorders, cancer, diabetes, atherosclerosis, and more. However, studies on their role in humans are very limited (144). More clinical studies are needed for these interesting byproducts of honeybees.

5.4 Fish Oils

Main byproducts of fish are fish oils. They include fish body oil and fish liver oil.

5.4.1 Fish Body Oil

Fish oil can be obtained from different species depending on the region of production. Fish used in fish oil preparation is harvested from cold water and includes sardines, salmon, herring, halibut, mackerel, and cod, among others. Methods to extract oil from fish include cooking, using sol-vents and, recently, by extraction by supercritical fluids, by enzymatic procedures, and by chemical or biological silages (145). The extraction of fish oil by wet-pressing is the most commonly used method for production on an industrial scale and is carried out in four stages: fish cooking, press-ing, decantation, and centrifugation (145). Extraction methods by supercritical fluids using carbon dioxide (CO_2), by enzymatic procedures, and by chemical or biological silages are called green extraction methods (146). Green extraction methods are designed with perseveration of the envi-ronment in mind, as well as improvement of oil extraction yield. However, these methods are still being developed (145–146). Fish oil, or more exactly fish body oil, is rich in omega-3 fatty acids

(DHA, EPA) and is used to manufacture fish oil supplements (capsule or liquid) for the prevention of chronic diseases such as CVDs, inflammatory diseases (rheumatism, asthma), neurodegenerative diseases, cancer, and more. In addition, fish oil has been broadly reported as a potential supplement to ameliorate the severity of some skin disorders such as photoaging, skin cancer, allergy, dermatitis, cutaneous wounds, and melanogenesis (147). However, excessive intake of fish oil supplements or omega-3 supplements can lead to hemorrhage, especially in combination with anticoagulant drugs (see Chapter 1 of this book) (148). Therefore, notify your doctor if you take fish oil or omega-3 supplements. Take note that the freshest and highest quality fish oils do not have a fishy odor or fishy taste, and do not contain mercury and other industrial contaminants.

5.4.2   Cod Liver Oil

Centuries ago, northern Europeans used cod liver oil to relieve some complaints such as rheumatism, aching joints, stiff muscles, as well as to protect them from the cold (149). Fish liver oil for human consumption is commonly obtained from fresh cod liver of *Gadus morhua* species by boiling water extraction (149–150). There are three categories of cod liver oils based on their color obtained: yellow, light-brown and brown. Only yellow and light-brown cod liver oils are used in therapeutics; the brown color must be discarded for human uses. The oil becomes darker in color due to oxidation by air.

Cod liver oil contains large amounts of vitamins A, D, saturated, monounsaturated, and various omega-3 fatty acids such as polyunsaturated fatty acids (PUFAs), including both eicosapentaenoic acid (EPA) and docosahexaenoic acid (DHA) (149–151). In fish oil, vitamins A and D are absent or in low amounts.

Because of its special components, cod liver oil is used in the treatment and prevention of various diseases from the twentieth century through today (149–151). Thanks to its vitamin D content, it is used to treat and prevent rickets in children, and osteoporosis and rheumatism in older people. Vitamin D not only prevents rickets but is also important for muscle function and may prevent Type 1 diabetes, hypertension, and many common cancers. Vitamin A is essential for the immune system, bone growth, night vision, cellular growth, testicular, and ovarian function (149). As cod liver oil contains both vitamin A and PUFAs (omega-3 fatty acids), recent studies have reported that cod liver oil may prevent the progression of glaucoma (151). Thanks to the presence of various fatty acids cited above, cod liver oil supplementation has been suggested to reduce cardiometabolic risk factors, have anticancer effects, and ameliorate cognitive impairment induced by chronic stress. Antibacterial, antiviral, and antifungal effects have also been associated with PUFAs (150). It has been reported that the unsaturated fatty acids' (FAs) potency increases with the degree of unsaturation, while esterified FAs are less effective than free FAs. Similarly, for cod liver oil, it has been shown that the extract of free FAs from cod liver oil is more potent than cod liver oil containing the same FAs in the form of triglycerides (150). Besides the strong antibacterial properties, free FAs also possess antiviral properties, and FAs extracted from cod liver oil have been shown to cause a significant reduction of herpes simplex virus type 1 activity. To date, the mechanisms by which FAs act as antibacterial agents have not been resolved, and this continues to be a subject of some research effort (150).

However, excessive intake of cod liver oil is not good for everyone and can cause diseases because vitamins A, D and fatty acids in excess are harmful to the health. Cod liver oil is probably best avoided by pregnant women, asthmatics, and people taking anticoagulants such as warfarin (149)

5.4.3   Other Byproducts of Fish

Some other main byproducts of fish used as foods are fish sauce and shark fin.

5.4.3.1   *Fish Sauce*

Fish sauce is an amber-colored salty liquid in Southeast Asian cuisine used as an important condiment for improving the taste of foods. Fish sauce is traditionally produced by using whole small or medium fish such as anchovies, sardines, mackerel, and catfishes with salt in a ratio of 1:1 to 3:1 and fermented in underground concrete tanks or earthenware between 6 and 12 months at ambient conditions (152). Fish proteins are gradually hydrolyzed into peptides and amino acids by both bacterial and fish proteinases during fermentation (152). Thus, microorganisms found during fish sauce production are generally classified as halophilic (salt-loving). The microbiological safety of these products therefore mainly depends on rapid adequate fermentation by lactic acid bacteria. Production does not include steps such as cooking or pasteurization, which kill bacteria. The fermented liquid is rich in fish soluble proteins, peptides, and amino acids that are characterized by umami tastes. Fish sauce has a very high concentration of salt (25–30%) that is harmful to people with CVDs, hypertension, edema, and kidney diseases.

5.4.3.2   Shark Fin

Dried fins of shark are another fish byproduct for preparing special soup in many Asian countries, especially in China, where shark fin is considered health-promoting. However, a recent publication revealed that shark fins found in the market were rich in mercury, methyl-mercury, and arsenic, and their levels frequently exceeded mercury limits established by local authorities (153). This finding is not surprising as it is well known that big fishes such as whale, shark, and tilefish are high in mercury. Mercury and methylmercury are very toxic to the brain and the central nervous system. Arsenic is toxic to the liver, skin, lungs, and kidneys. Moreover, sharks are endangered species. Therefore, limit or avoid the consumption of shark fins.

5.5   Krill Oils

In the last decade, krill oil has been receiving increasing attention due to its nutritional composition and functional potentials similar to those of fish oil. Krill are small crustaceans and are found in all oceans. Antarctic krill (*Euphausia superba*) is an important marine crustacean organism that lives in the Antarctic Ocean and has attracted strong research interest worldwide (154–157). Because krill oil contains the same omega-3 fatty acids, EPA and DHA, found in fish and fish oil, krill oil is viewed as a viable alternative to fish oil to deliver the health benefits associated with EPA and DHA (154–157). The current technologies used in krill oil production are solvent extraction, nonsolvent extraction, super/subcritical fluid extraction, and enzyme-assisted pretreatment extraction, which all greatly influence the yield and quality of the end-product (154). The nonsolvent process frequently used includes different stages such as cooking, decanting, pressing, and centrifuging. This method avoids the use of toxic solvents and can be realized in boat. Krill contains extremely high levels of active proteolytic enzymes, which would result in rapid autolysis of krill after catching. Thus, the processing of krill oil from fresh krill must take place on board soon after capture (154).

Krill oil is a unique lipid consisting of diverse lipid classes and is characterized by a high concentration (39–80%) of phospholipids (PLs) linked with eicosapentaenoic acid (EPA) and docosahexaenoic acid (DHA), primarily in the form of phosphatidylcholine (154–157). However, in krill oil, the EPA and DHA are not found in triglyceride form, contrary to fish oil (155). This form of fatty acid esterification with triglycerides (TGs) or phospholipids (PLs) has impact on the efficiency of absorption of the fatty acids into the blood and on serum lipid levels (156). Because PLs comprise the structure of cell membranes, long-chain omega-3 PUFAs in the form of PLs might facilitate the passage of fatty acids through the intestinal wall and increase the bioavailability of these fatty acids in krill oil, compared to when they are consumed from fish oil. The overall fatty acid composition in krill oil resembles that of fish oil, but the EPA content is higher. This makes the ratio between EPA and DHA different between krill oil and fish oil. Fish oil often has a ratio EPA/DHA of approximately 1:1, while krill oil has a ratio of 2:1 (156). These results suggest that EPA from krill oil may be more efficiently incorporated into plasma due to the high content of phospholipids and free fatty acids in this oil (157). In addition, krill oil also contains considerable amounts of bioactive minor components such as astaxanthin, sterols, tocopherols, vitamin A, flavonoids, and minerals

(154–157). Astaxanthin is a strong antioxidant and is dark reddish-orange in color which contributes to the pinkish pigmentation of the native krill (155).

Numerous studies have been performed to evaluate the health benefits of krill oil, including CVD prevention, anti-hyperlipidemia, co-treatment and prevention of inflammatory diseases (arthritis, asthma), neuroprotection, women's health, anti-obesity, anti-diabetic effects, and anti-cancer activities (154–157). Although the bioavailability of krill oil is greater than that of fish oil, krill oil is more costly than fish oil at the same dosage of EPA and DHA, and its research regarding some chronic diseases are still sparse.

An analog of krill oil named calanus oil is recently found in markets. This oil is obtained from a tiny crustacean, *Calanus finmarchicus*, which is a species of copepods belonging to zooplankton, and found in Nordic Seas and the northern Atlantic Ocean (Canada). Calanus oil has similar properties as krill oil.

At recommended dietary allowances (RDAs), side effects of krill oil are generally limited to mild gastrointestinal distress such as gas, flatulence, nausea, or gastrointestinal cramping (155). However, like fish oil, an excessive intake of krill oil may increase bleeding risk (epistaxis, cerebral hemorrhage), decrease blood pressure, or cause hypoglycemia.

In summary, when comparing efficiency of krill oil compared to fish oil, krill oil may have demonstrated some initial superiority to fish oil in terms of bioavailability and/or therapeutic effectiveness. However, these results should be confirmed by additional studies. Meanwhile, fish oil may continue to be the choice of many consumers for the prevention of some chronic diseases due to its low cost and its efficacy (155).

5.6 Velvet Antler

Velvet antlers are bony skeletal protuberances of deer skull and consist mainly of the protein collagen and the mineral calcium hydroxyapatite ($Ca_5(PO_4)_3OH$) (158). Antlers are covered in soft fuzzy skin like velvet fabric. They occur in most species of the deer family (Cervidae) such as deer, elk, caribou, and moose, and are grown and shed annually. Antlers typically occur only in males, and are functional only during the rutting (mating) season (158). In western countries, antlers are removed from the deer by local anesthesia with no harm coming to the animal before they solidify into solid bone. The antlers obtained are dried, then cut into slices or powdered. They are used as traditional medicine or food in East Asian countries (China, Korea, Japan) or as dietary supplement (capsule, tincture) in Western countries (158–161).

Antler is a simple extension of bone, so it is rich in calcium such as calcium phosphate (hydroxyapatite) integrated with smaller amounts of calcium carbonate and some other minerals like magnesium, selenium, and manganese (158–161). Velvet antlers are also rich in amino acids, polypeptides, proteins, and collagen, which are considered the most prominent bioactive components. Lipid fractions include phospholipids, lecithin, anti-inflammatory prostaglandins, fatty acids, and so on (158–159). Carbohydrates are represented by glycosamino-glycans including the most prominent chondroitin sulfate, and less-prominent glucosamine sulfate (158). Deer antler also has substantial amounts of gelatinous components such as glucosamine sulfate, chondroitin sulfate, and collagen (158–159). These compounds have been shown to benefit the joints in cases of osteoarthritis by providing substrate materials useful for regenerating the body's connective tissues (collagens) found in joints and sinews (158–159).

Claims made for velvet antler prepared by traditional Chinese medicine as well as for velvet antler supplements include: stimulation of the immune system, improvement of athletic performance, treatment of osteoarthrosis, reduction of stress and fatigue, enhancement of sexual functioning for both sexes, anti-inflammation, anti-cancer, prevention of some CVDs like hypertension, and more (158–160). However, claims made for velvet antler supplements do not appear to be based upon rigorous research from human trials, although for osteoarthritis the findings may have some promise (160). In some preliminary scientific research, velvet antler supplement may potentially have a role in bone diseases such as osteoporosis, bone development, and bone fracture healing rates (161). More clinical studies are needed for a precise evaluation of velvet antler used as dietary supplement (capsule, tincture) or as traditional medicine in the form of powder, slice, soup, or extraction liquid.

5.7 EDIBLE BIRD'S NEST

Edible bird's nest is another famous animal byproduct mostly consumed by Eastern Asians for festivities and also for its nutritional and medicinal values. It is sometimes referred to as the 'Caviar of the East'.

Edible bird's nest (EBN) or edible-nest swiftlet is made of solidified saliva of a small bird swiftlet (*Apodidae* family) which is found in Southeast Asia, from the Indian Ocean to the coastal regions of Malaysia, Thailand, Vietnam, Indonesia, Philippines, and Southeast China. The majority of EBN traded worldwide comes from two heavily exploited species, the White-nest swiftlet (*Aerodramus fuciphagus*) and the Black-nest swiftlet (*Aerodramus maximus*) (162–165). However, the nests of *A. fuciphagus* are preferred, more valuable, and heavily exploited, as they are mainly composed of salivary secretion (70–80%) with relatively small amounts of impurities (20–30%), such as feathers and droppings (163).

Saliva secreted from the swiftlet sublingual salivary glands is used as cement for building nests (163). The nests are built into the walls of inland, sea-side caves or houses over a period of approximately 35 days, and are mainly built by male swiftlets. The nests are used to protect their eggs and hatchlings. There are three different colors found in EBN in the market: white, orange, and red. The properties of their difference in color are not known (163).

The two major components of EBN formed by swiftlet's saliva are protein and carbohydrate, comprising 60% and 30% of the total mass, respectively (162–165). EBN also contains fat (<2%) and other nutrient components such as glycoproteins, amino acids, calcium, sodium, potassium, magnesium, and abundant sialic acid-containing sugar chains (162–165). The glycoprotein structure in EBN makes it different from other protein sources such as chicken and fish in term of solubility, functional properties, and bioactive compounds. The glycoproteins in bird's nest contain 9% sialic acid, about 5.3% glucosamine, 4.19 to 7.2% galactosamine, 5.03 to 16.9% galactose, and about 0.7% fucose (164). The most abundant amino acids are serine, threonine, aspartic acid, glutamic acid, proline, and valine. The micronutrients of EBN may be affected by seasonal variations and even breeding sites (163–164). This is because EBNs are produced by swiftlets whose diet is composed of food (insects) from the local environment.

Although many claims have been made on the therapeutic and health-promoting effects of EBN in folk medicine, scientific documentations regarding these effects are very limited in published literature because the nutrients in EBN are poor and uninteresting (162). Moreover, the mechanisms of action of EBN remain largely unknown and the tonic effects of EBN in folk medicine have never been scientifically proven (162). Several studies have found that EBN may enhance cell proliferation and differentiation, and various beneficial effects have been reported in vitro as well as in vivo, but still not in humans (162). While these studies point towards the potential use of EBN in the treatment or even prevention of several diseases, the mechanisms of action of EBN remain largely unknown; more explorations are needed. Until today, its tonic and therapeutic effects are still not recognized by any official health organizations. As edible bird's nest is very costly, some fake EBNs are found in the market. Adulterated or fake EBN may be hazardous to consume (166). In addition, many toxic chemicals used to clean and to preserve edible bird's nest are also eventually present in some marketed products.

5.8 SILKWORM (*BOMBYX MORI*)

Silkworm (*Bombyx mori*) is a domesticated insect which has been used for making silk for at least 5,000 years in China. Apart from silk production, *Bombyx mori* has many applications in biological and scientific research (167–168). The various stages during its life span include embryo, larva, pupa, and adult moth (167). Pupae are a source of proteins, vitamin B1, B2 and E, diapause hormone, amino acids, and more, and are used for antibacterial and antihistaminic preparations (168). As a source of animal protein and vitamins, the larvae and pupae can be used as food in some East Asian countries. In addition, silkworm is an excellent tool for drug screening and safety tests (167).

5.9 OTHER UTILIZATIONS OF ANIMAL BYPRODUCTS

Besides being used as animal source foods, wild and farmed animals are also used for manufacture of clothing and diverse objects. The skin and the fur of some animals like livestock, sheep, bison, alpaca, crocodile, lizard, boa, and so on are used as leather, wool, and fiber for clothing, shoe, and purse manufactures.

6 ANIMAL-BASED MEDICINES

Throughout human history, plants and animals in nature have been sourced as medicinal agents for the treatment of illness, and an impressive number of modern drugs have been isolated from natural sources including plants, animals, yeasts, fungi, bacteria, and so on.

6.1 IN WESTERN MEDICINE

Among 252 essential chemicals used as drugs that have been selected by the World Health Organization, 11.1% come from plants and 8.7% from animals (169). Among 150 prescription drugs currently in use in the United States, 27 have animal origin (169). In pharmaceutical industry, a number of medicines developed from animal sources or their byproducts are heparin, insulin, thyroid hormones, protamine, calcitonin, pituitary hormones, estrogens, chorionic gonadotropin, sex steroids, and more (170).

For example, heparin, an anticoagulant discovered in 1916 by Jay McLean from canine liver cells, is now prepared using porcine intestines and bovine lung (170). In 1921, three Canadian scientists named Frederick Banting, John Macleod, and Charles Best successfully purified insulin from a dog's pancreas. For this work, only Banting and Macleod received the Nobel Prize in Medicine in 1923. Insulin was then extracted from the pancreas of cattle and pigs and purified for treatment of diabetes in humans. In the 1980s, insulin was manufactured by genetic engineering from bacterium *Escherichia coli*, and also from yeast (170).

Further, protamine sulfate, a potent heparin antagonist, was derived from salmon sperm (170). It is also used to prepare long-acting insulin. Today, it is synthesized by recombinant DNA technology.

Calcitonin hormone, a polypeptide hormone of the human thyroid, was extracted from the ultimobranchial glands (thyroid-like glands) of fish, particularly Coho salmon (170). Salmon calcitonin resembles human calcitonin, but is more active. Calcitonin is used to treat postmenopausal osteoporosis, hypercalcemia, osteoarthritis, and Paget's disease. Moreover, it is a powerful analgesic agent and may be used to treat migraine and other pains, especially in elderly people. Calcitonin is now produced either by recombinant technology or by chemical peptide synthesis. In the 1970s, captopril, a potent angiotensin converting enzyme (ACE) inhibitor used for arterial hypertension and some cardiovascular diseases, was derived from a peptide in the venom of the Brazilian pit viper (170).

For over 60 years, eggs from chicken, hen or embryonic eggs have been used as support for virus inoculation in the preparation of different vaccines, especially influenza (flu) vaccines (170–171).

Chondroitin or glycosaminoglycan, a component of cartilage, is extracted from cartilaginous cow, pig, shark, fish, and bird tissues (171).

Glucosamine, an amino sugar, is extracted from exoskeletons of crustaceans and other arthropods. The mixture of glucosamine and chondroitin is a dietary supplement used for osteoarthritis therapy (171).

Honeybee venom and its major component melittin, an amphipathic 26-amino-acid-peptide, have demonstrated antitumoral effects in breast cancer, melanoma, non-small-cell lung cancer, glioblastoma, leukemia, ovarian, cervical, and pancreatic cancers, with higher cytotoxic potency in cancer cells compared to non-transformed cells (172).

Roscovitine, a new purine, is an inhibitor of cyclin-dependent kinase (CDK) present in starfish oocyte and was recently demonstrated to have potential therapeutic use against cancer, neurodegenerative diseases, cardiovascular disorders, viral infections, and parasitic protozoa (173).

Since the time of Hippocrates, bloodletting has been a popular remedy, and leeches (*Hirudo medicinalis*) played a key role. They became especially popular in the 1800s, when France and many other countries imported millions of leeches each year for medical purposes. Although the practice of bloodletting has been largely abandoned by Western medicine, leeches have nonetheless continued to be useful (170). Recently, extensive research on leech saliva unveiled the presence of a variety of bioactive peptides and proteins involving antithrombin (hirudin, bufrudin), antiplatelet (calin, saratin), factor Xa inhibitors (lefaxin), antibacterial (theromacin, theromyzin), and others. Consequently, leech has made a comeback as a new remedy for many chronic and life-threatening abnormalities, such as cardiovascular problems, diabetes mellitus, cancer, metastasis, and infectious diseases (174). In the twentieth century, leech therapy has established itself in plastic and microsurgery as a protective tool against venous congestion, and serves to salvage replanted digits (fingers, toes) and flaps (skin grafts). Many clinics for plastic surgery all over the world have begun to use leeches for cosmetic purposes (174). Leeches are also being used directly to preserve the viability of tissue grafts in the presence of significant vascular congestion. Despite the efficacious properties of leech therapy, the safety and complications of leeching are still controversial.

6.2 In Traditional Medicine

Since antiquity, traditional medicine has used an arsenal of plants and animals to cure illnesses and improve health. According to the World Health Organization, 80% of the developing world's rural population depends on traditional medicines for its primary healthcare needs (175).

Among traditional medicines, earthworms have been both sources of food consumption and medicinal cures in many countries for a very long time (176–178). Ayurveda, traditional Chinese medicine, and practices in Japan, Vietnam, and Korea have focused on earthworms as sources of food (176). Moreover, earthworms are important regulators of soil structure and dynamics of soil organic matter. Their activities are beneficial because they enhance soil nutrient cycling through the rapid incorporation of detritus into mineral soil (177). The medical value of earthworms has been known for centuries. Extracts prepared from earthworm tissues have been used for the treatment of numerous diseases, as they are valuable sources of proteins, peptides, enzymes, and physiologically active substances. Several studies have shown that the earthworm extracts contain different macromolecules which exhibit a variety of activities, such as antioxidative, antibacterial, anti-inflammatory, anticancer, and more. Preparation of earthworms are used to aid in the wound healing process. In some countries, earthworms are used as a part of healthy diet. They have very high nutritive value because their bodies contain a high percentage of various proteins. Earthworms are also used to feed animals (fish, chicken, etc.) (177). Some active proteins and compounds in earthworm include fibrinolytic enzymes, lumbrokinase, collagenase, superoxide dismutase, cholinesterase, glycosidases, catalases, metallothionein, calmodulin-binding protein, and other proteins (178). Besides, earthworm tissues contain lysenin, eiseniapore, antitumor protein, glycoprotein, gut mobility regulation peptide, antibacterial peptide, carbamidine, lumbritin, lumbrofobrim, terrestrolumbrolysin, purin, vitamin B, tyrosine, succinic acid, lauric acid, unsaturated fatty acid, and so on (178). These earthworm components have different pharmacological and clinical effects on different organs such as the nervous, cardiovascular, and respiratory systems, the blood, the uterus, and smooth muscle. They also have anticancer properties (178).

Blister beetles (also called Spanish fly) are insects of the order Coleoptera (beetles) of the family Meloidae that contains about 2,500 species. They can be found in certain areas of Europe and some eastern Asian regions such as Vietnam, Taiwan, Thailand, Korea, and China (179). In Europe, preparations made from dried blister beetle, called cantharides, have been used as aphrodisiac for over 2,000 years. Cantharides have been also used as vesicant. But its use has resulted in poisoning effects in humans (179). In 1810, the French pharmacist Pierre Robiquet isolated a crystalline compound known today as cantharidin from the dried Spanish fly or Cantharides (179). Earlier Chinese studies in twentieth century revealed that the dried bodies of the *Mylabris caragnae* or *Mylabris phalerata* possess antitumor properties and an increased number of leukocytes, but once again, the irritant effects on the urinary system reduce their uses (179). Cantharidin, a terpenoid, has been reported to be active against various human cancers, but with severe side effects such as nephrotoxicity (179–182). In order to reduce this toxicity, its demethylated analogue nor-cantharidin has been synthesized and used in cancer therapy (179–182). In China, nor-cantharidin, a synthetized compound, has been used to treat patients with hepatocellular carcinoma, breast cancer, colon cancer, gastric cancer, leukemia, and more, for many years (179–182). Nor-cantharidin has been shown to be ten times less nephrotoxic than its precursor, cantharidin (181–182). Nor-cantharidin also stimulates the bone marrow production of white cells, but without kidney toxicity (182). Nevertheless, nor-cantharidin is still not authorized to treat cancer in humans in Western countries.

7 DISCUSSION

Animal source foods (ASFs) have two origins: farm animals such as cattle and poultry, and wild animals like marine fish, shellfish, wild boars, and so on. Meat of these animals are divided into two groups: red meat and white meat. Red meat of beef, pork, horse, sheep, and rabbit is rich in energy, proteins, amino acids, iron, and vitamin B12, but they also contain bad fats – saturated fatty acids and cholesterol. Therefore, frequent consumption of red meat may cause hyperlipidemia, atherosclerosis, and risks of colon cancer. Processed red meats such as ham, sausage, bacon, and beef jerky are rich in saturated fats and preservatives like nitrates and salt, must be moderately consumed or avoided because they may cause cancer, CVD, and obesity. Besides meat, other animal organs such as heart, liver, brain, and kidney of pork and ox are also consumed. Heart, liver, and kidney of these farm mammals are rich in micronutrients, in particular, coenzyme Q10, vitamin A. In contrast, white meat like poultry, fish, and shellfish are high in good fats – unsaturated fatty acids like omega-3s – hence, they are considered better than red meat. Omega-3 fatty acids DHA and EPA in seafoods are active forms and are more useful than alpha-linolenic acid (ALA), an inactive form of omega-3 fatty acid found in poultry meat. DHA and EPA are necessary for heart and brain health. Wild seawater fish like salmon, mackerel, sardines, shads, and shellfish are the best source of essential macro- and micronutrients for all individuals, mostly in the elderly and children, as well as breastfeeding and pregnant women. Large fish like shark, swordfish, and tilefish must be avoided because they are high in mercury. Many health organizations, have recommended eating fatty fish at least two times a week for prevention of CVDs. In addition, the meat cooking mode also plays an important role in health and disease. In general, meat cooking by boiling, steaming, braising, and stewing is better than that by roasting, barbecuing, and frying because the direct contact of meat with a high heat source (flame) causes toxic compounds.

Milk and egg are good sources of essential macro- and micronutrients. Dairy products contain all essential nutrients for children and adults and play important roles in the prevention and treatment of some diseases in humans. Cheese, especially hard cheese, is rich in absorbable calcium. For the growth of children and for the prevention of bone diseases such as osteoporosis for the elderly and rickets for children, the best way is to consume dairy products regularly. Egg is also a complete food and contains all macro- and micronutrients. Lecithin, a specific phospholipid of egg yolk, is necessary for the functioning of brain, lungs, blood, bile, and more. However, egg is also rich in cholesterol. Therefore, a moderate intake of eggs is recommended for people with hypercholesterolemia and hyperlipidemia.

Vitamins A and B12 as well as iron, calcium, and omega-3 fatty acids like DHA and EPA are more absorbable in animals than those found in vegetables. Vitamin B12 does not exist in plants, except in seaweed. In addition, many drugs and supplements such as heparin, insulin, calcitonin, chondroitin, glucosamine, fish oil, and cod liver oil used in both modern and folk medicine are obtained by extraction of different insects and animal organs. More research is needed to find further drugs in the millions of animals and insects populating this planet.

8 REFERENCES

1. National Council of Educational Research and Training (NCERT). (2006). Chapter 4. Animal Kingdom, pp. 46–62. In: *Biology Textbook for Class 11*. http://ncert.nic.in/textbook/textbook.htm?kebo1=4-22.
2. Graham A. (2000). Animal Phylogeny: Root and Branch Surgery. *Curr. Biol.*, **10**(1): R36–R38.
3. Grosberg R.K., Vermeij G.J., Wainwright P.C. (2012). Biodiversity in Water and on Land. *Curr. Biol.*, **22**(21): R900–R903.
4. National Council of Educational Research and Training (NCERT). (2006). Chapter 7. Structural Organization in Animals, pp. 100–122. In: *Biology Textbook for Class 11*. http://ncert.nic.in/textbook/textbook.htm?kebo1=7-22.
5. Cuthill I.C., Allen W.L., Arbuckle K., Caspers B., Chaplin G., Hauber M.E., Hil G.E., Jablonski N.G., Jiggins C.D., Kelber A., Mappes J., Marshall J., Merrill R., Osorio D., Prum R., Roberts N.W., Roulin A., Rowland H.M., Sherratt T.N., Skelhorn J., Speed M.P., Stevens M., Stoddard M.C., Stuart-Fox D., Talas L., Tibbetts E., Caro T. (2017). The Biology of Color. *Science*. **357**(6350): eaan0221, 7 pages.
6. Mills M.G., Patterson L.B. (2009). Not Just Black and White: Pigment Pattern Development and Evolution in Vertebrates. *Semin. Cell Dev. Biol.*, **20**(1): 72–81.
7. Brenner M., Hearing V.J. (2008). The Protective Role of Melanin Against UV Damage in Human Skin. *Photochem. Photobiol.*, **84**(3): 539–549.
8. Larsen C.S. (2003). Animal Source Foods and Human Health During Evolution. *J. Nutr.*, **133**: 3893S–3897S.
9. Murphy S.P., Allen L.H. (2003). Nutritional Importance of Animal Source Foods. *J. Nutr.*, **133**(11): 3932S–3935S.
10. Schönfeldt H.C., Pretorius B., Hall N. (2013). The Impact of Animal Source Food Products on Human Nutrition and Health. *S. Afr. J. Anim. Sci.*, **41**(3): 394–412.
11. Neumann C., Harris D.M., Rogers L.M. (2002). Contribution of Animal Source Foods in Improving Diet Quality and Function in Children in the Developing World. *Nutr. Res.*, **22**: 193–220.
12. Khora S.S. (2014). Chapter 21. Health Risks Associated with Seafood, pp. 483–570. In: *Seafood Science: Advances in Chemistry, Technology and Applications*. Editor: Se-Kwon Kim. CRC Press, Taylor and Francis Group, Boca Raton, FL, September 16, 606 pages.
13. Costello C., Cao L., Gelcich S. (2019). *The Future of Food from the Sea*. World Resources Institute, Washington, DC. https://oceanpanel.org/sites/default/files/2019-11/19_HLP_BP1%20Paper.pdf.
14. Kim S-K., Venkatesan J. (2015). Chapter 1. Introduction to Seafood Science, pp. 1–13. In: *Seafood Science: Advances in Chemistry, Technology and Applications*. Editor: Se-Kwon Kim. CRC Press, Taylor and Francis Group, Boca Raton, FL.
15. Gunning D., Maguire J., Burnell G. (2016). The Development of Sustainable Saltwater-Based Food Production Systems: A Review of Established and Novel Concepts. *Water*, **8**(598), 37 pages.
16. Musick J.A., Musick S. (2011). *Sharks. FAO Fisheries and Aquaculture Reviews and Studies*. FAO, Rome, 13 pages. www.fao.org/fishery/docs/DOCUMENT/reviews%26studies/sharks.pdf.
17. Mahaffey K.R., Sunderland E.M., Chan H.M., Choi A.L., Grandjean P., Mariën K., Oken E., Sakamoto M., Schoeny R., Weihe P., Yan C.H., Yasutake A. (2011). Balancing the Benefits of n-3 Polyunsaturated Fatty Acids and the Risks of Methylmercury Exposure from Fish Consumption. *Nutr. Rev.*, **69**(9): 493–508.
18. Oken E., Choi A.L., Karagas M.R., Mariën K., Rheinberger C.M., Schoeny R., Sunderland E., Korrick S. (2012). Which Fish Should I Eat? Perspectives Influencing Fish Consumption Choices. *Environ. Health Perspect.*, **120**(6): 790–798.
19. Venugopal V., Gopakumar K. (2017). Shellfish: Nutritive Value, Health Benefits, and Consumer Safety. *Compr. Rev. Food Sci. Food Saf.*, **16**: 1219–1242.

20. Bordbar S., Anwar F., Saari N. (2011). High-Value Components and Bioactives from Sea Cucumbers for Functional Foods-A Review. *Mar. Drugs*, **9**(10): 1761–805.
21. Pangestuti R., Arifin Z. (2017). Medicinal and Health Benefit Effects of Functional Sea Cucumbers. *J. Tradit. Complement. Med.*, **8**(3): 341–351.
22. Hogan Z. (2011). Review of Freshwater Fish. Tenth Meeting of the Conference of the Parties. Bergen, November 20–25. www.cms.int/sites/default/files/document/inf_33_freshwater_fish_eonly_0.pdf.
23. Gilani N. (2019). What Is the Difference Between Freshwater Vs Saltwater Fish? November 22. https://sciencing.com/different-freshwater-vs-saltwater-fish-6307253.html.
24. Bloom D.D., Lovejoy N.R. (2014). The Evolutionary Origins of Diadromy Inferred from a Time-Calibrated Phylogeny for Clupeiformes (Herring and Allies). *Proc. Biol. Sci.*, **281**(1778): 20132081, 8 pages.
25. Cummings K., Jones H., Lopes-Lima M. (2016). Rapid Bioassessment Methods for Freshwater Molluscs, pp. 185–207. In: *Core Standardized Methods for Rapid Biological Field Assessment, Chapter: Rapid Bioassessment Methods for Freshwater Molluscs*. Editors: Trond H. Larsen. Conservation International, Arlington, VA.
26. Abouel-Yazeed A.M. (2013). Fatty Acids Profile of Some Marine Water and Freshwater Fish. *J. Arab. Aquac. Soc.*, **8**(2): 283–292.
27. Tasbozan O., Gokce M.A. (2017). Fatty Acids in Fish. Chapter 8, pp. 143–159. In: *Fatty Acids*. Editor: Angel Catala. InTech, June 21, 246 pages. doi:10.5772/68048. www.intechopen.com/chapters/54572.
28. United States Agency for International Development (USAID). (2016). Fishing for Food Security. The Importance of Wild Fisheries for Food Security and Nutrition, April, 56 pages. http://pdf.usaid.gov/pdf_docs/PA00M1T3.pdf.
29. Fisheries Research and Development Corporation. (2004). *What's So Healthy About Seafood? – A Guide for Seafood Marketers*. 2nd edition. Fisheries Research and Development Corporation, Deakin, Australia, 40 pages. www.wafic.org.au/wp-content/uploads/2016/12/Whats_so_healthy_booklet.pdf.
30. Gil A., Gil F. (2015). Fish, a Mediterranean Source of n-3 PUFA: Benefits Do Not Justify Limiting Consumption. *Br. J. Nutr.*, **113**: S58–S67.
31. Hellberg R.S., DeWitt C.A.M., Morrissey M.T. (2012). Risk-Benefit Analysis of Seafood Consumption: A Review. *Compr. Rev. Food Sci. Food Saf.*, **11**: 490–517.
32. Mozaffarian D., Rimm E.B. (2006). Fish Intake, Contaminants, and Human Health: Evaluating the Risks and the Benefits. *J.A.M.A.*, **296**(15): 1885–1899.
33. Bernstein A.S., Oken E., de Ferranti S. (2019). Fish, Shellfish, and Children's Health: An Assessment of Benefits, Risks, and Sustainability. *Pediatrics*, **143**(6): e20190, 25 pages.
34. Pham-Huy A.L., He H., Pham-Huy C. (2008). Free Radicals and Antioxidants in Disease and Health. *Int. J. Biomed. Sci. (IJBS)*, **4**(2): 89–96.
35. Burri L., Hoem N., Banni S., Berge K. (2012). Marine Omega-3 Phospholipids: Metabolism and Biological Activities. *Int. J. Mol. Sci.*, **13**(11): 15401–15419.
36. Shah M.M., Liang Y., Cheng J.J., Daroch M. (2016). Astaxanthin-Producing Green Microalga Haematococcus pluvialis: From Single Cell to High Value Commercial Products. *Front Plant Sci.*, **7**(531): 1–28.
37. European Food Safety Authority (EFSA). (2009). Scientific Opinion on Arsenic in Food. *EFSA J.*, **7**(10): 1351, 199 pages. https://efsa.onlinelibrary.wiley.com/doi/pdf/10.2903/j.efsa.2009.1351.
38. Stancheva M., Merdzhanova A. (2011). Fatty Acid Composition of Common Carp, Rainbow Trout and Grey Mullet Fish Species. *Agric. Sci. Technol.*, **3**(3): 285–289.
39. Norat T., Bingham S., Ferrari P., Slimani N., Jenad M., Mazuir M., Overvad K., Olsen A., Tjonneland A. (2005). Meat, Fish, and Colorectal Cancer Risk: The European Prospective Investigation into Cancer and Nutrition. *J. Natl. Cancer Inst.*, **97**(12): 906–916.
40. Van Huis A., Van Itterbeeck J., Klunder H., Mertens E., Halloran A., Muir G., Vantomme P. (2013). Edible Insects: Future Prospects for Food and Feed Security. By Food and Agriculture Organization of the United Nations, Rome. FAO Forestry Paper, N° 171, 201 pages.
41. Malomo G.A., Ihegwuagu N.E. (2017). Chapter 4. Some Aspects of Animal Feed Sampling and Analysis. In: *Ideas and Applications Toward Sample Preparation for Food and Beverage Analysis*. Editor: Mark T. Stauffer. IntechOpen. doi:10.5772/intechopen.70856.
42. Hanapi S.Z., Awad H.M., Sarip S.H.M., Aziz R., Sarmidi M.R., Ali S.I.S. (2012). Chapter 15. Animal Feed, pp. 421–444. In: *Biotechnology Development in Agriculture, Industry and Health: Current Industrial Application & Future Trends*, Volume 1. 1st edition. Editors: Zainul Akmar Zakaria, Wan Azlina Ahmad, Zainoha Zakaria. Penerbit Universiti Universiti Teknologi, Malaysia.

43. Daley C.A., Abbott A., Doyle P.S., Nader G.A., Larson S. (2010). A Review of Fatty Acid Profiles and Antioxidant Content in Grass-Fed and Grain-Fed Beef. *Nutr. J.*, **9**: 10, 12 pages.

44. Karsten H., Patterson P.H., Stout R., Crews G. (2010). Vitamins A, E and Fatty Acid Composition of the Eggs of Caged Hens and Pastured Hens. *Ren. Agric. Food Syst.*, **25**(1): 45–54.

45. Sapkota A.R., Lefferts L.Y., McKenzie S., Walker P. (2007). What Do We Feed to Food-Production Animals? A Review of Animal Feed Ingredients and Their Potential Impacts on Human Health. *Environ. Health Perspect.*, **115**(5): 663–670.

46. Centers for Disease Control and Prevention. (2018). Bovine Spongiform Encephalopathy (BSE), or Mad Cow Disease, October 9. www.cdc.gov/prions/bse/about.html.

47. Hilton D.A. (2006). Pathogenesis and Prevalence of Variant Creutzfeldt – Jakob Disease. *J. Pathol.*, **208**: 134–141.

48. Access Science Editors (January 2017). U.S. Bans Antibiotics Use for Enhancing Growth in Livestock. https://doi.org/10.1036/1097-8542.BR0125171.

49. Spellberg B., Hansen G.R., Kar A., Cordova C.D., Price L.B., Johnson J.R. (2016). Antibiotic Resistance in Humans and Animals, June 22, 15 pages. https://nam.edu/wp-content/uploads/2016/07/Antibiotic-Resistance-in-Humans-and-Animals.pdf.

50. Bennani H., Mateus A., Mays N., Eastmure E., Stärk K.D.C., Häsler B. (2020). Overview of Evidence of Antimicrobial Use and Antimicrobial Resistance in the Food Chain. *Antibiotics (Basel)*, **9**(2): 49, 18 pages.

51. Johnson R. (2015). The U.S.-EU Beef Hormone Dispute. Congressional Research Service (CRS) Report, January 14, 38 pages. https://fas.org/sgp/crs/row/R40449.pdf.

52. European Commission. (2019). The European Union and the United States Reach an Agreement on Imports of Hormone-Free Beef, June 14. https://ec.europa.eu/commission/presscorner/detail/en/ip_19_3012.

53. Speedy A.W. (2003). Global Production and Consumption of Animal Source Foods. *J. Nutr.*, **133**(11): 4048S–4053S.

54. Ndlovu L.R. (2010). The Role of Foods of Animal Origin in Human Nutrition and Health. Chapter 5, pp. 77–91. In: *The Role of Livestock in Developing Communities: Enhancing Multifunctionality*. Editors: Frans Swanepoel, Aldo Stroebel, Siboniso Moyo. http://ir.nust.ac.zw/xmlui/handle/123456789/261.

55. Keeton J.T., Dikeman M.E. (2017). 'Red' and 'White' Meats – Terms That Lead to Confusion. *Anim. Front.*, **7**(4): 29–33.

56. Williams P. (2007). Nutritional Composition of Red Meat. *Nutr. Diet.*, **64** (Suppl. 4): S113–S119.

57. Luciano F.B. (2009). The Impacts of Lean Red Meat Consumption on Human Health: A Review. *CyTA – J. Food*, **7**(2): 143–151.

58. Schönfeldt H.C., Hall N. (2012). Red Meat in Nutrition and Health. Editors: Professor Catherine M. Champagne, Doctor Ingrid van Heerden. Institute of Food, Nutrition and Well-being University of Pretoria, Hatfield Pretoria, South Africa, 76 pages.

59. Wolk A. (2017). Potential Health Hazards of Eating Red Meat (Review). *J. Intern. Med.*, **281**(2): 106–122.

60. International Agency for Research on Cancer (IARC) of the World Health Organization (WHO). (2015). Monographs Evaluate Consumption of Red Meat and Processed Meat. *Press Release*, N° 240, October 26. www.iarc.fr/en/media-centre/pr/2015/pdfs/pr240_E.pdf.

61. Bouvard V., Loomis D., Guyton K.Z., Grosse Y., El Ghissassi F., Benbrahim-Tallaa L., Guha N., Mattock H., Straif K. (2015). Carcinogenicity of Consumption of Red and Processed Meat. *The Lancet Oncol.*, **16**(16): 1599–1600.

62. Larsson S.C., Orsini N. (2014). Red Meat and Processed Meat Consumption and All-Cause Mortality: A Meta-Analysis. *Am. J. Epidemiol.*, **179**(3): 282–289.

63. Pan A., Sun Q., Bernstein A.M., Schulze M.B., Manson J.E., Stampfer M.J., Willett W.C., Hu F.B. (2012). Red Meat Consumption and Mortality. Results From 2 Prospective Cohort Studies. *Arch. Intern. Med.*, **172**(7): 555–563.

64. Cross A., Leitzmann M.F., Gail M.H., Hollenbeck A.R., Schatzkin A., Sinha R. (2007). A Prospective Study of Red and Processed Meat Intake in Relation to Cancer Risk. *PLoS Med.* (Public Library of Science), **4**(12): e325, 1973–1984.

65. Taylor E.F., Burley V.J., Greenwood D.C., Cade J.E. (2007). Meat Consumption and Risk of Breast Cancer in the UK Women's Cohort Study. *Brit. J. Cancer.*, **96**: 1139–1146.

66. Zhu H., Yang X., Zhang C., Zhu C., Tao G., Zhao L., Tang S., Shu Z., Cai J., Dai S., Qin Q., Xu L., Cheng H., Sun X. (2013). Red and Processed Meat Intake Is Associated with Higher Gastric Cancer Risk: A Meta-Analysis of Epidemiological Observational Studies. *PLoS One* (Public Library of Science) **8**(8): e70955, 1–10.

67. McAfee A.J., McSorley E.M., Cuskelly G.J., Moss B.W., Wallace J.M.W., Bonham M.P., Fearon A.M. (2010). Red Meat Consumption: An Overview of the Risks and Benefits. *Meat Sci.*, **84**: 1–13.
68. Truswell A.S. (2002). Meat Consumption and Cancer of the Large Bowel. *Eur. J. Clin. Nutr.*, **56**: S19–S24.
69. Micha R., Wallace S.K., Mozaffarian D. (2010). Red and Processed Meat Consumption and Risk of Incident Coronary Heart Disease, Stroke, and Diabetes Mellitus. A Systematic Review and Meta-Analysis. *Circulation*, **121**: 2271–2283.
70. Micha R., Michas G., Mozaffarian D. (2012). Unprocessed Red and Processed Meats and Risk of Coronary Artery Disease and Type 2 Diabetes – An Updated Review of the Evidence. *Curr. Atheroscler. Rep.*, **14**(6): 515–524.
71. Arshad M.S., Zulfiqar A., Faqir M., Saeed F., Khan M.I., Sohaib M. (2015). Red Meat Consumption: A Threat Towards Cardiovascular Diseases. *Pak. J. Food Sci.*, **25**(2): 86–91.
72. Pan A., Sun Q., Bernstein A.M., Schulze M.B., Manson J.E., Willett W.C., Hu F.B. (2011). Red Meat Consumption and Risk of Type 2 Diabetes: 3 Cohorts of US Adults and an Updated Meta-Analysis. *Am. J. Clin. Nutr.*, **94**(4): 1088–1096.
73. Vergnaud A-C., Norat T., Romaguera D., Mouw T., May A.M., Travier N., Luan J., Wareham N., Slimani N. (2010). Meat Consumption and Prospective Weight Change in Participants of the EPIC-PANACEA Study. *Am. J. Clin. Nutr.*, **92**(2): 398–407.
74. Astrup A., Clifton P., Layman D.K., Mattes R.D., Westerterp-Plantenga M.S. (2010). Meat Intake's Influence on Body Fatness Cannot Be Assessed Without Measurement of Body Fat. *Am. J. Clin. Nutr.*, **92**(5): 1274–1275; author reply 1275–1276.
75. Rouhani M.H., Salehi-Abargouei A., Surkan P.J., Azadbakht L. (2014). Is There a Relationship Between Red or Processed Meat Intake and Obesity? A Systematic Review and Meta-Analysis of Observational Studies. *Obes. Rev.*, **15**(9): 740–748.
76. Key T.J., Fraser G.E., Thorogood M., Appleby P.N., Beral V., Reeves G., Burr M.L., Chang-Claude J., Frentzel-Beyme R., Kuzma J.W., Mann J., McPherson K. (1999). Mortality in Vegetarians and Non-Vegetarians: Detailed Findings from a Collaborative Analysis of 5 Prospective Studies. *Am. J. Clin. Nutr.*, **70**(3): 516s–524s.
77. Qian F., Riddle M.C., Wylie-Rosett J., Hu F.B. (2020). Red and Processed Meats and Health Risks: How Strong Is the Evidence? *Diabetes Care*, **43**: 265–271.
78. Rohrmann S., Linseisen J. (2016). Processed Meat: The Real Villain? *Proc. Nutr. Soc.*, **75**(3): 233–241.
79. Marangoni F., Corsello G., Cricelli C., Ferrara N., Ghiselli A., Lucchin L., Poli A. (2015). Role of Poultry Meat in a Balanced Diet Aimed at Maintaining Health and Wellbeing: An Italian Consensus Document. *Food Nutr. Res.*, **59**, Art. 27606, 1–11.
80. Soriano-Santos J. (2010). Chapter 25: Chemical Composition and Nutritional Content of Raw Poultry Meat, pp. 467–489. In: *Handbook of Poultry Science and Technology, Volume 1: Primary Processing.* Editors: Isabel Guerrero-Legarreta, Y.H. Hui. John Wiley & Sons, Inc., Hoboken, NJ, 788 pages.
81. Kralik G., Kralik Z., Grčević M., Hanžek D. (2018). Chapter 4. Quality of Chicken Meat. In: *Animal Husbandry and Nutrition.* Editors: Banu Yücel, Turgay Taşkin. IntechOpen. www.intechopen.com/books/animal-husbandry-and-nutrition/quality-of-chicken-meat.
82. Underwood R. (2018). Chapter 5. Food and Dairy Technology. In: *Bioprocesses in Food Industry.* ED-Tech Press, London, UK, 348 pages.
83. Gibbs R.A., Rymer C., Givens D.I. (2010). Long-Chain n-3 PUFA: Intakes in the UK and the Potential of a Chicken Meat Prototype to Increase Them. *Proc. Nutr. Soc.*, **69**: 144–155.
84. Yang W.S., Wong M.Y., Vogtmann E., Tang R.Q., Xie L., Yang Y.S., Wu Q.J., Zhang W., Xiang Y.B. (2012). Meat Consumption and Risk of Lung Cancer: Evidence from Observational Studies. *Ann. Oncol.*, **23**: 3163–3170.
85. Norat T., Bingham S., Ferrari P., Slimani N., Jenad M., Mazuir M., Overvad K., Olsen A., Tjonneland A., Clavel F., Boutron-Ruault M.C., Kesse E., Boeing H., Bergmann M.M., Nieters A., Linseisen J., Trichopoulou A., Trichopoulos D., Tountas Y., Berrino F., Palli D., Panico S., Tumino R., Vineis P., Bueno-de-Mesquita H.B., Peeters P.H., Engeset D., Lund E., Skeie G., Ardanaz E., González C., Navarro C., Quirós J.R., Sanchez M.J., Berglund G., Mattisson I., Hallmans G., Palmqvist R., Day N.E., Khaw K.T., Key T.J., San Joaquin M., Hémon B., Saracci R., Kaaks R., Riboli E. (2005). Meat, Fish, and Colorectal Cancer Risk: The European Prospective Investigation into Cancer and Nutrition. *J. Natl. Cancer Inst.*, **97**(12): 906–916.
86. Yeung R.M.W., Morris J. (2001). Consumer Perception of Food Risk in Chicken Meat. *Nutr. Food Sci.*, **31**(6): 270–278.

87. John E.M., Stern M.C., Sinha R., Koo J. (2011). Meat Consumption, Cooking Practices, Meat Mutagens, and Risk of Prostate Cancer. *Nutr. Cancer*, **63**(4): 525–537.

88. Sun Y., Liu B., Snetselaar L.G., Robinson J.G., Wallace R.B., Peterson L.L., Bao W. (2019). Association of Fried Food Consumption with All Cause, Cardiovascular, and Cancer Mortality: Prospective Cohort Study. *BMJ.*, **364**: k5420, 9 pages.

89. Gadiraju T.V., Patel Y., Gaziano J.M., Djoussé L. (2015). Fried Food Consumption and Cardiovascular Health: A Review of Current Evidence. *Nutrients*, **7**(10): 8424–8430.

90. Food and Agriculture Organization (FAO) of the United Nations. (2017). Milk Composition. Edited: September 2017. www.fao.org/dairy-production-products/products/milk-composition/en/.

91. Ballard O., Morrow A.L. (2013). Human Milk Composition: Nutrients and Bioactive Factors. *Pediatr. Clin. North Am.*, **60**(1): 49–74.

92. Wijesinha-Bettoni R., Burlingame B. (2013). Chapter 3. Milk and Dairy Product Composition, pp. 41–102. In: *Milk and Dietary Products in Human Nutrition.* Editors: Ellen Muehlhoff, Anthony Bennett, Deirdre McMahon. Food and Agriculture Organization of the United Nations, Rome. www.fao.org/3/i3396e/i3396e.pdf.

93. Haug A., Hostmark A.T., Harstad O.M. (2007). Bovine Milk in Human Nutrition – A Review. *Lipids Health Dis.*, **6**(25): 1–16.

94. Pereira P.C. (2014). Milk Nutritional Composition and Its Role in Human Health. *Nutrition*, **30**: 619–627.

95. Guetouache M., Guessas B., Medjekal S. (2014). Composition and Nutritional Value of Raw Milk. *Issues Biol. Sci. Pharm. Res.*, **2**(10): 115–122.

96. Visioli F., Strata A. (2014). Milk, Dairy Products, and Their Functional Effects in Humans: A Narrative Review of Recent Evidence. *Adv. Nutr.*, **5**: 131–143.

97. Lee S.H.F., Zulkipli I.N., David S.R., Ahmad S.R., Ja'afar F., Lim Y.C., Rajabalaya R. (2018). A Review on Milk and Its Biological Effects on Human Health: Neurological Conditions, Cardiovascular Diseases and Cancer. *Int. J. Food Sci. Nutr.*, **3**(6): 84–89.

98. Park Y.W. (2009). Chapter 1. Overview of Bioactive Components in Milk and Dairy Products, pp. 3–12. In: *Bioactive Components in Milk and Dairy Products.* Editor: Young W. Park. Wiley-Blackwell, Hoboken, USA, 426 pages.

99. Pietrzak-Fiecko R., Anna M., Kamelska-Sadowska A.M. (2020). The Comparison of Nutritional Value of Human Milk with Other Mammals' Milk. *Nutrients*, **12**(1404), 18 pages.

100. Fardet A., Rock E. (2018). In Vitro and in Vivo Antioxidant Potential of Milks, Yoghurts, Fermented Milks and Cheeses: A Narrative Review of Evidence. *Nutr. Res. Rev.*, **31**(1): 52–70.

101. Thorning T.K., Raben A., Tholstrup T., Soedamah-Muthu S.S., Givens I., Astrup A. (2016). Milk and Dairy Products: Good or Bad for Human Health? An Assessment of the Totality of Scientific Evidence. *Food Nutr. Res.*, **60**(32527): 1–11.

102. Cormick G., Belizán J.M. (2019). Calcium Intake and Health. *Nutrients*, **11**(7): 1606, 16 pages.

103. Tunick M.H., Van Hekken D.L. (2015). Dairy Products and Health: Recent Insights. *J. Agric. Food Chem.*, **63**(43): 9381–9388.

104. Pellegrino L., Masotti F., Cattaneo S., Hogenboom J.A., de Noni I. (2013). Chapter 16. Nutritional Quality of Milk Proteins, pp. 515–538. In: *Advanced Dairy Chemistry Volume 1A: Proteins: Basic Aspects.* Editors: Paul L.H. McSweeney, Patrick F. Fox. 4th edition. Springer Science, Berlin, Germany.

105. Gómez-Gallego C., Gueimonde M., Salminen S. (2018). The Role of Yogurt in Food-Based Dietary Guidelines. *Nutrition Reviews*, **76** (Suppl. 1): 29–39.

106. Chandan R.C., Gandhi A., Shah N.P. (2017). Chapter 1. Yogurt: Historical Background, Health Benefits, and Global Trade, pp. 3–29. In: *Yogurt in Health and Disease Prevention.* Editor: Nagendra P. Shah. Academic Press, Elsevier, New York, USA, 542 pages.

107. Kwak H-S., Ganesan P., Hong Y-H. (2012). Chapter 14. Nutritional Benefits in Cheese, pp. 269–289. In: *Cheese: Types, Nutrition and Consumption.* Editor: Richard D. Foster. Nova Science Publishers, New York.

108. Walther B., Schmid A., Sieber R., Wehrmüller K. (2008). Cheese in Nutrition and Health. *Dairy Sci. Technol.* **88**: 389–405.

109. Macwan S.R., Dabhi B.K., Parmar S.C., Aparnathi K.D. (2016). Whey and Its Utilization. *Int. J. Curr. Microbiol. Appl. Sci.*, **5**(8): 134–155.

110. Alberts B., Johnson A., Lewis J., Raff M., Roberts K., Walter P. (2002). Eggs. In: *Molecular Biology of the Cell.* 4th edition. Garland Science, New York. www.ncbi.nlm.nih.gov/books/NBK26842/.

111. Belitz H-D., Grosch W., Schieberle P. (2009). Chapter 11. Eggs, pp. 546–561. In: *Food Chemistry.* Springer, Berlin, Heidelberg. https://doi.org/10.1007/978-3-540-69934-7_12.

112. Réhault-Godbert S., Guyot N., Nys Y. (2019). The Golden Egg: Nutritional Value, Bioactivities, and Emerging Benefits for Human Health. *Nutrients*, **11**(3): 684, 26 pages.

113. Griffin B.A. (2016). Eggs: Good or Bad? *Proc. Nutr. Soc.*, **75**(3): 259–264.
114. Nimalaratne C., Wu J. (2015). Hen Egg as an Antioxidant Food Commodity: A Review. *Nutrients*, **7**(10): 8274–8293.
115. Benedé S., Molina E. (2020). Chicken Egg Proteins and Derived Peptides with Antioxidant Properties. *Foods*, **9**(6): 735, 16 pages.
116. McNamara D.J. (2015). The Fifty Year Rehabilitation of the Egg. *Nutrients*, **7**(10): 8716–8722.
117. Blesso C.N. (2015). Egg Phospholipids and Cardiovascular Health. *Nutrients*, **7**(4): 2731–2747.
118. Spitzer H. (2016). An Analysis of Bacterial Contamination of Chicken Eggs and Antimicrobial Resistance. All College Thesis Program, 2016. https://digitalcommons.csbsju.edu/honors_thesis/27.
119. Magriplis E., Mitsopoulou A.V., Karageorgou D., Bakogianni I., Dimakopoulos I., Micha R., Michas G., Chourdakis M., Chrousos G.P., Roma E., Panagiotakos D., Zampelas A. (2019). Frequency and Quantity of Egg Intake Is Not Associated with Dyslipidemia: The Hellenic National Nutrition and Health Survey (HNNHS). *Nutrients*, **11**(5): 1105, 11 pages.
120. Fuller N.R., Sainsbury A., Caterson I.D., Markovic T.P. (2015). Egg Consumption and Human Cardio-Metabolic Health in People with and Without Diabetes. *Nutrients*, **7**(9): 7399–7420.
121. Mott M.M., McCrory M.A., Bandini L.G., Cabral H.J., Daniels S.R., Singer M.R., Moore L.L. (2019). Egg Intake Has No Adverse Association with Blood Lipids or Glucose in Adolescent Girls. *J. Am. Coll. Nutr.*, **38**(2): 119–124.
122. Shin J.Y., Xun P., Nakamura Y., He K. (2013). Egg Consumption in Relation to Risk of Cardiovascular Disease and Diabetes: A Systematic Review and Meta-Analysis. *Am. J. Clin. Nutr.*, **98**(1): 146–159.
123. Tran L.N., Barraj L.M., Heilman J.M., Scrafford C.G. (2014). Egg Consumption and Cardiovascular Disease Among Diabetic Individuals: A Systematic Review of the Literature. *Diabetes Metab. Syndr. Obes.*, **7**: 121–137.
124. Caubet J.C., Wang J. (2011). Current Understanding of Egg Allergy. *Pediatr. Clin. North Am.*, **58**(2): 427–443.
125. Sun C., Liu J., Yang N., Xu G. (2019). Egg Quality and Egg Albumen Property of Domestic Chicken, Duck, Goose, Turkey, Quail, and Pigeon. *Poult. Sci.*, **98**(10): 4516–4521.
126. Tolik D., Polawska E., Charuta A., Nowaczewski S., Cooper R. (2014). Characteristics of Egg Parts, Chemical Composition and Nutritive Value of Japanese Quail Eggs. A Review. *Folia Biologica (Kraków)*, **62**: 287–292.
127. Bledsoe G.E., Bledsoe C.D., Rasco B. (2003). Caviars and Fish Roe Products. *Crit. Rev. Food Sci. Nutr.*, **43**(3): 317–356.
128. Khan K.A., Ghramh H.A., Ahmad Z., El-Niweiri M.A.A., Mohammed M.E.A. (2021). Honey Bee (Apis Mellifera) Preference Towards Micronutrients and Their Impact on Bee Colonies. *Saudi J. Biol. Sci.*, **28**(6): 3362–3366.
129. Ediriweera E.R., Premarathna N.Y. (2012). Medicinal and Cosmetic Uses of Bee's Honey – A Review. *Ayu.*, **33**(2): 178–182.
130. Wakgari M., Yigezu G. (2021). Honeybee Keeping Constraints and Future Prospects. *Cogent Food Agric.*, **7**: 1872192, 31 pages.
131. Jaganathan S.K., Mandal M. (2009). Antiproliferative Effects of Honey and of Its Polyphenols: A Review. *J. Biomed. Biotechnol.*, Art. 830616, 13 pages.
132. Kunugi H., Mohammed Ali A. (2019). Royal Jelly and Its Components Promote Healthy Aging and Longevity: From Animal Models to Humans. *Int. J. Mol. Sci.*, **20**(19): 4662, 26 pages.
133. Samarghandian S., Farkhondeh T., Samini F. (2017). Honey and Health: A Review of Recent Clinical Research. *Pharmacognosy Res.*, **9**(2): 121–127.
134. Alvarez-Suarez J.M., Gasparrini M., Forbes-Hernández T.Y., Mazzoni L., Giampieri F. (2014). The Composition and Biological Activity of Honey: A Focus on Manuka Honey. *Foods*, **3**: 420–432.
135. Cianciosi D., Forbes-Hernández T.Y., Afrin S., Gasparrini M., Reboredo-Rodriguez P., Manna P.P., Zhang J., Bravo Lamas L., Martínez Flórez S., Agudo Toyos P., Quiles J.L., Giampieri F., Battino M. (2018). Phenolic Compounds in Honey and Their Associated Health Benefits: A Review. *Molecules*, **23**: 2322.
136. Ahmed S., Sulaiman S.A., Baig A.A., Ibrahim M., Liaqat S., Fatima S., Jabeen S., Shamim N., Othman N.H. (2018). Honey as a Potential Natural Antioxidant Medicine: An Insight into Its Molecular Mechanisms of Action. *Oxid. Med. Cell Longev.*, Art. 8367846, 19 pages.
137. Alvarez-Suarez J.M., Giampieri F., Battino M. (2013). Honey as a Source of Dietary Antioxidants: Structures, Bioavailability and Evidence of Protective Effects Against Human Chronic Diseases. *Curr. Med. Chem.*, **20**(5): 621–638.
138. Mandal M.D., Mandal S. (2011). Honey: Its Medicinal Property and Antibacterial Activity. *Asian Pac. J. Trop. Biomed.*, **1**(2): 154–160.

139. Kwakman P.H.S., Zaat S.A.J. (2012). Antibacterial Components of Honey. *Crit. Rev. IUBMB Life*, **64**(1): 48–55.

140. Erejuwa O.O., Sulaiman S.A., Wahab M.S. (2014). Effects of Honey and Its Mechanisms of Action on the Development and Progression of Cancer. *Molecules*, **19**(2): 2497–2522.

141. Ramadan M.F., Al-Ghamdi A. (2012). Bioactive Compounds and Health-Promoting Properties of Royal Jelly: A Review. *J. Func. Foods*, **4**: 39–52.

142. Bălan A., Moga M.A., Dima L., Toma S., Elena Neculau A., Anastasiu C.V. (2020). Royal Jelly-A Traditional and Natural Remedy for Postmenopausal Symptoms and Aging-Related Pathologies. *Molecules*, **25**(14): 3291, 22 pages.

143. Pasupuleti V.R., Sammugam L., Ramesh N., Gan S.H. (2017). Honey, Propolis, and Royal Jelly: A Comprehensive Review of Their Biological Actions and Health Benefits. *Oxid. Med. Cell. Longev.* **2017**: 1259510, 21 pages.

144. Kocot J., Kiełczykowska M., Luchowska-Kocot D., Kurzepa J., Musik I. (2018). Antioxidant Potential of Propolis, Bee Pollen, and Royal Jelly: Possible Medical Application. *Oxid. Med. Cell Longev.*, **2018**: 7074209.

145. Bonilla-Mendez J.R., Hoyos-Concha J.L. (2018). Methods of Extraction Refining and Concentration of Fish Oil as a Source of Omega-3 Fatty Acids. *Corpoica Cienc. Tecnol. Agropecu.*, **19**(3): 645–668.

146. Ivanovs K., Blumberga D. (2017). Extraction of Fish Oil Using Green Extraction Methods: A Short Review. *Energy Procedia*, **128**: 477–483.

147. Huang T.H., Wang P.W., Yang S.C., Chou W.L., Fang J.Y. (2018). Cosmetic and Therapeutic Applications of Fish Oil's Fatty Acids on the Skin. *Mar. Drugs*, **16**(8): 256, 20 pages.

148. Smutna M., Kruzikova K., Marsalek P., Kopriva V., Svobodova Z. (2009). Fish Oil and Cod Liver as Safe and Healthy Food Supplements. *Neuro Endocrinol. Lett.*, **30** (Suppl. 1): 156–162.

149. Griffing G.T. (2008). Mother Was Right About Cod Liver Oil. *Medscape J. Med.*, **10**(1): 8.

150. Ilievska B., Loftsson T., Hjalmarsdottir M.A., Asgrimsdottir G.M. (2016). Topical Formulation Comprising Fatty Acid Extract from Cod Liver Oil: Development, Evaluation and Stability Studies. *Mar. Drugs.*, **14**(6): 105, 11 pages.

151. Huang W.B., Fan Q., Zhang X.L. (2011). Cod Liver Oil: A Potential Protective Supplement for Human Glaucoma. *Intl. J. Ophthalmol.*, **4**(6): 648–651.

152. Gowda S.G.S., Narayan B., Gopal S. (2016). Bacteriological Properties and Health Related Biochemical Components of Fermented Fish Sauce: An Overview. *Food Rev. Int.*, **32**: 203–229.

153. Garcia Barcia L., Argiro J., Babcock E.A., Cai Y., Shea S.K.H., Chapman D.D. (2020). Mercury and Arsenic in Processed Fins from Nine of the Most Traded Shark Species in the Hong Kong and China Dried Seafood Markets: The Potential Health Risks of Shark Fin Soup. *Mar. Pollut. Bull.*, **157**: 111281.

154. Xie D., Gong M., Wei W., Jin J., Wang X., Wang X., Jin Q. (2019). Antarctic Krill (*Euphausia Superba*) Oil: A Comprehensive Review of Chemical Composition, Extraction Technologies, Health Benefits, and Current Applications. *Compr. Rev. Food Sci. Food Saf.*, **18**: 514–534.

155. Kwantes J., Grundmann O. (2014). A Brief Review of Krill Oil History, Research, and the Commercial Market. *J. Diet. Suppl.*, **12**. doi:10.3109/19390211.2014.902000.

156. Ulven S.M., Holven K.B. (2015). Comparison of Bioavailability of Krill Oil Versus Fish Oil and Health Effect. *Vasc. Health Risk Manag.*, **11**: 511–524.

157. Sung H.H., Sinclair A.J., Lewandowski P.A., Su X.Q. (2018). Postprandial n-3 PUFA Response to Krill Oil and Fish Oil Consumption in Healthy Women: A Randomised Controlled, Single-Dose, Crossover Study. *Asia Pac. J. Clin. Nutr.*, **27**(1): 148–157.

158. Kawtikwar P.S., Bhagwat D.A., Sakarkar D.M. (2010). Deer Antlers – Traditional Use and Future Perspectives. *Indian J. Tradit. Knowl.*, **9**: 245–251.

159. Sui Z., Zhang L., Huo Y., Zhang Y. (2014). Bioactive Components of Velvet Antlers and Their Pharmacological Properties. *J. Pharm. Biomed. Anal.*, **87**: 229–240.

160. Gilbey A., Perezgonzalez J.D. (2012). Health Benefits of Deer and Elk Velvet Antler Supplements: A Systematic Review of Randomised Controlled Studies. *N. Z. Med. J.*, **125**(1367): 80–86.

161. Chen J., Yang Y., Abbasi S., Hajinezhad D., Kontulainen S., Honaramooz A. (2015). The Effects of Elk Velvet Antler Dietary Supplementation on Physical Growth and Bone Development in Growing Rats. *Evid. Based Complement Alternat. Med.*, **2015**: 819520, 10 pages.

162. Wong R.S. (2013). Edible Bird's Nest: Food or Medicine? *Chin. J. Integr. Med.*, **19**(9): 643–649.

163. Chua L.S., Zukefli S.N. (2016). A Comprehensive Review on Edible Bird Nests and Swiftlet Farming. *J. Integr. Med.*, **14**(6): 415–428.

164. Babji A.S., Nurfatin M.H., Etty Syarmila I.K., Masitah M. (2015). Secrets of Edible Bird Nest. Edible Bird Nest Is the Most Highly Priced Agricultural Product of South-East Asia. What Is Edible Bird Nest Really? *Utar Agr. Sci. J.*, **1**(1): 32–37.

165. Daud N., Yusop S., Babji A., Lim S.J., Sarbini S., Yan T. (2019). Edible Bird's Nest: Physicochemical Properties, Production, and Application of Bioactive Extracts and Glycopeptides. *Food Rev. Int.*: 1–20.

166. Lee T.H., Wani W.A., Koay Y.S., Kavita S., Tan E.T.T., Shreaz S. (2017). Recent Advances in the Identification and Authentication Methods of Edible Bird's Nest. *Food Res. Int.*, **100**(Pt 1): 14–27.

167. Soumya M., Harinatha Reddy A., Nageswari G., Venkatappa B. (2017). Silkworm (Bombyx Mori) and Its Constituents: A Fascinating Insect in Science and Research. *J. Entomol. Zool. Stud.*, **5**(5): 1701–1705.

168. Singh K.P., Jayasomu R.S. (2002). Bombyx Mori – A Review of Its Potential as a Medicinal Insect. *Pharm. Biol.*, **40**(1): 28–32.

169. Costa-Neto E.M. (2005). Animal-Based Medicines: Biological Prospection and the Sustainable Use of Zoo-Therapeutic Resources. *An. Acad. Bras. Ciênc. (Annals of the Brazilian Academy of Sciences)*, **77**(1): 33–43.

170. Bozoghlanian V., Butteri M. (2015). The Diverse and Promising World of Animal Derived Medications. *Pharos Alpha Omega Alpha Honor Med. Soc.*, **78**(1): 16–22. http://alphaomegaalpha.org/pharos/PDFs/2015-1-Bozoghlanian-Butteri.pdf.

171. Queensland Health, Australia. (2013). Guideline for the Use of Medicines and Pharmaceuticals of Animal Origin. Document n° QH-GDL-954: 2013. www.health.qld.gov.au/__data/assets/pdf_file/0024/147507/qh-gdl-954.pdf.

172. Duffy C., Sorolla A., Wang E., Golden E., Woodward E., Davern K., Ho D., Johnstone E., Pfleger K., Redfern A., Iyer K.S., Baer B., Blancafort P. (2020). Honeybee Venom and Melittin Suppress Growth Factor Receptor Activation in HER2-Enriched and Triple-Negative Breast Cancer. *NPJ Precis. Onc.*, **4**: 24.

173. Norez C., Vandebrouck C., Bertrand J., Noel S., Durieu E., Oumata N., Galons H., Antigny F., Chatelier A., Bois P., Meijer L., Becq F. (2014). Roscovitine Is a Proteostasis Regulator That Corrects the Trafficking Defect of F508del-CFTR by a CDK-independent Mechanism. *Br. J. Pharmacol.*, **171**(21): 4831–4849.

174. Abdualkader A.M., Ghawi A.M., Alaama M., Awang M., Merzouk A. (2013). Leech Therapeutic Applications. *Indian J. Pharm. Sci.*, **75**(2): 127–137.

175. Alves R.R.N., Alves R.N. (2011). The Faunal Drugstore: Animal-Based Remedies Used in Traditional Medicines in Latin America. *J. Ethnobiol. Ethnomed.*, **7**(9): 1–43.

176. Cooper E.L., Balamurugan M., Huang C-Y., Tsao C.R., Heredia J., Tommaseo-Ponzetta M., Paoletti M.G. (2012). Earthworms Dilong: Ancient, Inexpensive, Noncontroversial Models May Help Clarify Approaches to Integrated Medicine Emphasizing Neuroimmune Systems. *Evid. Based Complement. Alternat. Med.*, Article ID 164152, 11 pages.

177. Grdisa M., Grsic K., Grdisa M.D. (2013). Earthworms – Role in Soil Fertility to the Use in Medicine and as a Food. *Invertebrate Surviv. J.*, **10**: 38–45.

178. Sun Z. (2015). Earthworm as a Biopharmaceutical: From Traditional to Precise. *Eur. J. BioMed. Res.*, **1**(2): 28–35.

179. Galvis C.E.P., Mendez L.Y.V., Kouznetsov V.V. (2013). Cantharidin-Based Small Molecules as Potential Therapeutic Agents. *Chem. Biol. Drug Des.*, **82**: 477–499.

180. Zhang Q-Y., Yue X-Q., Jiang Y-P., Han T., Xin H-L. (2017). FAM46C Is Critical for the Anti-Proliferation and Pro-Apoptotic Effects of Nor-Cantharidin in Hepatocellular Carcinoma Cells. *Sci. Rep.*, **7**, Article number: 396: 1–10.

181. Hsieh C-H., Clifford Chao K.S., Liao H-F., Chen Y-J. (2013). Norcantharidin, Derivative of Cantharidin, for Cancer Stem Cells. *Review. Evid. Based Complement. Alternat. Med.*, Article ID 838651, 11 pages.

182. Massicot F., Dutertre-Catella H., Pham-Huy C., Liu X-H., Duc H.T., Warnet J-M. (2005). *In Vitro* Assessment of Renal Toxicity and Inflammatory Events of Two Protein Phosphatase Inhibitors Cantharidin and Nor-Cantharidin. *Basic Clin. Pharmacol. Toxicol.*, **96**: 26–32.

7 Fungi and Water

1 FUNGI

1.1 Fungi Description

Fungi including mushrooms, molds, and yeasts are eukaryotic organisms as vegetable or animal species, but are classified as a separate kingdom because fungal cell walls contain rigid chitin and glucans that are not found in animal, vegetal, or bacterial species (1–8). Eukaryotic cells are cells that contain a nucleus and other organelles enclosed within membranes. In other words, the fungal kingdom comprises a hyper diverse clade of heterotrophic eukaryotes characterized by the presence of a chitinous cell wall, the loss of phagotrophic capabilities, and cell organizations that range from completely unicellular monopolar organisms to highly complex syncytial filaments (containing several nuclei) that may form macroscopic structures (8). Mushrooms like morels, button mushroom, and puffballs are macroscopic multicellular fungi, while molds are a large group of microscopic multicellular fungi. Molds are characterized by filamentous forms named hyphae. Many fungi occur not as hyphae but as unicellular forms called yeasts, which are invisible to the naked eye and reproduce by budding (2–4).

Feeding usually occurs through the mycelia. Fungi feed on dead and living materials of plants and animals for their growth. For the mode of nutrition, fungi are either saprophytes, parasites, or symbiotics (3–5). When they obtain their foods (energy) from nonliving organic substrates such as dead and decaying matters, in this case, they are called saprophytes. When they obtain their foods from living organic material by absorption of nutrients through their cell wall, they are named parasites. When they grow in association with other living organisms like plants or animals, they are called symbionts (3–5). Fungi are essentially aerobic organisms. Many fungi are also associated with trees symbiotically because they are linked with the tree roots, an association benefiting both the fungi and the trees. This particular type of association between fungi and the roots of plants is known as a mycorrhiza (2–3). Some fungi have very specific associations and will grow only with one kind of tree; for example, the bolete grows only under alders. Other fungi may be found in association with several different trees (2–4). Chanterelles, for example can be found linked with birch, pine, oak, and beech trees. Fungi together with bacteria are ecologically important decomposers for the process of decay (3). They are essential for nutrient recycling by transforming dead materials like dead plants or animals in the soil into a form of fertilizer. Without fungi and bacteria, the world would be very dirty and uninhabitable.

The mode of reproduction of fungi is characterized by the formation of spores, and can be either asexual or sexual (2). However, yeasts cannot produce spores – they reproduce by budding. Asexual methods include fragmentation, somatic budding, or fission. Most yeasts reproduce asexually by mitosis, and many do so by the asymmetric division process known as budding (2). Reproductive sexual methods include gametic copulation, gametangium copulation, somatic copulation, gamate-gametangium copulation, and spermatization (4).

The spores of fungi have the same role as the seeds of plants. Each spore can give birth to a fungus. An ordinary mushroom can release millions of spores from the gills under the mushroom cap into the air.

There are about 200,000 fungus species found worldwide, among 1–1.5 million estimated species (4, 9). They are one of the most important groups of organisms on this planet. The kingdom Fungi is divided into four major phyla or divisions: Chytridiomycota, Zygomycota, Ascomycota,

DOI: 10.1201/9781003220817-7

and Basidiomycota (1, 4–8). The two fungal phyla that produce large, visible fruit bodies are the Ascomycota and Basidiomycota. The Ascomycota contains at least 40,000 different species worldwide, including morels and truffles, cup fungi, and most of the lichens, as well as microscopic molds and yeasts (10). The group Basidiomycota, also known as basidiomycetes, contains from 30,000 to 35,000 different species and includes many familiar fungi, including edible and poisonous mushrooms, bracket fungi, chanterelles, and so on (10). Lichens are not fungi but arise from algae or cyanobacteria and live in common with some fungi.

Fungi have cell walls similar to plants and are different from animals. The fungal cell wall is composed of chitin that gives shape, form, and rigidity to fungi. It protects against mechanical injury, prevents osmotic lysis, and provides passive protection against the ingress of potentially harmful macromolecules (2–3). Chitin is a polymer of N-acetyl-D-glucosamine. The major polysaccharides of the cell wall matrix consist of non-cellulosic glucans such as glycogen-like compounds, mannans (polymers of mannose), chitosan (polymers of glucosamine), and galactans (polymers of galactose). Small amounts of fucose, rhamnose, xylose, and uronic acids may be present (2). Glucan refers to a large group of D-glucose polymers having glycosidic bonds. Insoluble β-glucans are apparently amorphous in the cell wall. Yeast cell wall is composed of three layers and is about 200- to 600-nm thick. Its inner surface is chitinous, and its outer layer contains α-glucan (2). In addition to chitin, glucan, and mannan, cell walls may contain lipid, protein, chitosan, acid phosphatase, α-amylase, protease, melanin, and inorganic ions such as phosphorus, calcium, and magnesium (2). The fungal wall also protects cells against mechanical injury and blocks the ingress of toxic macromolecules. The fungal cell wall is also essential to prevent osmotic lysis. Even a small lesion in the cell wall can result in extrusion of cytoplasm due to the internal (turgor) pressure of the protoplast. The cell membrane of a fungus has a unique sterol and ergosterol (3).

Yeasts and mushrooms are the third source of foods and medicines for humans after plants and animals, while molds are the source of many drugs and antibiotics. Some fungi or their extracts are used as drugs in traditional and modern medicines. Some chemicals have pharmacological and therapeutic effects, such as penicillin, ciclosporins, and statins, which have saved millions of humans since being discovered during the twentieth century. Recently, plectasin, an antibiotic isolated from the saprophytic fungus *Pseudoplectania nigrella*, was especially active against *Streptococcus pneumoniae*, including strains resistant to conventional antibiotics (11). PSK or Polysaccharide-Krestin, an anticancer drug isolated from *Trametes (Coriolus) versicolor* mushroom; lentinan, a polysaccharide obtained from shiitake mushroom; and lovastatin, or monacolin K, an anti-cholesterol drug, isolated from the red yeast rice (RYR), are some examples of drugs recently isolated from diverse fungi (10–13). However, some mushrooms such as dead cap (*Amanita phalloides*) or fly agaric (*Amanita muscaria*) are very toxic and deathly. More than 100 fungi such as *Candida albicans, Pneumocystis, Aspergillus, Blastomyces,* and *Coccidioides* are responsible for human infection (4, 14). Fungi must meet four criteria to infect humans: growth at human body temperatures, circumvention or penetration of surface barriers, lysis and absorption of tissue, and resistance to immune defenses, including elevated body temperatures (14). Nevertheless, the potent human immune system evolved in interaction with potential fungal pathogens, so few fungi meet all four conditions for a healthy human host. Paradoxically, the advances of modern medicine have made millions of people newly susceptible to fungal infections by disrupting immune defenses (14).

Fungi are an important source of proteins, polysaccharides (β-glucans), ergosterol, amino acids, enzymes, and other nutrients. Mycoprotein has some advantages over protein from animal or milk origin; it has a high-protein but low-fat content, and this fat is cholesterol-free. Fungi have different sterols from those of animals and have also high levels of dietary fiber and a low degree of allergenicity (12). β-glucans are immunomodulators for the prevention of cancer and infection. Ergosterol is a precursor of vitamin D2. Under the action of UV or sunlight, ergosterol is transformed into vitamin D2, an analog of vitamin D3 in humans. However, fungi are not rich in energy. Many yeasts and molds have been used to elaborate fermented foods (rice alcohol, wine, beer, cheese, yogurt, etc.) throughout the world since ancient times.

1.2 MUSHROOMS

Mushrooms are macro-fungi with diverse sizes depending on their varieties. A classical mushroom has a stem (or stipe), a cap (pileus), and gills (lamellae, sing) on the underside of the cap. These three parts form the fruiting body which can be either epigeous (above ground) or hypogeous (below ground) and large enough to be seen with naked eye and to be picked by hand (5, 10, 13–16). The gills, formed by hundreds of thin folds, produce microscopic spores that spread across the ground for the development of new mushrooms. There are two types of mushrooms: edible mushrooms and inedible or poisonous mushrooms. Edible mushrooms are an important natural source of food and medicine for humans since antiquity. They are also consumed for their specific aroma and texture (13–15). Edible mushrooms are either collected from nature or more commonly cultivated and harvested under defined conditions with rigorous quality control on size, shape, tenderness, and palatability (10). In general, all species of mushrooms take several days to form primordial fruiting bodies. Mushroom picking generally takes place in autumn because mushrooms prefer this season to develop.

From a taxonomic point of view, mainly basidiomycetes but also some species of ascomycetes belong to mushrooms. The basidiomycetes contain mushrooms, bracket fungi and boletes; the ascomycetes include truffles and morels (5, 13–16). Mushrooms generally belong to basidiomycetes, which harbors numerous mushroom species with a diversity of metabolites of nutraceutical and therapeutic significance (10). Mushrooms constitute at least 14,000 and perhaps as many as 22,000 known species (16–18). The number of mushroom species on the earth is estimated to be around 140,000, suggesting that only 10% are known (16). Assuming that the proportion of useful mushrooms among the undiscovered and unexamined mushrooms will be only 5%, this still implies 7,000 yet undiscovered species that will be of possible benefit to humankind (16). Even among known species the proportion of well-investigated mushrooms is very low.

1.2.1 Edible Mushrooms

Edible fungi include wild and cultivated mushrooms. Wild edible mushrooms are mushrooms naturally living in the wild such as forests, woods, or meadows, and are collected by professionals who can distinguish edible versus inedible or poisonous mushrooms. Wild edible fungi have been hunted and consumed by people for thousands of years. The archaeological record reveals edible species associated with people living 13,000 years ago in Chile, but it is in China where the eating of wild fungi is first reliably noted, about 2,500 years ago (5). Wild edible mushrooms are often researched for their nutritional value and their specific taste and aroma. They are also occasionally taken for their medicinal value and are known as medicinal mushrooms. Some edible mushrooms commonly harvested from the wild are: truffles, bolete, chanterelles, matsutake (pine mushroom), maitake, blewit, saffron milk cap, and more (10, 14). Some wild edible mushrooms like truffle and matsutake are very costly due to their specific taste, aroma and nutrients, and their rarity in nature (10, 14).

Mushrooms that grow under professional care are called cultivated mushrooms. They are commonly cultivated and harvested under defined conditions with rigorous quality control by a professional or industry. Almost all edible cultivated mushrooms sold in the market are grown indoors under controlled conditions. There are nearly a hundred species of fungi that can be cultivated (5). All are saprobic: they feed on dead or decaying organic matter. Some of the best-known cultivated mushrooms for culinary uses are white button mushroom (*Agaricus bisporus*), shiitake (*Lentinula edodes*), oyster (Pleurotus spp.), morel, black trumpets, and wood ear (5, 10, 14).

Wild edible and cultivated mushrooms are consumed as a delicacy, and particularly for their specific aroma and texture. Besides being culinary delicacies, edible mushrooms are also known for their nutritional and medicinal values, which have been supported by numerous recent studies (10). Some mushrooms, such as shiitake, reishi, maitake, Auricula judas, cordyceps, and *Trametes (Coriolus) versicolor* mushroom, have medicinal actions such as immunomodulator or anticancer properties (13, 15–17). They are mostly used in traditional medicine as well as in recent research.

Concerning nutrition values, polysaccharides such as β-glucans and glycoproteins or polysaccharide-protein complexes are the two main constituents of wild or cultivated mushrooms, while the lipid content is low (5, 10, 13, 15–20). Chitin, glycogen, β-glucans, mannitol, and trehalose are typical carbohydrate constituents. Mushroom fruiting bodies, in general, on a dry weight basis, contain about 55% carbohydrate, 32% protein, and 2% fat, and the rest is minerals (10). They contain all essential amino acids for humans, including lysine, valine, leucine, and methionine whose levels are nutritionally favorable. Their nitrogen content may vary between 15–40% of dry weights, while, mushrooms contain more than 90% water and a very low quantity of fat and soluble sugars (10, 13, 15). Mushrooms are a rich source of ergocalciferol (vitamin D2), water-soluble vitamins of group B (riboflavin or B2, niacin or B3, pantothenic acid or B5), and minerals (selenium, copper, phosphorus, zinc, magnesium, potassium, calcium). The vitamin D2 content of a mushroom depends on its exposure to sunlight. When exposed to sunlight or UVB light, even after harvesting, ergosterol (a provitamin D) in mushrooms is converted to vitamin D2 which is essential for the absorption of calcium (5, 10, 13, 15–20). However, the contents of omega-3 fatty acid, vitamin C, and sodium are negligible (10, 15). In addition, fibers are also present in this food. Fiber helps to lower cholesterol and is important for the digestive system. Mushrooms are very low in calories and fat, are cholesterol-free, and may be helpful to obese and hyperlipidemic people (10).

Polysaccharides and their beta-glucans are the best known and most potent mushroom derived substances with immunomodulator, antitumor, and anti-inflammatory properties (10, 15–21). Beta-D-glucans are a type of polysaccharide of D-glucose monomers linked through beta-glycosidic bonds. They are viscous, soluble dietary fiber, and abundantly found in the cell walls of mushrooms, yeasts, and cereals (mainly oat and barley) (see Chapter 1 of this book). Beta-glucans in mushrooms and yeasts have immunomodulator and anti-cancer properties, while those in cereals (oat and barley) have anti-hypercholesterolemia and anti-diabetes actions. Diverse structures of beta-glucans can proceed from different sources. For instance, β-glucan obtained from mushrooms and yeasts consists of β-(1,3) and (1,6) linkages, while β-glucans present in cereals (oat and barley), are polysaccharides of glucose residues with β-(1,3) and β-(1,4) linkages (21–23). Yeast β-glucans have β (1, 6) branches that are further intricate with additional β (1, 3) regions. These diversities in beta-glucan structures are why they have different therapeutic functions (21–23). High molecular weight glucans appear to be more effective than those of low molecular weight (10). The extraction of β-glucans from oat and barley is difficult, therefore, the β-glucan supplements present in the market is obtained from baker's yeast *Saccharomyces cerevisiae*. Therefore, for the prevention of hypercholesterolemia and diabetes, it is superior to consume oat and barley food, rather than β-glucan dietary supplements. Some β-glucans isolated from specific mushrooms and used as anticancer drugs are lentinan, a polysaccharide obtained from shiitake mushroom, and PSK, or Polysaccharide-Krestin, an anticancer drug isolated from *Trametes (Coriolus) versicolor* mushroom. Polysaccharides of some other medicinal mushroom species also show good results (13, 16, 17).

Many studies show that mushrooms possess various bioactivities, such as antioxidant, anti-inflammatory, anticancer, immunomodulatory, antimicrobial, hepatoprotective, and antidiabetic properties; therefore, mushrooms have attracted increasing attention in recent years, and could be developed into functional food or medicines for the prevention and treatment of several chronic diseases, such as cardiovascular diseases, cancer, diabetes mellitus, and neurodegenerative diseases (18–20). The low energy content of mushrooms, in concert with high proportions of indigestible fiber, specific β-glucans, and antioxidative and flavor constituents, provoke increasing interest of both researchers and consumers in recent years (15). However, mushrooms are not staple foods because they are not rich in energy (10).

Avoid eating raw and old mushrooms because of the potential presence of some toxins, parasites, and microbes, which are destroyed by cooking. In addition, the cell wall of mushrooms is rigid due to the presence of chitin, which is not broken by the human digestive system, but only by heating. Cooking will break down the fungal cell wall and release its nutrients into the food preparation, making it digestible and healthy. Excessive intake of mushrooms such as white buttons mushrooms can cause indigestion, flatulence, digestive troubles, and so on.

In brief, mushrooms are considered a source of nutraceuticals in nutrient balancing. They may strengthen the human immune system, enhance the body's natural resistance, and prevent some diseases. Some common edible mushrooms the most widely consumed and/or used as medicines are cited as follows.

1.2.1.1 Wild Edible Mushrooms

Some wild mushrooms frequently consumed are: truffle, matsutake (pine mushroom), morel, chanterelles, bolete, and maitake (13, 15). Truffle and matsutake are precious wild mushrooms because of their specific taste, aroma, and nutrients, and their rarity in nature.

1.2.1.1.1 Truffle Amongst all the edible mushrooms, wild edible truffles have been regarded worldwide as a great delicacy because of their unique flavor and high nutritional value. Therefore, truffles are taken as type of precious food and, amongst all other mushrooms, are the world's most expensive mushrooms (24–26). Truffles are hypogeous ascomycetes fungi growing underground in a depth between five and ten cm. Taxonomically, edible truffles belong to the genus Tuber (family Tuberaceae and Pezizaceae), and to the order Pezizales. In general, truffles have no stalk, no gills, with firm, dense, and woody features, and mycelium that grows underground (24, 26). Truffles are ectomycorrhizal, having symbiotic root association. Truffles establish a symbiotic interaction with host organisms, predominantly with the roots of various trees, both gymnosperms and angiosperms, such as hazel, poplar, pine, eucalyptus, and oak (24). For example, the black truffle in the Périgord region (France) grows in close association with the roots of oak trees (25). Because truffles produce their sexual fruiting bodies underground, the dispersal of their spores relies on insects and mammals. As truffles grow underground, their forage is mainly realized by specialists in autumn with the aid of special pigs or dogs.

More than 100 different kinds of wild truffle species are known worldwide, and new species are being discovered consistently (24–25). Not all truffles are edible but those of genus Tuber serve as a food source. Most culinary-grade truffles found in northern temperate forests of Europe, Australia, New Zealand, Asia, and North America generally belong to genus Tuber (24). On the other hand, desert truffles growing in arid and semi-arid regions such as Syria, Iraq, Kuwait, Saudi Arabia, Morocco, Egypt, South Africa, and Tunisia generally belong to the genus Terfezia and Tirmania (24). Among the edible truffles, black and white truffles are the most highly prized in French, Spanish, northern Italian, and Greek cuisines (24). Each kilogram of truffles varies between 600–6,000 €, depending on species (25). White truffles include *Tuber magnatum*, *T. borchii*, *T. maculatum*, *T. oregonense*, *T. latisporum*, *T. japonicum*, and *Tirmania nivea*. Among them, *T. magnatum*, generally found in Italy and eastern Europe, is the highest cost truffle species. Black truffles include *Tuber melanosporum*, *T. aestivum*, *T. brumale*, *T. uncinatum*, *T. indicum*, *T. himalayense*, and *Terfezia claveryi* (24–25). Terfezia and Tirmania are also called desert truffles, as these fungi are found in the arid and semi-arid areas of the Mediterranean (25).

Concerning the nutritional profiles of truffles, scientists found that they varied from species to species. Two main components present in truffles are aroma and nutritive chemicals. Truffles are appreciated worldwide as valuable foodstuffs due to their distinctive flavor. The aroma of truffles can range from mild to intense and can vary from garlicky, pungent, vanilla-like, creamy, musky, earthy, to dusty. Among hundreds of active aroma compounds in truffles, 2-methylbutanal, 3-methylbutanal, dimethyl disulphide (DMDS), and dimethyl sulphide (DMS) are the most common natural aroma compounds (24–25). Apart from being aromatic, the biochemical composition of truffles encompasses multiple nutritional and medicinal benefits. Truffles are rich in various types of essential nutrients including carbohydrates, proteins, fats, minerals, lipids, and amino acids. In addition, they are rich in phenolics, terpenoids, polysaccharides, and phytosterols, which are related to their antitumor, antioxidant, antibacterial, hepatoprotective, anti-inflammatory, and immunomodulatory properties (24–25). Truffles also contain different minerals including silicon, potassium, calcium, magnesium, manganese, sodium, iron, phosphate, sulfur, copper, zinc, and aluminum (25–26).

In summary, truffles are valuable foods due to their special aromatic flavors that lend to various dishes and confectioneries, though scientific investigations into their nutritional and varied biological activities are still very limited. Although different truffle species have been shown to have similar nutritional properties, such as being high in protein, it must be noted that truffles are not a major contributor to the human diet (25). Some truffle species are still a puzzle to scientists as their chemical and biological functions have not been thoroughly investigated. Besides their special aromatic properties, the potential therapeutic activities of truffles have not been determined and accepted by the medical community (25).

1.2.1.1.2 Matsutake Matsutake or pine mushroom (matsu = pine, take = mushroom) is a Japanese common name for the edible ectomycorrhizal mushroom *Tricholoma matsutake*, living in symbiosis exclusively with the root of some pine trees in Japan (27–29). *Tricholoma matsutake*, a genus of Basidiomycete fungi belonging to the order Agaricales, family Tricholomataceae, is a white to brownish wild edible mushroom with a broad stem and an umbrella cap 2 to 8 inches in size (5–20 cm). It grows in many parts of Asia (Japan, China, North Korea, South Korea, Russia, and Bhutan), Europe (Turkey, Sweden, Finland, Norway, Germany, Czechoslovakia, Austria, Switzerland, and Italy), and North Africa (Algeria and Morocco) (27–28). Wild matsutake is a traditional delicacy in Japan. Matsutake has become one of the most widely known edible mycorrhizal mushrooms in the world. This is due to its unique flavor, high commercial value, and wide natural distribution (28). The characteristic aroma of a freshly picked, unopened matsutake fruitbody can be preserved not more than three days under optimal conditions during transport (29). In spite of vast research, the cultivation of matsutake has been mostly unsuccessful. Commercial demand is therefore met by harvesting the fruiting bodies that naturally occur during autumn in forests of coniferous trees, mainly *Pinus densiflora* (27). After truffles, matsutake are one of the most expensive wild edible mushrooms in the world. Matsutakes harvested in Japan are pricier than those found in other countries (China, Canada, the United States, Scandinavia).

Tricholoma matsutake has two kinds of chemical compounds: volatile compounds and fixed compounds. The main volatile compounds in *T. matsutake* fruiting bodies are (E)-2-octenal, phenylacetaldehyde, 3-octanone, methyl cinnamate, benzaldehyde, and 1-octen-3-ol (30). Kinds and levels of volatile compounds from different geographical areas vary. Volatile compounds, chemical compositions, and nutritional values of *T. matsutake* vary with age and geographical origin and can serve as chemical indicators for classification of *T. matsutake* from different geographical areas and at different stages of maturity (30). Concerning fixed compounds of *T. matsutake*, the dominant compounds are proteins, fibers, amino acids, and carbohydrates. The fat content is low, with a predominance of oleic and linoleic acids (31). The mushroom is especially rich in glutamic acid, alanine, aspartic, and leucine (30–31). *T. matsutake* has good amounts of minerals, especially potassium. In addition, many bioactive molecules have been isolated from *T. matsutake* such as nuclease, polysaccharide, laccase, and α-galactosidase (32). These substances with diverse biological activities are beneficial to human health and are useful in the environment (31–32). Some preliminary research found that *T. matsutake* had some biological effects such as anti-hypertension, anti-microorganism, anti-tumor, and immunostimulant (32–33). In brief, *T. matsutake* is a delicious edible mushroom rich in some nutrients with some potentially beneficial health effects.

1.2.1.1.3 Chanterelle (Cantharellus Cibarius) The chanterelle *Cantharellus cibarius* is the most well-known species of the genus Cantharellus (family Cantharellaceae, division Basidiomycota). It is a yellow or orange and funnel-shaped ectomycorrhizal mushroom that grows at different altitudes, with different kinds of trees, in hardwood forests throughout Europe. Chanterelle lives in symbiosis with pine, oak, hornbeam, and spruce (34–36). It is a wild edible mushroom and cannot be cultivated without its host (36). It is known as the Girolle in France, Capo gallo in Italy, Yumurta mantari in Turkey, and simply as Chanterelle or Golden chanterelle in Britain. Chanterelle is also found in North America, Asia, Mexico, and Africa. Chanterelle is harvested from summer to fall in Europe (34–36).

In cookery, *Cantharellus cibarius* is widely consumed due to its aroma, taste, firmness, and crunchiness of its fruiting bodies. It is highly appreciated for its wonderful fruity, apricot-like aroma, being particularly prized for cooking throughout Europe. It can be used to make tasty soups, omelets, risotto dishes, or sauces to be served with chicken or fish. Chanterelle mushrooms are widely consumed in western Europe, Asia, and Central America (34–36).

Concerning nutrients, chanterelle contains a great number of carbohydrates and proteins and a low amount of fat and fatty acids. It also rich in vitamins (B1, B2, B5, B6, C) – especially vitamin D2 (ergocalciferol) – as well as minerals (34–36). Besides, chanterelle is also a source of phytochemicals and antioxidants such as indole, in addition to phenolic compounds, fatty acids, amino acids, carotenoids, and enzymes. Due to the presence of these compounds, chanterelle may have immunomodulatory, anti-inflammatory, antioxidant, antiviral, antimicrobial, and antigenotoxic properties (34–36). However, scientists have suggested that chanterelle may possess potent insecticidal properties that are harmless to humans and yet protect the mushroom body against insects and other potentially harmful organisms (34). Concerning toxic metallic elements (mercury, lead, cadmium, silver) among mineral constituents, their contents found are much below the tolerance limits (37). However, the presence of toxic metals in *C. cibarius* depends on the collection site. For example, toxic metals such as arsenic, lead, barium, chromium, lithium, rubidium, and strontium were found at higher values in chanterelle from polymetallic soils of Yunnan in China, while lower values were measured in fruiting bodies from Poland (38). In brief, chanterelle is a delicious wild mushroom with a specific aroma for culinary purposes. It contains some significant and interesting nutrients for human health. Its medicinal values are not yet recognized for therapeutic uses.

1.2.1.1.4 Morels Morels are edible mushrooms of the genus Morchella, in the order Pezizales, division Ascomycota. Morels have a cone-shape cap that forms a honeycomb appearance. They are also called sponge mushrooms. Due to difficulties in cultivation, morels are harvested in the wild, mainly in temperate regions of the Northern hemisphere such as China, the Himalaya, India, Turkey, Mexico, and the United States, where they typically fruit for only a few weeks each spring (39–41). Their various habitats include hardwood and coniferous trees, roads and road cuts, excavation, lightly burned grassy areas, and swampy ground; though its favorite habitat is in areas destroyed by fire (39–41). Morels can form ectomycorrhiza or saprophytic relationships with deciduous or coniferous trees in temperate regions (40–41). Outdoor cultivation is currently very limited, and only three cases of its domestication have been reported in Israel, the United States, and China (39, 41). Therefore, all fresh or dry morels sold in the market are of wild origin. Morel fruiting bodies differ in shape, color, taste, edibility, chemical composition, and bioactivity (39). Though Morchella as a genus is fairly easy to recognize, species differentiation within genus is markedly difficult, and more than 25 varieties of them are identified today with Latin binomials (39–41). Based on gross morphology, the species of Morchella were initially placed into three groups: black or smoked morels, yellow morels, and semi-free capped morels or white morels (41). Some well-known black morels are *Morchella conica*, *M. angusticeps*, *M. elata*, and *M. vulgaris*; while yellow morels include *Morchella esculenta*, *M. crassipes*, and *M. deliciosa*; and white morels are *M. analotica* and *M. rufobrunnea*. The yellow morel *Morchella esculenta* and the black morel *M. conica* are the most studied species in regard to nutritional and phytochemical composition, due to their wide consumption (39).

Due to their desirable flavor and short fruiting season, morels have become the world's most prized edible fungi. Fresh or dried morels are highly appreciated worldwide among gastronomists for their rich unique aroma, noticeable umami taste, delicate flavor, and meaty texture

(39–41). Morels are cooked with vegetables and are considered as significant as meat and fish in Tibet and India (39).

Morel's health benefits are attributed mainly to polysaccharides as the active compounds, and to various phytochemicals, mainly phenolic compounds, tocopherols, ascorbic acid, and vitamin D. Its nutritional composition includes sugar, amino acid, fatty and organic acid, and mineral profile (39). *Morchella esculenta*, the most consumed morel, is highly nutritious, delicious, and healthy. It is rich in protein, polysaccharides, carbohydrates, and vitamins, particularly vitamins B, C, D, and A. It also contains minerals and possesses low calories, fats, and cholesterol. *Morchella esculenta* also contains minerals (magnesium, calcium, iron, zinc, copper, potassium, sodium, phosphorus, manganese), and a variety of aromatic compounds including phenols, alcohols, aldehydes, acids, ketones, terpenes, esters, and carbamic acid (40).

Morels have been in use in traditional medicine for centuries, due to their health-related benefits, and current research has demonstrated their antioxidative and anti-inflammatory bioactivities, in addition to immunostimulatory and anti-tumor properties (39). *M. esculenta* extract was found to be active against *Escherichia coli*, *Bacillus mesentericus*, and *Bacillus subtilis*. Polysaccharide from *M. esculenta* have strong antibacterial and anti-actinomycete powers (40). The galactomannan polysaccharide isolated from *M. esculenta* demonstrated immunostimulatory activity (40). However, *M. esculenta* and some other morel species can be poisonous if eaten raw, producing many adverse reactions (39–40). Some of the edible morel species contain toxic substances which might cause fatigue, dizziness, difficulty breathing, some neurologic effects such as ataxia and visual disturbances, and even ultimate death, if excessively consumed (39–40). To avoid these side effects, morel mushrooms as well as other edible mushrooms should never be eaten raw; they must be well-cooked before consumption.

In brief, wild edible morel mushrooms are delicious foods, rich in nutrients, with potential health benefits. To avoid some adverse reactions due to consumption of morels, these mushrooms must be well-cooked before use.

1.2.1.1.5 Bolete or Porcini Mushroom The bolete or porcini mushroom (*Boletus edulis*) is the most well-known species among at least 25 species of the genus Boletus (family Boletaceae, division Basidiomycota). It is a wild edible mycorrhyzal fungus that grows in association with a wide variety of trees, including both conifers and broad-leaved species (42–46). Bolete is a macro-fungus with large brown cap which can grow up to 14 inches (35 cm) in diameter and 6.6 pounds (3 kg) in weight, and produces fruiting bodies from the soil in summer and autumn. It exists in the market as fresh or dried form. The last one is the most consumed worldwide. Bolete occurs in temperate zone forests throughout the northern hemisphere (North America, Europe, Near East, Afghanistan, China, etc.) (42–46).

Porcini mushroom has a reputation of being like 'vegetable meat', with its hypertrophic fruiting body, pleasant aroma, and unique taste. It is used widely in a number of cuisines, especially in Europe. The strong, distinctive flavor of this mushroom has been appreciated since Roman times (42–43).

Porcini mushrooms are low in fat and energy but rich in proteins, fibers, polyphenols, flavones carbohydrates, vitamins, minerals (especially selenium), ergosterol (precursor of vitamin D2), and alkaloids, which are nutritionally useful and medicinally beneficial, including antioxidant, antiviral, anti-tumor, antifungal, and immunomodulator effects (42–46). Porcini mushrooms are traditionally believed to have numerous medicinal properties, including the removal of freckles and blemishes, and the treatment of dog bites using a salve from boletes (43). In brief, wild edible *boletus edulis* is one of the most appreciated mushroom species due to its exceptional flavor and high nutritional value, especially high content of proteins, polyphenols, antioxidants, vitamins, and minerals, in comparison to other mushrooms (46).

1.2.1.1.6 Maitake Maitake is the Japanese name for the edible mushroom *Grifola frondosa* species belonging to the genus Grifola, family Meripilaceae, division Basidiomycetes. Maitake is the Japanese name that means 'dancing mushroom' because in Japanese, *mai* means dance and *take* means mushroom. It is a recognized culinary and medicinal polypore mushroom with a diverse number of physiologically active compounds (47–51). Maitake mainly occurs in the northern temperate forests of Asia, Europe, and eastern North America. In Japan, it is found in the northern part (47–50). Wild maitake is characterized by a large fruiting body with overlapping caps and heavy mass (clumps may weigh many pounds), and often grows at the base of stumps and on the roots of dead or dying deciduous trees such as oaks, elms, persimmons, and more (47, 50). Maitake has been eaten as food in Japan and China since antiquity. People also used it to make medicine. Maitake cultivation is a recent development. Since the mid-1980s, maitake is commercially cultivated in Japan and elsewhere for use as a dietary supplement (47, 49–50).

Wild maitake (*Grifola frondosa*) is served only at top-class restaurants because of its good flavor, crisp texture, and excellent aroma and taste. It goes well with both Asian and European dishes (47, 50). Its edible fruit bodies consist of approximately 86% water and 14% dry matter, of which carbohydrates represent 59%, crude protein 21%, crude fiber 10%, crude fat 3%, and ash 7% (49). Its primary active compounds are polysaccharides, glycoproteins, and proteins. Scientists found that polysaccharides in *Grifola frondosa* have a typically basic structure of a 1,6-β-branched 1,3-β-D-glucan and heteroglycan, or heteroglycan-protein complex which is the major biologically active component (49, 51). So, maitake has dramatic health-promoting potential (47). It also contains monosaccharides such as d-xylose, d-fucose, d-mannose, l-arabinose, uronic acid, and galactose (51).

Medicinal effects of *G. frondosa* are numerous, including its anti-cancer activity, immune stimulation, effects on angiogenesis, effects on lipid metabolism, and antidiabetic activity (47–51). Several glucans isolated from *G. frondosa* have been patented in Japan as potential immunomodulating and anti-cancer agents, and maitake extract is sometimes recommended to cancer patients (48–49). In Asia, maitake extracts are recommended medicinally for a number of diseases, including arthritis, hepatitis, and human immunodeficiency virus (HIV) (47–48). In addition, maitake might have anti-obesity, anti-hyperlipemia, and antihypertension properties (47, 50). A *G. frondosa* polysaccharide-based drug was developed in China and used as an adjunctive therapeutic drug for cancer treatment by the State Food and Drug Administration (SFDA) in 2010 (51). There are eight fungal glycan-based drugs; some of them must be injected in order to be effective in vivo, but some can also be taken orally as an adjunctive drug for cancer therapy (51). However, the therapeutic effects of *G. frondosa* are still under investigation and are not recognized by official healthcare organizations such as the FDA and WHO. Maitake may be the most promising medicinal mushroom supplement, though currently less well-known than shiitake and reishi (47).

1.2.1.2   Cultivated Mushrooms
Some cultivated mushrooms frequently consumed are: white button mushroom, almond mushroom, shiitake mushroom, oyster mushroom, and Auricula judas.

1.2.1.2.1   White Button Mushroom (Agaricus Bisporus)
Agaricus bisporus is a species of the genus Agaricus, family Agaricaceae, phyllium Basidiomycete. It is also called white button mushroom, white mushroom, button mushroom, table mushroom, portobello mushroom, cremini mushroom, Paris mushroom, Italian mushroom, and Swiss brown mushroom (52–55). *A. bisporus* is an edible mushroom native to grasslands in Europe and North America. Wild *A. bisporus* appears in fields and compost piles between May and September (52). It is now one of the most widely cultivated mushrooms in the world (53–54). Historically, it was first cultivated in the Paris area (France) in 1707 by cultivar strains originated in Western Europe, and for this reason, the species is also widely known as Paris mushroom (52, 54). It is now easily cultivated indoors (cellar) on special culturing substrates called compost, which are mainly composed of straw, horse manure, and gypsum (calcium sulfate) (52, 54, 56). Cultivated white button mushroom is now the most consumed worldwide, especially in the United States and Australia. The original wild form has a brownish cap and dark brown gills, while the familiar cultivated form has a white cap, stalk, and flesh, and brown gills (53). Caps of both forms are hemispherical in shape and measure a few centimeters in diameter.

Cultivated white button mushroom (A. bisporus) is well known for its luscious taste and aroma. Thanks to its nutritional value and its flavorful taste, it is used as food for preparing dishes in cuisine and processed food in food industries (52, 54). The most important qualities of A. bisporus are its dietetic and medicinal properties. A. bisporus is a rich source of nutrients such as dietary fiber (chitin), amino acids (alanine, aspartic acid, glutamic acid, arginine, leucine, lysine, phenylalanine, serine, proline, tyrosine, threonine), unsaturated fatty acids including linoleic and linolenic acids, easily digestible proteins, sterols, phenolic and indole compounds, and vitamins, especially ergosterol (provitamin D2) and B1, B2, B6, B7, and C. A. bisporus is also a rich source of selenium, zinc and other elements such as magnesium, copper, iron, potassium, sodium, calcium, phosphorus, sulfur, and manganese (52–55). It also contains other bioactive compounds such as ergothioneine, flavonoids, glucans, and agaritine. Agaritine and its derivatives, which chemically belong to hydrazine, are the main aromatic compounds of this mushroom (54). Phenolic and flavonoid compounds are represented by myricetin and catechin (54). Cultivated white button mushrooms must be exposed to sunlight or UV lamp to transform ergosterol into bioactive vitamin D2. White button mushroom cell walls contain a mixture of fibers and matrix components that are rich in chitin (a crosslinked polymer of N-acetylglucosamine) and other polysaccharides such as β-D-glucans and mannans. One of the most significant compounds found in fruiting bodies of A. bisporus is lovastatin, a statin drug used in the treatment of hypercholesterolemia (52). Some studies have revealed that raw A. bisporus, along with some other edible mushrooms, contains small amounts of carcinogenic hydrazine derivatives, including agaritine and gyromitrin (52, 55). These compounds were shown to induce adenomas and adenocarcinomas in the lungs and to cause bladder and stomach cancer in mice (54). However, when cooked or stored at 5°C, these carcinogenic compounds were reduced significantly and did not cause cancer with moderate consumption (53, 54). Moreover, agaritine displays antiviral activity, for example, as a potent inhibitor of HIV protease (52). Thanks to the presence of different nutrients cited above, fruiting bodies of A. bisporus have antioxidant, immunomodulatory, antibacterial, anti-inflammatory, antitumor, hypoglycemic, and hypocholesterolemic activities (52–55). However, excess consumption of this mushroom may cause flatulence and indigestion because it is rich in fibers and chitin. Button mushroom must be well cooked before consumption for the liberation of its nutrients into food preparation and the destruction of microorganisms and toxins (carcinogen hydrazine derivatives) potentially present.

1.2.1.2.2 Almond Mushroom (A. Subrufescens)   Another species of *Agaricus bisporus* is *Agaricus subrufescens*, also known as the 'almond mushroom' (57–59). Since its discovery in 1893, *A. subrufescens* has been cultivated throughout the world, especially in Brazil, hence, it is also called *Agaricus brasiliensis* (57, 59). This mushroom was discovered in North America and later South America. However, it has also been found outside America, in Europe, Hawaii, and Thailand, where it grows under forest trees and in parks and gardens (57). Cultivation of *A. subrufescens* generally follows that of *Agaricus bisporus*. Despite this, the cultivation of the button mushroom has a much shorter cultivation cycle and a much higher yield (58). Therefore, the two species can be grown using similar technology; however, the results are not the same. Raw materials for growing almond mushroom consist typically of a cereal straw (wheat, barley, rice) (58). Almond mushroom is a medium-sized mushroom, forming caps of 7.5–12 cm in diameter. A mature cap is dark brown and shaped like an inverted, truncated cone with a smooth surface (59). *A. subrufescens* is known as the 'almond mushroom' due to its almond-like taste (57, 59). It is rich in polysaccharides (glucomannans, riboglucans), agaritine, sodium pyroglutamate, and other healthy nutrients (57). Almost 48% of total dry matter consists of crude protein and 18% of carbohydrates, but the lipid content is only 0.5% (57, 59). The fruiting bodies of *A. subrufescens* contain high levels of minerals like potassium, phosphorus, calcium, magnesium, and zinc. However, a minute amount of toxic cadmium has also been detected (57). The bioactive compounds isolated from *A. subrufescens* are mainly polysaccharides such as riboglucans, β-glucans and glucomannans (59). This mushroom has been used as a medicinal food for the prevention of cancer, diabetes, hyperlipidemia, arteriosclerosis, hypertension, and viral hepatitis. It is known to stimulate the immune system (57, 59).

1.2.1.2.3 Shiitake Shiitake is the Japanese name of the edible mushroom *Lentinus edodes*, a species of the genus Lentinus, belonging to Agaricomycetes class in Basidiomycota phylum. *L. edodes* (shiitake) has been renowned in Japan and China as a food and medicine for thousands of years. The cultivation of shiitake is likely quite ancient (60). Nowadays, shiitake is the second most cultivated mushroom in the global market after white button mushroom (*Agaricus bisporus*), and its value is attributed not only to its nutritional potential but also to possible therapeutic applications (60–66). In Asia, the main cultivation materials of *L. edodes* are hard wood or its sawdust (64). Wild *L. edodes* grows in abundance on fallen wood of a wide variety of deciduous trees in warm, moist climates, such as shii, oak, chestnut, beech, and maple (61–62). Shiitake has a brownish to dark-brown cap and white stem with a distinctly smoky taste (61–62). Fresh and dried shiitake are important ingredients in Chinese and Japanese cuisine, with heat cooking. Shiitake has recently gained popularity in North America, Europe, and elsewhere for its nutritional and medicinal values (61).

Lentinus edodes (shiitake) is the source of several well-studied preparations with proven pharmacological properties, especially the polysaccharide lentinan, eritadenine, shiitake mushroom mycelium, and culture *Lentinus edodes* mycelium (LEM) extract (60–65). Lentinan is a high molecular weight polysaccharide extracted from cell walls of the fruiting body, containing only glucose molecules with mostly β-(1–3)-glucose linkages in the regularly branched backbone, and β-(1–6)-glucose side chains (60, 62). Lentinan has strong immunostimulant and anti-cancer properties because it can suppress the growth of cancer cells and induce them to apoptosis (60–65). Lentinan has been approved as a drug for clinical use in cancer treatments, especially gastric cancer, in combination with oral fluoropyrimidines in several countries, including Japan and Korea (65). Lentinan may exert a synergistic action with anti-cancer monoclonal antibodies by activating complement systems through the mechanism of antibody-dependent cytotoxicity and complement-dependent cytotoxicity (65). Lentinan is also used for cardiovascular diseases (CVDs) and to combat infections. However, it has not yet been approved by the Food and Drug Administration in the United States.

Eritadenine, 2(R), 3(R)-dihydroxy-4-(9-adenyl)-butyric acid, is a secondary metabolite produced mainly by *L. edodes*. Eritadenine lowers blood cholesterol levels (62). In addition, *L. edodes* has shown to contain medicinal compounds, including polysaccharides, terpenoids, sterols, and lipids, which are effective in treating various tumors and infections, among other activities which are still being studied (61). Antibacterial and antifungal properties of Shiitake extracts have also been reported (63).

The dietary fibers present in *L. edodes* (Shiitake) consist of soluble and insoluble structures. The water-soluble structures contain β-glucans and proteins. The non-soluble structures extract salts with acids or alkalis, and contain polyuronide (acidic polysaccharide), hemicellulose, and β-glucan chains with heterosaccharide, lignin, and chitin (61). They also provide a nutritionally significant content of vitamins (B1, B2, B12, C, D, and E) and minerals. The aroma components include alcohols, ketones, sulfides, alkanes, and fatty acids, among others. The characteristic aroma compound of shiitake has been identified as 1,2,3,5,6-Pentathiepane (61). The consumption of raw or undercooked shiitake mushroom can cause allergic dermatitis, likely caused by lentinan, a heat-inactivated beta-glucan polysaccharide (66).

In brief, recent scientific studies found that *L. edodes* has immune-modulating, antitumor, antiviral, and cholesterol-regulating effects (60–65). More randomized, double-blind, controlled studies are needed for the use of shiitake in the treatment of cancer and other diseases such as infections and CVDs.

1.2.1.2.4 Oyster Mushroom Oyster mushroom or *Pleurotus ostreatus* is a species of the genus *Pleurotus* belonging to *Polyporaceae* family, Agaricomycetes class in the Basidiomycota phylum. It is a cultivated edible mushroom marketed worldwide due not only to its nutritional and medicinal values but also to its easy cultivation (67–73). There are about 40 species of the genus *Pleurotus* and all are edible. About ten species are commercially cultivated (67). Among different cultivated mushrooms in the world market, oyster mushroom occupies third position, after white button mushroom (first) and Shiitake (second) (68). *Pleurotus* species have an oyster shaped cap; hence, the name oyster mushroom (68). Their shell-like cap is about 5–20 cm in diameter (1.9–7.8 inches), fleshy, with eccentric or lateral stipe; and their color can be white, cream, yellow, pink, brownish, or dark gray (69). Oyster mushroom was first cultivated in 1917 in Germany by Flank (69). *Pleurotus* species can be cultivated at a wide range of temperatures (12–32°C) from temperate to tropical regions (67–69, 73). They can grow saprophytically on various types of lignocellulosic uncomposted agro-wastes like agricultural wastes, forest residues, and industrial byproducts (67–69, 72–73). Thus, most organic matters containing cellulose, hemicellulose, and lignin can be used as oyster mushroom substrate for cultivation; rice and wheat straw, paddy straw, cottonseed hulls, corncob, sugarcane bagasse, sawdust, waste paper, and leaves (73). Moreover, oyster mushroom grows faster than other edible mushrooms (72). Therefore, the cost of oyster mushroom production is lower than that of other cultivated mushrooms, and people in developing countries can afford it as food. Wild *Pleurotus* species often appear on a wide array of forest and live as saprotrophs. They prefer dead wood or dying hardwood trees and are preeminent wood decomposers (71). This action benefits the forest by making it cleaner. Several species can attack nematodes or bacterial colonies in living trees by killing and digesting them for the obtention of nitrogen compounds such as proteins and amino acids for the growth of the mushroom (71).

Oyster mushroom is consumed by people worldwide, due to its taste, flavor, high nutritional values, and medicinal properties (67–73). It is generally rich in polysaccharides, proteoglycans, proteins with essential amino acids, fatty acids, dietary fibers, phenolics, flavonoids, important minerals, and some vitamins. Thanks to the polysaccharide-protein complex, *Pleurotus* has been reported to have some pharmacological potentials such as antioxidant, anticancer, anti-inflammation, anti-hypercholesterolemia, anti-hypertensive, anti-diabetic, antibacterial, hepato-protective, and anti-allergic activities (67–73). Thus, *Pleurotus* can act as functional food (71). In brief, oyster mushroom and some *Pleurotus* species are inexpensive and a good source of nutrients, especially polysaccharide-protein complex; they can be used for the protection of some chronic diseases and the maintenance of health.

1.2.1.2.5   Jelly Ear or Wood Ear (Auricularia Auricula-Judae)   The botanical name of jelly ear or wood ear or black ear is *Auricularia auricula-judae*. It belongs to the genus *Auricularia* of *Auriculariaceae* family, Agaricomycetes class, and Basidiomycota phylum. The genus *Auricularia* is comprised of 10 to 15 species and sourced as either wild or cultivated edible mushrooms (74–76). Among them, *Auricularia auricula-judae*, *A. fuscosuccinea*, and *A. polytricha* are grown mostly in Asian countries (74). *Auricularia auricula-judae* is an edible mushroom and a traditional medicine in China as well as the fourth largest cultivated mushroom species in the world after *Agaricus bisporus* (white button mushroom), *Lentinus edodes* (Shiitake), and *Pleurotus ostreatus* (oyster mushroom) (74–75). This mushroom was cultivated in China since antiquity (74, 76–77). It is now cultivated in China and East Asia. China is the first producer of cultivated ear mushroom in the world for culinary and medicinal uses, mostly in dried form (74–77). Cultivation of *Auricularia* species is carried out by using compost and agro-waste products and involves two important methods like spawn production and fruiting body production (76–77).

The fruiting body of *A. auricula-judae* is distinguished by its noticeably ear-like shape, brown to black-brown coloration, and width of about 3–8 cm (1.2–3.1 in) (74, 77). The species has a soft, gelatinous, elastic texture when fresh, but its dried form is hard and brittle. It is a saprophytic mushroom and can be found throughout the year in temperate regions worldwide, where it grows upon both dead and living wood, especially the wood of elder tree (*Sambucus nigra*) (74, 77). Fresh and dried ear mushroom is edible, but not edible when raw. It should be thoroughly washed before cooking. It is used for culinary recipes and traditional medicine since antiquity mostly in East

Asian countries such as China, Japan, and so on (74–77). It has a mild flavor and its dried form is rehydrated before cooking for soups and sauces. However, it is not widely consumed in the West (Europe, USA) (74, 77).

The nutritional content of edible *Auricularia* varies according to species. On average, the nutritional value of 100 g of *A. auricula-judae* dried fruiting body includes 81 g of carbohydrate, 8.1 g of protein, 6.9 g of crude fiber, 1.5 g of fat, and the rest of vitamins (thiamin, riboflavin, ascorbic acid, vitamin D2), and minerals (74, 76). Pharmacological compounds in *A. auricula-judae* include non-starch polysaccharides, polysaccharide-protein, and polysaccharide-peptide complexes (76). Most of them belong to β-glucans which are crucial for their therapeutic action. The β-glucans of *A. auricula-judae* showed potent antitumor properties in mice implanted with Sarcoma 180 tumors (74, 76). They could also reduce the glucose levels in diabetic mice. Another study reported that this mushroom may be effective in stopping platelet binding *in vitro* and is considered an anticoagulant. Research has shown that *A. auricula-judae* can be used to lower cholesterol levels (74). Moreover, it may be used as complementary medicine or dietary supplements for anticancer, and may have hepatoprotective, immune-potentiating, and hypo-cholesterolemic properties (74). However, extracts of *A. auricula-judae* are still not applied in modern therapy. More researches are needed to confirm these preliminary observations.

1.2.1.3 Medicinal Mushrooms

Some medicinal mushrooms include Lingzhi or Reishi, Yun zhi or *Trametes (Coriolus) versicolor* and *Cordyceps sinensis*. They are used in Asian traditional medicine and are the subjects of much modern academic research.

1.2.1.3.1 Lingzhi or Reishi
Lingzhi or Reishi is the Chinese or Japanese name, respectively, of the species *Ganoderma lucidum* which is a medicinal mushroom of the genus Ganoderma, family Ganodermataceae, division Basidiomycetes (78). Worldwide, more than 250 Ganoderma species have been described. However, in therapeutic practices and literature citations, Ganoderma usually refers to the species of *G. lucidum* with popular name Lingzhi or Reishi (79). It is a large, dark mushroom with a glossy exterior and a woody texture (78–79). This mushroom is too tough to be used in cuisine (79). Lingzhi has been recognized as a medicinal mushroom for over 2,000 years (78–79). The fruiting body and mycelium are used as traditional medicine in China, Japan, Korea, and Vietnam since antiquity, and now are prepared as dietary supplements in capsule or powder forms. This annual mushroom grows on a wide variety of dead or dying trees, especially oak, maple, elm, and plum trees (78–79). In the past, *G. lucidum* grew in small quantities only in the wild; therefore, it was very expensive. Artificial cultivation of this valuable mushroom was successfully achieved in 1970s, and since 1980, production of *G. lucidum* has developed rapidly, particularly in China (78–79).

The fruiting body, mycelia, and spores of *G. lucidum* contain approximately 400 different bioactive compounds, which mainly include triterpenoids, polysaccharides, nucleotides, sterols, steroids, fatty acids, proteins, peptides, and trace minerals (79). Polysaccharides, peptidoglycans, and triterpenes are three major physiologically active constituents in *G. lucidum*. At least 140 different triterpenes have been identified in *G. lucidum* (78–79). More than 100 types of polysaccharides such as β-D-glucans, hetero-polysaccharides, and glycoprotein have been isolated from the fruiting body, spores, and mycelia (78–79). However, the amount and percentage of each component can be very diverse in natural and cultivated products. When 11 randomly selected samples of commercial lingzhi products purchased in Hong Kong shops were evaluated for the two major active components, triterpenes and polysaccharides, it was found that the triterpene content ranged from undetectable to 7.8%, and the polysaccharide content varied from 1.1–5.8% (78). Such variations can occur for several reasons, including differences in the species or strains of mushroom used, and differences in production methods. That may explain the contradictory results found in human therapies with this mushroom (78).

G. lucidum has been reported to have a number of pharmacological effects including immu-nostimulant, anti-atherosclerotic, anti-inflammatory, analgesic, antitumor, antibacterial, antiviral (including anti-HIV), antioxidative, anti-aging, anti-ulcer, sleep promoting, hypolipidemic, hypo-glycemic, hepatoprotective, radioprotective, and antifibrotic properties observed in laboratory experiments (78–79). Different components from *G. lucidum* were proven to enhance the prolifera-tion and maturation of T and B lymphocytes, splenic mononuclear cells, NK cells, and dendritic cells in culture in vitro and in animal studies. Some clinical assays reported the beneficial effects of *G. lucidum* in the treatment and cotreatment of leukemia, carcinoma, hepatitis, and diabetes (78). However, some reviews in 2016 did not find sufficient evidence to justify the use of *G. lucidum* as a first-line treatment for cancer (80–81). It remains uncertain whether *G. lucidum* helps prolong long-term cancer survival. However, *G. lucidum* could be administered as an alternative adjunct to con-ventional treatment in consideration of its potential of enhancing tumor response and stimulating host immunity. *G. lucidum* was generally well tolerated by most participants, with only a scattered number of minor adverse events. No major toxicity was observed across the studies (80–81). Indeed, *G. lucidum* could have better effects when used in combination with other classic anti-cancer drugs instead of used alone, but this also requires more research to confirm. Concerning the use of reishi in treatment of cardiovascular disease in people with Type 2 diabetes mellitus, a 2015 Cochrane review did not support the use of *G. lucidum* for treatment of cardiovascular risk factors in these patients due only to a small number of randomized controlled trials (82). More clinical investiga-tions and analytical controls of different reishi species found in the market are needed because this interesting *G. lucidum* dietary supplement contains a lot of beneficial active compounds which can vary enormously batch by batch depending on species origin and preparation.

1.2.1.3.2 Yun Zhi or Kawaratake or Coriolus Versicolor   Yun zhi or Kawaratake is the Chinese or Japanese name, respectively, of the mushroom species *Coriolus versicolor*, *Trametes versi-color*, or *Polyporus versicolor*, which belongs to the genus Coriolus, family Polyporaceae, order Polyporales and division Basidiomycotina (83–86). In North America, *C. versicolor* is commonly known as 'turkey tail' mushroom because the upper surface of its cap is velvety and attractively marked with concentric zones of varying colors – brown, yellow, gray, greenish, or black – and resembles a turkey tail (84). It is a polypore mushroom found throughout the world, but mostly in temperate Asia, North America, and Europe (83, 85). This mushroom rises up from lignocellulosic wastes. In nature, *C. versicolor* occurs as a mushroom body, but it can also be grown as mycelial biomass in submerged culture in bioreactors (84).

The fruiting body of *C. versicolor* is harvested for its nutritional and medicinal values. The bracket or shelf mushroom body in the wild or the mycelial biomass collected from submerged fermentation could all be used for this purpose (83–85). Yun zhi or Kawaratake mushroom prepa-rations such as dried powdered tea has been employed in Chinese and Japanese traditional medi-cine practices since antiquity for general health-promoting effects, endurance, and longevity (85). Nowadays, scientists found that the main bioactive components of *C. versicolor* are the polysac-charopeptides (PSPs), which are isolated from the mycelium as well as fermentation broth (85). *Coriolus versicolor* contains two bioactive polysaccharopeptides (PSPs) derived from two different strains of this mushroom: COV-1 (PSP) and CM101 (polysaccharide Krestin, PSK) (83–87). Both products (PSP and PSK) are obtained from the extraction of *C. versicolor* mycelia. PSK and PSP are Japanese and Chinese products, respectively. Both products have similar physiological activities but are structurally differently (84). Both products are obtained by batch fermentation. After extensive clinical trials, PSK was approved for therapeutic use in Japan in 1977, and by 1985, it ranked 19th on the list of the world's most commercially successful drugs (84). PSP appeared on the market about ten years after PSK. These two polysaccharides, polysaccharopeptide (PSP) and polysaccharopep-tide Krestin (PSK), isolated from *C. versicolor*, were used as supplements to support chemotherapy and radiotherapy of cancers due to their immunostimulatory properties (83–87). In Japan, PSK was approved for use in combination with chemotherapy to prolong survival of patients with gastric cancer (resected cases) or colorectal cancer (curatively resected cases), and to prolong remission of patients with small-cell lung carcinoma (87). With regard to its antitumor properties, PSK acts directly on tumor cells, as well as indirectly in the host to boost cellular immunity. Furthermore, it seems that these polysaccharides, PSK and PSP, may also act as prebiotics by stimulating the growth and/or activity of probiotic bacteria in the colon (83). In addition to clinically tested PSK and PSP, numerous other extract preparations of *C. versicolor* are on the market as nutraceuticals and traditional medicines. Nutraceutical polysaccharopeptide preparations are sold worldwide in the form of capsules, ground biomass tablets, syrups, food additives, and teas (86). *C. versicolor* polysaccharopeptides appear to be nontoxic in prolonged use and are claimed to benefit general health (84).

The clinical effectiveness of PSK has been demonstrated for various cancers. In patients with gastric or colorectal cancer, combined use of PSK with postoperative adjuvant chemotherapy prolongs survival, and this effect has been confirmed in multiple meta-analyses (87). For small-cell lung carcinoma, PSK in conjunction with chemotherapy prolongs the remission period. In addition, PSK has been shown to be effective against various other cancers, reduce the adverse effects of chemotherapy, and improve quality of life. Future studies should examine the effects of PSK under different host immune conditions and tumor properties, elucidate the mechanism of action exhibited in each situation, and identify biomarkers (87). In brief, PSP is an immunostimulant, while PSK has anticancer activity and can be used as adjuvant for chemotherapy and post cancer operation.

1.2.1.3.3 Cordyceps Sinensis   *Cordyceps*, the name given to the fungi on insects, has been known and used as a medication in China for over 300 years (88). *Cordyceps sinensis* or *Ophiocordyceps sinensis*, of the division Ascomycetes, family Ophiocordycipitaceae, is a fungal parasite living primarily on the head of the larva of one particular species of moth, *Hepialus armoricanus* Oberthur (Lepidoptera), but is occasionally found growing on other moth species (88–92). In China, this fungus is usually called 'Dong Chong Xia Cao', which means 'winter worm, summer grass', or more precisely 'worm in winter, grass in summer' (88, 90–91). This name explains the particular life cycle of the fungus *Cordyceps sinensis* (90). In late autumn, the fungus parasitizes larvae of moths belonging to the order Lepidoptera. The infected larva is converted into a sclerotium covered by the intact exoskeleton of the insect to withstand the winter, which is regarded as 'winter worm'. In the late spring or summer of the next year, a clavate stroma of the fungus grows from the sclerotium and emerges from the ground appearing as an herb, which is regarded as 'summer grass' (90). This fungus consists of two parts: a black part which is the fruiting body or stroma, and a yellowish-brown part which is the caterpillar corpus or larva (91). The larva body resembles a silkworm, and is three to five cm in length and three to eight mm in diameter. The stroma is slenderly cylindrical, and measures four to seven cm in length and about three mm in diameter (91). *C. sinensis* is endemic to alpine habitats above 3,000 m of the Himalaya region including Tibet, Yunnan, Sichuan, Gansu, and Qinghai in China (90–91).

In Traditional Chinese Medicine, *C. sinensis* has long been used as an herbal tonic and aphrodisiac, as well as to slow aging and to prevent infections, colds, flues, and many other diseases (89–90).

Recently, many bioactive constituents of *C. sinensis* have been reported, such as polysaccharides, cordycepin, cordycepic acid, guanosine (a nucleotide), mannitol, aminophenol, unsaturated fatty acids, metals, and ergosterol (88–91). Recent studies have demonstrated that the chemical constituents extracted from *Cordyceps* have various pharmacological actions, such as immunomodulating, nephroprotective, hepatoprotective, inflammatory effects, antioxidant, anti-aging, and antiapoptotic properties (88–92). However, safety concerns associated with the daily consumption of Cordyceps fungi or related products are still being debated (92). On the one hand, the known compounds from these fungi such as adenosine analogs cordycepin and pentostatin have demonstrated different beneficial and pharmaceutical activities, but on the other hand, dose-dependent cytotoxicities, neurological toxicities, and/or toxicological effects have also occurred in humans and animals (92). The possibility of mycotoxin production by Cordyceps fungi has not been completely ruled out (92). Based on the known compounds and putative mycotoxins that might be produced by Cordyceps fungi, safety assessments and more research are still required to alleviate concerns when consuming these costly fungi as dietary supplements (92).

Due to the scarcity of this resource and immaturity of artificial cultivation, it has not been possible to fully meet the needs of medical use (88). So, be careful when purchasing these expensive mushrooms, especially *Cordyceps sinensis*, because there are numerous counterfeit or modified products in the market and their pharmacological properties and medicinal uses are still not officially approved by healthcare organisms. More research is required to discover the full extent of the activity of *Cordyceps*, mostly in clinical study, and to determine the exact quantity of active compounds as well as the potential presence of toxic substances (arsenic, mycotoxins, etc.) found in each Cordyceps variety in the market.

1.2.1.3.4 Pseudoplectania Nigrella and Plectasin   Recently, a novel antibiotic called plectasin has been isolated from a fungus, the saprophytic ascomycete *Pseudoplectania nigrella*, also called ebony cup, hairy black cup, or black false plectania. The fungus *P. nigrella* is an inedible small black saprophytic ascomycete (about two cm) found on the floor of pine forests in Europe, North America, and other temperate countries (13). Plectasin is a peptide composed of 40 amino acids that fold into an α-β-β structure stabilized by three disulfide bonds (93). In vitro, plectasin was especially active against Gram-positive bacteria such as *Streptococcus pneumoniae*, including strains resistant to conventional antibiotics (13, 93). In vivo, plectasin showed extremely low toxicity in mice, and cured them of experimental peritonitis and pneumonia caused by *S. pneumoniae* as efficaciously as vancomycin and penicillin (13). Importantly, it does not show any cytotoxicity to mammalian cells such as murine L929 fibroblasts, human erythrocytes, and THP-1 monocytes (93). These findings show the therapeutic potential of plectasin as a novel source of antimicrobial agents (13, 93). Thus, plectasin is a potential alternative for conventional antibiotics, and is now being commercialized as antimicrobial.

The list of different wild and cultivated edible mushrooms cited here is not exhaustive. There are still hundred of other fungi used as food and/or medicine around the world. More research are needed to explore the immense forest of mushrooms.

1.2.2 Poisonous Mushrooms

Poisonous mushrooms are fungi that can cause toxic effects, diseases, or eventually death to those who consume them. Mushroom poisoning, named mycetism or mycetismus, most commonly occurs after foraging and consumption of misidentified wild mushrooms in nature (94–97). The most common reason for this misidentification is close resemblance in terms of color and general morphology of the toxic mushroom species with an edible species (95). These accidents are often due to the collection of wild mushrooms by amateur foragers in the forest, meadow, or home garden. For this reason, never solely identify any mushroom based on pictures in a book or website; always consult a competent mycological expert for the identification of a new wild mushroom before consumption (95). Also, always buy mushrooms at the store or market; not from an amateur seller.

The symptoms of mushroom poisoning can vary from slight gastro-intestinal troubles and vomiting to life-threatening organ failure (liver, kidneys) resulting in death (94–97). The incubation period can vary from one day to several weeks after which serious symptoms may occur, during which time the toxins attack the kidney or liver (95). Generally, gastrointestinal (GI) troubles are the first symptoms reported in all cases of mushroom poisoning and include nausea (86.6%), vomiting (79.8%), and diarrhea (21.1%) (94). Moderate to severe acute hepatic failure is also observed (94). In the past, some have promoted reliance on an initial time to development of GI symptoms to predict prognosis. Specifically, a latency of less than six hours to development of GI symptoms was utilized to predict that ingestion of a mushroom would produce toxicity (94). However, this practice has limitations. Conversely, GI symptoms occurring more than six hours after ingestion remain concerning for a possible serious clinical course and potential death (94). Beside GI symptoms, other adverse effects such as liver failure, bradycardia, chest pain, seizures, intestinal fibrosis, renal failure, erythromelalgia, and rhabdomyolysis are also observed (97). The symptoms and the gravity of fungal poisoning vary with each poisonous fungus and its quantity ingested.

Among 140,000 known species of mushroom worldwide, approximately 100 of them are poisonous to humans, with new toxic species continually being identified (94, 96–97). There are numerous mushroom poisonings in different countries each year with several hundred death cases (94).

Poisonous mushrooms contain a variety of different toxic compounds named mycotoxins that can differ markedly in toxicity (95). Mycotoxins are secondary metabolites produced by mushrooms and include different chemical groups like amatoxin, phallotoxin, muscarine, ibotenic acid, psilocybin, psilocin, ergotamine, coprine, and so on, that can be highly toxic or fatal to humans (95–97).

Mushrooms of the genus Amanita are the most toxic and often deadly. For example, the species *Amanita phalloides* (known as 'death cap') causes the most fatalities in the world (94). The toxic agents of different amanitas are amatoxins. The pathogenicity of mushrooms depends on cyclopeptide toxins, and reports indicate that amatoxins account for 90% of fatal mushroom poisonings and have their most significant impact on the liver (95). For the rapid detection of amatoxins in urine samples of intoxicated people, a rapid immunoassay called lateral flow immunoassay (LFIA) has been recently developed (98). Urine is sampled directly without the need for any pretreatment, detection from urine is completed in ten min, and the results are read by the eye, without the need for specialized equipment (98). Mushroom poisonings occur every year between June and December, the period of mushroom harvesting (95). Some well-known poisonous mushrooms will be described as follows.

1.2.2.1 Amanita Mushroom Poisoning

The genus Amanita belonging to the family *Amanitaceae* has many toxic species including *Amanita phalloides* (death caps), *A. pantherina* (panther cap), *A. citrina* (false death cap), *A. muscaria* (fly agaric), *A. ibotengutake* (Japanese ringed-bulb amanita), *A. smithiana* (North American Lepidella), *A. proxima* (Mediterranean Amidella), *A. virosa*, *A. verna*, *A. bisporigera*, *A. ocreata*, *A. suballiacea*, *A. tenuifolia* and *A. hygroscopica* (94–96). The species *Amanita phalloides* (death caps) may be the deadliest of all mushrooms in the world, and is responsible for the majority of fatalities caused by mushroom poisoning (96). The toxins involved belong to the amatoxin and phallotoxin complexes (95–97). Amatoxins are bicyclic octapeptides and powerful thermostable poisons. The most potent amatoxin is α-amanitine, and is among the nine amatoxins that have been recognized (97). Ataxia, motor depression, euphoria, dizziness, gastrointestinal disturbances, drowsiness, muscle twitches, and changes in insight, feelings, and mood are common symptoms associated with amatoxin poisoning (97). Phallotoxin includes phalloin, phalloidin, phallisin, phallacidin, phallacin, and phallisacin (96). Phallotoxin causes alterations of enterocytes cellular membrane, while amatoxin inhibits protein synthesis at a transcriptional level within enterocytes, hepatocytes, and proximal renal tubular cells. After ingestion of *A. phalloides* (death caps), these toxins tend to accumulate in the liver, damaging it severely (95). Amatoxin causes necrosis of liver cells with mortality rates ranging from about 10% to 20%. Only a minority of patients need liver transplantation (96). Poisoning by *A. phalloides* (death caps) is a medical emergency requiring immediate hospitalization.

In addition, some species of amanita genus like *Amanita pantherina* and *A. muscaria* have hallucinogenic effects (96). They contain two constituents called ibotenic acid and muscimol which are responsible for the hallucinogenic effects. Ibotenic acid is a powerful agonist of N-methyl-D-aspartic-acid receptor and muscimol is a potent gamma-aminobutyric acid A agonist (96). The intoxications caused by *A. muscaria* were long believed to be due to muscarine, but it was demonstrated that muscarine is present in small amounts. People around the world have intentionally eaten *A. muscaria* or *A. pantherina* to evoke euphoria and hallucinations (96). The most common symptoms of intoxication are dizziness, drowsiness, motor depression, ataxia, changes in mood, gastrointestinal disturbances, and muscle twitches (96). Fatality due to *Amanita pantherina* and *A. muscaria* poisoning is rare. In most cases recovery is complete after 24 hours. The treatment is mainly symptomatic. Cholinesterase inhibitors, benzodiazepines, or phenobarbitone can be used in case of seizures (96).

1.2.2.2   Clitocybe Mushroom Poisoning

The genus *Clitocybe* has different species such as *C. amoenolens, C. acromelalga, C. dealbata, C. rivulosa, C. candicans, C. cerussata*, and *C. phyllophila*. They are poisonous mushrooms due to the presence of muscarine in their chemical composition (96). The symptoms appear 15 minutes to 2 hours after ingestion and include gastrointestinal problems, miosis, hypersecretion, and in severe cases bradycardia, collapses, and death (96). Symptoms of muscarinic syndrome include increased pulse rate, headache, nausea, vomiting, diarrhea, dizziness, blurred vision, lachrymation, sweating, salivation, perspiration, reduced heart rate, lowering of blood pressure, and asthmatic-like breathing (95–97). Most patients recover within 24 hours, except in cases when the heart has stopped. The treatment of this poisoning is symptomatic, and atropine can be administered to counteract the effects of muscarine (95–97).

1.2.2.3   Inocybe Mushroom Poisoning

There are approximately 40 species belonging do Inocybe genus in China, and they are known to be inedible (96). Some species including *Inocybe asterospora, I. fastigiata* f. subcandida, *I. gobeyi*, and *I. lilacina* have neurotoxic and psychotropic effects due to the presence of biogenic amines such as muscarine and aeruginacin (96). Poisoning symptoms caused by Inocybe mushrooms are similar to those caused by Clitocybe because both genera contain muscarine (96).

1.2.2.4   Psilocybe Mushroom Poisoning

Species of genus Psilocybe are known due to their psychedelic effects caused by psilocybin (96–97). Some mushrooms containing psylocibin are: *P. semilanceata, P. Mexicana, P. bohemica, P. cubensis*, and *P. baeocistis* (96–97). They are commonly known as 'magic mushrooms'. Magic mushrooms are hallucinogens, but cannot cause addiction. The symptoms of intoxication occur 30 minutes after ingestion of fresh or dried mushroom and start with anxiety, nausea, vertigo, and asthenia. Neurosensorial symptoms consist of visual problems (mydriasis), disorientation, motor incoordination, tachycardia, and hypertension (96–97). Recovery is complete 4 to 12 hours after ingestion. The need of hospitalization is rare and in exceptional cases myocardial infarction may occur in adult patients, while children may present hyperthermia, seizures, and coma (96–97).

The list of poisonous mushrooms cited here is not exhaustive. There are still 100 toxic fungi in nature. Therefore, to avoid poisoning, do not consume wild mushrooms collected by an amateur.

1.3   YEASTS

1.3.1. Description

Yeasts are primitive fungi. They are eukaryotic unicellular microorganisms that are classified, along with mushrooms and molds, as members of the kingdom Fungi (99–101). Evolution of yeasts is diverse; therefore, yeasts are classified into two separate phyla, Ascomycota or sac fungi and Basidiomycota or higher fungi (99, 100). They include about 1,500 identified species; among them, *Saccharomyces cerevisiae* and *Candida albicans* are the most well-known (101–102). Yeasts have existed for hundreds of millions of years. Yeast sizes vary from 3–4 μm to 40 μm in diameter (99–103). Yeasts are invisible to the naked eye. Their reproduction is asexual by budding (case of *Saccharomyces*) or by mitosis (case of *Schizosaccharomyces*). Yeast cells can also reproduce sexually. In sexual reproduction most yeasts form asci, which contain up to eight haploid ascospores (101).

1.3.2 Yeast Habitat

Yeasts are widely dispersed in nature in a variety of habitats. They are commonly found on the skins of fruits and berries as white powder, especially sugary fruits (such as grapes, peaches, apples, etc.), and exudates from plants (such as plant saps or cacti) (99–103). They are also found on the surfaces of leaves and flowers, and are carried in the air by wind. Some yeasts are found in association with soil and insects (102–103). For example, *Saccharomyces cerevisiae* is insect-borne, and was detected in several different insects, such as wasps and *Drosophila* species (103).

Yeasts are also found on the surface of the skin (mostly skin between toes) and in the mouth, vagina, and intestinal tracts of humans, where they may live symbiotically or as parasites and normally cause no ill effects. However, when the host is ill or stressed, yeast will develop and cause infection (101–102).

1.3.3 Chemical Composition of Yeast

Yeast is a rich source of proteins, enzymes, nucleic acids, all essential amino acids, all vitamins of B group (except vitamin B12), niacin, folic acid, and many minerals (selenium, chromium, iron, zinc, phosphorus). Yeast contains 40 to 50% protein and is rich in antioxidants, aromas, colors, and flavors (101–104). The cell wall of yeasts, especially of *Saccharomyces cerevisiae*, contains different beta-glucans, mannoproteins, and chitin (105). Wall composition and organization vary during growth and development. Both beta-glucans and chitin are polysaccharides. Beta-glucans are soluble fibers, whereas chitin is a special insoluble fiber found in mushroom, yeast cell walls, and shells of crustaceans and insects (105). Chitin is similar to cellulose in vegetables. Beta-glucans in yeasts and mushrooms are strong immunostimulant and may have antitumor activity, while beta-glucans in cereals (oat, barley) decrease blood levels of LDL cholesterol and lipids. Due to its composition rich in nutrients, yeast, especially *S. cerevisiae*, is also used as dietary supplements (101–102).

1.3.4 Yeast Uses

Yeast is used in food preparations since antiquity such as alcohol production, bread making, dairy products, sauce preparation, and more. The most well-known and commercially significant yeasts are the related species and strains of *Saccharomyces cerevisiae*.

1.3.4.1 Alcoholic Beverage Production

The production of alcoholic beverages dates back thousands of years, after the discovery of wine residue in a pottery jar in Iran, around 5,400–5,000 BC (103).

The fermentation of sugars by yeast is accompanied by the production of alcohol or ethanol (CH_3CH_2OH) and carbonic gas (CO_2) (101–104, 106–108). The aim of the production of alcohol by yeast is to kill other microorganisms (bacteria, viruses) which are eventually present in its environment (food), because alcohol is toxic for these microorganisms, and thus eliminate competition and protect its food (103).

Yeasts are able to rapidly convert sugars to ethanol at both anaerobic and aerobic conditions (106). Yeast has long been utilized to ferment the sugars of rice, wheat, barley, and corn to produce alcoholic beverages such as wine, beer, cider, rum, vodka, whisky, brandy, and sake, and also biofuel in various industries (101–104, 106–108). Fermentation can take place either from a spontaneous development of the raw material microflora, or from the addition of a pure yeast culture (103). Nowadays, most yeasts used in baking and fermentation are cultivated yeasts (101–103). However, spontaneous fermentation of must is due to wild yeasts which are present on grape skin and in the vineyard. Cultivated yeast *S. cerevisiae* has only been used in winemaking since eighteenth century in Europe. Before this date, all alcoholic beverages were fermented on local wild yeast (101–103). In wine production, the use of sulfite is to kill bacteria, molds, and yeasts possibly present in grapes (101). Yeast fermentation of sugars not only produces ethanol and carbon dioxide but a range of minor but sensorially important volatile metabolites which gives wine its distinct character. These volatile metabolites, which comprise esters, higher alcohols, carbonyls, volatile fatty acids, and sulfur compounds, are derived from sugar and amino acid metabolism. The aroma and flavor profile of wine is due to the choice of yeast for fermentation (107). In the production of several types of beers including lagers, there are two major types of brewing yeast, top-fermenting ale yeast and bottom-fermenting lager yeast (101). Top-fermenting yeast such as *S. cerevisiae* rises to the surface of the brewing vessel during fermentation, and is used for the production of different types of beers like ales, stouts, porters, and wheat beers. *S. carlsbergensis* is a bottom-fermenting yeast and is used to make lager beer (101). In modern brewing many of the original top fermentation strains have been modified to become bottom fermenters (101). Each type of beer has its own prevailing aroma triggered either by the yeast strain chosen or by parameters used during fermentation (108).

1.3.4.2   Bread Making

The practice of bread making is one of the oldest biochemistry processes in the world, and is estimated to have begun around 10,000 years old in Egypt and northwestern China (103). In the baking industry, *S. cerevisiae* is used to expand or raise dough. Bakers use yeast as a leavening agent in the rising of dough for baking. A secondary role of yeast is to give flavor and aroma to bread (109).

1.3.4.3   Other Culinary Uses

In addition to these traditional uses, yeasts are also used in the preparation of dairy products (probiotic milk, cheese, yogurt, kefir, etc.), and different soy and fish sauces (108–110).

In addition, yeast has a nutty, cheesy flavor making it an ideal cheese substitute for vegans. Yeast is also used in the food industry for production of food additives including colorants, antioxidants, and flavor enhancers (104). Yeasts reduce the levels of bitter and astringent polyphenols and alkaloids in cocoa beans, and develop flavor to the chocolate obtained by fermentation (103). In East Asia, yeasts are used for the preparation of different soy and fish sauces (111–112).

1.3.4.4   In Petrochemical Industry and Environment Protection

In the fermentation industry, yeast is also used for the production of biofuel. This industry uses yeast to transform sugars in plants (corn, sugar cane, sugar beet, cereals), and algal biomass (microalgae and macroalgae) into ethanol (biofuel) for the functioning of machine motors (102–103). Biofuel or green fuel is less harmful to the atmosphere and human health than classic petroleum fuel. In addition, some yeasts have potential applications in the field of bioremediation (102). For example, the yeast *Yarrowia lipolytica* can degrade palm oil and other hydrocarbons, such as alkanes, fatty acids, fats, and oils. *Saccharomyces cerevisiae* has potential to bioremediate toxic pollutants like arsenic, mercury, and lead from industrial effluent and mining waste (102).

1.3.4.5   In Medicine

As yeasts are very rich in essential amino acids, minerals, beta-glucan, and the B vitamins (except B_{12}), many dried cultured yeasts – such as brewer's yeasts, usually *S. cerevisiae* – have been used to prepare dietary supplements. In addition, yeasts have probiotic properties (102, 110, 113). Probiotics are helpful microorganisms which are useful for health and the prevention of diseases, particularly for the digestive tract (110). Probiotics include bacterial strains and yeasts (see Chapter 9 of this book). Some yeasts used as probiotics are *Saccharomyces cerevisiae*, *Saccharomyces boulardii*, and *Monascus purpureus* (102, 110, 113). These probiotics are used to prepare probiotic milk and dairy products for disease prevention by maintaining and restoring the natural flora in the gastrointestinal tract (102, 110). *Saccharomyces boulardii*, a tropical yeast found on the outer skin of lychee and mangosteen fruits, is used as probiotic and medicine for the treatment of some intestinal infections such as diarrhea caused by bacteria or prolonged antibiotic therapy (113). However, excessive intake of probiotics can cause flatulence and indigestion (110). In addition, beta-(1, 3), (1, 6)- glucan extracted from baker's yeasts is used as an immunostimulant and tumor preventive agent and is sold as supplement (102).

1.3.4.6 In Fundamental Cellular Biology and Drug Production

Yeasts are the model organism for studying genetics and cell biology. Due to the high degree of similarity between yeast genes and human genes, as well as its easy manipulation and obtention, yeast is now a model system for the study of DNA, human genetic diseases, and fundamental cellular biology (99–103).

Saccharomyces cerevisiae is a unicellular fungus, possessing a nuclear genomic DNA of 12,068 kilobases organized in 16 chromosomes (103). Its genome contains about 6,000 genes, of which 5,570 are predicted to be protein-encoding genes. *S. cerevisiae* is a model organism, a valuable tool for all aspects of basic research. Unlike other model organisms though, such as *Escherichia coli*, or *Caenorhabditis elegans*, *S. cerevisiae* is concomitantly also a most valuable species for a variety of industrial applications (103).

Yeast is becoming the organism of choice to identify drug targets and to study the mode of action of various pharmaceutical products. Nowadays, various drugs have been produced from various genetically engineered yeast species (114–116). *Saccharomyces cerevisiae* remains the predominant yeast species used in synthetic biology, primarily due to its well-characterized genome, well-understood physiology, powerful homologous recombination machinery, and a well-developed set of synthetic biology tools (114). However, other nonconventional yeast species are also used, such as *Pichia pastoris* and *Pichia angusta* for the production of protein, or *Yarrowia lipolytica* for the production of high levels of lipids (114). Yeasts are often used in the production of pharmaceuticals including antiparasitic, anticancer compounds, biopharmaceuticals such as insulin, interferon, vitamin supplements, artemisinic acid, opioids, probiotics, antioxidants (resveratrol, astaxanthin, lycopene, etc.), antimicrobials, some drugs for diarrhea, and vaccines (114–116). In addition, yeast is commonly used in the production of organic acids (arachidonic acid, docosahexaenoic acid, eicosapentaenoic acid), amino acids, enzymes (invertase, lactase), and therapeutic proteins (116). One of the limitations regarding the use of yeast is, however, that it performs high-mannose type N-glycosylation. This confers a short half-life of the modified protein in vivo, which can lead to reduced efficacy for therapeutic use (115).

1.3.5 Some Harmful Yeasts

Some yeasts such as *Candida albicans* and *Candida auris* are harmful to the human body and cause infections.

1.3.5.1 Candida Albicans

The yeast-like fungus, *Candida albicans*, is commonly found in the mouth, vagina, and intestinal tract of humans. *C. albicans* is a normal inhabitant of humans and may live symbiotically or as parasites. Normally, it does not cause ill effects in healthy hosts (101). However, when the defense systems of the hosts are weak, such as under chemotherapy, immunosuppressive medication, antibiotic therapy, or when the hosts have other diseases, Candida will develop and causes infection in the mouth, vagina, and intestinal tract (99–101). Candidiasis of the mucous membranes of the mouth is known as thrush and is also the cause of white tongue, diaper rash, and thrush of the mouth and throat. Candidiasis of the vagina is called vaginitis. *C. albicans* also causes severe disease in persons with compromised immune systems such as Acquired Immuno-Deficiency Syndrome (AIDS) or cancer (101).

Occasional candidiasis can occur in a majority of people and can be treated by local antiseptic, antifungal drugs, or by foods rich in terpenoids, and antiseptic phenolic or sulfur compounds such as galangal, ginger, turmeric, garlic, onion, and more. Fermented foods such as milk probiotic, yogurt, and kefir stimulate the immune system and may prevent the development of Candida. Except Candida, white tongue may be caused by other factors such as bacterial infection, poor buccal hygiene, oral steroid treatment, dry mouth, smoking, and alcoholism. However, if *Candida albicans* pass through blood into internal organs such as the lungs and uterus, an emergency treatment is needed.

1.3.5.2   Candida Auris

Candida auris, a novel Candida species first reported in Japan in 2009, is an emerging multi-drug-resistant fungus associated with severe invasive infections worldwide and high mortality rates (117–119). *C. auris* can cause nosocomial transmission by forming adherent biofilms on venous catheter, or other lines entering the body; therefore, a high number of related hospital outbreaks have been reported worldwide (119). Variable antifungal susceptibility profiles and the development of resistance following antifungal exposure have been observed (117). Moreover, high virulence, difficulty in microbiological identification, multi-drug resistance profile, and rapid global spread with several reported outbreaks, have led the healthcare and scientific communities to consider *C. auris* as one of the most serious emerging pathogens (118). The emergence of multidrug-resistant *Candida auris* advocates and amplifies the vigilance of early diagnosis and appropriate treatment of fungal infections. More research are needed to find an efficacious therapy against this pathology caused by the dangerous yeast *Candida auris*.

1.4   MOLDS

1.4.1   Description

Unlike unicellular yeasts, molds are multicellular fungi, typically characterized by the presence of a network (mycelium) of threadlike filaments called hyphae (10, 120–121). Molds are visible to the eye and may appear cottony, velvety, granular, or leathery, and may be white, gray, black, brown, yellow, greenish, or other colors (120). Some types of molds are called mildew. Technically, mold and mildew are the same type of fungi (120). Molds and mildews are usually saprophytes (i.e., they gather their food from dead, moist organic matter) (120–121). Mildew is often used to describe a specific mold fungus that grows on plants and is characterized by a downy, whitish, or silvery appearance. Mildew is also sometimes used to describe mold growing on textiles, leather, or building exteriors (121). Molds exist in both indoor and outdoor environments. Indoors, molds generally grow on the skin of old fruits, tubers, and vegetables, as well as on the surface of meat products; while mildews prefer wet surfaces such as wall papers, carpets, bathroom walls, basement walls, kitchen, and windows. Mold reproduces via the production and dispersion of spores which can be sexual or asexual (10, 120). Spores are volatile and invisible to the eyes. Moisture is the essential condition for the survival and growth of mold and its spores. In general, most molds require fairly wet conditions, lasting for many days, to extensively colonize an environment (120). When mold spores in the air meet a surface where moisture is present, spores can germinate to form a new mold. Mold spores can survive longer than molds in dry and harsh environments. When the right growing conditions (moisture, food, temperature) are available, mold spores will develop into mold (120–121). Molds absorb their nutrients through their cell wall following the release of catalytic enzymes which digest organic macromolecules such as sugars, lipids, and proteins in the extracellular environment (10). The resulting small molecules such as glucose, amino acids, and fatty acids are then absorbed by diffusion into the fungi cells (10). The presence of mold indoors is due to the penetration of mold and spore from the exterior environment through windows, doors, shoes, and clothes of inhabitants of the house. Indoor mold can cause health problems (allergy, asthma, rhinitis, etc.) for some types of inhabitants, and can destroy foods, organic surfaces, and objects where it grows, such as wood, carpets, and wallpaper (10, 120).

Outdoors, molds are essential to the processes of decay that play important roles in the ecosystem as they digest organic matter, such as dead leaves, trees, dead animals, and insects, helping to prevent accumulation of nature's debris (120–121). It would be impossible to eliminate molds from our environment. They are essential for natural recycling. Together with other fungi and bacteria, molds help make this world clean and livable. In addition, some molds can be used to prepare foods (cheese, tofu, soybean sauce).

1.4.2   Molds and Diseases

People are exposed to molds and their invisible volatile spores every day and everywhere, both indoors and outdoors. Molds are generally not harmful to healthy humans (122). Inhalation is considered the primary way that people are exposed to mold because invisible mold spores are always present in outdoor and indoor air. People may also be exposed to mold through the skin. In some cases, people may be exposed to mold through their diet (122). There are more than 100,000 species of molds; approximately 2 dozen can cause health problems in humans (123). The most common indoor molds mostly in damp houses and buildings are: *Penicillium*, *Cladosporium*, *Aspergillus*, *Alternaria*, *Ulocladium*, *Geomyces pannorum*, *Sistronema brinkmannii*, *Trichophyton tonsurans*, *Malassezia furfur*, *Psilocybe cubensis*, and *Stachybotrys chartarum* (also known as black mold) (120, 122, 124).

Mycotoxins are secondary metabolites produced by microfungi (molds, yeasts) that are capable of causing disease and death in humans and animals. Growth of fungi in human hosts leads to diseases collectively called mycoses, while dietary, respiratory, dermal, and other exposures to toxic fungal metabolites named mycotoxins produce the diseases collectively called mycotoxicosis (125). Mycoses range from merely annoying (e.g., athlete's foot) to life-threatening (e.g., invasive aspergillosis). The fungi that cause mycoses can be divided into two categories: primary pathogens (e.g., *Coccidioides immitis* and *Histoplasma capsulatum*) and opportunistic pathogens (e.g., *Aspergillus fumigatus* and *Candida albicans*) (125). In general, primary pathogens affect healthy individuals with normal immune systems, while opportunistic pathogens produce illness in debilitated or immunocompromised hosts – in atopic subjects. The majority of human mycoses are caused by opportunistic fungi (125). In contrast to mycosis, mycotoxicosis is a disease caused by mycotoxins that are toxic compounds present in molds. Mycotoxins are analogous to pesticides or heavy metal residues in foods and can cause disease to everybody (125). The symptoms of a mycotoxicosis depend on the type of mycotoxin; the amount and duration of the exposure; the age, health, and sex of the exposed individual; and many poorly understood synergistic effects involving genetics, dietary status, and interactions with other toxic insults (125).

Many molds produce numerous protein or glycoprotein allergens capable of causing allergic reactions in certain people. These allergens are found in the spores, as well as in the molds (120).

1.4.2.1 Molds and Allergy

Some people may have health problems after contact with certain mold and spore species. However, these diseases caused by molds are not observed in everyone living in the same place. Only some atopic individuals – for example, people with high levels of immunoglobulin E (IgE) in the blood – will react to certain molds and spores, causing allergic symptoms such as asthma, sneeze, runny nose, nasal and sinus congestion, sore throat, eye irritation, blurred vision, chronic cough, skin rash, bronchopulmonary aspergillosis, and hypersensitivity pneumonitis (122, 126). It is estimated that approximately 10% of the population have IgE antibodies to common inhalant molds (126). The evidence indicates that mold, spore, dampness, and mold odor in the home are determinants of developing asthma, mostly in children (127–128). A study conducted by scientists of the National Institute of Environmental Health Sciences (NIEHS) shows that mold exposure during the first year of life may increase the risk of childhood asthma (122). Exposure to mold in a work building is also associated with incidence and exacerbations of occupational asthma (127). Mold exposure is also the cause of allergic rhinitis (127). According to the U.S. Department of Housing and Urban Development (HUD), residents, especially people with atopic diseases (asthma, rhinitis, eczema), must keep the house clean and dry and avoid using carpeting, wall papers, and wooden ceilings in areas of the home that may become wet, such as kitchens, bathrooms, and basements (122). The presence of aquariums and ornamental plants in the home can also become a source for mold growth. This is why some asthmatic people observed that since they moved out of their moist home, their asthmatic disease improved considerably, or disappeared completely. In general, bodily reactions against molds and spores like sneeze, rhinitis, or asthma occur to some hypersensitive people and not to everybody. However, other compounds such as pollen, acarid, dusts, odors, and some fruits and foods can also cause these allergic reactions. Evidently, molds, their volatile invisible spores and dampness, are one of multiple causes of asthma. The prevalence of indoor molds is around 5–10% in cold climates, and 10–30% in moderate and warm climates (128). In all cases, asthmatic and atopic people must pay attention to the potential presence of molds and dampness in their habitation, and seek to eliminate them for the prevention of their disease because molds may aggravate the disease. The relationship between severity of asthma and total dampness and mold growth is now well known (126–128).

For the elimination of molds and volatile spores in indoor environments, some essential oils such as clove oil, tea tree oil, oregano, thyme, and lemon are considered potential antifungal agents (129). It is the same for essential oils obtained from heartwood, marjoram, cinnamon, lemon basil, caraway, fir, peppermint, pine, cedar leaf, and manuka (129). These essential oils are considered superior to chemical fungicides (129). In all cases, the best way is to keep the indoors dry, and to clear all materials that can promote mold and spore growth. The use of fungicides or essential oils may not solve mold problems completely.

1.4.2.2   Molds and Occupational Diseases

Occupational mycoses are professional forms of extrinsic allergic alveolitis. They are all inflammatory reactions caused by breathing high concentrations of mold spores and other antigenic organic matter (130). Some forms of these human diseases have been associated particularly with exposure to high concentrations of *Aspergillus* spores, including farmer's lung, malt worker's lung, compost lung, and bird fancier's lung. Malt worker's lung, one of the best known of these, is an occupational mycosis encountered during beer manufacture correlated with inhalation of high levels of *Aspergillus clavatus* and *A. fumigatus* spores from contaminated barley (130).

1.4.2.3   Molds and Aflatoxins

Aflatoxins are mycotoxins which are the secondary metabolites produced primarily by the molds *Aspergillus flavus* and *A. parasiticus* (131–134). These species are crucial in the pathogenesis of human diseases. Aspergillus species are ubiquitously found in soil and decaying plants, and their spores are transferred via air currents and insects to crops and food storages (131–134). The various food products contaminated with aflatoxins include cereals like maize, sorghum, pearl millet, rice, and wheat; oilseeds such as groundnut, soybean, sunflower and cotton; spices like chilly, black pepper, coriander, turmeric, and ginger; tree nuts such as almonds, pistachio, walnuts, and coconut; and milk and milk products (131). Aflatoxins belongs to a group of difuranocoumarins (125, 131). There are about 18–20 known aflatoxins (AF) such as AFs B1, B2, G1, G2, and M1 (131, 132). Among these, aflatoxin B1 (AFs B1) has been by far the most studied, followed by AFG1 and AFM1 (131–135). Ingestion of contaminated food is the main source of exposure to aflatoxins, which adversely affect the health of both humans and animals. Aflatoxins can cause acute or chronic toxic effects such as hepatotoxic, carcinogenic, mutagenic, immunotoxic, or teratogenic diseases, infections, and growth impairment in hosts (131–135). Molecular aflatoxins affect DNA mutations, postranslation peptides chains modification, proteins and nucleic acids methylation, and the formation of free radicals (134). Although aflatoxins have primarily been associated with cancers, it is now well established that they cause various other acute and chronic diseases of the kidneys, the pancreas, the bladder, the central nervous system, and the bone – most of which are severe. Additionally, despite the additive effects for carcinogenicity between aflatoxin B1 and hepatitis viruses B and C, and the hepatotoxic algal microcystins, the mechanisms of this synergy remain unclear (132).

Aspergillus growth can occur on food at any point in the pre- or post-harvest stage, making it difficult to control contamination. Additionally, high temperatures and humidity favor fungal growth, so countries that have these environmental conditions, namely sub-Saharan Africa and Southeast Asia, often experience greater contamination (133). Therefore, hepatic cancer is mainly observed in these countries due to the simultaneous presence of Aspergillus molds and hepatitis viruses B and C. Aflatoxins are also responsible for the malabsorption of various nutrients, thus leading to nutritional deficiencies, immune dysfunction, malnutrition, and stunted growth, and hence the development of protein deficiency diseases like kwashiorkor and marasmus in infants (131). Chronic consumption of aflatoxin-contaminated foods is a common problem in both humans and animals worldwide, especially in poor developing nations of Southeast Asia and sub-Saharan Africa, where inferior harvesting, processing, and storage of foods allows for growth of molds (131). Very high concentrations of aflatoxins are most often found in nutritive seeds such as maize, millet nuts, and cereal grains in Africa, and rice in China and Southeast Asia (131). To prevent or remove contamination of aflatoxins in food products, many strategies are proposed such as drying, packaging, storage in proper and closed places without humidity and high temperature, and the use of preservatives and pesticides (133).

1.4.2.4   Molds and Diseases of Livestock

According to FAO, at least 25% of the world's food crops are contaminated with mycotoxins, of which the most well-known are aflatoxins (135). Ruminant diets could be contaminated by several mycotoxigenic fungi that increase and diversify the risk of mycotoxin exposure in these animals (136). Therefore, cows infected by mycotoxins are also sources of mold contamination for humans. For the prevention of mold in forage, forage must be kept in dry and closed places, and potentially treated by fungicides. If straw has been infected by mold, the best option is the destruction of the infected straw.

1.4.3   Molds for Food Processing

Molds have been used in food processing and fermentation since ancient times throughout the world (14, 137–138). As food processors, filamentous fungi participate in various aspects during the elaboration of some products, contributing to ripening, preventing the growth of undesirable molds and bacteria, and providing products with characteristic flavors and colors (14). In Western countries, different mold species are used for ripening various types of cheese (e.g., Roquefort, Camembert, etc.), enzyme production, and dairy waste management (137). The majority of molds involved in these fermentations belong to the genera *Penicillium, Aspergillus, Rhizopus, Amylomyces*, and *Mucor*. Species of *Neurospora, Monascus*, and *Actinomucor* are also involved in some fermentations (14, 137–138). Species of *Aspergillus* and *Penicillium* are typically used in temperate areas (Europe, North America, China, Japan) for the production of cheese, meat, and soy sauce, whereas *Rhizopus, Amylomyces*, and *Mucor* are predominantly used in tropical regions (Indonesia, India) for making temped (a Javanese fermented soy food), or tapai (an Austronesian fermented rice food) (14).

1.4.3.1   Molds for Cheese, Meat and Citric Acid Processing

In Western countries, almost exclusively species of the genus *Penicillium* are used in the ripening processes of different cheese products, dry-fermented sausages, and smoke/dry-cured hams, all of them from animal origin, whereas mold species like *Aspergillus, Mucor, Rhizopus* and *Neurospora* are used in Asia in the elaboration of foods of plant origin such as soybeans, rice, and wheat (14). Certain types of cheeses ripened by Penicillium include roquefort, camembert, brie, gorgonzola, and stilton (14, 137–138).

Penicillium camemberti is the mold used for the preparation of all white-mold cheeses, especially French camembert and Brie cheeses (14, 137–138). *Penicillium roqueforti* is one of the most frequently isolated fungi on cheese due to particular physiological features that allow it to colonize the inner part of the product, playing a crucial role in the ripening of the so-called blue cheeses such as Roquefort, Gorgonzola, Stilton Blue, and Danish Blue cheeses (14). These cheeses have strong and pungent flavors. Roquefort is a sheep milk cheese made in the South of France. Its strong proteolytic and lipolytic activities are responsible for the typical organoleptic features of these cheeses. In addition, during the ripening process *P. roqueforti* produces andrastins (A-D), compounds with antitumoral properties which inhibit the protein farnesyltransferase enzyme (14). *Penicillium solitum* is found on naturally fermented lamb meat on the Faroe Islands, and may be used as a starter culture. This species does not produce any known mycotoxins (138). On other meat products, *Penicillium nalgiovense* and few strains of *Penicillium chrysogenum* are used, especially for mold-fermented salami

(138). However, *P. nalgiovense* was originally found on cheeses from Nalzovy (Czech Republic), and may be used for fermenting cheeses too. *Fusarium domesticum*, a mold species, has been used for cheese fermentations (cheese smear) (138). *Fusarium venenatum* A 3/5 (first identified as *F. graminearum*) is being used extensively for mycoprotein production in Europe (138). Mycoprotein has some advantages over protein from animal or milk origin because it has a high-protein but low-fat content, and also has high levels of dietary fiber and a low degree of allergenicity (14). Finally, some fungi can be used to produce food colorants, including *Epicoccum nigrum* and *Penicillium purpurogenum*, but these fungi are not used directly for food fermentation (138).

Aspergillus niger is used in the food industry to produce citric acid. *A. niger* is superior to other microorganisms like yeasts (*Candida tropiclaus*, *C. oleophilis*, etc.), bacteria (*Bacillus subtilis*, etc.), or other molds (*Penicillium glaucum*) for the production of citric acid because of its ease of preparation and its cheaper costs (139–140). Citric acid is also obtained by chemical synthesis. Citric acid is commonly used in food, cosmetic, and pharmaceutical industries (130, 139–140).

1.4.3.2 Molds for Asian Food Processing

Asian cuisines are rich in fermented foods mostly obtained from plant origin such as soybeans, rice, and wheat (14). Soy sauce, miso, tempeh, oncom, and sufu are among the most popular fermented foods consumed in East Asia (14). *Aspergillus oryzae* and *A. sojae*, sometimes called koji molds, are used in the production of miso and soya sauce fermentations. In Japan, *Aspergillus oryzae* and *A. niger* are also used for production of sake and awamori liquors, respectively (138). *Aspergillus acidus* is used for fermenting Puerh tea. *Rhizopus oligosporus* is used in the fermentation process of Tempeh in Indonesia (138). Miso, a Japanese fermented paste, is obtained from soybean, rice, barley, or rye fermented by *Aspergillus oryzae* or koji mold (14).

1.4.4 Molds for Medicine Production

Molds occupy an important place in the production of many famous drugs since the beginning of the twentieth century, such as the antibiotic penicillin, the immunosuppressant cyclosporins, and the anti-cholesterol statins.

1.4.4.1 Penicillins, Cephalosporins, Griseofulvin for Infectious Diseases

In the twentieth century, three main antibiotic drugs isolated from molds for the treatment of infectious diseases included: penicillins, cephalosporins, and griseofulvin.

1.4.4.1.1 Penicillins The first major contribution of molds began back in 1928, when Alexander Fleming, a bacteriologist at the Saint Mary's Hospital in London, discovered in a petri dish seeded with *Staphylococcus aureus* that a compound produced by a mold killed the bacterium (140–143). The contaminated mold found in this petri dish was *Penicillium notatum* and the product secreted by this mold was called penicillin (140–143). Thus, for keeping their foods against bacteria which can consume their foods, molds produce active agents which are used to destroy bacteria living together in the same milieu. These results stimulated Fleming's interest, leading him to study the sensitivity of several bacterial strains to this substance; he found that several human pathogenic species of Gram-positive bacteria (staphylococcus, streptococcus, pneumococcus, and gonococcus) were sensitive to penicillin (142). Penicillin was not introduced into clinical practice until 1941, when Florey, Chain, and their colleagues had been successful in extracting enough of it (143). In 1945, Fleming, Florey, and Chain were awarded the Nobel Prize of Medicine for this discovery (142). After World War II, penicillin was the antibiotic most widely used for the treatment of infections such as pneumonia, syphilis, streptococcal infections of the pharynx, scarlet fever, diphtheria, bacterial meningitis, and septicemia (140, 143). Penicillin belongs to non-ribosomal peptide antibiotics (140). The basic structure of penicillin includes a nucleus (6-aminopenicillanic acid) and side chain (143). In the natural penicillin (penicillin G), the side chain is benzyl (143). All penicillins are β-lactam antibiotics (143). Natural penicillins include penicillin G (benzylpenicillin) and penicillin V (phenoxymethylpenicillin) (143). Penicillin G is only given by intravenous or intra-muscular injections and is more active than Penicillin V, which is taken orally. Penicillin G is the drug of choice for infections caused by pneumococci, streptococci, meningococci, staphylococci, gonococci, *Treponema pallidum* (bacterium of syphilis), and many other spirochetes, clostridia, and *Bacteroides* (143).

Semisynthetic penicillins include amoxicillin, ampicillin, cloxacillin, oxacillin, carbenicillin, and more. These antibiotics have greater activity than penicillin G against Gram-negative bacteria, but they are inactivated by beta-lactamases. These drugs are given orally to treat common urinary tract infections with enteric Gram-negative bacteria or infections of the respiratory tract (sinusitis, otitis, bronchitis) (143). Ampicillin is ineffective against *Enterobacter, Pseudomonas*, and indole-positive *Proteus* infection (143).

1.4.4.1.2 Cephalosporins Cephalosporin compounds were first isolated from the mold *Cephalosporium acremonium* (nowadays this fungus is known as *Acremonium* chysogenum) from a sewage outfall in Sardinia in 1948 by Italian scientist Giuseppe Brotzu (142, 144). Cephalosporins have bactericidal properties, and their structure contains a β-lactam ring, as do penicillins (144). Cephalosporins are β-lactam antibiotics. Cephalosporins can be administrated by oral, intramus-cular, or intravenous mode. The cephalosporin antibiotics interfere with cell-wall synthesis of bac-teria, leading to the breakdown of infectious bacteria (144). Cephalosporins are classified into five generations according to their microbial spectrum (142, 144). Each generation contains about some cephalosporin compounds and has preferential antimicrobial activity against Gram + or Gram – bacteria. Some cephalosporins can be active against both kinds of Gram bacteria (144).

Cephalosporins of the first generation include: Cefazolin, Cephalothin, Cephalexin, Cefadroxil, Cephapirin, and Cephradine. They are active against Gram-positive microorganisms like staphylo-coccus and streptococcus. They also have a small Gram-negative spectrum (144).

Cephalosporins of the second generation are: Cefamandole, Cefuroxime, Cefotetan, Cefaclor, Cefoxitin, Cefmetazole, Cefprozil, Cefpodoxime, and Loracarbef. They are more active against Gram-negative bacteria (*Haemophilus influenzae, Enterobacter aerogenes*) when compared with the first generation, but their spectrum against Gram-positive bacteria is less when compared with the first generation (144).

Cephalosporins of the third generation include: Cefotaxime, Cefoperazone, Ceftriaxone, Ceftizoxime, Ceftazidime, and Cefixime. They are effective against both Gram-positive and Gram-negative bacteria, but their optimal activity is mostly against Gram-negative bacteria (144).

Cephalosporins of the fourth generation only include Cefepime, an extended-spectrum antibiotic that is resistant to beta-lactamases (144).

Cephalosporins of the fifth generation are: Ceftaroline and Ceftobiprole. They enhance activity against methicillin-resistant *Staphylococcus aureus* (144).

Here are some examples of the antimicrobial activity of some cephalosporins. Cefadroxil, cephradine, cefaclor, and cephalexin are used orally for the therapy of both acute and chronic upper and lower respiratory tract infections associated with *Haemophilus influenzae, Streptococcus pyo-genes, Klebsiella, Streptococcus pneumoniae*, and *S. aureus* (144). Cefoxitin is more potent against the *Bacteroides fragilis* species and many Gram-negative and Gram-positive bacteria. Cefoxitin is also used in the treatment of pelvic and intraabdominal infections and is frequently employed as a preventive agent in patients subjected to pelvic or colorectal surgery (144).

1.4.4.1.3 Griseofulvin Griseofulvin is an antifungal antibiotic produced by various species of the mold *Penicillium* such as *Penicillium griseofulvum, Penicillium nigricans, Penicillium jancz-weskii*, and *Penicillium patulum* (145–146). Among different *Penicillium* species, *Penicillium gris-eofulvum* was found to be the best for the griseofulvin production in submerged shake culture (145). Griseofulvin is used mostly to treat fungal infections of the skin, hair, and nails such as tinea capitis, athlete's foot, onychomycosis (fungal infection of the nail), tinea manuum (fungal infection of the hand skin), and tinea corporis (fungal infection of the trunk, arm and leg skin), following topical application or oral administration (146–147). Tinea capitis is a common fungal infection of the hair of the scalp affecting predominately prepubertal children (146). The efficacy of griseofulvin in the treatment of tinea capitis is improved when used in combination with selenium sulfide shampoo (147). Griseofulvin is pregnancy category X and should never be used in pregnant women due to its embryotoxic effects (146, 147). Patients should wait at least a month after completion of treatment with griseofulvin before becoming pregnant (147). In an in vitro study of murine spermatocyte, a dose-dependent increase in chromosomal abnormalities has been observed in spermatocytes treated with griseofulvin. Therefore, men are warned against fathering a child for six months after receiving treatment (146). Griseofulvin is an inducer of cytochrome P-450 and thus interacts with medications that metabolize via the P-450 system. One such drug is warfarin. When taken with griseofulvin, warfarin's anticoagulation effect decreases (147). In addition, griseofulvin increases the effects of alcohol and may cause a disulfiram-like reaction (147). Headaches and gastrointestinal upsets are the most common side effects (146–147). Do not use this drug in a person who has a hypersensitivity to this antibiotic. Contraindications also include patients with hepatic failure and porphyria cutanea tarda (147). Briefly, consult a doctor before taking griseofulvin.

1.4.4.2 Cyclosporine for Organ Transplantation and Auto-Immune Diseases

The cyclopeptide cyclosporine, also called cyclosporin A (CsA), was first isolated from the filamentous fungus (mold) *Tolypocladium inflatum* for its antifungal antibiotic and was later developed as an immunosuppressant drug in the early 1970s (148–150). This white mold was isolated from soil samples collected in Hardanger Vidda (Norway) and Wisconsin (USA) (150). CsA was first investigated as an antifungal antibiotic, but Borel et al. discovered its immunosuppressive activity in 1976, and it was approved for clinical use in 1983 (150). More than 30 analogs of CsA have been identified with different biological activities, including immunosuppressive, antifungal, antiviral, and antiparasitic properties (149).

Cyclosporine is a cyclic peptide of 11 amino acids. It is now used to prevent rejection of organ transplantation (kidney, bone marrow, heart, liver), and to treat some autoimmune diseases in humans such as rheumatoid arthritis, psoriasis, and severe atopic dermatitis (148–150). Its main immunosuppressive activity is to lower the activity of T lymphocytes. However, cyclosporine has different side effects in which nephrotoxicity and hepatotoxicity are the most important (148–156). To prevent these side effects, a therapeutic monitoring control of ciclosporin A in the blood of the patient during treatment is necessary (157–158). Some analogs of ciclosporin A such as ciclosporins C, D, G, and some ciclosporin A metabolites M1, M17, and M21 have been evaluated for their immunosuppressive effects and their nephrotoxicity in comparison with ciclosporin A (151–152, 156, 159–161). Our studies found that ciclosporin A was the strongest immunosuppressant, then ciclosporin G; in contrast, the immunosuppressive effects of the others (Ciclosporins C and D, metabolites M1, M17, M21) were much weaker than ciclosporin A or insignificant (159–160). Regarding nephrotoxicity, ciclosporin A was more toxic than its analogs and its metabolites (151–152). However, the hepatotoxicity of CsA and its analog ciclosporin G were about the same (156). In brief, the discovery of cyclosporines opens a new era of immunotherapy and organ transplantation.

1.4.4.3 Statins, Red Yeast Rice for Hypercholesterolemia, and Cardiovascular Diseases

1.4.4.3.1 Statins Statins are other drugs extracted from some molds such as *Penicillium citrinum* (a blue green mold), *Penicillium brevicompactum*, and *Aspergillus terreus* (162). Statins are now used to lower LDL cholesterol (bad cholesterol), total cholesterol and lipids in blood for the treatment of atherosclerosis, and the prevention of cardiovascular accidents by inhibiting the enzyme HMG-Coenzyme A reductase, which is responsible for the synthesis of cholesterol in the body (162–164). The first statin, compactin, from the mold *Penicillium citrinum*, was discovered by the scientist and teacher Akira Endo, born in 1933 in Japan (162–164). In the rabbit, monkey, and dog, compactin was shown to lower plasma cholesterol. The prototype compound compactin was developed by Sankyo, and was shown to be highly effective in reducing concentrations of total and LDL cholesterol in the plasma of patients with heterozygous familial hypercholesterolemia (162–164). However, clinical trials of compactin were stopped because of concerns about serious animal toxicity (164). In 1978, Alberts, Chen, and others at Merck Research Laboratories found a potent inhibitor of HMG-CoA reductase in a fermentation broth of the mold *Aspergillus terreus* (162–164). They named their discovery mevinolin and later named it officially as lovastatin (164). Compactin and lovastatin have similar chemical structures (162–163). Lovastatin, the first statin developed, produced a significant mean reduction in LDL cholesterol, had few adverse effects, and was marketed in 1987 (164). Since lovastatin was commercialized, six statins, including two semi-synthetic statins (simvastatin and pravastatin) and four synthetic statins (fluvastatin, atorvastatin, rosuvastatin and pitavastatin), have been introduced to the market (162, 164).

In animals, statins produce significant toxicity at high doses: increases in hepatic transaminases, atypical focal hyperplasia of the liver, cataracts, vascular lesions in the central nervous system (CNS), skeletal muscle toxicity, testicular degeneration, and more (164). Fortunately, except for rare cases of myopathy and marked but asymptomatic increases in hepatic transaminases, none of the adverse effects found in animals occur at human therapeutic doses (162–164). Muscle complaints or myalgia are common in statin users, occurring in about 7% of statin users (164). Cerivastatin was introduced in 1998 but was withdrawn in August 2001 by the manufacturer because of a large number of reports of rhabdomyolysis, of which more than 50 cases were fatal (164). In 2010, the British Medical Journal published a study that statins may raise cataract and kidney risk (164). Therefore, the use of statins must be prescribed by physicians only.

Thanks to his discovery of the first statin named 'compactin', isolated from the mold *Penicillium citrinum* in 1970's, the Japanese scientist Akira Endo received the Japan Prize in 2006, the Massry Prize (United States) in 2006, and the Albert Lasker-DeBakey Clinical Medical Research Award (United States) in 2008 (162–164). He is now distinguished Professor Emeritus at Tokyo University of Agriculture and Technology (162). Endo's discovery opened the door to a new era in preventive cardiology (164).

1.4.4.3.2 Red Yeast Rice Red yeast rice, also called red mold rice, is a fermented food product obtained by the fermentation of steamed rice with a nonpathogenic red mold named *Monascus purpureus* (165–166). The appellation of red yeast rice is not correct because *Monascus purpureus* is a mold, and not a yeast. Other species of the *Monascus* genus, such as *M. ruber*, *M. anka*, and *M. pilosus*, are also used for red mold rice production (166). The *Monascus* genus belongs to family Monascaceae, class Eurotiomycetes in Ascomycota. Red mold rice is a dried red powder. It has been used in China and other Asian countries (Japan, Korea, Vietnam, Indonesia, Thailand) since antiquity as a traditional medicine for promoting blood circulation, rejuvenating the body, and restoring stomach balance (165–166). Due to its high contents of red colorants and other chemical compounds, it has been also used as food additive, food preservative, and food coloring agent to enhance the color of salted meats (Peking duck, char siu), fish sauces, and soybean products (166).

Red yeast rice, a Chinese dietary supplement, has gained popularity because of its properties as a natural statin. This fermented rice product is used as a medicinal food to improve blood circulation by decreasing cholesterol and triglyceride levels (165–168). The supplement contains varying amounts of natural monacolins as a result of the different strains of *Monascus purpureus* used in fermentation. There are 14 different naturally occurring monacolins in red yeast rice. One of these, monacolin K, is the most abundant in this mold, and is structurally identical to lovastatin, a statin obtained from *Aspergillus terreus* (167–168). Monacolins lower cholesterol by inhibiting HMG-CoA (5-hydroxy-3 methylglutarylcoenzyme A) reductase, the rate-limiting step for cholesterol synthesis in the liver (167). In 2007, the FDA warned consumers to avoid red yeast rice supplements promoted on the Internet (Red Yeast Rice, Red Yeast Rice/Policosonal Complex, and Cholestrix) to lower cholesterol because of the possibility of myopathy, leading to kidney impairment (167). Red mold rice and statins have similar potential side effects, including liver toxicity and muscle damage, because monacolins in red mold rice and conventional statins have the same chemical structures (167–168). Patients should only take red mold rice under the supervision of a physician and should have laboratory monitoring at least twice a year to evaluate lipid parameters and liver function (167–168).

In conclusion, red yeast rice is an over-the-counter supplement that has been used in China for centuries and has lipid-lowering effects. Unlike most herbal supplements, it has been fairly well studied and shown to be effective and safe in several randomized placebo-controlled clinical trials (168). For this reason, it has been used as an example of a traditional Chinese medication that is effective and may play a role in contemporary Western medicine. Because it is an unregulated supplement, different products are not standardized. For example, the exact levels of monacolin are unknown, and some commercial supplements have been found to contain high levels of the toxin citrinin, a potentially nephrotoxic byproduct of fermentation (168). Until regulation and standardization improve, its use will remain controversial (168).

1.4.5 Molds for Other Uses

Aspergillus niger is used in the industrial production of gluconic acid, which is an additive in certain metal cleaning applications, as well as for the therapy for calcium and iron deficiencies (130). *A. terreus* is used for itaconic acid production, a synthetic polymer (130). *Aspergillus oryzae* is fermented for kojic acid production which is used for skin whitening and as a precursor for synthesis of flavor enhancers (130).

1.5 DISCUSSION ABOUT FUNGI

Fungi are extraordinary eukaryotic organisms which are neither plants nor animals, and play important roles on this planet. Fungi are both friends and foes towards humans, animals, and plants. Without fungi, other organisms cannot live normally. Fungi are strong decomposers, essential for natural recycling, helping to maintain ecology and equilibrated life on earth. Fungi include mushrooms, yeasts, and molds, the first of which are macro-organisms and the other two, microorganisms. Yeasts are single cells while molds are multi-cells in the form of filaments.

Mushrooms are the type of fungi best used as foods and medicines since antiquity. However, until today, only about 10% of mushrooms among 140,000 estimated mushroom species have been exploited (15). They are rich in nutrients such as proteins, amino acids, vitamins (vitamin D2, B group), beta-glucans, enzymes, and minerals. Due to their special aroma and flavor, some wild mushrooms like matsutake and truffle are very costly. White button mushroom is the most consumed worldwide. Some other mushrooms such as reishi, shiitake, and maitake are used in traditional medicine. However, some wild mushrooms like death cap, deadly webcap, and destroying angel are deadly poisons. Mushrooms must be cooked before eating because heating destroys chitin cell membrane to liberate nutrients into the food.

Yeasts are mainly used in food fermentation for the processing of alcohol beverages such as wine, beer, cider, rum, liquor, and so on. They are also used for baking bread and cakes and making dairy products like cheese, yogurt, and cream. Yeasts are also used in medicine for preparing β-glucan (an immunostimulant), B group vitamins, and amino acids, because yeasts are rich in these nutrients. Some yeasts can produce various drugs such as insulin, interferon, probiotics, and some vaccines. Some yeasts are used to treat intestinal troubles. However, yeasts like *Candida albicans* are pathogens that can cause oral and vaginal infections.

Molds are often the source of allergic reactions such as sneeze, running nose, and asthma in certain allergic people. Some molds such as *Aspergillus flavus* can produce aflatoxins that are toxic and carcinogenic. Molds are used in the fermentation of foods for making alcohol, soybean sauce, fermented sausages, and more. Molds are also the source of a number of medicines such as penicillin, cephalosporins, griseofulvin, ciclosporins, and statins. Much more scientific investigations are needed to explore the vast and mysterious kingdom of fungi for the discovery of new medicines and nutrients in the future.

2 WATER

2.1 ROLE OF WATER

Water is essential for human life as well as for all living organisms like microbes, fungi, animals, and plants, although water does not furnish energy for their activity. Water is a macronutrient and constitutes about 60–70% of human body weight, and this level can vary with sex, age, size, and activity of each individual (169–172). All cells, tissues and organs need water for their functioning and activity. An adult needs about two to three liters of water in different forms (pure water, beverages, soup, fruit liquid, etc.) a day to maintain the good functioning of all organs according to size, sex, age, activity, and the climate where this person lives (169–172). Body fluid levels also vary according to gender and age (170). Males have more lean tissue and thus a higher percentage of body weight as fluid than females. The amount of body fluid as a percentage of total weight decreases with age. Water comprises from 75% body weight in infants to 55% in elderly, and is essential for cellular homeostasis and life (170, 172). This decrease in total body water is, in part, a result of the loss of lean tissue that can occur as people age. For example, an adult contains about 37–45 l of water. Adult males are composed of about 60–70% water and females are composed of about 55–60% water (170).

On average, a sedentary adult should drink 1.5 l of water per day; male adults need 3.0 l/day, female adults need 2.2 l/day (171). Male adolescents aged 9–13 years need 1.8 l l/day; those aged 14–18 years need 2.6 l/day. Female adolescents aged 9–13 years need 1.6 l/day; those aged 14–18 years need 1.8 l/day (171). Infants 7–12 months old need 0.6/l day; children 1–3 years old need 0.9 l/day; and children 4–8 years old need 1.2 l/day (171).

As stated, daily water output for adults averages 2.5 liters. The body loses about 400 milliliters of its daily water output through exhalation. Another 500 milliliters are lost through our skin. Urine accounts for about 1,500 milliliters of water output, and feces account for roughly 100 milliliters of water output (169).

Every cell in the body contains fluid. When cells lose their fluid, they quickly shrink and die. On the other hand, when cells take in too much fluid, they swell and burst apart (170). About two-thirds of the body's fluid is held within the walls of cells and is therefore called intracellular fluid. The remaining third of the body's fluid is referred to as extracellular fluid because it flows outside of the cells (170). There are two types of extracellular fluid: interstitial fluid and intravascular fluid. Interstitial fluid flows between the cells that make up a particular tissue or organ, such as muscle fibers or the liver (170). Intravascular fluid is the water in the bloodstream and lymph. Plasma is specifically the extracellular fluid portion of blood that transports blood cells within the body's arteries, veins, and capillaries (170).

Water regulates our body temperature and helps our digestion, circulation, and excretion. Without water, we would die within a few days, while without food we can live for a week or more (169, 170, 172). According to the 'rule of threes', a person can survive three minutes without oxygen, three days without water, and three weeks without food (169). Functions of water in the human body may include four types: transportation of all nutrients and their metabolites (waste products), medium for biological and chemical reactions, temperature regulation, and lubricant or shock absorber (169, 171). In addition, water intake may be important for disease prevention and health promotion (172). Increased risk for colon cancer was linked with low water intake (169, 173). A recent publication in 2020 reported that women with breast cancer consumed less water and total fluids compared with controls, suggesting that higher water intake may decrease breast cancer risk (173). In addition, drinking more water or fruit juices like orange juice and eating more vegetable fibers (date fruit, prune) may prevent constipation. Drinking more water may also decrease high blood pressure. When age advances to 80 years, the percentage of water in our bodies decreases to about 45–50%. Loss in body water plays a role in the aging process, and is accelerated by dehydration. To avoid the acceleration of aging, keeping hydrated may slow down this process (169). However, keep in mind that excessive water intake can cause diseases and even death due to the breakdown of homeostasis – the disruption of equilibrium between water and other essential nutrient levels (electrolytes) in the body and cells. This phenomenon is called water intoxication or water poisoning which is due to overconsumption of water without appropriate replacement of electrolytes. Maintaining a constant level between water and other nutrients in the body is essential for the good functioning of all organs (169). The regulation of water balance is very precise, as a loss of 1% of body water is usually compensated within 24 h (171). Both water intake and water losses are controlled to reach water balance. Healthy adults regulate water balance with precision, but young infants and elderly people are at greater risk of dehydration. Dehydration can affect consciousness and can induce weakness, hypotonia of ocular globes, speech incoherence, orthostatic hypotension, and tachycardia. Human water requirements are due to numerous factors that modify water needs such as climate, physical activity, diet, age, disease, and so on (171).

Some main organs and tissues rich in water are: blood (78% water), brain (75%), rectum (90%), sweat (98–99%), and saliva (99.5%) (169). Water is also the main constituent of mucus in the nose, eyes, and digestive tracts, and is the lubricating fluid between bone joints. Our body can produce around 300 milliliters of water per day through metabolic processes, but the quantity of this endogenous water is insufficient (169). Too little or too much water in the body will create a disturbance in the functioning of all cells and organs. One mechanism to help ensure the body maintains water balance is thirst (169). Thirst is the result of a complex communication between the brain and different cells in the body, especially cells in the mouth. Sensory proteins in cells detect the modification of water and salt levels in different tissues and organs such as mouth, blood, heart, and kidneys, and then send signals to the brain by stimulating the feeling to drink (169). For example, when food contains too much salt, the body needs more water to maintain homeostasis by ordering the brain to create a thirst sensation in the mouth. The 'thirst center' or 'thirst coordinator' is located in the hypothalamus, a mini-organ of the brain. In older people the thirst mechanism becomes weakened and as age advances, there is a higher risk for dehydration (169). Other mechanisms for the maintenance of water balance are aimed at controlling the water volume of urine. The amount of water filtered from the blood and excreted as urine is dependent upon the amount of water in blood and the electrolyte composition of blood. The regulation of water output involves complex communication between the kidneys, hypothalamus, and endocrine glands (169). Moreover, water plays an important role in the thermoregulation of our body. Too low or too high temperatures stop the activities of enzymes and the functioning of metabolism (169). Normal temperature of the body is 37° C or 98.6° F. When the temperature is high, perspiration occurs by liberating heat via sweat through the skin. Water on the skin's surface evaporates, thereby cooling the body. This must be balanced with water input. Drinking more water is also necessary when the weather is too hot (169). Elderly people, infants, and children are most vulnerable to heat and thirst. Dehydration decreases blood volume and is a primary cause of heat stroke (169–170). Dehydration is due to heavy exercise or exposure to high environmental temperatures, when the body loses significant amounts of water through increased sweating and breathing (170). However, elderly people and infants can get dehydrated even when inactive, as their risk for dehydration is much higher than that of healthy young and middle-aged adults. Heat stroke is a potentially fatal heat illness characterized by failure of the body's heat regulating mechanisms. Symptoms include rapid pulse; hot, dry skin; high temperature; and loss of consciousness (170). The 2003 heatwave caused the death of about 15,000 elderly people in France, mostly elderly people living alone (174). Infants excrete urine frequently, causing them to respond more dramatically to heat and cold and to lose more body water than older children (170). Therefore, never leave infants and young children alone in the car.

2.2 TYPES OF WATER

Water that is safe to drink or to prepare food is called potable water or drinking water. In developed countries, two main types of drinking water or potable water are: tap or municipal water, and bottled water comprising natural mineral water, spring water, and other treated drinking water.

2.2.1 Tap or Municipal Water

Tap water or municipal water comes from lakes, rivers, underground stream, large wells, or reservoirs. Water is then processed, disinfected, and purified at treatment plants. The kind of treatment applied by a public water system varies with source type and quality. Public drinking water systems use various methods of water treatment to provide safe drinking water for their communities. Today, the four steps in water treatment used by community water systems (mainly surface water treatment) include: coagulation and flocculation; sedimentation; filtration; and disinfection (175–176).

In the coagulation and flocculation step, chemicals with a positive charge are added to the water. The positive charge of these chemicals neutralizes the negative charge of dirt and other dissolved particles in the water. When this occurs, the particles bind with the chemicals and form larger particles, called floc (175–176).

In the sedimentation step, floc settles to the bottom of the water supply, due to its weight.

In the filtration step, once the floc has settled to the bottom of the water supply, the clear water on top will pass through filters of varying compositions (sand, gravel, and charcoal) and pore sizes, in order to remove dissolved particles, such as dust, parasites, bacteria, viruses, and chemicals (175–176).

The last step is disinfection. Disinfectants used in tap water treatment are chlorine or chloramine. Chlorination is added in order to kill any remaining parasites, bacteria, and viruses, and to protect the water from germs when it is piped to homes and businesses (175–176). However, chlorination is less effective at removing protozoa, such as *Giardia lamblia*. Chlorine-resistant protozoa and viruses are instead removed by extensive filtration methods (169).

Water may be treated differently in different communities depending on the quality of the water that enters the treatment plant. Typically, surface water requires more treatment and filtration than ground water because lakes, rivers, and streams contain more sediment and pollutants and are more likely to be contaminated than ground water (175). After preparation, tap water obtained is controlled, adjusted, or eliminated for the quantity of minerals and undesirable compounds. After control, water is then piped to residential homes and industries. In most cases, this tap water is used for drinking, for food and beverages preparation, or for other domestic purposes (washing, cleaning, watering plants, etc.).

In some areas, fluoride is added to tap water in an adequate amount to prevent dental caries and some bone diseases owing to the absence or the insufficiency of fluoride levels in the original water (175). High fluoride levels are toxic to the organism, especially to the bone. In contrast, lack of fluoride also damages bone formation, especially teeth. An analysis is necessary for the control of fluoride levels in tap water, bottled waters, and other products containing fluoride (raw materials for pharmaceuticals, tea) (177–178). Fluoridation of community drinking water to prevent dental caries is considered one of the ten most important public health achievements of the twentieth century (179). Most tap water in industrialized countries is potable and controlled bacteriologically and chemically by a competent laboratory. In the United States, water treatment plants routinely check water supplies for hazardous chemicals, minerals, and other contaminants under the controls of the Environmental Protection Agency (EPA). Because of these efforts, the United States has one of the safest water systems in the world (170). However, in developing countries, the quality of tap water leaves much to be desired. In addition, many areas in the world do not yet have tap water. Therefore, a number of infectious diseases such as cholera, dysentery, and so on are still observed in developing countries due to lack of money and competent technicians to produce tap water.

2.2.2   Bottled Water

Bottled water comprises natural mineral water, spring water, artesian water, and other treated water. In the United States, bottled water is under the control of the Food and Drug Administration (FDA) because it is sold as food in the market, while tap water is controlled by the Environment Protection Agency (EPA) (169, 180). For bottled water, the FDA adheres to the same quality standards as those set by the EPA for tap water. Therefore, the contaminant levels set by the EPA for tap water are not different for bottled water; although there is much less testing, monitoring, and oversight of bottled water in comparison to tap water. Similar to tap water, the source and treatment of bottled water determines its taste and quality (169). In the United States, bottled water is often treated and filtered by different methods than those used for tap water, and thus its taste and appearance may differ (170). Most bottling plants use an ozone treatment instead of chlorine to disinfect water, and many people feel this process leaves the water tasting better than water treated with chlorine (170). Bottled water is taken from either surface water or groundwater sources.

2.2.2.1   Natural Mineral Water

According to the Food Standards Agency in the United Kingdom (180), natural mineral water is water originating in an underground water table, deposit, or aquifer, which emerges or is extracted from a source tapped at one or more natural or bore exits. It must come from an officially recognized spring, be microbiologically wholesome (i.e., free of parasites, pathogenic microorganisms) and have been protected from all risk of pollution both at source and during its processing (180–181). Water must be bottled at source. Natural mineral water is analyzed by its chemical and microbiological composition and may not be treated in any way that alters these properties. In the UK, disinfection of natural mineral water is not permitted (180). However, the use of ozone-enriched air treatment is only allowed as prescribed by the regulations (182). The composition, temperature and other essential characteristics must remain stable over time. In addition, natural mineral water must provide certain information about the mineral composition on its labels (180). As reported in the European legislation (2009/54/EC Directive) natural mineral waters are 'originated from an aquifer or underground reservoir, spring from one or more natural or bore sources and have specific hygienic features and, eventually, healthy properties' (181). They are different from drinking water because of their spring purity and conservation, their constant levels of minerals, and certain healthy effects (181). According to the US FDA, natural mineral water does have at least 250 parts per million (ppm) total dissolved solids (181). In Europe, however, by law, there is no upper or lower limit for mineral contents in natural mineral water; as opposed to tap drinking water, which is strictly regulated as regards the fixed residue at 180°C (181). European bottled waters generally contain higher mineral levels than North American tap water sources and North American bottled waters (182). Significant differences exist between North American and European standards regulating the bottled water industry. The US Food and Drug Administration requires that 'mineral waters' contain between 500 and 1,500 mg/L of total dissolved solids, a combination of the dissolved minerals. In Europe, however, water with any level of mineralization is considered 'mineral water' (182). In addition, the European Economic Community Mineral Water Regulations prohibit the processing and treatment of any water bottled from a source (182). Mineral waters are also classified by other physical parameters, like pH, temperature, and hardness. With regard to pH, mineral waters are classified as acid water (pH<7) or alkaline water (pH>7). By temperature, mineral waters may be cold (<20°C at source), hypothermal (20–30°C at source), mesothermal waters (30–40°C at source) and hyperthermal waters (>40°C at source). Hardness indicates the presence of alkaline earth metals. Mineral waters may be very soft (0–100 mg/L of CaCO3), soft (100–200 mg/L of CaCO3), hard (200–300 mg/L of CaCO3), or very hard (>300 mg/L of CaCO3) (181). Mineral composition enables classification of natural mineral waters as bicarbonate mineral waters, sulphate mineral waters, chloride mineral waters, calcium mineral waters, magnesium mineral waters, fluoride mineral waters, ferrous mineral waters, and sodium-rich mineral waters (181). The levels of these minerals in natural mineral water are important for health and diseases. For example, a high or low level of fluoride in water can cause disease. It is the same for other minerals like sodium, iron, chloride, sulphate, and so on. Therefore, in the United States, the levels of these minerals in natural mineral water must comply with FDA norms, and must be indicated on the label of each water bottle. According to the European Legislation (2009/54/EC Directive), physical and chemical characterization is used to classify different mineral waters based on the analysis of main parameters (181). North American bottled waters were grouped into spring waters or mineral waters, according to their label. Because all European bottled waters are labeled 'mineral waters', they were grouped into low, moderate, or high mineralization waters. Precise definitions of mineralization levels vary from country to country. In general, low mineralization indicates less than 200 mg/L of Ca^{2+}, Mg^{2+}, and Na^+; moderate mineralization indicates between 200 and 700 mg/L of these minerals; and high mineralization indicates more than 700 mg/L (182).

2.2.2.2 Spring and Artesian Water

Spring water is natural mineral water obtained from a spring. A spring is groundwater obtained from rain and melted snow that seeps into the ground and forms a water table. By gravity, pressure, or other forces, the groundwater flows along paths of least resistance, often emerging as springs wherever the water table intersects the land surface, such as the side of a hill, a valley bottom, or other excavation (183). A spring may emanate from water saturated soil or porous rock, from a fracture, fissure, or cave, or along a contact zone between two rock types of different permeability (183). In brief, a spring is a place at which water flows from groundwater or an aquifer to the land surface. Spring water is bottled at source and satisfies most of the exploitation conditions, microbiological criteria, and some of the labelling requirements that apply to natural mineral water (180). Spring water must also comply for all physical, chemical, and microbiological parameters. However, spring water does not have to contain the same 250 ppm mineral quantity as natural mineral water. For this reason, some spring waters contain very little minerals, while others may contain a lot. Indeed, mineral quantity in spring water is source dependent (180). Artesian water is spring water, but this groundwater is under enough pressure to rise naturally above the land surface through an underground well. The word artesian comes from the Artois town in France. Artesian water must meet all requirements that apply to spring water.

2.2.2.3 Other Bottled Water

Bottled drinking water means drinking water which is bottled, and is neither described as spring water or natural mineral water. It can come from different sources, including municipal tap water or filtered water. Filtered water is tap water that runs through carbon or micron filters to remove the chlorine before being treated by ozone (O_3) and bottled. Bottled drinking water must also comply for physical, chemical, and microbiological parameters as cited previously regarding spring water (180). Recently, a new type of bottled water is marketed and named alkaline water. There are two types of bottled alkaline water: artificial alkaline water and natural alkaline water. The description and role of alkaline water have been covered in the Chapter 4 of this book.

2.2.2.4 Advantages and Inconveniences of Bottled Water and Tap Water

Many studies have focused attention on the safety of bottled mineral water, in particular on the migration of chemicals such as plasticizers and endocrine disruptors from plastic containers to water. Plasticizers (additives used to impart flexibility and handling properties to several kinds of plastics) and endocrine disruptors (chemicals that interfere with function of the endocrine system) are the main compounds involved in adverse effects on human health (181).

For some ancient houses built before the first World War, indoor water pipes were often covered with lead in their interior surface to avoid rust. These lead pipes caused chronic lead poisoning, called saturnism, when the pH of water becomes acidic, because normally, lead is not soluble in water at neutral or alkaline pH. In the case where the lead pipe cannot be removed from these ancient houses, municipal water is delivered by bottle for drinking and cooking, while tap water is reserved for bathing and sanitary use only.

Although bottled water may taste better than tap water, there is no evidence that the quality of bottled water is safer than that of tap water. However, in developing countries, tap water is not rigorously controlled; the use of imported bottled water or boiled tap water is necessary to preserve health and to prevent infectious diseases, especially for tourists.

Tap water in the United States costs, on average, much less than one cent per gallon, while bottled water is upwards of three dollars per gallon (169). Moreover, bottled water uses more resources and produces more waste in comparison to tap water. Iowa State University reports that in the United States alone, the making of plastic bottles for bottled water consumption uses more than 1.5 million barrels of oil every year, which is more than the fuel required for 100,000 cars (169). Plastic is very harmful to the lives of animals and the environment. In industrialized countries, tap water is considered safe to drink.

2.3 MINERAL COMPOSITION OF TAP WATER AND BOTTLED WATER

The mineral composition of potable water like tap water, natural mineral water, and spring water consists of two kinds of elements: macro-elements and micro-elements. Macro-elements are Calcium, Magnesium, Phosphor, Natrium, Potassium, and Chlorine. Micro-elements include Iron, Fluor, Manganese, Selenium, Copper, Zinc, Chrome, Bore, Molybdenum, Vanadium, Nickel, Cobalt, and Lithium. Natural mineral water is richer in macro- and micro-minerals than spring water and municipal water (184–185). The overall pH range of natural water is between 6 and 8, except Waikea Hawaiian spring water and Iceland spring water, both with pH 8.8 (184–185). In general, all drinking waters are beneficial to our health not only for the supply of precious potable water but also extra dietary minerals like calcium, magnesium, and other trace essential nutrients such as selenium, copper, zinc, fluorine, and iron that we all need plenty of each and every day. However, some people prefer bottled natural mineral water because its mineral content and its pH are guaranteed and labeled. Minerals such as calcium and magnesium in natural mineral and spring waters are in soluble form and are easily absorbed by the digestive tract; in contrast, the same minerals in tablets are often insoluble salts, hence less absorbable. Calcium, phosphate, and fluorine are constituent minerals of bone and teeth and necessary for their growth, while magnesium, iron, zinc, selenium, copper, and so on, are essential for the activity of cells and enzymes.

2.4 OTHER DRINKING WATERS

In some rural areas and developing countries, two other sources of drinking water frequently used are well water and rainwater.

2.4.1 Well Water

People in rural areas may obtain their water from private or municipal wells. The mineral composition of well water and natural mineral water is similar because both are groundwater. Water from wells generally requires less treatment than surface water such as from rivers and lakes. The water well must be dug far from homes and cultivation areas to avoid harmful substances. In industrialized countries, testing well water is a relatively simple process. A sample of water from the well is analyzed by an accredited laboratory (186). In the United States, approximately 13 million American rural households obtain their water from private wells (186). However, in developing countries, well water is not controlled due to lack of money and technical competence; therefore, a number of diseases, like infectious diseases (cholera, gastroenteritis, hepatitis, parasites, etc.) and chemical poisoning (arsenic, nitrate, pesticides, etc.) have been observed (187). To disinfect contaminated well water, the use of chlorine is the best way, but the excess of chlorine is also harmful to the health. To eliminate toxic chemicals, a specific filter can be used. However, this treatment of well water in developing countries needs materials and competent technicians.

2.4.2   Rainwater

Rainwater is water that has been obtained from rain. Rain is water precipitated from clouds which is caused by the evaporation of water from lakes, rivers, seas and ocean into the sky. Therefore, rainwater contains not only water but also other water-soluble solid and gas products that are present in the original water and in the atmosphere. The quantity of constituents and the quality of rainwater vary with each area as well as with the mode of collection and storage. For example, rainwater in an area near the sea is richer in iodine and salt than rainwater in land far from the sea. Theoretically, rainwater is better than natural surface water such as rivers and lakes. But rainwater can contain toxic compounds due to air pollution and bacteria from the excrements of birds or insects deposited on the roofs of a building or home. Direct consumption of collected rainwater without any form of purification or treatment is strongly discouraged by the World Health Organization due to evidence of microbiological and chemical contamination from both atmospheric deposition and rooftop run-off (188). However, in developing countries, access to safe drinking water is a major problem. In the face of decreasing water sources, rainwater harvesting may be seen as one of the most appropriate alternatives for supplying freshwater at a household or community level. Rainwater has received increased attention worldwide as an alternative source of potable and non-potable water for rural areas and developing countries (189).

2.5   Water in Traditional Medicine

Since antiquity, traditional Greco-Roman medicines have used sea water and source water (spring water) from specific areas by bathing for the treatment or relief of some chronic diseases like gout, rheumatism, psoriasis, eczema, stress, and asthma (190–198). The therapy using natural source freshwater by bathing is called balneology or balneotherapy, spa therapy or thermal cure; while that using sea water by bathing is named thalassotherapy (190–198). The natural source water with its mineral contents penetrates the skin through pores, then stimulates circulation and boosts the action of certain minerals with some organs in the body. It is usually practiced at spas – places or resorts with natural source water; therefore, it is also called spa therapy. Thermalism or thermal cure is therapy using spring water at its source by bathing and sometimes accompanied by drinking (197–198). However, bathing in a specific sea for the treatment of specific diseases is called thalassotherapy. Nowadays, the two types of traditional natural water therapy, including thalassotherapy and spa therapy or thermalism, still remain popular in many European countries such as France, Italy, Spain, Greece, Switzerland, Germany, Belgium, Israel, but are going into decline especially in the Anglo-Saxon world (191).

2.5.1   Thalassotherapy

Thalassotherapy is bathing in sea water of a specific sea for the treatment of chronic diseases such as rheumatism, arthrosis, asthma, dermatological, and so on, or for their prophylaxis in healthy individuals (193–195). The bathing is performed either directly in the open-air sea or in a bath or pool containing this sea water. The repeated immersion of the body in warm seawater, and/or the application of marine mud, or algae of the sea station are some practices often used in thalassotherapy for the therapy of some diseases. The marine climate (air and sun) of the sea place is also another factor for health and wellness promotion (195). The Dead Sea in the Middle East is the saltiest natural lake and seaside station, well-known throughout the world for thalassotherapy of skin diseases such as psoriasis, psoriatic arthritis, and some other skin diseases (eczema, acne) (193–195). The Dead Sea is rich in magnesium, sodium, calcium, potassium, bromide, iodine, and selenium. In addition, the air of these sea stations is also rich in iodine and bromine. Other areas such as the Mediterranean basin, the Black Sea (Bulgaria, Ukraine, Russia), and some ocean coasts in France, Germany, Estonia, Brazil, Romania, Japan, and New Zealand have become more well-known stations in thalassotherapy (193).

2.5.2 Balneotherapy, Spa Therapy, or Thermal Cure

Balneotherapy or spa therapy or thermal therapy is bathing in natural thermal mineral waters for the treatment of some chronic diseases such as chronic low back pain, rheumatism, gout, psoriasis, atopic dermatitis, pruritus, acne, stress, asthma, and more (191, 197–198). Bathing in thermal springs, sometimes accompanied by drinking, was a common practice in ancient Greece and Rome for the treatment of different chronic diseases. Today, this traditional therapy is still used in many European countries and Japan for the treatment of some chronic diseases cited above.

Thousands of health resort areas have developed around these hot springs. Spa resorts are differentiated according to their location (sea side, mountain area) and the chemical composition of their mineral water. Each spring has its own characteristics and related therapeutic properties (192). Spa resorts are also classified as being low mineralized (0.6–2 g/l), mildly mineralized (>2–10 g/l), or highly mineralized (>10 g/l) (196). Water temperature is described as being cold (<20°C), hypothermal (20–30°C), thermal (>30–40°C), or hyperthermal (>40°C) (196). Absorption of minerals through the skin seems to be limited. The dermatological therapeutic effect would therefore appear to lie in a local interaction between the mineral water and the structure of the skin surface. The effects of spa therapy are due to three categories: mechanical, thermal, and chemical (196). For the mechanical effects, the immersion allows the patient to mobilize joints and strengthen muscles with minimal discomfort. This hydrostatic effect is increased when the water is more concentrated in salt. Hydrostatic pressure also causes displacement of fluids from the extremities to the trunk, thus causing hemodilution and increased diuresis. It has been shown that immersion for 1 hour increases water excretion by about 50% (196). For the thermal effect, the hot water causes superficial vasodilation, and it has been shown to reduce vascular spasm and stasis in the nail bed and conjunctiva (196). Anti-inflammatory and immunomodulatory effects have been attributed to thermal baths and spa therapy. The heat stimulates the body to release a range of immunomodulatory mediators such as β-endorphin, enkephalin, and irisin (198). Regarding the chemical effect, the composition and physical properties of various spa waters play a role in the efficacy of thermal therapy for each type of illness. These properties include salty, sulfurous, carbonic, radon-rich, selenium-rich, arsenical, and ferruginous, among others. It is still not clear which elements are essential and what is the ideal concentration of each element in order to attain an optimal response to treatment (196). In general, the sum of the cations of Na^+, K^+, Ca^+, and Mg^+ and the anions of SO_4^{2-}, Cl^-, and HCO_{3-} of these natural spring waters must exceed one g/l, and sulfur in the form of sulfate radical is the main chemical component of spring water (191). The amounts of gas NH_3, NO, and NO_2 must be negligible, and the waters must be bacteria-free. Some elements, such as iodine, require contents of one mg/l or more (191). Thanks to its unique composition of minerals, each thermal water might play a different role in the treatment of each type of disease.

In thermal therapy, the body is immersed in a bath or a pool containing spring water directly collected at the source at a warm temperature during a period of time fixed by the therapist. Water jet showers can be used at the end of this bath. Depending on the illness, other types of treatment may be accompanied, such as inhalation of fumes of mineral water, drinking or oral rinse of natural mineral water, or covering the body with mud (mud bath). Steam baths, saunas, and whirlpools are standard equipment in many spa resorts, with the main objective being to relax and strengthen the body and mind, and to prevent development of disease (196).

For the efficacy of thermal therapy, the results varied with the concerned disease and the thermal station. Therapeutic effects of thermal waters are due to the combination of chemical, physical, immunological, and microbiological properties. Dermatologic diseases frequently treated by balneotherapy with a high rate of success are psoriasis and atopic dermatitis (198). Other conditions treated by balneotherapy include acne vulgaris, lichen planus, pruritus, rosacea, seborrheic dermatitis, and xerosis (198). However, for non-specific chronic low back pain, the effect of thermal therapy on short-term pain reduction is not superior to any control treatment except for ultra-sound treatment (197). Low back pain is another non-inflammatory musculoskeletal disease that benefits from short and long-term effects of spa therapy (196).

2.5.3 Contraindication in Thermalism and Thalassotherapy

General contraindications for thermalism and thalassotherapy should also be considered (196). These contraindications include severe psychiatric conditions, acute alcoholic states, cardiac dysrhythmias, epilepsy, inadequate balance, severe varicose veins, open wounds, and hypersensitivity to mineral baths (197). Furthermore, hyperthermic immersion might produce potentially dangerous cardiovascular effects, such as ectopic beats and excessive tachycardia (196). Some diseases such as contagious infection, kidney stone, gallstone, and more, are contraindicated in thermalism and thalassotherapy. These therapies are also not recommended to pregnant women or those breastfeeding. A consultation with a doctor before these therapies is necessary. Although, many publications reported some benefits of thalassotherapy in psoriasis treatment, or of thermal therapy for the relief of rheumatic pain, the effectiveness of these methods of traditional therapy is not widely accepted by many healthcare professionals.

2.7 Discussion About Water

Water is the chief source of food and also the essential nutrient for every living organism on this planet. Among different beverages, tap water and bottled mineral water are the most consumed worldwide, mostly in industrialized countries. They are safe to drink and also contain most essential minerals for the body. Keeping the right level of water in the body is important to maintain health and to avoid many diseases. Too little or too much water in the body will disrupt homeostasis and create a disturbance in the functioning of all cells and organs. However, the lack of potable tap water in developing countries is also the source of many illnesses and infectious diseases. The use of well water or rainwater in these countries also needs competent technicians and financial support. It is important to resolve the problems of water scarcity in many areas of this planet due to absence of water sources.

The use of some specific seawater and natural mineral water (spring water) by bathing, called thalassotherapy and thermalism, respectively, are traditional therapies still used in Europe today for the treatment of rheumatism, gout, psoriasis, and asthma. Their therapeutic effects depend on the source of each natural water. However, these traditional therapies are not recognized by modern medicine.

3 REFERENCES

1. Guarro J., Gené J., Stchigel A.M. (1999). Developments in Fungal Taxonomy. *Clin. Microbiol. Rev.*, **12**(3): 454–500.
2. McGinnis M.R., Tyring S.K. (1996). Introduction to Mycology. In: *Medical Microbiology*. 4th edition. Editor: S. Baron. University of Texas Medical Branch at Galveston, Galveston, TX. www.ncbi.nlm.nih.gov/books/NBK8125/.
3. Cole G.T. (1996). Chapter 73: Basic Biology of Fungi. In: *Medical Microbiology*. 4th edition. Editor: S. Baron. University of Texas Medical Branch at Galveston, Galveston, TX. www.ncbi.nlm.nih.gov/books/NBK8099/.
4. Karki G. (2017). Fungi: Characteristics and Classification, August 15. www.onlinebiologynotes.com/fungi-characteristics-classification/.
5. Boa E. (2004). Wild Edible Fungi. A Global Overview of Their Use and Importance to People. In: *Non-Wood Forest Products*. Food and Agriculture Organization of the United Nations, Rome, 157 pages. www.fao.org/3/a-y5489e.pdf.
6. Tedersoo L., Sánchez-Ramírez S., Kõljalg U., Bahram M., Doring M., Schigel D., May T., Ryberg M., Abarenkov K. (2018). High-Level Classification of the Fungi and a Tool for Evolutionary Ecological Analyses. *Fungal Divers.*, **90**: 135–159.
7. Cavalier-Smith T. (2001). What Are Fungi? In: *Systematics and Evolution. The Mycota (A Comprehensive Treatise on Fungi as Experimental Systems for Basic and Applied Research)*, Volume 7A. Editors: D.J. McLaughlin, E.G. McLaughlin, P.A. Lemke. Springer, Berlin, Heidelberg. https://doi.org/10.1007/978-3-662-10376-0_1.

8. Naranjo-Ortiz M.A., Gabaldon T. (2019). Fungal Evolution: Diversity, Taxonomy and Phylogeny of the Fungi. *Biol. Rev.*, **94**: 2101–2137.

9. Blackwell M. (2011). The Fungi: 1, 2, 3. . . 5.1 Million Species? *Am. J. Botany*, **98**(3): 426–438.

10. Rahi D.K., Malik D. (2016). Diversity of Mushrooms and Their Metabolites of Nutraceutical and Therapeutic Significance. *J. Mycol.*, Article ID 7654123, 18 pages.

11. Mygind P.H., Fischer R.L., Schnorr K.M., Hansen M.T., Sonksen C.P., Ludvigsen S., Raventos D., Buskov S., Christensen B., De Maria L., Taboureau O., Yaver D., Elvig-Jørgensen S.G., Sørensen M.V., Christensen B.E., Kjærulff S., Frimodt-Moller N., Lehrer R.I., Zasloff M., Kristensen H-H. (2005). Plectasin Is a Peptide Antibiotic with Therapeutic Potential from a Saprophytic Fungus. *Nature*, **437**(13): 975–980.

12. Chávez R., Fierro F., García-Rico R.O., Laich F. (2011). Chapter 5. Mold-Fermented Foods: Penicillium spp. as Ripening Agents in the Elaboration of Cheese and Meat Products, pp. 73–98. In: *Mycofactories.* Editor: Ana Lucia Monterio Durao Leitão. Bentham Science Publishers Ltd, Portugal.

13. Rathee S., Rathee D., Rathee D., Kumar V., Rathee P. (2012). Mushrooms as Therapeutic Agents. *Braz. J. Pharmacog.*, **22**(2): 459–474.

14. Köhler J.R., Hube B., Puccia R., Casadevall A., Perfect J.R. (2017). Fungi That Infect Humans. *Microbiol. Spectrum*, **5**(3): 29 pages. FUNK-0014–2016.

15. Kalac P. (2009). Chemical Composition and Nutritional Value of European Species of Wild Growing Mushrooms: A Review. *Food Chem.*, **113**: 9–16.

16. Rai M., Tidke G., Wasser S.P. (2005). Therapeutic Potential of Mushrooms. *Nat. Prod. Rad.*, **4**(4): 246–257.

17. Wasser S.P. (2002). Medicinal Mushrooms as a Source of Antitumor and Immunomodulating Polysaccharides. *Appl. Microbiol. Biotechnol.*, **60**: 258–274.

18. Lindequist U., Niedermeyer T.H.J., Julich W-D. (2005). The Pharmacological Potential of Mushrooms. *ECAM (Evidence-Based Complementary and Alternative Medicine)*, **2**(3): 285–299.

19. Elsayed E.A., El Enshasy H., Wadaan M.A., Aziz R. (2014). Mushrooms: A Potential Natural Source of Anti-Inflammatory Compounds for Medical Applications. *Mediators Inflamm.*, **2014**: 805841, 15 pages.

20. Zhang J.J., Li Y., Zhou T., Xu D.P., Zhang P., Li S., Li H.B. (2016). Bioactivities and Health Benefits of Mushrooms Mainly from China. *Molecules*, **21**(7): 938, 16 pages.

21. Chaichian S., Moazzami B., Sadoughi F., Kashani H.H., Zaroudi M., Asemi Z. (2020). Functional Activities of Beta-Glucans in the Prevention or Treatment of Cervical Cancer. *J. Ovarian Res.*, **13**(24): 1–12.

22. Rahar S., Swami G., Nagpal N., Nagpal M.A., Singh G.S. (2011). Preparation, Characterization, and Biological Properties of β-Glucans. *J. Adv. Pharm. Technol. Res.*, **2**(2): 94–103.

23. Novak M., Vetvicka V. (2008). β-Glucans, History, and the Present: Immunomodulatory Aspects and Mechanisms of Action. *J. Immunotoxicol.*, **5**(1): 47–57.

24. Lee H., Nam K., Zahra Z., Farooqi M.Q.U. (2020). Potentials of Truffles in Nutritional and Medicinal Applications: A Review. *Fungal Biol. Biotechnol.*, **7**: 9, 17 pages.

25. Wang S., Marcone M.F. (2011). The Biochemistry and Biological Properties of the World's Most Expensive Underground Edible Mushroom: Truffles. *Food Res. Int.*, **44**: 2567–2581.

26. Enshasy H.E., Elsayed E.A., Aziz R., Wadaan M.A. (2013). Mushrooms and Truffles: Historical Biofactories for Complementary Medicine in Africa and in the Middle East. *Evid Based Complement. Alternat. Med.*, **2013**, Article ID 620451, 10 pages.

27. Yamanaka T., Yamada A., Furukawa H. (2020). Advances in the Cultivation of the Highly-Prized Ectomycorrhizal Mushroom Tricholoma Matsutake. *Mycoscience*, **61**: 49–57.

28. Wang Y., Yu F., Zhang C., Li S. (2017). Tricholoma Matsutake: An Edible Mycorrhizal Mushroom of High Socioeconomic Relevance in China. *Scientia Fungorum*, **46**: 55–61.

29. Palmén J. (2016). Matsutake: Mushroom of the Year – or Millenium? *Fungi*, **8**(5): 41–48.

30. Li Q., Zhang L., Li W., Li X., Huang W., Yang H., Zheng L. (2016). Chemical Compositions and Volatile Compounds of *Tricholoma Matsutake* from Different Geographical Areas at Different Stages of Maturity. *Food Sci. Biotechnol.*, **25**: 71–77.

31. Liu G., Wang H., Zhou B., Guo X., Hu X. (2010). Compositional Analysis and Nutritional Studies of *Tricholoma Matsutake* Collected from Southwest China. *J. Med. Plants Res.*, **4**(12): 1222–1227.

32. Geng X., Tian G., Zhang W., Zhao Y., Zhao L., Wang H., Ng T.B. (2016). A Tricholoma Matsutake Peptide with Angiotensin Converting Enzyme Inhibitory and Antioxidative Activities and Antihypertensive Effects in Spontaneously Hypertensive Rats. *Sci. Rep.*, **6**(24130): 1–9.

33. Hou Y., Ding X., Hou W., Zhong J., Zhu H., Ma B., Xu T., Li J. (2013). Anti-Microorganism, Anti-Tumor, and Immune Activities of a Novel Polysaccharide Isolated from Tricholoma Matsutake. *Pharmacogn. Mag.*, **9**(35): 244–249.

34. Kozarski M., Klaus A., Vunduk J., Zizak Z., Niksic M., Jakovljevic D., Vrvic M.M., Van Griensven L.J.L.D. (2015). Nutraceutical Properties of the Methanolic Extract of Edible Mushroom Cantharellus Cibarius (Fries): Primary Mechanisms. *Food Funct.*, **6**: 1875–1886.

35. Vlasenko V., Turmunkh D., Ochirbat E., Budsuren D., Nyamsuren K., Samiya J., Ganbaatar B., Vlasenko A. (2019). Medicinal Potential of Extracts from the Chanterelle Mushroom, Cantharellus Cibarius (Review) and Prospects for Studying Its Strains from Differs Plant Communities of Ultra-Continental Regions of the Asia. *BIO Web of Conferences*, **16**(00039): 1–4. https://doi.org/10.1051/bioconf/20191600039.

36. Muszyńska B., Kała K., Firlej A., Sułkowska-Ziaja K. (2016). Cantharellus Cibarius – Culinary-Medicinal Mushroom Content and Biological Activity. *Acta Pol. Pharm.*, **73**(3): 589–598.

37. Falandysz J., Drewnowska M. (2015). Macro and Trace Elements in Common Chanterelle (Cantharellus Cibarius) Mushroom from the European Background Areas in Poland: Composition, Accumulation, Dietary Exposure and Data Review for Species. *J. Environ. Sci. Health B.*, **50**(5): 374–387.

38. Falandysz J., Chudzińska M., Barałkiewicz D., Drewnowska M., Hanć A. (2017). Toxic Elements and Bio-Metals in Cantharellus Mushrooms from Poland and China. *Environ. Sci. Pollut. Res.*, **24**(12): 11472–11482.

39. Tietel Z., Masaphy S. (2018). True Morels (Morchella) – Nutritional and Phytochemical Composition, Health Benefits and Flavor: A Review. *Crit. Rev. Food Sci. Nutr.*, **58**(11): 1888–1901.

40. Sushant Sud Vd., Khyati S. Sud Vd. (2017). A Review of Toxic Effects and Aphrodisiac Action of Morchella Esculenta (Wild Morel-Guchhi Mushroom) – A Himalayan Delight. *Eur. J. Pharm. Med. Res.*, **4**(8): 726–730.

41. Du X.H., Zhao Q., Yang Z.L. (2015). A Review on Research Advances, Issues, and Perspectives of Morels. *Mycology*, **6**(2): 78–85.

42. Li X.P., Li J., Li T., Liu H., Wang Y. (2020). Species Discrimination and Total Polyphenol Prediction of Porcini Mushrooms by Fourier Transform Mid-Infrared (FT-MIR) Spectrometry Combined with Multivariate Statistical Analysis. *Food Sci. Nutr.*, **8**(2): 754–766.

43. Ciesla W.M. (2002). Chapter 9. Non-Wood Products from Organisms Associated with Temperate Broad-Leaved Trees. In: *Non-Wood Forest Products from Temperate Broad-Leaved Trees. Non-Wood Forest Products 15.* FAO, Rome. www.fao.org/3/y4351e/y4351e0d.htm#bm13.

44. Dentinger B.T.M., Ammirati J.F., Both E.E., Desjardin D.E., Halling R.E., Henkel T.W., Moreau P-M., Nagasawa E., Soytong K., Taylor A.F., Watlingm R., Moncalvo J-M., McLaughlin D.J. (2010). Molecular Phylogenetics of Porcini Mushrooms (Boletus Section Boletus). *Mol. Phylogenet. Evol.*, **57**: 1276–1292.

45. Vamanu E., Nita S. (2013). Antioxidant Capacity and the Correlation with Major Phenolic Compounds, Anthocyanin, and Tocopherol Content in Various Extracts from the Wild Edible Boletus Edulis Mushroom. *Biomed Res. Int.*, **2013**: 313905.

46. Jaworska G., Pogoń K., Skrzypczak A., Bernaś E. (2015). Composition and Antioxidant Properties of Wild Mushrooms Boletus Edulis and Xerocomus Badius Prepared for Consumption. *J. Food Sci. Technol.*, **52**(12): 7944–7953.

47. Mayell M. (2001). Maitake Extracts and Their Therapeutic Potential. A Review. *Altern. Med. Rev.*, **6**(1): 48–60.

48. Ulbricht C., Weissner W., Basch E., Giese N., Hammerness P., Rusie-Seamon E., Varghese M., Woods J. (2009). Maitake Mushroom (Grifola Frondosa): Systematic Review by the Natural Standard Research Collaboration. *J. Soc. Integr. Oncol.*, **7**(2): 66–72.

49. Svagelj M., Berovic M., Gregori A., Wraber B., Simcic S., Boh B. (2012). Immunomodulating Activities of Cultivated Maitake Medicinal Mushroom Grifola Frondosa (Dicks.: Fr.) S.F. Gray (Higher Basidiomycetes) on Peripheral Blood Mononuclear Cells. *Int. J. Med. Mushrooms*, **14**(4): 377–383.

50. Zhuang C., Wasser S.P. (2004). Medicinal Value of Culinary-Medicinal Maitake Mushroom *Grifola Frondosa* (Dicks.: Fr.) S.F. Gray (Aphyllophoromycetideae). *Review. Int. J. Med. Mushrooms,* **6**(4): 287–314.

51. He Y., Zhang L., Wang H. (2019). The Biological Activities of the Antitumor Drug Grifola Frondosa Polysaccharide. *Prog. Mol. Biol. Transl. Sci.*, **163**: 221–261.

52. Muszynska B., Kala K., Rojowski J., Grzywacz A., Opoka W. (2017). Composition and Biological Properties of *Agaricus Bisporus* Fruiting Bodies – a Review. *Pol. J. Food Nutr. Sci.*, **67**(3): 173–181.

53. Dhamodharan G., Mirunalini S. (2010). A Novel Medicinal Characterization of *Agaricus Bisporus* (White Button Mushroom). *Pharmacologyonline*, **2**: 456–463.

54. Bhushan A., Kulshreshtha M. (2018). The Medicinal Mushroom *Agaricus Bisporus*: Review of Phytopharmacology and Potential Role in the Treatment of Various Diseases. *J. Nat. Sci. Med.*, **1**: 4–9.

55. Blumfield M., Abbott K., Duve E., Cassettari T., Marshall S., Fayet-Moore F. (2020). Examining the Health Effects and Bioactive Components in Agaricus Bisporus Mushrooms: A Scoping Review. *J. Nutr. Biochem.*, **84**: 108453.

56. Munshi N.A., Dar G.H., Ghani M.Y., Kauser S., Mughal N. (2010). *Button Mushroom Cultivation*. Shere-Kashmir University of Agricultural Sciences and Technology of Kashmir, Shalimar, India, 28 pages. file:///C:/Users/NOUVEA~1/AppData/Local/Temp/sk-mushroom.pdf.

57. Wisitrassameewong K., Karunarathna S.C., Thongklang N., Zhao R., Callac P., Moukha S., Ferandon C., Chukeatirote E., Hyde K.D. (2012). Agaricus Subrufescens: A Review. *Saudi J. Biol. Sci.*, **19**: 131–146.

58. Pardo-Giménez A., Pardo J.E., Dias E.S., Danny Lee Rinker, Caitano C.E.C., Zied C.D. (2020). Optimization of Cultivation Techniques Improves the Agronomic Behavior of *Agaricus Subrufescens*. *Sci. Rep.*, **10**: 8154, 9 pages.

59. Lisiecka J., Sobieralski K., Siwulski M., Jasińska A. (2013). Almond Mushroom *Agaricus Brasiliensis* (Wasser et al.). Properties and Culture Conditions. *Acta Sci. Pol.*, **12**(1): 27–40.

60. Hobbs C.R. (2000). Medicinal Value of Lentinus Edodes (Berk.) Sing. (Agaricomycetideae). A Literature Review. *Int. J. Med. Mushrooms*, **2**: 287–302.

61. Finimundy T., Dillon A., Henriques J., Ely M. (2014). A Review on General Nutritional Compounds and Pharmacological Properties of the *Lentinula Edodes* Mushroom. *Food Nutr. Sci.*, **5**: 1095–1105.

62. Bisen P.S., Baghel R.K., Sanodiya B.S., Thakur G.S., Prasad G.B. (2010). Lentinus Edodes: A Macrofungus with Pharmacological Activities. *Curr. Med. Chem.*, **17**(22): 2419–2430.

63. Ziaja-Sołtys M., Radzki W., Nowak J., Topolska J., Jabłonska-Ryś E., Sławinska A., Skrzypczak K., Kuczumow A., Bogucka-Kocka A. (2020). Processed Fruiting Bodies of Lentinus Edodes as a Source of Biologically Active Polysaccharides. *Appl. Sci.*, **10**: 470, 12 pages. doi:10.3390/app10020470.

64. Chen L., Gong Y., Cai Y., Liu W., Zhou Y., Xiao Y., Xu Z., Liu Y., Lei X., Wang G., Guo M., Ma X., Bian Y. (2016). Genome Sequence of the Edible Cultivated Mushroom *Lentinula Edodes* (Shiitake) Reveals Insights into Lignocellulose Degradation. *PLoS One*, **11**(8): e0160336, 12 pages.

65. Ina K., Kataoka T., Ando T. (2013). The Use of Lentinan for Treating Gastric Cancer. *Anticancer Agents Med. Chem.*, **13**: 681–688.

66. Stephany M.P., Chung S., Handler M.Z., Handler N.S., Handler G.A., Schwartz R.A. (2016). Shiitake Mushroom Dermatitis: A Review. *Am. J. Clin. Dermatol.*, **17**: 485–489.

67. Paul C., Roy T., Das N. (2017). Potentiality of Oyster Mushroom (Pleurotus Spp.) in Medicine- A Review. *Ann. Food Process Preserv.*, **2**(2): 1014, 8 pages.

68. Patel Y., Naraian R., Singh V.K. (2012). Medicinal Properties of Pleurotus Species (Oyster Mushroom): A Review. *World J. Fungal & Plant Biol.*, **3**(1): 1–12.

69. Oloke J.K., Adebayo E.A. (2015). Effectiveness of Immunotherapies from Oyster Mushroom (Pleurotus Species) in the Management of Immunocompromised Patients. *Int. J. Immunol. Special Issue: Immunotherapy*, **3**(2–1): 8–20.

70. Waktola G., Temesgen T. (2020). Pharmacological Activities of Oyster Mushroom (Pleurotus Ostreatus). *Novel Res. Microbiol. J.*, **4**(2): 688–695.

71. Adebayo E.A., Oloke J.K. (2017). Oyster Mushroom (Pleurotus Species); A Natural Functional Food. *J. Microbiol. Biotech. Food Sci.*, **7**(3): 254–264.

72. Dicks L., Ellinger S. (2020). Effect of the Intake of Oyster Mushrooms *(Pleurotus ostreatus)* on Cardiometabolic Parameters-A Systematic Review of Clinical Trials. *Nutrients*, **12**(4): 1134.

73. Tesfay T., Godifey T., Mesfin R., Kalayu G. (2020). Evaluation of Waste Paper for Cultivation of Oyster Mushroom (*Pleurotus ostreatus*) with Some Added Supplementary Materials. *AMB Expr.*, **10**: 15, 8 pages.

74. Sekara A., Kalisz A., Grabowska A., Siwulski M. (2015). *Auricularia* Spp. – Mushrooms as Novel Food and Therapeutic Agents – A Review. *Sydowia*, **67**: 1–10.

75. Zhao Y., Wang L., Zhang D., Li R., Cheng T., Zhang Y., Liu X., Wong G., Tang Y., Wang H., Gao S. (2019). Comparative Transcriptome Analysis Reveals Relationship of Three Major Domesticated Varieties of *Auricularia Auricula-Judae*. *Sci. Rep.*, **9**: 78, 13 pages.

76. Bandara A.R., Rapior S., Mortimer P.E., Kakumyan P., Hyde K.D., Xu J. (2019). – A Review of the Polysaccharide, Protein and Selected Nutrient Content of Auricularia, and Their Potential Pharmacological Value. *Mycosphere*, **10**(1): 579–607.

77. Priya R.U., Geetha D., Darshan S. (2016). Biology and Cultivation of Black Ear Mushroom – *Auricularia* Spp. *Adv. Life Sci.*, **5**(22): 10252–10254.

78. Wachtel-Galor S., Yuen J., Buswell J.A., Benzie I.F.F. (2011). Chapter 9. Ganoderma Lucidum (Lingzhi or Reishi): A Medicinal Mushroom. In: *Herbal Medicine: Biomolecular and Clinical Aspects*. 2nd edition. Editors: I.F.F. Benzie, S. Wachtel-Galor. CRC Press/Taylor & Francis, Boca Raton, FL.

79. Wasser S.P. (2005). Reishi or Ling Zhi (Ganoderma lucidum), pp. 603–622. In: *Encyclopedia of Dietary Supplements*. Marcel Dekker Publisher, New York. doi:10.1081/E-EDS-120022119.

80. Jin X., Ruiz Beguerie J., Sze D.M., Chan G.C. (2016). Ganoderma Lucidum (Reishi Mushroom) for Cancer Treatment. *Cochrane Database Syst. Rev.*, **4**: CD007731.

81. Santesso N., Wieland L.S. (2016). Ganoderma Lucidum (Reishi Mushroom) for the Treatment of Cancer. *Eur. J. Integr. Med.*, **8**(5): 619–620.

82. Klupp N.L., Chang D., Hawke F., Kiat H., Cao H., Grant S.J., Bensoussan A. (2015). *Ganoderma Lucidum* Mushroom for the Treatment of Cardiovascular Risk Factors (Review). *Cochrane Database Syst. Rev.* (2), Art. No: CD007259, 38 pages.

83. Cruz A., Pimentel L., Rodríguez-Alcalá L.M., Fernandes T., Pintado M. (2016). Health Benefits of Edible Mushrooms Focused on Coriolus Versicolor: A Review. *J. Food Nutr. Res.*, **4**(12): 773–781.

84. Cui J., Chisti Y. (2003). Polysaccharopeptides of Coriolus Versicolor: Physiological Activity, Uses, and Production. *Biotechnol. Adv.*, **21**: 109–122.

85. Habtemariam S. (2020). *Trametes Versicolor* (Synn. *Coriolus Versicolor*) Polysaccharides in Cancer Therapy: Targets and Efficacy. *Biomedicines*, **8**(5): 135.

86. Saleh M.H., Rashedi I., Keating A. (2017). Immunomodulatory Properties of Coriolus Versicolor: The Role of Polysaccharopeptide. *Front. Immunol.*, **8**(1087): 1–12.

87. Maehara Y., Tsujitani S., Saeki H., Oki E., Yoshinaga K., Emi Y., Morita M., Kohnoe S., Kakeji Y., Yano T., Baba H. (2012). Biological Mechanism and Clinical Effect of Protein-Bound Polysaccharide K (KRESTIN): Review of Development and Future Perspectives. *Surg. Today*, **42**: 8–28.

88. Yue K., Ye M., Zhou Z., Sun W., Lin X. (2013). The Genus Cordyceps: A Chemical and Pharmacological Review. *J. Pharm. Pharmacol.*, **65**(4): 474–493.

89. Das G., Shin H-S., Leyva-Gómez G., Prado-Audelo M.L.D., Cortes H., Singh Y.D., Panda M.K., Mishra A.P., Nigam M., Saklani S., Chaturi P.K., Martorell M., Cruz-Martins N., Sharma V., Garg N., Sharma R., Patra J.K. (2021). Cordyceps Spp.: A Review on Its Immune-Stimulatory and Other Biological Potentials. *Front. Pharmacol.*, **11**: 602364, 31 pages.

90. Wang X.L., Yao Y.J. (2011). Host Insect Species of Ophiocordyceps Sinensis: A Review. *Zookeys*, **127**: 43–59.

91. Liu H-J., Hua H-B., Chu C., Li Q., Li P. (2011). Morphological and Microscopic Identification Studies of Cordyceps and Its Counterfeits. *Acta Pharm. Sin. B*, **1**(3): 189–195.

92. Chen B., Sun Y., Luo F., Wang C. (2020). Bioactive Metabolites and Potential Mycotoxins Produced by *Cordyceps* Fungi: A Review of Safety. *Toxins (Basel)*, **12**(6): 410.

93. Wan J., Li Y., Chen D., Yu B., Zheng P., Mao X., Yu J., He J. (2016). Expression of a Tandemly Arrayed Plectasin Gene from Pseudoplectania Nigrella in Pichia Pastoris and its Antimicrobial Activity. *J. Microbiol. Biotechnol.*, **26**(3): 461–468.

94. Graeme K.A. (2014). Mycetism: A Review of the Recent Literature. *J. Med. Toxicol.*, **10**(2): 173–189.

95. Ukwuru M.U., Muritala A., Eze L.U. (2018). Edible and Non-Edible Wild Mushrooms: Nutrition, Toxicity and Strategies for Recognition. *J. Clin. Nutr. Metab.*, **2**: 2, 9 pages.

96. Lima A.D.L., Costa Fortes R., Garbi Novaes M.R.C., Percário S. (2012). Poisonous Mushrooms: A Review of the Most Common Intoxications. *Nutr. Hosp.*, **27**(2): 402–408.

97. Jo W.S., Hossain M.A., Park S.C. (2014). Toxicological Profiles of Poisonous, Edible, and Medicinal Mushrooms. *Mycobiology*, **42**(3): 215–220.

98. Bever C.S., Swanson K.D., Hamelin E.I., Filigenzi M., Poppenga R.H., Kaae J., Cheng L.W., Stanker L.H. (2020). Rapid, Sensitive, and Accurate Point-of-Care Detection of Lethal Amatoxins in Urine. *Toxins*, **12**(123), 10 pages.

99. Kurtzman C.P., Fell J.W., Boekhout T. (2011). *The Yeasts: A Taxonomic Study*. 5th edition. Elsevier, Amsterdam, 2354 pages.

100. Kurtzman C.P., Mateo R.Q., Kolecka A., Theelen B., Robert V., Boekhout T. (2015). Advances in Yeast Systematics and Phylogeny and Their Use as Predictors of Biotechnologically Important Metabolic Pathways. *FEMS Yeast Res.*, **15**(6): 1–17.

101. Schneiter R. (2004). Genetics, Molecular and Cell Biology of Yeast. Université de Fribourg, Suisse, January, 85 pages. www.unifr.ch/biochem/assets/files/schneiter/cours/Yeast/YeastGenetics.pdf.

102. Phale S. (2018). Yeast: Characteristics and Economic Significance. *J. Bioprocess Biotech.*, **8**: 5.

103. Parapouli M., Vasileiadis A., Afendra A.S., Hatziloukas E. (2020). *Saccharomyces Cerevisiae* and Its Industrial Applications. *AIMS Microbiol.*, **6**(1): 1–31.

104. Abbas C.A. (2006). Chapter 10. Production of Antioxidants, Aromas, Colours, Flavours, and Vitamins by Yeasts, pp. 285–334. In: *The Yeast Handbook. Yeasts in Food and Beverages*. Editors: Amparo Querol, Graham H. Fleet. © Springer-Verlag, Berlin Heidelberg, 453 pages.

105. Orlean P. (2012). Architecture and Biosynthesis of the Saccharomyces Cerevisiae Cell Wall. *Genetics*, **192**: 775–818.

106. Dashko S., Zhou N., Compagno C., Piskur J. (2014). Why, When and How Did Yeast Evolve Alcoholic Fermentation? *FEMS Yeast Res.*, **14**(6): 826–832.

107. Swiegers J.H., Bartowsky E.J., Henschke P.A., Pretorius I.S. (2005). Microbial Modulation of Wine Aroma and Flavour. *Aust. J. Grape Wine Res.*, **11**: 139–173.

108. Pires E.J., Teixeira J.A., Brányik T., Vicente A.A. (2014). Yeast: The Soul of Beer's Aroma – A Review of Flavour-Active Esters and Higher Alcohols Produced by the Brewing Yeast. *Appl. Microbiol. Biotechnol.*, **98**(5): 1937–1949.

109. Ali A., Shehzad A., Khan M.R., Shabbir M.A., Amjid M.R. (2012). Yeast, Its Types and Role in Fermentation During Bread Making Process-A Review. *Pak. J. Food Sci.*, **22**(3): 171–179.

110. Madhavi B.R. (2016). Probiotic Milk – A Review. *Res. Rev. J. Food Dairy Technol. (RRJFPDT)*, **4**(3): 1–11.

111. Gao P., Xia W., Li X., Liu S. (2019). Use of Wine and Dairy Yeasts as Single Starter Cultures for Flavor Compound Modification in Fish Sauce Fermentation. *Front Microbiol.*, **10**: 2300, 13 pages.

112. Devanthi P.V.P., Gkatzionis K. (2019). Soy Sauce Fermentation: Microorganisms, Aroma Formation, and Process Modification. *Food Res. Int.*, **120**: 364–374.

113. McFarland L.V. (2010). Systematic Review and Meta-Analysis of *Saccharomyces Boulardii* in Adult Patients. *World J. Gastroenterol.*, **16**(18): 2202–2222.

114. Walker R.S.K., Pretorius I.S. (2018). Applications of Yeast Synthetic Biology Geared Towards the Production of Biopharmaceuticals. *Genes (Basel)*, **9**(7): 340, 22 pages.

115. Nielsen J. (2013). Production of Biopharmaceutical Proteins by Yeast: Advances Through Metabolic Engineering. *Bioengineered*, **4**(4): 207–211.

116. Nandy S.K., Srivastava R.K. (2018). A Review on Sustainable Yeast Biotechnological Processes and Applications. *Microbiol. Res.*, **207**: 83–90.

117. Jeffery-Smith A., Taori S.K., Schelenz S., Jeffery K., Johnson E.M., Borman A., *Candida Auris* Incident Management Team, Manuel R., Brown C.S. (2018). *Candida Auris*: A Review of the Literature. *Clin. Microbiol. Rev.*, **31**: e00029–17, 18 pages.

118. Cortegiani A., Misseri G., Fasciana T., Giammanco A., Giarratano A., Chowdhary A. (2018). Epidemiology, Clinical Characteristics, Resistance, and Treatment of Infections by *Candida Auris*. *J. Intensive Care*, **6**: 69, 13 pages.

119. Lone S.A., Ahmad A. (2019). Candida Auris-the Growing Menace to Global Health. *Mycoses*, **62**(8): 620–637.

120. Ashley P., Williams E. (U.S. Department of Housing and Urban Development Office of Healthy Homes and Lead Hazard Control). (2006). Healthy Homes Issues: Mold. Version 3.37 pages, March. www.hud. gov/sites/documents/DOC_12483.PDF.

121. Parrott K. (2009). *Mold Basics*. Virginia Polytechnic Institute and State University. www.pubs.ext. vt.edu/content/dam/pubs_ext_vt_edu/2901/2901-7019/2901-7019_pdf.pdf.

122. National Institute of Environmental Health Sciences. (2020). Mold, January 17. www.niehs.nih.gov/ health/topics/agents/mold/index.cfm.

123. Campbell A.W. (2016). Molds and Mycotoxins: A Brief Review. *Altern. Ther. Health Med.*, **22**(4): 8–11.

124. Kuhn D.M., Ghannoum M.A. (2003). Indoor Mold, Toxigenic Fungi, and Stachybotrys Chartarum: Infectious Disease Perspective. *Clin. Microbiol. Rev.*, **16**(1): 144–172.

125. Bennett J.W, Klich M. (2003). Mycotoxins. *Clin. Microbiol. Rev.*, **16**(3): 497–516.

126. Bush R.K., Portnoy J.M., Saxon A., Terr A.I., Wood R.A. (2006). The Medical Effects of Mold Exposure. *J. Allergy Clin. Immunol.*, **117**: 326–333.

127. Caillaud D., Leynaert B., Keirsbulck M., Nadif R. (2018). Indoor Mould Exposure, Asthma and Rhinitis: Findings from Systematic Reviews and Recent Longitudinal Studies. *Eur. Respir. Rev.*, **27**: 170137, 18 pages.

128. Quansah R., Jaakkola M.S., Hugg T.T., Heikkinen S.A.M., Jaakkola J.J.K. (2012). Residential Dampness and Molds and the Risk of Developing Asthma: A Systematic Review and Meta-Analysis. *PLoS One*, **7**(11): e47526.

129. Whiley H., Gaskin S., Schroder T., Ross K. (2018). Antifungal Properties of Essential Oils for Improvement of Indoor Air Quality: A Review. *Rev. Environ. Health*, **33**(1): 63–76.

130. Bennett J.W. (2017). Aspergillus: Molecular Biology and Genomics. In: *Brewing Microbiology: Current Research, Omics and Microbial Ecology*. Editors: Nicholas A. Bokulich, Charles W. Bamforth. Caister Academic Press, June, 332 pages.

131. Bbosa G.S., Kitya D., Lubega A., Ogwal-Okeng J., Anokbonggo W.W., Kyegombe D.B. (2013). Chapter 12. Review of the Biological and Health Effects of Aflatoxins on Body Organs and Body Systems, pp. 239–265. In: *Aflatoxins: Recent Advances and Future Prospects*. Editor: Mehdi Razzaghi-Abyaneh. IntechOpen, London, UK.

132. Benkerroum N. (2020). Chronic and Acute Toxicities of Aflatoxins: Mechanisms of Action. *Int. J. Environ. Res. Public Health*, **17**(2): 423, 28 pages.

133. Rushing B.R., Selim M. (2019). Aflatoxin B1: A Review on Metabolism, Toxicity, Occurrence in Food, Occupational Exposure, and Detoxification Methods. *Food Chem. Toxicol.*, **124**: 81–100.

134. Kowalska A., Walkiewicz K., Kozieł P., Muc-Wierzgoń M. (2017). Aflatoxins: Characteristics and Impact on Human Health. *Postepy Hig Med Dosw (Online).*, **71**: 315–327.

135. Eskola M., Kos G., Elliott C.T., Hajšlová J., Mayar S., Krska R. (2020). Worldwide Contamination of Food-Crops with Mycotoxins: Validity of the Widely Cited 'FAO Estimate' of 25%. *Crit. Rev. Food Sci. Nutr.*, **60**(16): 2773–2789.

136. Gallo A., Giuberti G., Frisvad J.C., Bertuzzi T., Nielsen K.F. (2015). Review on Mycotoxin Issues in Ruminants: Occurrence in Forages, Effects of Mycotoxin Ingestion on Health Status and Animal Performance and Practical Strategies to Counteract Their Negative Effects. *Toxins (Basel)*, **7**(8): 3057–3111.

137. Awasti N., Anand S. (2020). The Role of Yeast and Molds in Dairy Industry: An Update, pp. 243–262. In: *Dairy Processing: Advanced Research to Applications*. Editors: J. Minj, V.A. Sudhakaran, A. Kumari. Springer, Singapore. https://doi.org/10.1007/978-981-15-2608-4_12.

138. Bourdichon F., Casaregola S., Farrokh C., Frisvad J.C., Gerds M.L., Hammes W.P., Harnett J., Huys G., Laulund S., Ouwehand A., Powell I.B., Prajapati J.B., Seto Y., Schure E.T., Van Boven A.V., Vankerckhoven V., Zgoda A., Tuijtelaars S., Hansen E.B. (2012). Food Fermentations: Microorganisms with Technological Beneficial Use. *Int. J. Food Microbiol.*, **154**: 87–97.

139. Show P.L., Oladele K.O., Siew Q.Y., Zakry F.A.A., Lan J.C-W., Ling T.C. (2015). Overview of Citric Acid Production from *Aspergillus Niger. Front. Life Sci.*, **8**(3): 271–283.

140. Pham J.V., Yilma M.A., Feliz A., Majid M.T., Maffetone N., Walker J.R., Kim E., Cho H.J., Reynolds J.M., Song M.C., Park S.R., Yoon Y.J. (2019). A Review of the Microbial Production of Bioactive Natural Products and Biologics. *Front Microbiol.*, **10**, Art. 1404, 27 pages.

141. Demain A., Martens E. (2017). Production of Valuable Compounds by Molds and Yeasts. *J. Antibiot.*, **70**: 347–360.

142. Muñiz C.C., Zelaya T.E.C., Esquivel G.R., Fernández F.J. (2007). Penicillin and Cephalosporin Production: A Historical Perspective. *Microbiologia*, **49**(3–4): 88–98.

143. Kadurina M., Bocheva G., Tonev S. (2003). Penicillin and Semisynthetic Penicillins in Dermatology. *Clin. Dermatol.*, **21**: 12–23.

144. Nath A.P., Balasubramanian A., Ramalingam K. (2020). Cephalosporins: An Imperative Antibiotic Over the Generations. *Int. J. Res. Pharm. Sci.*, **11**(1): 623–629.

145. Venkata Dasu V., Panda T. (1999). Studies on Production of Griseofulvin. *Bioprocess Eng.*, **21**: 489–495.

146. Alkeswani A., Cantrell W., Elewski B. (2019). Treatment of Tinea Capitis. *Skin Appendage Disord.*, **5**: 201–210.

147. Olson J.M., Troxell T. (2020). Griseofulvin. In: *StatPearls [Internet]*. StatPearls Publishing, Treasure Island, FL, January 2021. www.ncbi.nlm.nih.gov/books/NBK537323/.

148. Tedesco D., Haragsim L. (2012). Cyclosporine: A Review. *J. Transplant.*, **2012**, Article ID 230386, 7 pages.

149. Yang X., Feng P., Yin Y., Bushley K., Spatafora J.W., Wang C. (2018). Cyclosporine Biosynthesis in Tolypocladium Inflatum Benefits Fungal Adaptation to the Environment. *mBio9*, **9**(5): e01211–18, 14 pages.

150. Survase S.A., Kagliwal L.D., Annapure U.S., Singhal R.S. (2011). Cyclosporin A. A Review on Fermentative Production, Downstream Processing and Pharmacological Applications. *Biotechnol. Adv.*, **29**: 418–435.

151. Sadeg N., Pham-Huy C., Martin C., Warnet J.M., Claude J.R. (1993). Effect of Cyclosporin A and Its Metabolites and Analogs on Lipid Peroxidation in Rabbit Renal Microsomes. *Drug Chem. Toxicol.*, **16**: 165–174.

152. Sadeg N., Pham-Huy C., Martin C., Warnet J.M., Claude J.R. (1994). In Vitro Comparative Study on Nephrotoxicity of Cyclosporin A, Its Metabolites M1, M17, M21, and Its Analogues: Cyclosporins C and D in Suspensions of Rabbit Renal Cortical Cells. *Drug Chem Toxicol.*, **17**: 93–111.

153. Massicot F., Pham- Huy C., Martin C., Thevenin M., Warnet J.M., Claude J.R. (1991). Inhibitory Effects of a Platelet Activating Factor-Antagonist 48740RP in Cyclosporin-Induced Nephrotoxicity in the Rat as Assessed by Renal Glutathione Metabolism Parameters. *Arch. Toxicol. Suppl.*, **14**: 213–217.

154. Massicot F., Lamouri A., Martin C., Pham-Huy C., Warnet J.M., Claude J.R. (1997). Preventive Effects of Two PAF-Antagonists, PMS 536 and PMS 549, on Cyclosporin-Induced LLC-PK1 Oxidative Injury. *J. Lipid Mediat. Cell Signal.*, **15**: 203–214.

155. Massicot F., Martin C., Dutertre-Catella H., Ellouk-Achard S., Pham- Huy C., Warnet J.M., Claude J.R. (1997). Modulation of Energy Status and Cytotoxicity Induced by FK506 and Cyclosporin A in a Renal Epithelial Cell Line. *Arch. Toxicol.*, **71**(8): 529–531.

156. Ellouk-Achard S., Martin C., Pham- Huy C., Duc H.T., Thevenin M., Dutertre-Catella H., Warnet J.M., Claude J.R. (1997). Implication of CYP 3A in the Toxicity of Cyclosporin G (CsG), Cyclosporin A (CsA) and FK506 on Rat Hepatocytes in Primary Culture. *Arch. Toxicol.*, **71**(7): 437–442.

157. Sadeg N., Pham-Huy C., Postaire M., Lebrec H., Broyer M., Gagnadoux M.F., Fischer A., Claude J.R., Hamon M. (1989). Study of Cyclosporine Blood Levels in Patients After Kidney or Bone-Marrow Transplantation. Comparison Between the Two Methods, Fluorescent Polarization Immunoassay and Radioimmunoassay (in French). *Ann. Pharm. Fr.*, **47**: 5–15.

158. Sadeg N., Pham-Huy C., Postaire M., Claude J.R., Hamon M. (1991). Clinical Utility of Cyclosporine Concentrations Determined in Recipients of Small-Bowel Transplant by HPLC and Fluorescence Polarization Immunoassay. *Clin. Chem.*, **37**(2): 291.

159. Sadeg N., Pham-Huy C., Rucay P., Righenzi S., Halle-Pamenko O., Claude J.R., Bismuth H., Duc H.T. (1993). In Vitro and in Vivo Comparative Studies on Immunosuppressive Properties of Cyclosporines A, C, D and Metabolites M1, M17, and M21. *Immunopharmacol. Immunotoxicol.*, **15**(2–3): 163–177.

160. Saada V., Pham-Huy C., Voisin J., Righenzi S., Rucay P., Claude J.R., Duc H.T. (1996). Comparative Evaluation of in Vitro and in Vivo Immunosuppressive Potential of Cyclosporin G with Cyclosporin A and FK-506. *Int. J. Immunopharmacol.*, **18**(1): 79–87.

161. Pham-Huy C., Sadeg N., Becue T., Martin C., Mahuzier G., Warnet J-M., Hamon M., Claude J.R. (1995). In Vitro Metabolism of Cyclosporin A with Rabbit Renal or Hepatic Microsomes: Analysis by HPLC-FPIA and HPLC-MS. *Arch. Toxicol.*, **69**(5): 346–349.

162. Endo A. (2010). A Historical Perspective on the Discovery of Statins. *Proc. Jpn. Acad. Ser. B Phys. Biol. Sci.*, **86**(5): 484–493.

163. Steinberg D. (2006). An Interpretive History of the Cholesterol Controversy, Part V: The Discovery of the Statins and the End of the Controversy. *J. Lipid Res.*, **47**: 1339–1351.

164. Hajar R. (2011). Statins: Past and Present. *Heart Views*, **12**(3): 121–127.

165. Shi Y-C., Pan T-M. (2011). Beneficial Effects of Monascus Purpureus NTU 568-Fermented Products: A Review. *Appl. Microbiol. Biotechnol.*, **90**: 1207–1217.

166. Zhu B., Qi F., Wu J., Yin G., Hua J., Zhang Q., Qin L. (2019). Red Yeast Rice: A Systematic Review of the Traditional Uses, Chemistry, Pharmacology, and Quality Control of an Important Chinese Folk Medicine. *Front. Pharmacol.*, **10**: 1449.

167. Klimek M., Wang S., Ogunkanmi A. (2009). Safety and Efficacy of Red Yeast Rice (Monascus purpureus) as an Alternative Therapy for Hyperlipidemia. *P&T® (Pharmacy and Therapeutics)*. **34**(6): 313–317.

168. Becker D.J., Gordon R.Y. (2011). The Lipid-Lowering Properties of Red Yeast Rice. *AMA J. Ethics (American Medical Association Journal of Ethics)*, **13**(6): 365–368.

169. Zimmerman M., Snow B. (2012). Chapter 7: Nutrients Important to Fluid and Electrolyte Balance, pp. 335–402. In: *An Introduction to Nutrition*, 812 pages. https://2012books.lardbucket.org/pdfs/an-introduction-to-nutrition.pdf.

170. Thompson J.L., Manore M.M., Vaughan L.A., Editors (2011). Chapter 9. Nutrients Involved in Fluid and Electrolyte Balance, pp. 323–355. In: *The Science of Nutrition*. 2nd edition. Pearson Benjamin Cummings, San Francisco, 942 pages.

171. Jequier E., Constant F. (2010). Water as an Essential Nutrient: The Physiological Basis of Hydration. *Eur. J. Clin. Nutr.*, **64**: 115–123.

172. Popkin B.M., D'Anci K.E., Rosenberg I.H. (2010). Water, Hydration and Health. *Nutr. Rev.*, **68**(8): 439–458.

173. Keren Y., Magnezi R., Carmon M., Amitai Y. (2020). Investigation of the Association Between Drinking Water Habits and the Occurrence of Women Breast Cancer. *Int. J. Environ. Res. Public Health*, **17**: 7692, 11 pages.

174. Vandentorren S., Bretin P., Zeghnoun A., Mandereau-Bruno L., Croisier A., Cochet C., Riberon J., Siberan I., Declercq B., Ledrans M. (2006). August 2003 Heat Wave in France: Risk Factors for Death of Elderly People Living at Home. *Eur. J. Public Health*, **16**(6): 583–591.

175. Centers for Disease Control and Prevention (CDC). (2015). Water Treatment, January 20. www.cdc.gov/healthywater/drinking/public/water_treatment.html.

176. Bowyer J.L. (2018). Environmental Impacts of Tap vs. Bottled Water. Dovetail Partners Consuming Responsibly Report No. 1, September 10. www.mwra.state.ma.us/monthly/wscac/2018/113018-Dovetail ConsumeRespIWater.pdf.

177. Pham-Huy C., Nadji F., Postaire M., Hamon M. (1991). Determination of Fluorides and Fluorophosphates in Drugs, Toothpastes and Mineral Waters by Gas Liquid Chromatography. *Ann. Pharm. Fr.*, **49**(3): 139–150. French.

178. Bouygues-de-Ferran A.M., Pham-Huy C., Postaire M., Hamon M. (1991). Determination of Trace Amounts of Fluoride in Raw Materials for Pharmaceuticals by Gas-Liquid Chromatography. *J. Chromatogr. A*, **585**(2): 289–295.

179. Everett E.T. (2011). Fluoride's Effects on the Formation of Teeth and Bones, and the Influence of Genetics. *J. Dent. Res.*, **90**(5): 552–560.

180. Burden R. (Food Standards Agency, U.K.). (2007). The Natural Mineral Water, Spring Water and Bottled Drinking Water (England) Regulations 2007 No. 2785 (as amended). Revised July 2010. www.legislation.gov.uk/uksi/2007/2785/pdfs/uksi_20072785_en.pdf.

181. Quattrini S., Pampaloni B., Brandi M.L. (2016). Natural Mineral Waters: Chemical Characteristics and Health Effects. *Clin. Cases Miner. Bone Metab.*, **13**(3): 173–180.

182. Azoulay A., Garzon P., Eisenberg M.J. (2001). Comparison of the Mineral Content of Tap Water and Bottled Waters. *J. Gen. Intern. Med.*, **16**(3): 168–175.

183. Glazier D.S. (2009). Springs, pp. 734–755. In: *Encyclopedia of Inland Waters.* Editor: Gene E. Likens. Academic Press, 2250 pages. ISBN 9780123706263. https://doi.org/10.1016/B978-012370626-3.00259-3.

184. Rosborg I., Nihlgård B., Ferrante M. (2015). Mineral Composition of Drinking Water and Daily Uptake. Chapter 2, pp. 25–31. In: *Drinking Water Minerals and Mineral Balance.* Editor: I. Rosborg. Springer International Publishing, Switzerland.

185. Olivares M., Uauy R. (2005). Essential Nutrients in Drinking Water. Chapter 4, pp. 41–60. In: *Nutrients in Drinking Water.* World Health Organization, Geneva, 186 pages.

186. Association of Public Health Laboratories (APHL, USA). (2019). Private Well Sampling and Testing. A Guide for Public Health Laboratories, 31 pages. www.aphl.org/aboutAPHL/publications/Documents/EH-Nov2019-Private-Well-Water-Testing-Guide.pdf.

187. Ramirez E., Robles E., Gonzalez M.E., Martinez M.E. (2010). Microbiological and Physicochemical Quality of Well Water Used as a Source of Public Supply. *Air, Soil Water Res.*, **3**: 105–112.

188. Adler I., Campos L.C., Hudson-Edwards K.A. (2011). Converting Rain into Drinking Water: Quality Issues and Technological Advances. *Water Sci. Technol. Water Supply*, **11**(6): 659–667.

189. Amin M.T., Alazba A.A. (2011). Probable Sources of Rainwater Contamination in a Rainwater Harvesting System and Remedial Options. *Aust. J. Basic & Appl. Sci.*, **5**(12): 1054–1064.

190. Maraver F., Karagulle M.Z., Editors (2012). *Medical Hydrology and Balneology: Environmental Aspects.* UCM, Balnea, N° **6**, 465 pages.

191. Bender T., Karagülle Z., Bálint G.P., Gutenbrunner C., Bálint P.V., Sukenik S. (2005). Hydrotherapy, Balneotherapy, and Spa Treatment in Pain Management. *Rheumatol. Int.*, **25**(3): 220–224.

192. van Tubergen A., van der Linden S. (2002). A Brief History of Spa Therapy. *Ann. Rheum. Dis.*, **61**: 273–275.

193. Charlier R.H., Chaineux M-C.P. (2009). The Healing Sea: A Sustainable Coastal Ocean Resource: Thalassotherapy. *J. Coastal Res.*, **25**(4): 838–856.

194. Halevy S., Sukenik S. (1998). Different Modalities of Spa Therapy for Skin Diseases at the Dead Sea Area. *Arch. Dermatol.*, **134**: 1416–1420.

195. Munteanu C., Munteanu D. (2019). Thalassotherapy Today. *Balneo Res. J.*, **10**(4): 440–444.

196. Nasermoaddeli A., Kagamimori S. (2005). Balneotherapy in Medicine: A Review. *Environ. Health Prev. Med.*, **10**(4): 171–179.

197. Wittenwiler S., Stoop R., Hohenauer E., Clijsen R. (2018). Thermal Therapy in Patients Suffering from Non-Specific Chronic Low Back Pain – A Systematic Review. *Int. J. Clin. Med.*, **9**: 294–314.

198. Cacciapuoti S., Luciano M.A., Megna M., Annunziata M.C., Napolitano M., Patruno C., Scala E., Colicchio R., Pagliuca C., Salvatore P., Fabbrocini G. (2020). The Role of Thermal Water in Chronic Skin Diseases Management: A Review of the Literature. *J. Clin. Med.*, **9**(9): 3047, 19 pages.

8 Lifestyle and Diet

1 DEFINITION OF LIFESTYLE AND DIET

Lifestyle can also be written as life-style or life style (1–2). Different definitions of lifestyle are found in the literature. According to Dictionary.com, lifestyle is the habits, attitudes, tastes, moral standards, economic level, and more, that together constitute the mode of living of an individual or group (1). From the Collins Dictionary, the lifestyle of a particular person or group of people is the living conditions, behavior, and habits that are typical of them or chosen by them (2).

In the field of sociology, lifestyle is a mode of living chosen by an individual, a society, or a nation, and is shaped by its economic, geographical, political, cultural, and religious context (3). Lifestyle reflects the characteristics of individuals or inhabitants of a region in a particular time and place. It includes day-to-day behaviors and functions of individuals in jobs, activities, fun, and diet (3). An individual can, in the form of different practices, express him- or herself through their choice of lifestyle (4). Lifestyle may also include opinions of an individual or a group of individuals regarding the environment, philosophy, religion, health, politics, and so on. In brief, lifestyle is the manner of living, being, and thinking of a person or a society. Examples include the lifestyles of city-dwellers and villagers, of rich and poor countries, of religious believers and non-believers, and so on.

In the field of health, lifestyle includes choice of foods, physical activity, leisure, sleeping duration, and the use of alcohol, cigarettes, abuse drugs (cocaine, heroin, etc.). It also includes choice of diet, habitation, temperament, and behaviors with family, coworkers, friends, and neighbors (3–4). For example, the choice of meal preparation such as cooking at home, eating at a restaurant, buying packaged food or fast food, may influence the health. Daily physical activities such as walking, jogging, cycling, gymnastic, dancing, and oriental gymnastics like tai-chi and yoga can play a role in health maintenance or disease development. The lifestyle of a society may influence the lifestyle of an individual. For example, in a country where there are many public transits such as bus, metro, bicycle, public health is often better than that of a country where people always go to work by individual car or motorcycle. The environment and climate also play an important role in health and disease. The pollution in industrialized countries is the main cause of numerous dreadful diseases such as cancer, cardiovascular diseases, pulmonary affection, and so on. Indeed, the healthy lifestyle of an individual first depends on his or her proper lifestyle choice, and secondarily on his or her environment. Individual genetic factors also play a role in health and disease, but are of lesser importance than his or her daily lifestyle.

In recent decades, lifestyle as an important factor of health has gained more interest by researchers. According to the World Health Organization (WHO), 60% of related factors to individual health and quality of life are correlated to lifestyle (3). The habits of eating, moving, working, thinking, entertaining, and sleeping play important roles in health and disease. Therefore, lifestyle and lifespan of an individual as well as of a population are closely linked. For a similar situation (race, economy, geography, climate, environment), the difference in health and disease between individuals mainly depend on the choice of lifestyle. However, many people in this world cannot chose their lifestyle due to poverty, and lack of food, water, medicines, and hygiene in their countries or their environment. However, this does not mean that rich individuals or people in rich countries live healthier or have longer lifespans than poor people. For example, pollution due to the emission of toxic gas from factories, mines, and cars, is a main concern of people living in rich industrialized countries today.

DOI: 10.1201/9781003220817-8

2   LIFESTYLE IN HEALTH AND DISEASE

There are two forms of lifestyle: healthy lifestyle (or good habits) and unhealthy lifestyle (or bad habits). The choice between these two forms of lifestyle depends on the habits of each individual and also on those of his or her environment, including family, society, nation, climate, economy, religion, and so on. In other terms, the lifestyle of a person or a community encompasses habits of choosing foods and physical activities that are suitable for him, her, or them. An individual can, in the form of different practices, express him- or herself through many lifestyles; for example, choice of food and drink, choice of physical activities (sport, dance, walking), choice of leisure, and more (4). For food and drink, each individual has the choice between 'good' foods and 'bad' foods. The choice between these two eating modes depends not only on the money, the available time, and the scientific knowledges of each person, but also on the influence of his or her family, society, or religion. It is important to realize that many other lifestyle and environmental factors, in addition to nutrition, influence health and well-being, but nutrition is a major, modifiable, and powerful factor in promoting health, preventing and treating disease, and improving quality of life (5).

Lifestyle is not only a public health issue; it is also a medical and clinical care issue. Lifestyle medicine is not just about preventing chronic disease but also about treating it, often more effectively and less expensively than relying only on drugs and surgery (6). Lifestyle intervention is often more effective in reducing cardiovascular disease, hypertension, heart failure, stroke, cancer, diabetes, obesity, dementia, and all-cause mortality than almost any other medical intervention (6). Lifestyle is the best medicine when applied correctly. Our lifestyle and environment influence the fundamental biological mechanisms in our body leading to disease development (6). For example, tobacco smokes, car smokes, industrial pollution, and barbecue meat, can change gene expression leading to cancer. The distinction between risk factors and causes of a disease is an important thing for a doctor to do. High blood pressure, hypercholesterolemia, hyperglycemia, are common signs of disease, and are called biological markers or risk factors. Among different causes of these biological marker anomalies, lifestyle may be the first question to ask (6). For example, bad diet, lack of exercise, insomnia, smoking, alcoholism, and stress may be the cause of hypertension, diabetes, atherosclerosis, and so on. Typically, doctors treat 'risk factors' for disease such as giving a list of medications to lower high blood pressure, elevate blood sugar, and high cholesterol (6). However, in many cases, changing lifestyle may resolve these problems. The INTERHEART study, published in the famous scientific journal *The Lancet* in 2004, followed 30,000 people and found that changing lifestyle could prevent at least 90% of all heart disease (6). In other words, unhealthy lifestyle is often the underlying cause of many chronic diseases. According to a recent cohort study in the United Kingdom (7) among older adults without cognitive impairment or dementia, both an unfavorable lifestyle and high genetic risk were significantly associated with higher risk of dementia. A favorable lifestyle was associated with a lower dementia risk among participants with a high genetic risk. Briefly, favorable lifestyle means no tobacco smoking, healthy diet, regular physical activity, and moderate alcohol consumption, and an unfavorable lifestyle is the opposite of the previous definition (7).

2.1   HEALTHY LIFESTYLE

As mentioned previously, a healthy lifestyle encompasses a nutrient-rich diet, regular physical activity, adequate sleep, and good choice of hobby. It avoids tobacco, drugs of abuse (heroin, cocaine, cannabis), and limits alcohol drink, fast foods, packaged foods, sugary drinks, and over-the-counter medicines or dietary supplements. It also supports the environment, limits the use of pesticides, plastic bags, and so on. Many public health organizations recommend the importance of healthy lifestyles because they may prevent or cure some chronic diseases such as cardiovascular diseases, cancer, diabetes, obesity, and more (3, 6, 8–10).

2.1.1 Food Choice

Eating does not mean satisfying the mouth or filling the stomach. The choice of foods and eating modes determines to a great extent the health and the disease of an individual as well as of a population. According to the World Health Organization (WHO 2002), many diseases such as cardiovascular disease (CVD), ischemic stroke, diabetes, and some specific cancers, which until recently were common only in high-income countries, are now becoming the dominant sources of morbidity and mortality worldwide (8). In addition, rates of cancers and CVD among migrants from low-risk to high-risk countries almost always increase dramatically. In traditional African societies, for example, CVD is virtually nonexistent, but rates among African Americans are similar to those among Caucasian Americans (8). These striking changes in rates within countries over time and among migrating populations indicate that the primary determinants of these diseases are not genetic but environmental factors, including diet and lifestyle (8). Therefore, choice of food plays an important role in the prevention or the apparition of some chronic diseases (8–10).

2.1.1.1 *Fruit and Vegetable Choice*

Many public health organizations in the world recommend that all people consume five or more fruits and vegetables per day in order to maintain health and to avoid chronic diseases such as CVDs, obesity, and cancer. Fruits and vegetables are well known to be rich in vitamins, minerals, and antioxidants. These compounds fight or neutralize the excess of free radicals produced by the body through oxidative stress, which is the cause of numerous diseases. To prevent these diseases, the first recommendation is to eat fruits and vegetables regularly. Unfortunately, many people on this planet, even in rich and developed countries, do not know or do not have the habits to consume fruits and vegetables regularly each day. For example, some statistics revealed that the difference in lifestyle between France and the United States regarding the consumption of fruits and vegetables is the following: about 44% of French people consume more than five servings of fruits and vegetables per day, whereas approximately 24% of Americans do this (11). In addition, about 70% of the French drink less than one glass of sweetened beverage per day; only 37% of Americans meet this guideline (11). As a result, among French adults, 17% are obese, and among American adults, 34% are obese (11). These rates of obesity track well with deaths from coronary heart disease. The French retain their position of having one of the lowest incidence of CVD in the world (men: 73 per 100,000; women: 17 per 100,000, the lowest in the world), and the United States remains in the middle of a 37-country comparison (men: 174 per 100,000; women: 73 per 100,000) (11). Americans rank right behind Eastern Europe, China, Scotland, Ireland, and England. This rank has not changed over the past 15 years, despite the enormous time and effort that has been directed toward improving the health of Americans (11). This difference in health between these two developed populations is mainly due to habits of food consumption. However, in recent years in the United States, fruit and vegetables have become a cornerstone of healthy dietary recommendations; the 2015–2020 U.S. Dietary Guidelines for Americans recommend that fruit and vegetables constitute one-half of the plate at each meal (12). Fruit and vegetables include a diverse collection of plant foods that vary in their energy, nutrient, and dietary bioactive contents. They have potential health-promoting effects beyond providing basic nutrition needs in humans (12). Therefore, World Health Organization (WHO) recommends eating ≥400 g per day of fruits and vegetables, not counting potatoes and other starchy tubers such as cassava (13). Many epidemiological studies have shown that high intakes of fruit and vegetables are associated with a lower risk of chronic inflammatory diseases; particularly, cardiovascular disease, Type 2 diabetes, premature mortality, and certain cancers of the mouth, pharynx, larynx, esophageal, stomach, colon, and lungs (12–13).

In comparison with omnivorous people, vegetarians and vegans are at reduced risk of certain health conditions, including heart disease, diabetes, hypertension, cancer, and obesity (14). However, vegans need vitamin B-12 supplements because plant foods (except algae and seaweed) do not contain vitamin B12 (14). Therefore, no individual food or food group has all of the nutrients needed to support life. However, consuming a mixture of plant and animal source foods is optimal for achieving nutrient intakes required for growth, development, reproduction, and longevity, because humans are omnivorous (12).

Many health organizations such as the American Institute for Cancer Research, the American Heart Association, and the US Department of Agriculture Food and Nutrition Service have advocated eating 'the rainbow' of healthy food-based colors (15). In nature, many fruits and vegetables have different colors and/or flavors. Some of these colored or flavored fruits and vegetables are considered a good source of antioxidant compounds; for example, anthocyanins, an antioxidant group of phenolic compounds are responsible for red, blue, and purple colors in fruits and vegetables (16–20). Carotenoids, another antioxidant group, are associated with red or orange colors, while chlorophyll antioxidants present in leaf and peel give green color to fruits and vegetables (16). Therefore, consumers must include various colors on their plate to obtain various antioxidants, vitamins, and minerals.

The roles of fruits and vegetables in health and disease are now well known, however, the choice of fruits and vegetables for consumption is a subject that is still not well understood by a majority of the population. Most fruits and vegetables have different colors and savors. For example, grapefruit has in general three colors: dark red, pink, and green. Which color among them is better for health? Keep in mind that the color of an organic compound depends on the conjugated systems of the double bonds present in its chemical structure. In other word, conjugated systems have unique properties that give rise to strong colors (21). Conjugation is possible by means of alternating single and double bonds (21). Regarding the chemical structure of an antioxidant, the number of double bonds or conjugated double bonds in side chain and/or in heterocyclic ring plays an important role in its antioxidant activity. Therefore, the colors of fruits, tubers, and leaves, are in relation to their antioxidant activity. In general, the more pronounced the color, the higher the antioxidant activity. For example, blackberry contains more antioxidants than strawberry; black or red grapes are richer in resveratrol, a red polyphenol antioxidant, than green grape; yellow or purple sweet potatoes are better for health than white sweet potatoes, and so on. However, if you prefer savor and flavor, many green grapes are sweeter and more delicious than dark grapes. So, the choice between these grapes depends on your preference: health or pleasure. White sweet potatoes and colored sweet potatoes give the same calories, or energy, to the body, but colored sweet potatoes may defend the organism against free radicals for disease prevention more efficaciously than white sweet potatoes. In general, for the same fruit or vegetable with different colors, choose the one that is the most colorful. However, among different colored fruits, the choice depends on the biological role of each colored antioxidant present in this fruit. For example, yellow sweet potato is rich in carotenoid antioxidants which are used to prevent eye diseases and cancer; while purple sweet potato is rich in anthocyanin, a flavonoid polyphenol antioxidant, which is used to prevent CVDs, cancer, and so on. Red or pink fruits are generally high in lycopene, such as tomatoes, watermelon, cherry, gac (*Momordica cochinchinensis*), rosehip, papaya, pink guava, strawberry, pomegranate, pink grapefruit, and persimmon. Red cabbage and red kale contain more red anthocyanin antioxidants than green varieties. Various colored fruits and vegetables are described in Chapter 5 of this book.

The aroma and taste of fruits and vegetables are also due to the chemical compounds containing double bonds. For example, chili pepper, bell pepper, curcuma, galangal, ginger, and pepper containing many compounds rich in double bonds such as terpenoids and flavonoids, are strong antioxidants. These spicy vegetables are well known for the prevention and treatment of some chronic diseases such as CVDs, neurodegenerative diseases, inflammatory diseases, and cancer. Therefore, a diet containing multicolor fruits and different fragrant and spicy vegetables is considered a good choice.

Fruits and vegetables are not only rich in antioxidants, but also in vitamins and minerals. Most vitamins such as vitamin C, all vitamins of B group except vitamin B12, carotenoids, vitamins E and K are present in fruits and vegetables. All minerals (calcium, potassium, magnesium, selenium, phosphate, etc.) are also found in fruits and vegetables because most minerals are in soil. Many well-known diseases such as scurvy and beriberi are due to inadequate consumption of fruits and vegetables.

Nuts such as walnut, almond, cashew, peanut, pistachio, pecan, macadamia, Brazil nut, chestnut, and ginkgo nut are used mostly in cuisine or roasted as snack food. Nuts have a high oil content – mostly essential monounsaturated and polyunsaturated fatty acids – and are an excellent source of protein and amino acids, especially L-arginine. Regular consumption of nuts may reduce incidence of cardiovascular diseases. However, peanuts and walnuts can cause allergies in some people which can be particularly severe, even life-threatening, principally in young children (see Chapter 5).

Moreover, fruits and vegetables are rich in soluble and insoluble fibers that are necessary for the digestion and the prevention of diseases. The skins or peels of some fruits such as apple, grape, plum, prune, lemon, lime, and kiwi contain more vitamins, antioxidants, and insoluble fibers than their flesh or pulp, and are edible; therefore, do not discard them – eat them. Insoluble fibers in fruits and vegetables are called prebiotics. Prebiotic fibers are not digested in the small intestine, but are fermented in the large intestine where they are served as food for beneficial colon bacteria that are called probiotics. The roles of probiotics and prebiotics are described in Chapter 9 of this book.

The natural vitamins, minerals, and antioxidants present in food, especially in vegetables, fruits, nuts, mushrooms, are better than their corresponding synthetic compounds. For example, selenium is an essential mineral for the activities of many enzymes in the body. In some areas where soil is poor in selenium, a supplementation of this mineral in tablets is given to the population of this area. However, many poisonings of selenium are observed in people after selenium supplement intake. In contrast, when selenium is mixed with fertilizers for wheat or rice culture, the selenium poisoning does not occur because wheat or rice plants have transformed mineral selenium in soil into organic selenium which is more easily absorbed and eliminated by the human body. It is the same for mineral iodine in fortified salt, and organic iodine in sea foods. Japanese people are the highest consumers of iodine from seaweeds in the world. They eat about two to three mg of iodine per day from sea foods; about three times the Tolerable Upper Intake Level of iodine, without any toxicity because iodine in seaweeds and other sea foods is in organic form; hence, it is easily eliminated from the body (22). Another example has been cited in the scientific literature between vitamin E supplement and vitamin E in food. Some studies observed that vitamin E supplement was associated with a higher risk of stroke (23–24). However, one large clinical study suggested that vitamin E from foods, not supplements, may reduce the risk of death from stroke in postmenopausal women (23). In addition, there is a phenomenon called synergistic effect between many nutrients in fruits and vegetables. A vitamin used alone is less effective than the same vitamin in the presence of other vitamins or coenzymes. For example, a vitamin of B group used alone is less effective than the same vitamin used in the presence of other B group vitamins. For this reason, taking a B-complex vitamin, which includes all the B vitamins, is better than taking any vitamin B alone. Eating natural foods rich in vitamin B1 is the best choice, because in cereals and fruits, this vitamin is often accompanied with other vitamins of B group. So, avoid white rice without bran and replace it by brown or normal rice due to the presence of many vitamins of B group in bran.

Consuming fresh local fruits and vegetables is better than purchasing the same imported products from distant countries because many vitamins and antioxidants are easily deteriorated with time. Purchase organic fruits and vegetables, especially if they will be consumed entirely, such as grapes, berries, apricot, cherry, apple, lettuce, broccoli, tomato, and celery. In addition, canned fruits and canned vegetables are not good for health with regular consumption because they contain preservatives and their nutrients may be destroyed or diminished with time. It is the same for dried fruits and vegetables, excepted for some products that need heat to become edible or preserved such as cassava flour, seeds, nuts, prune, and date. Indeed, regular consumption of fresh fruits and vegetables are very necessary for the maintenance of health and the prevention of dreadful diseases. That is why many healthcare organizations around the world have intensely recommended eating five or more fruits and vegetables every day.

2.1.1.2   Meat Choice

There are many types of meat in the market such as beef, pork, poultry, fish, and seafoods. From a scientific point of view, meat is classified into two categories: red meat and white meat. Red meat is any meat obtained from mammalian animals such as beef, pork, lamb, veal, and goat; while white meat includes poultry, fish, and seafoods. In general, this classification is based on the concentration of myoglobin in the muscle fiber (25). Myoglobin is a complex protein like hemoglobin in red blood cells.

Concerning the choice of meat, many studies have revealed that white meat is better than red meat because white meat contains less saturated fats or bad fats than red meat (26–28). Some red meats are high in saturated fats, which raise blood cholesterol, especially LDL or bad cholesterol, thereby increasing the risk of CVDs, diabetes, and colon cancer (26–28). Moreover, red meats are often used to make processed meat like spam, sausage, saucisson, bacon, and so on. Processed meat is not only rich in saturated fats but also high in salt, nitrates, and preservatives, which can cause high blood pressure, colon cancer, CVDs, and more. The evidence-based conclusion is that high consumption of red meat, and especially processed meat, is associated with an increased risk of several major chronic diseases and preterm mortality (27–29). However, red meat is rich in calories, proteins, amino acids, vitamin B12, and iron. These nutrients are necessary for hematopoiesis, the development of muscle, and growth in young people. Red meat is a good source of vitamin B12, which does not exist in plants. So, moderate consumption of fat-free red meat, and avoiding frequent eating of processed meat like sausage, ham, and bacon, are the best choices to maintain good health and avoid many harmful diseases.

Fish and seafood are also a good source of energy for the body and contain a number of vitamins, especially vitamins A and D, fatty acids, antioxidants (astaxanthin), and minerals. In general, fish in saltwater is better than fish in freshwater because the first is higher in omega-3 fatty acids than the latter (30–31). Seafood like fish and crustaceans are rich in omega-3 unsaturated fatty acids such as docosahexaenoic acid (DHA) and eicosapentaenoic acid (EPA), which play an important role in health promotion and chronic disease prevention like cardiovascular disease, neurodegenerative disease, inflammatory disease, diabetes, and cancer. Moreover, seafood is good for brain development of the fetus and for pregnant women, because the brain needs DHA and EPA omega-3 unsaturated fatty acids for its functioning. Well-cooked whole sardines are also a good choice for bone health because they are rich in calcium, phosphate, and vitamin D. Many people in the world such as Inuit, Japanese, and Mediterranean populations have less incidence of cardiovascular diseases than others because their favorite foods are seafood. However, excessive intake of fish and shellfish can increase bleeding risks like epistaxis, cerebral hemorrhage, or cause hypoglycemia or hypotension, as observed in Inuit people who only eat seafood. Many international health organizations (World Health Organization, American Heart Association, Food and Agriculture Organization) have recommended to consume fatty fish, especially sea fish, at least two times a week for the prevention of cardiovascular and inflammatory diseases (31). On the other hand, seafood can contain toxic compounds such as mercury and industrial pollutants (dioxins and polychlorinated biphenyls, PCBs) when they are caught in sea near industrial zones or volcanoes (32). Therefore, the choice of seafood is important. In general, wild and small fishes such as salmon, sardine, anchovy, Atlantic mackerel, and Alaskan pollock, harvested in large oceans, are considered safe (33). Fish oil, a natural extract from sea fish, is often used as dietary supplement for the prevention of CVDs and inflammatory diseases such as asthma, rheumatoid arthritis, and more (34). An excess of fish oil or omega-3 fatty acids capsules is also harmful to the body because they can cause hemorrhage. Consult a doctor when using fish oil with other medicines to avoid incompatibility between them.

Poultry meat from chicken, duck, turkey, and goose is good food because it is not high in energy, but is rich in digestible proteins, and low in saturated or bad fats. In addition, it contains many vitamins of B-group, and minerals, especially zinc, selenium and copper and alpha-linoleic acid (ALA), a precursor of omega-3 unsaturated fatty acid. Poultry meat is suitable for overweight and obese people and the elderly. Poultry meat may also prevent cardiovascular diseases and Type 2 diabetes mellitus (35). Moreover, it is cheaper than beef, pork, and fish. However, poultry skin is richer in saturated fats or bad fats than poultry meat. So, discard poultry skin when consuming poultry meat. Besides meat, some organs of mammals (beef, pork) and poultry such as liver, heart, kidney, and stomach are edible and delicious. The levels of some nutrients such as coenzyme Q10 from these organs are found higher than those in corresponding meats. Coenzyme Q10, present in liver and heart of beef and pork, is more active than its synthetic supplement. It is a nutrient necessary for elderly people because its production in the human body decreases with age. Coenzyme Q10 is necessary for the activity of muscle, especially for heart activity.

Among different types of meat, fish and seafoods are the best meats of choice for everybody because they are low in saturated fats and rich in omega-3 fatty acids and other nutrients and minerals for the prevention of many chronic diseases, especially CVDs and inflammatory diseases such as asthma and rheumatoid arthritis.

The choice of different meats (beef, pork, poultry, fish, seafoods) often depends on the habits of an individual, but also on the lifestyle of a population or the laws of some religions. For example, people in Western countries prefer cow meat; beefsteak is the favorite dish for people in these countries. However, Chinese people tend to like pork meat; Japanese prefer fish and seafood; country dwellers choose poultry or freshwater fish. The choice of meat type may have an influence on the health of an individual or a population. Japanese and Mediterranean people have the longest lifespans in the world because their preferred foods are sea foods. Some religions in the world ban the consumption of certain meats (36). Indeed, the choice of meat type and processed meat plays an important role in the health of an individual as well as a population.

2.1.1.3   Egg Choice

Eggs sold in the market are mainly obtained from chicken and duck. All eggs are particularly rich in proteins, fats, cholesterol, lecithin (a glycerophospholipid), and many essential vitamins and minerals such as choline, lutein, zeaxanthin, vitamin A, vitamin B12, iron, and selenium. In general, duck eggs are bigger than chicken eggs; hence, duck eggs provide more nutrients than chicken eggs. That is why duck eggs have more fats and cholesterol than chicken eggs (37–38). On the other hand, duck eggs have approximately six times more vitamin B12 and about two times more iron than chicken eggs, making them a good food for treating anemia. The problem of egg intake is linked to the presence of cholesterol in yolk. However, most experimental, epidemiologic, and clinical studies to date have indicated very little association between a high egg intake and an increase in plasma total-cholesterol and cardiovascular disease or mortality in the general population (39–40). Egg remains a food product of high nutritional quality for adults including elderly people and children, and is extensively consumed worldwide. Most healthy people can eat up to seven chicken eggs a week with no increase in their risk of heart disease (41). However, for people who have diabetes, hypercholesterolemia, or heart disease, their daily egg intake is limited to three chicken eggs a week. A chicken egg weighs about 50 g, while a duck egg is about 70 g. Because eggs are cheap and rich in essential nutrients, moderation of egg intake is recommended for normal people. Indeed, choice of egg type (chicken egg or duck egg) and quantity of consumption depend on your cholesterol levels. More details of egg are described in Chapter 6 of this book.

2.1.1.4   Milk and Dairy Product Choice

Milk is a complete liquid food that Nature has designed for the growth of babies of all mammals, whether human or animal. Human milk contains not only all necessary nutrients but also all defensive materials such as antibodies, immune cells for the protection of babies against microbes during the first months of their life (42). Therefore, breastfeeding is the best choice for the nourishment of a baby. In a majority of countries in the world, humans continue to consume milk and its byproducts beyond infancy by using the milk of other animals such as cow, sheep, goat, and yak as a drink, or its byproducts like cheese, yogurt, and kefir as foods. However, many people in East Asia never consume milk from animals, from their infancy to adult life. That could explain their smaller size among adults and their frequent bone diseases like bone fractures, osteoporosis, and osteoarthritis in elderly people, because milk is the best source of soluble calcium, phosphate, magnesium, and other minerals and vitamins, especially vitamin D2, which are used for bone formation (43–45). Recently, many East Asian children and adults begin to change their lifestyle by drinking milk and eating cheese, yogurt, and so on, like other people in the world. Indeed, milk and dietary products are not only necessary for babies and children for their growth and their health, but also for adults and elderly people for the prevention of many diseases, in particular, bone diseases. Among dairy products, hard cheeses such as parmesan, gouda, cheddar, gruyere, Emmental, and pecorino, are the richest sources of calcium. Calcium in milk and hard cheese is better than calcium supplement found over the counter, because it is easily absorbable and cannot cause hypercalcemia or side effects, as often seen with calcium supplement. The use of calcium supplement must be managed by a physician in order to avoid its eventual side effects. Drinking a bowl of milk and a bit of cheese or yogurt each day is a good habit for health maintenance and disease prevention. Yogurt, cheese, and kefir are not only rich in nutrients but also contain many good bacteria called probiotics that are necessary for the good functioning of the digestive tract, especially the large intestine (46–47). However, whole cow's milk is rich in fats, therefore, people with hyperlipidemia or hypercholesterolemia are recommended to replace whole milk with fat-free or semi-skimmed milk.

Briefly, milk and dairy products are necessary for body growth, health maintenance, and disease prevention for everybody, and breastfeeding is the best nourishment for babies. In some Asian countries where the habits of consuming milk and dairy products are absent, the governments of these countries should encourage their populations to change their lifestyle by regularly consuming dairy products from infancy to old age for the sake of their health and their form.

2.1.1.5   Water Choice

In industrialized countries, there are two main types of potable water: tap water and bottled water (see Chapter 7). The latter includes natural mineral water and spring water. Tap water and bottled water contain a quantity of essential soluble minerals such as sodium, potassium, calcium, magnesium, iron, phosphate, chloride, fluoride, and more (48–51). Their composition and purity are controlled by health care offices. In general, tap water is often used to cook, while bottled water is destined to drink. For bottled water, natural mineral water is, in general, higher in minerals than spring water. The choice between these two types of bottled water depends on the preference of each individual and the availability of each bottled water type in the market. Maintaining the right level of water in the body is crucial to survival and to maintaining health. Too little or too much water in the body will create a disturbance in the functioning of all cells and organs. A male adult needs about 3 liters of water a day in different forms (pure water, beverages, soup, fruit liquid, etc.); a female adult needs average 2.2 liters/day, and a child 1 liter/day (49). The quantity of water consumed depends on the size, sex, age, physical activity, disease, and the climate where a person lives (49). Therefore, an appropriate supply of water is needed for health maintenance. In certain cases, water intake may decrease high blood pressure, diminish fever, or treat constipation. Drinking more water is necessary for the elderly and for people engaging in physical activity, especially during periods of hot weather. In industrialized countries, tap water has the same quality of hygiene and nutrients (minerals) as bottled mineral water. However, in developing countries, tap water does not exist or is not rigorously controlled; therefore, epidemics of cholera or dysentery are still observed in these areas.

2.1.1.6   Beverages

Beverages, or drinks, are artificial liquids and mainly include tea, coffee, fruit juices, soft drinks, energy drinks, and alcoholic drinks. Besides pure water, tea and coffee infusion are the drinks most consumed worldwide.

Tea is described in Chapter 4 of this book. Tea is primarily consumed in Asia, in particular in China, Japan, Korea, Vietnam, and India. The habitants of these countries drink about one to two liters of tea infusion a day. However, people in Western countries drink only about one to two cups of tea a day. People drink tea due not only to its aromatic flavor and thirst-quenching property, but also to its perceived health benefits. Tea is rich in polyphenols/catechins belonging to the flavan-3-ol class of flavonoids (50). These compounds may prevent numerous pathologies such as cancer, cardiovascular disorders, neurodegenerative diseases, dental caries, obesity, diabetes, and more. In addition, they are promising compounds in exhibiting antiviral activities against viruses such as influenza, hepatitis, herpes simplex virus, and HIV (human immunodeficiency viruses) (50–53). Tea has a slight stimulant effect, and is used to fight somnolence. Green tea is better than black tea and oolong tea because it contains more catechin antioxidants than the others. Bottled iced tea has no catechin antioxidants, contrary to tea infusion recently prepared, because catechins are easily oxidized by air with time (50).

Coffee is described in Chapter 4 of this book. It is an infusion of milled roasted coffee beans. Coffee contains two main compounds, chlorogenic acids and caffeine, as well as many minor compounds such as vitamins, minerals, alkaloids, and phenolic compounds (54–56). Caffeine or trimethylxanthine is a bitter purine alkaloid; while chlorogenic acids belong to a group of phenolic compounds. Coffee consumption may help prevent some chronic diseases such as Type 2 diabetes mellitus, Parkinson's disease, and liver disease. However, coffee consumption may cause high blood pressure, tachycardia, palpitation, and plasma homocysteine. For adults consuming moderate amounts of coffee (3–4 cups/d providing 300–400 mg/d of caffeine), there is little evidence of health risks and some evidence of health benefits. Excessive intake of coffee and tea can cause insomnia, palpitation, and hypertension due to caffeine. Do not take coffee during dinner to avoid insomnia.

Fruit juices are obtained from natural fruits and are divided into two groups: pure fruit juice and diluted fruit juice in syrup. Pure fruit juice does not have the same nutrients as corresponding whole fruit because some vitamins, antioxidants, and labile nutrients can disappear with time, such as vitamin C, polyphenols, some amino acids, and so on. However, from a health point of view, pure fruit juice is better than diluted juice because the latter is not only a diluted solution, but also contains sugar and preservatives which can cause obesity, excess weight gain, diabetes, and more.

Soft drinks, also called sparkling soft drinks, are not good for health and may cause many diseases such as obesity, diabetes, and dental caries with frequent consumption (see Chapter 4). Like soft drinks, energy drinks are non-alcoholic beverages containing caffeine, taurine, vitamins, herbal supplements, and sugar or sweeteners known to have stimulant properties. Consumption of alcohol is generally harmful to the body and will be discussed below. In brief, the choice of a drink, its quantity and frequency of consumption, depends on the habits of an individual and the lifestyle of a community. Keep in mind that your health depends not only on what is on your plate, but also what is in your cup.

2.1.1.7 Cooking Mode Choice

There are two main types of cooking: moist-heat cookery and dry heat cookery (57–64) (see chapter 4). The first mode uses water for heating foods such as boiling, simmering, steaming, braising, and stewing; while the second uses direct fire or oil for cooking like grilling, barbecuing, roasting, frying, and baking (57–64). From a health point of view, the first mode is better than the later. By dry-heat methods, the food obtained could contain toxic compounds formed during their preparation. The fumes produced by barbecuing or grilling are also carcinogenic and may cause lung cancer in cookers if regularly exposed. Frequent consumption of fried foods may cause obesity, CVDs, hypercholesterolemia, diabetes, and more. Boiling, steaming, simmering, and braising are the best choices for cooking meat and vegetables. For leafy vegetables, do not overcook them, and remember to eat the water used to cook vegetables because many nutrients in vegetables can pass into this liquid (63). Cooking at home is better than eating in restaurants because you can choose good quality foods, such as organic foods, fresh vegetables, wild fish, and so on. Consumers should pay attention to the role of cooking in health and disease (64).

2.1.2 Physical Activity

Physical activity plays an important role in health maintenance and disease prevention. It contributes to a healthy lifestyle (65–74). Physical activity means body movement or exercise. Physical activity is defined as any bodily movement, produced by skeletal muscles, that requires energy (65). Body movement requires more energy than resting. Walking, running, dancing, swimming, cycling, aerobics, climbing stairs, housework, gardening, tai chi, and yoga, are a few forms of body movement (65, 66). At any age, exercise plays a main role in health and well-being. Any body movement that works your muscles requires more energy than resting. Physical activity is not only reserved for athletes, children, and adults, but also for the elderly. Depending on the age, intensity of physical activity varies from simple walking to running or jogging, from simple movement like dance, aerobics, tai chi, and yoga to intensive sports like athletics, tennis, and so on (10, 65, 66). Among different physical activities, walking is the best choice for maintaining good health and preventing diseases from children to the elderly. Moreover, walking is economic and easy to practice everywhere and anytime. Indeed, the human body is built to move, and major systems, including the skeletal, muscular, metabolic, circulatory, digestive, and endocrine systems, do not develop and function properly unless stimulated by frequent physical activity. As such, physical activity has both a preventive and therapeutic effect across several diseases and conditions and contributes to quality of life in many ways (65–72). In general, normal individuals of all ages must do at least 30 minutes of moderate-intensity physical activity each day, 5 or more days a week (67–70). This level of physical activity should be maintained throughout adulthood in order to reduce the risk of chronic disease, and should be continued into old age for as long as capabilities allow, in order to counteract age-related losses in muscle and bone, deterioration of the cardiovascular system, and to decrease the risk of osteoporotic fractures (68). However, excessive physical activity is also not good for health and can cause diseases or even death.

2.1.2.1 Roles of Physical Activity in Health and Disease

Physical activity contributes to preventing cardiovascular diseases, cancer, and diabetes and has significant health benefits for heart, body, and mind (65–72). Physical activity reduces symptoms of depression and anxiety and enhances thinking, learning, and judgment skills (70). Physical activity ensures healthy growth and development in young people. Briefly, it improves overall well-being. Globally, one in four adults do not meet the global recommended levels of physical activity. Up to five million deaths per year could be avoided if the world's population was more active. People who are insufficiently active have a 20–30% increased risk of death compared to people who are sufficiently active. More than 80% of the world's adolescent population is insufficiently physically active (70). In addition, physical activity can modify body form favorably by decreasing fat mass and increasing lean mass (68). In contrast, physical inactivity is a modifiable risk factor for cardiovascular disease and a widening variety of other chronic diseases, including diabetes mellitus, cancer (colon and breast), obesity, hypertension, bone and joint diseases (osteoporosis and osteoarthritis), and depression (69, 70). For example, physically inactive middle-aged women (engaging in less than one hour of exercise per week) experienced a 52% increase in all-cause mortality, a doubling of cardiovascular related mortality, and a 29% increase in cancer-related mortality compared with physically active women (69). Inactivity is described as a 'silent killer'. It is evident that sedentary behavior, such as sitting or lying down for long periods to watch TV, use a computer, or drive a car, is bad for health (66).

2.1.2.1.1 Physical Activity and Cardiovascular Disease

For the cardiovascular system, physical activity can reduce resting blood pressure and increase capacity to carry blood in the coronary arteries. Regular physical activity can also exert beneficial effects on the body's capacity to form and break down blood clots, and it produces favorable changes in plasma lipid profile (68). Men maintaining an active lifestyle halve their risk of dying from, or contracting, serious heart diseases such as heart attack, angina pectoris. For women, the reduction in risk is between 30–40% (65).

A moderate-intensity aerobic activity for 150 minutes a week (25–30 min a day) can lower the risks of cardiovascular diseases (CVD) including hypertension and hypercholesterolemia for normal people (67). For people with cardiac issues, normal walking or slight aerobic activity done regularly may help the heart work better. It also may reduce the risk of a second heart attack in people who have already had heart attacks. Physical activity reduces the risk of CVD in a dose-dependent manner. Benefits are seen with regular moderate-intensity physical activity like walking; however, more intense exercise, like running for long periods, can increase risk of CVD further (68). Vigorous aerobic activity may not be safe for people who have CVD. Ask your doctor what types of physical activity are safe for you, especially if you have cardiac issues.

2.1.2.1.2 Physical Activity and Type 2 Diabetes For Type 2 diabetes (T2D), there is good evidence that being physically active improves blood glucose control and prevents or delays the onset of T2D. For example, in a study of almost 6,000 men, it was found that for every 500 calories expended weekly in leisure time physical activity, the risk of developing T2D was reduced by 6%. In a cohort of over 34,000 women, it was found that any level of physical activity reduced the risk of T2D compared with being sedentary (65). Physical activity independently reduces the risk of Type 2 diabetes by 33–50%. Those who are at high risk of T2D (e.g., the obese and those with impaired glucose tolerance) can benefit most from physical activity (68). Physical activity improves the ability of the liver, skeletal muscle, and fat cells to respond to insulin, known as insulin sensitivity. For example, exercise training for 16 weeks by older men resulted in a significant improvement of insulin sensitivity and fasting glycemia (65).

2.1.2.1.3 Physical Activity and Overweight and Obesity It is evident that greater physical activity is associated with less weight gain for young and adult people. It is likely that for many people, 45–60 minutes of moderate-intensity physical activity a day is necessary to prevent obesity (68). Physical activity alone is insufficient to cause weight loss, however, when combined with calorie-restricted diets, physical activity not only increases weight loss but also improves body form, maintaining metabolically active muscle, while increasing fat loss. It is obvious that a combination of regular physical activity and good diet allows for better reduction of obesity and overweight than any method used alone (65).

2.1.2.1.4 Physical Activity and Cancer Concerning cancer risk, physical activity has been shown to reduce the risk of a number of cancers. It is well established that physical activity reduces the risk of colon cancer (especially in men) and breast cancer (especially in post-menopausal women) (68–71). The 2018 the US Physical Activity Guidelines Advisory Committee found strong evidence that physical activity is associated with a lower risk of several additional cancer sites, including endometrial, bladder, esophageal adenocarcinoma, kidney, and gastric (71). There is also consistent evidence that physical activity reduces the risk of lung and endometrial cancers and some indication that physical activity can reduce the risk of advanced prostate cancer (68–70). Given this evidence, physical activity will play an increasingly important role in population-based cancer prevention efforts (71). Routine physical activity, whether occupational or leisure, is often associated with reductions in the incidence of overall risk of cancer. However, the evidence of a preventive effect is strongest for colon and breast cancer. Physically active men and women exhibited a 30–40% reduction in the relative risk of developing colon cancer, and physically active women a 20–30% reduction in the relative risk of developing breast cancer, compared to their inactive counterparts (68–71). Mechanisms by which physical activity may reduce cancer include: reducing inflammation (for example, reducing long-term inflammation of the gut, which may help reduce colon cancer); an improvement in the function of the immune system, which enables the individual to fight the cancer; and improved hormone balance, which reduces the use of hormones by cancer cells to grow and spread, such as in breast cancer (65). Most health care professionals encourage adults to adopt and maintain physical activity at recommended levels to lower risks of multiple cancers (71).

2.1.2.1.5   Physical Activity and Bone Health and Osteoporosis   For bone health and osteo-porosis risk, physical activity habits, particularly during growth periods including puberty, have a long-lasting effect on bone health in childhood. Activities such as running or skipping are the most effective in increasing bone strength for children. In older adults, slight physical activity such as walking, tai chi, and yoga, is important to counteract age-related decrease in bone mass. Physical activity can decrease the risk of osteoporotic fractures in older people, particularly if the activity increases muscle strength, balance, and co-ordination (68). Moreover, it produces strong muscles, tendons, ligaments, and healthy joints. Keeping active in old age reduces the risk of hip fractures and falls, and helps maintain functional ability such as lifting, carrying, and climbing stairs, which are necessary for independent living (65). Regular physical activity ensures growing during child-hood, and the maintenance of musculoskeletal health during adulthood and old age.

2.1.2.1.6   Physical Activity and Mental Health and Sleep   For mental health and sleep, there is good evidence that physical inactivity increases the risk of clinical depression. In con-trast, physical activity such as dance, tai chi or yoga has an important beneficial effect on anx-iety. Physical activity such as collective sport (tennis, ping-pong, football, etc.) is important for psychological well-being and can reduce the symptoms of depression by boosting mood and self-esteem. There is evidence that even small amounts of physical activity can improve sleep, cognitive function, and reactivity to stress (65, 68, 70). Regular physical activity can also improve mental acuity and help to fight insomnia. It has been shown to improve academic performance in young people and to contribute to the maintenance of thinking, learning, and judgement skills in adults. In older adults, keeping active can improve mental functioning, and delay or prevent the onset of dementia (65).

A recent cohort study found that living a healthy lifestyle including regular physical activity, no smoking, a healthy diet, and moderate alcohol consumption was associated with a reduced demen-tia risk across all genetic risk groups (7). In brief, physical activity plays important roles in health maintenance and disease prevention, especially in overweight, cardiovascular diseases, mental health, sleep, and so on. The success of this activity depends on the type of exercise chosen and the lifestyle of each individual such as choice of diet, hobby, and environment.

2.1.2.2   Physical Activity Types

According to each age group and health category, there are different physical activity or exercise types. Physical activities that move the legs and arms are the basic exercises necessary for the func-tioning of all organs, especially for the heart. In general, exercise and physical activity include four basic categories: aerobic exercise or endurance, strength or weight training, stretching or flexibility, and balance (73, 74). Most people tend to focus on one activity or type of exercise conforming to their age or healthy state. When engaging in regular physical activity, it is important for you to know the benefits of the physical activity type that you choose (75).

2.1.2.2.1   Aerobic Exercise or Endurance   Aerobic exercise or endurance involve steady, rhyth-mic movement of the legs and arms. Such activities include brisk walking, running, swimming, bicycling, stair climber and dancing. Aerobic exercise, which speeds up heart rate and breathing, is important for many body functions. It gives heart and lungs a workout, increases endurance, and improves overall fitness (75). Strengthening endurance makes it easier to perform many daily activities. Regular aerobic exercise conditions the heart to pump blood to the whole body (74–76). Aerobic exercise also helps relax blood vessel walls, lower blood pressure, burn body fat, lower blood sugar levels, reduce inflammation, boost mood, and raise 'good' HDL cholesterol. Combined with weight loss, it can lower 'bad' LDL cholesterol levels, too. Over the long term, aerobic exercise reduces your risk of heart disease, stroke, Type 2 diabetes, breast and colon cancer, depression, and falls (73). Endurance or aerobic exercises include: moderate-intensity aerobic activity and vigorous-intensity aerobic activity. Moderate-intensity aerobic activity causes a slight increase in breathing and heart rate. Examples include: brisk walking (5 km/hr), leisure cycling (<16 km/hr), leisure swimming, playing doubles tennis, and line-dancing. Vigorous-intensity aerobic activity causes heart rate to increase significantly (75). Examples of vigorous-intensity physical activity include: jogging or running, swimming continuous laps, playing singles tennis, rollerblading at a fast pace, playing basketball or football, and skipping with a rope (75). These activities can vary in intensity between individuals depending on the effort put in and their fitness levels. Aerobic exercise also helps relax blood vessel walls, lower blood pressure, burn body fat, lower blood sugar levels, reduce inflammation, boost mood, and raise 'good' HDL cholesterol. Combined with weight loss, it can lower 'bad' LDL cholesterol levels, too. Over the long term, aerobic exercise reduces your risk of heart disease, stroke, Type 2 diabetes, breast and colon cancer, depression, and falls. Aim for 150 minutes per week of moderate-intensity activity. Choose normal walking, brisk walking, dancing, cycling, swimming, jogging, or step aerobics according to your age and your state of health (73). Do the aerobic activity in segments of at least ten minutes. You do not have to do the 20 or 30 minutes in one go (74). If you are unhealthy, consult a doctor before choosing a type of exercise cited previously.

2.1.2.2.2 Strength or Weight Training   Strength or weight training increases muscle mass, boosts metabolism, improves balance, and makes bones stronger. Strength training can be done at home, or in a gym or fitness center (75, 76). Strength or weight training is muscle-strengthening activity which increases muscular fitness and bone strength. Such activities should work all the major muscle groups of the body such as the legs, hips, back, chest, abdomen, shoulders, and arms (75). Weight training allows to increase the metabolism and to prevent weight gain for old people. Strength training, such as weightlifting, helps make bones stronger, improves balance, and increases muscle strength. All of this helps prevent osteoporosis and lowers the risk of hip fractures from falls (76). Strength training has also been shown to lessen arthritis pain. In general, strength training can be done easily at home with a minimum of time. Two 30-minute sessions a week of weight training is enough to increase muscle mass and bone density. Muscle mass is lost when as age climbs. Strength training builds it back. Strengthening the muscles not only makes the body stronger, but also stimulates bone growth, lowers blood sugar, assists with weight control, improves balance and posture, and reduces stress and pain in the lower back and joints (73). Consult a physical therapist who can design a strength training program. It will likely include body weight exercises like squats, push-ups, and lunges and exercises involving resistance from a weight, a band, or a weight machine (73). Consult a doctor before strength training or exercise with weight if you are unhealthy.

2.1.2.2.3 Stretching or Flexibility Exercise   Stretching helps maintain flexibility. Flexibility exercises stretch the muscles and can help the body stay limber (73). When you are young, your muscles are stronger and more flexible than when you are old. Aging leads to a loss of flexibility in the muscles and tendons because muscles shorten and no longer function properly. That increases the risk for muscle cramps and pain, muscle damage, strains, joint pain, falling, and it also makes it tough to get through daily activities (73). Likewise, stretching the muscles routinely makes them longer and more flexible, which increases your range of motion and reduces pain and risk of injury. Aim for a program of stretching every day, or at least three or four times per week (73). Warm up your muscles first, with a few minutes of dynamic stretches such as marching in place or arm circles. Then perform static stretches (holding a stretch position for up to 60 seconds) for the calves, the hamstrings, hip flexors, quadriceps, and the muscles of the shoulders, neck, and lower back. However, do not practice these exercises excessively into the painful range – that tightens the muscle and is counterproductive (73). Consult a physical therapist to explain various excercises.

2.1.2.2.4 Balance Exercise   Balance exercise is recommended especially for the elderly. This type of exercise is supple and easy to do. Having good balance is important for many everyday activities, such as going up and down stairs. Improving your balance makes you feel steadier on your feet and helps prevent falls, a common problem in older people (73). When we get older, our vision, our inner ear, and our leg muscles and joints tend to break down. Training balance regularly can help prevent and reverse these losses (73). Many senior centers and gyms offer balance-focused exercise classes such as tai chi or yoga. It is never too early to start this type of exercise, even if you feel you do not have balance problems (73). You can also go to a physical therapist, who can determine your current balance abilities and prescribe specific exercises to target your areas of weakness. Typical balance exercises include standing on one foot, walking heel to toe, tai chi, or yoga. The physical therapist may also have you focus on joint flexibility, walking on uneven surfaces, and strengthening leg muscles with exercises such as squats and leg lifts. Get the proper training before attempting any of these exercises at home (75).

2.1.2.3 Mind-Body Exercises and Health Benefits

Mind-body exercises may improve body function and health, since the nervous system affects the endocrine and immune systems while performing these mind-body exercises. Tai Chi, Qigong and Yoga are considered the most popular mind-body exercises, ranked by the 2002–2012 National Health Interview Surveys as the top three of the ten most common complementary health approaches in practice (77). In addition, Unipedal standing therapy or Dynamic Flamingo therapy may be also a mind-body exercise for the prevention of falls in the elderly.

2.1.2.3.1 Tai Chi and Health Benefits
Tai Chi translates to mean, 'Grand Ultimate', and in the Chinese culture, it represents an expansive philosophical and theoretical notion which describes the universe in the spontaneous state of dynamic balance between mutually interactive phenomena including the balance of light and dark, movement and stillness, and waves and particles (78). Tai Chi is a traditional Chinese healing/martial art combining martial art movement with Qi (vital energy) circulation, breathing, and stretching techniques (77). Tai Chi exercise consists of a series of graceful movements with deep and slow diaphragmatic breathings performed while standing. Tai Chi movement has been shown to have both physical and psychosocial benefits for different populations (77). Tai Chi is known as an effective intervention for balance enhancement and falls prevention among the elderly, and there is a growing interest in safe, alternative forms of exercise across all age groups (78). Tai Chi practices not only improve lung health and capacity in people affected by lung disease such as chronic obstructive pulmonary disease (COPD), asthma or lung cancer, but can also help one cope with the stress, anxiety and depression that unfortunately sometimes accompany a lung disease (79). Tai chi, sometimes called 'moving meditation', improves balance by moving the body slowly, gently, and precisely, while breathing deeply. Other benefits from practicing Tai Chi may include: improvements in bone and heart health, relief of pain and stiffness from osteoarthritis, better sleep, and improvements in overall wellness (78–79). Although these therapeutic effects have not been recognized by healthcare professionals, Tai Chi is still an accessible exercise that is convenient for the elderly.

2.1.2.3.2 Qigong and Health Benefits
Qigong or Qi-gong exercise, similar to Tai Chi, is a traditional Chinese practice for millenia and consists of a series of breath practices with body movement and meditation to attain a deeply focused and relaxed state (77). Qi means the circulating life force or the enhancement of the life essence or energy (78). The literal translation from the Chinese 'qi' is 'gas', 'air', or 'breath'. Qi is often translated as 'life energy', 'life force', or 'energy flow' (80). Gong (or kung) means work, cultivation, or practice. Qi is the conceptual foundation of traditional Chinese medicine in acupuncture, herbal medicine, and Chinese physical therapy.

Simply speaking, Qigong exercise is used to cultivate the balance and harmony of vital energy in the human body (77). According to the National Institute of Health (NIH) Research Report, considerable scientific evidence supports the health benefits of practicing Qigong and Tai Chi in various populations with different characteristics such as age, gender, and occupation (77). From the perspective of Western thought and science, Qigong practices activate naturally occurring physiological and psychological mechanisms of self-repair and health recovery (78). The Qigong practices generally tested in health research incorporate a range of simple movements (repeated and often flowing in nature), or postures (standing or sitting), and include a focused state of relaxed awareness and a variety of breathing techniques that accompany the movements or postures. A key underlying philosophy of the practice is that any form of Qigong has an effect on the cultivation of balance and harmony of Qi, positively influencing the human energy complex (Qi channel) which functions as a holistic, coherent and mutually interactive system (78). In Chinese medicine, Qigong exercises may be very useful as an intervention strategy for adults with different forms of arthritis (80). In Western medicine, some evidence of Qigong practice was observed in the prevention of body falls in the elderly, and in the improvement of life and health in subjects suffering from chronic arthritis (78).

2.1.2.3.3 Yoga and Health Benefits Yoga, a mind-body exercise, is an important part of health and spiritual practices in Indo-Tibetan traditions that have become increasingly more common in Western society (81–82). It involves a combination of muscular activity and an internally directed mindful focus on awareness of the self, the breath, and energy (77, 81–84). Yoga brings balance and health to the physical, mental, emotional, and spiritual components of the individual. It plays an important role in the improvement of physical and mental health, particularly stress-related illnesses. Yoga is unique because it incorporates physical activity, breathing, and meditation (81–84). Yoga is another excellent option for low-impact exercise. The practice of yoga is made up of two essential parts: performing physical poses, called asana, while being mindful of breathing techniques, called pranayama. Both parts are beneficial for maintaining physical and mental fitness (79). Yoga breathing (pranayama) can rapidly bring the mind to the present moment and reduce stress (81–82). According to a recent review article, it can be concluded that yoga interventions were effective in reducing depression (83). Yoga is both a form of meditation in itself and a preparation for deep meditation. Breath work can affect longevity mechanisms in ways that overlap with meditation, and in other ways that are different from, but that synergistically enhance, the effects of meditation. Some lung clinical studies have demonstrated the use of yoga breathing in the treatment of depression, anxiety, post-traumatic stress disorder, and for victims of mass disasters (82). Yoga is also efficacious in the treatment of tobacco addiction and drug abuse. By inducing stress resilience, breath work enables us to rapidly and compassionately relieve many forms of suffering (82). Yoga breathing may improve lung health and some lung diseases such as chronic obstructive pulmonary disease and asthma (81). Moreover, yoga practice may lower blood pressure and improve many chronic cardiac complications, such as myocardial ischemia, congestive cardiac failure, and impairment of diastolic function (81). Yoga is generally safe in healthy people. However, if you are unhealthy or you have a special disease such as cardiovascular diseases, lung disease, cancer, arthritis, and so on, consult your health care provider before starting yoga. In Western medicine, yoga is not considered to be an official treatment of any disease, but to be used as complementary therapy for certain ailments such as mental diseases, addiction and for health maintenance in the elderly. Some studies comparing the effects of yoga and classic forms of exercise seem to indicate that, in both healthy and diseased populations, yoga may be as effective as or better than classic exercise such as aerobic practice because yoga combines body exercise with mind practice at the same time (82–84).

2.1.2.3.4 Unipedal Standing Therapy or Dynamic Flamingo Therapy and Fall Prevention In Dynamic Flamingo therapy, the patient stands on one leg so that the load applied to the femoral head of the supporting side is approximately 3-fold greater than that applied when standing on two legs. Standing on one leg for one minute is considered equivalent to about one hour of walking. This therapy should be useful for preventing femoral neck fractures by promoting increased mineralization, improving standing balance, and preventing falls in the elderly (85–86). Be careful when you practice this exercise because you can fall. Therefore, for the first exercises, you can lean on a wall or a chair to avoid fall. Repeat this exercise 3 times for 30 sec. to 1 min. a day. For the elderly, this exercise is not easy to perform. Dynamic Flamingo therapy might prevent falls for the elderly, but was not shown to be statistically significant in the prevention of hip fracture (86). This therapy is a method based on Wolff's laws and Pauwels' lever arm theory (1980) for increasing bone mineral density at the femoral neck (85).

Briefly, mind-body exercises such as Tai Chi, yoga, Qigong, and so on, might improve, enhance, or strengthen the integrative health and well-being of all kinds of people, especially the elderly.

2.1.2.4   Duration of Physical Exercise

For the duration of each exercise type, the Physical Activity Guidelines for Americans recommends adults get 150 minutes (2 hours and 30 minutes) of moderate physical activity every week or 20 minutes of vigorous-intensity aerobic activity 3 or more days a week (74, 87–88). Do the aerobic activity in segments of at least 10 minutes. You do not have to do the 20 or 30 minutes in one go. Strength training should be included in a routine as two 30-minute sessions per week. The 150 minutes can be spread out through the week – like exercising for 20–25 minutes every day or working out for 50 minutes 3 times per week (74, 87–88).

Older adults should do multicomponent physical activity that includes balance training as well as aerobic and muscle-strengthening activities. When older adults cannot do 150 minutes of moderate-intensity aerobic activity a week because of chronic diseases, they should be as physically active as their abilities and conditions allow (87).

Women during pregnancy and the postpartum period should do at least 150 minutes of moderate-intensity aerobic activity a week. Preferably, aerobic activity should be spread out throughout the week (87).

Children and adolescents ages 6 through 17 years should do 60 minutes (1 hour) or more of moderate-to-vigorous physical activity daily (87).

It should be noted that a long duration of any exercise type is harmful to health and an excessive practice of sports and gymnastics can cause death. Many sportspersons or athletes have gone faint or died after long durations of hard competition or training. It is the same for construction workers. A break is necessary for any physical exercise or manual work. The intensity of most physical activity should be moderate. Examples include walking, running, skipping, playing on the playground, playing tennis, or biking. Vigorous-intensity aerobic activity like running, jumping jacks, and fast swimming should be included about three days a week for young people.

2.1.2.5   Precautions and Risks of Physical Activity

Healthy adults generally do not need to consult a health care provider before becoming physically active. However, the risk of heart problems due to physical activity is higher for children and young adults who have congenital heart problems such as hypertrophic cardiomyopathy, congenital heart defects, and myocarditis (89). For middle-aged and older adults, the risk of heart problems due to physical activity is related to coronary heart disease (CHD). People who have CHD are more likely to have a heart attack when they are exercising vigorously than when they are not. The risk of heart problems due to physical activity is related to your fitness level and the intensity of the activity you are doing (89). For chronic diseases and the elderly, the consultation of a specialist doctor or health care provider is necessary before any exercise practice (77). Before you start planning a routine of regular physical activities for yourself, it is important for you to know the types of physical activity that you should engage in and the benefits they provide (77). For example, aerobic activity makes you breathe harder and your heart beat faster, as a result, increases heart and lung fitness. Moreover, you can combine classical aerobic activity with mind-body exercises such as Tai Chi, Yoga, or Qigong. Some statistical results revealed that social sports such as playing tennis, ping-pong, volleyball, and football regularly might expand lifespan about nine, six, and five years, respectively; while solitary sports like jogging, swimming or solo cycling might prolong lifespan about four or three years only (90). Collective or social sport like tennis and football is better than solitary sport such as solo cycling, solo walking, because collective sport stimulates not only our muscle, heart, lungs, and so on, but also our brain, eyes, our mood, our intelligence. However, to play a collective sport, you must have a partner or a team with you and a court or a special place for this sport in your town. Therefore, these conditions limit the choice of these collective sports. Jogging, biking, walking, and dancing remain the most popular sports for everyone. Moreover, these sports are free and can be practiced in any moment of the day. Hence, it is well known that people who exercise are likely to live longer than sedentary or unsociable people.

Yet the physical activity of an individual is also influenced by the lifestyle of their people or nation. Therefore, many diseases are often seen in one country, but are rare in others, despite these countries have the similar economic levels, health care structures and even races. For example, about 65% of French people walk briskly 7 days/week; only about 50% of Americans walk briskly 5 days/week. This same cross-cultural comparison showed that the French spend 1.69% of time walking versus 0.63% for Americans (11). The French move around regularly, using bikes and public transportation to go to work or to other occupations; while Americans prefer to use their private cars because public transportation is rare in some US areas. This American lifestyle leads to sedentary habits. Among French adults, 17% are obese, and among American adults, 34% are obese. Thus, the French retain their position of being among the lowest in the world for CHD and the United States remains in the middle of a 37-country comparison (11). In conclusion, physical activity is as important as choice of food to maintain health and prevent disease.

2.1.3 Sleep in Health and Disease
Sleep is vital for the functioning and repair of all organs and tissues in the body and for the maintenance of good health and well-being throughout life. Getting enough sleep helps support healthy brain function and maintain physical health. In babies, sleep is important for the development of the brain. In children and teenagers, sleep is necessary for their growth and their school activities. Insufficient or poor sleep quality can affect the memory and the behavior of an adult. Sleep loss can also increase the risks of road traffic accidents and some chronic diseases.

2.1.3.1 Physiology and Roles of Sleep
Sleep is an extremely complicated process. It is a state of reversible unconsciousness in which the brain is in a relative state of rest and less responsive to external stimuli. However, the brain is reactive primarily to internal stimuli (91–93). Sleep results from the inhibition of wake-promoting systems by homeostatic sleep factors such as adenosine and nitric oxide and GABAergic neurons in the preoptic area of the hypothalamus, resulting in large-amplitude, slow electroencephalogram (EEG) oscillations (93). We are functionally blind during sleep with no response to visual stimuli and a decreased threshold of response to auditory stimuli. Natural sleep is divided into two distinct states: non-rapid eye movement (NREM) sleep, and rapid eye movement (REM) sleep, with different mechanisms and electrophysiological characteristics to each state (91–93). NREM sleep is subdivided into several stages, numbered 1 to 3 (92). Each phase and stage represent the relative depth of sleep and offers unique characteristics in brain wave, muscle tones, and eye movement patterns. As the name implies, NREM is characterized by an absence of eye movements and REM is characterized by rapid eye movements. Sleep begins with a short NREM stage 1 phase, followed by NREM stage 2, then NREM stage 3, then finally into REM. NREM accounts for approximately 75–80% of total sleep and REM accounts for the remaining 20–25% of sleep. The progression through the stages of sleep occurs in this order of events on repeat throughout the night for varying lengths of time (92). Rapid eye movement (REM) is the phase of sleep responsible for dreaming. It is characterized by total body voluntary muscle paralysis (except for the extraocular muscles). This paralysis is thought to be a mechanism to prevent neural stimulus from dreams to manifest in actual muscular impulses during sleep (92). Natural wakening usually occurs from REM sleep. Subjects woken from REM sleep are much more likely to recall dream content than those awakened from NREM sleep. NREM dreams are generally vague and formless in contrast to REM dreams (91).

Many different neurotransmitters, neuromodulators, and hormones have an important role in regulation of sleep and wakefulness. These substances include: acetylcholine, adenosine, alpha melanocyte-stimulating hormone (alpha-MSH), cholecystokinin, dopamine, gamma-aminobutyric acid (GABA), ghrelin, glutamate, glycine, insulin, histamine, hypocretin (orexin), leptin, melatonin, melanin-concentrating hormone (MCH), norepinephrine, neuropeptide Y (NPY), prostaglandins, somatotrophin, serotonin, and thyrotropin (99). Little is known about the effect of vitamins and minerals on sleep (94).

The exact purpose of sleep has not been fully elucidated. There are several prominent theories to explain the roles of sleep including the Inactivity theory, Energy conservation theory, Restoration theory, and the Brain plasticity theory (92). The theory of inactivity is explained by the fact that the body needs rest to be able to start again. Energy conservation theory posits that the main function of sleep is to reduce a person's energy demand during part of the day. This theory is supported by the fact that the body has decreased metabolism of up to 10% during sleep. The restorative theory states that sleep allows for the body to repair and replete cellular components necessary for biological functions that become depleted throughout an awake day. This is backed by findings that many functions in the body, such as muscle repair, tissue growth, protein synthesis, and the release of many hormones for growth occur primarily during sleep. Brain plasticity theory is that sleep is necessary for neural reorganization and growth of the brain's structure and function. It is clear that sleep plays an important role in the development of the brain in infants and children (92).

2.1.3.2 Duration of Sleep

Age has a major effect on the duration of sleep and the ratio of NREM/REM sleep. Neonates sleep 16–18 h per day (91). Their sleep is widely distributed throughout the day with REM sleep accounting for 50% of total sleep time (TST). This may be even greater in premature babies. By the age of 2 years, children should sleep 10 h per day, mainly at night with one or two naps during the daytime, and REM sleep declines to 20–25% of TST. Adults aged 26 to 64 years normally sleep 7–9 h per day with 15–20% REM sleep (91, 95). For people aged ≥65 years, total sleep time decreases to about 6–7 h per day, although sleep is more fragmented with more frequent and longer awakenings (decreased sleep efficiency) with less REM sleep and more NREM sleep (96). Night-time sleep may be decreased if naps are taken during the day (91, 95). However, sleep duration of adults still depends on cultural, social, psychological, behavioral, pathophysiological, and environmental influences. Long sleep duration over nine hours per day may be associated with obstructive sleep apnea, heart disease, and failing health with increased risk of mortality, or may represent a symptom of early 'latent' disease preceding a formal diagnosis (95). Some researchers found a significant association between deviations in sleep duration and both mortality and adverse cardiovascular problems. Sleep duration above the recommended level of seven to eight hours was associated with a moderate degree of harm compared with sleeping less than the suggested duration (95).

2.1.3.3 Sleep Disorders

Sleep disorders are a large and under-recognized problem in many parts of the world. Based on the international classification of sleep disorders (ICSD), the most frequent and often the most severe are obstructive sleep apnea (OSA), narcolepsy, restless legs syndrome (RLS), periodic limb movement disorder, insomnia, parasomnias, circadian rhythm disorders including jet lag and shift work, and sudden infant death syndrome (94). However, the major research focuses on insomnia, obstructive sleep apnea, and restless legs syndrome since they are among the most highly prevalent sleep disorders and there are established links between them and other health conditions (94).

2.1.3.3.1 Sleep Loss   Sleep loss is an important factor in the global burden of disease with collateral effects on cardiovascular and mental health as well as injury and violent death through road or work accidents (96). The term sleep loss denotes voluntary and involuntary short sleep hours, insomnia, and other sleep disorders that result in the attenuation of the benefits of sleep (96). Sleep loss appears to favor the development of a proinflammatory state with increased risk of vascular damage such as stroke, myocardial infarction, and overall mortality. This is based on research over the last decade linking short sleep hours, insomnia, and sleep apnea to the development of vascular pro-inflammatory factors and subsequent heart disease (96). Sleep loss impacts cellular mechanisms of learning and memory occurring during NREM sleep and REM sleep (93).

2.1.3.3.2 Insomnia   Insomnia is a type of sleep loss. Insomnia, defined as insufficient quantity or quality of sleep, is the most prevalent sleep disorder. Approximately 50% of adults complain of occasional insomnia, and 10–15% of chronic insomnia (93, 97). Insomnia can involve difficulty falling asleep, staying asleep, or poor quality of sleep. Insomnia commonly leads to daytime sleepiness, lack of energy, lethargy, cognitive impairment, and a general feeling of being unwell, both mentally and physically. Mood swings, irritability, and anxiety are common associated symptoms (93, 97). Insomnia may even precipitate or accompany the development of psychiatric disorders.

2.1.3.3.3 Obstructive Sleep Apnea   Obstructive Sleep Apnea (OSA) is one of the three forms of sleep apnea which is characterized by short pauses in breathing or abnormally low breathing while asleep. Sleep apneas are divided into three categories: central, obstructive, and complex (a combination of obstructive and central sleep apneas). Central sleep apnea involves dysfunction of the central respiratory control centers in the brain (93). The most common type of sleep apnea is Obstructive Sleep Apnea (OSA). OSA is a breathing disorder that occurs during sleep, characterized by a partial or complete blockage of the upper airway. OSA is caused by the collapse of soft tissue and muscles in the upper airway between the hard plate and the larynx (98, 99). The apneic moment is usually terminated by a slight arousal, as well as an increase in sympathetic tone, as airway patency is re-established. OSA affects nearly 7% of the general population (93). Untreated OSA is associated with long-term health consequences including cardiovascular disease, metabolic disorders, cognitive impairment, and depression. Common symptoms include excessive daytime sleepiness, fatigue, non-refreshing sleep, nocturia, morning headache, irritability, and memory loss. Untreated OSA is also associated with lost productivity and workplace and motor vehicle accidents resulting in injury and fatality (99).

Other sleep disorders include restless legs syndrome (RLS), hypersomnia, and narcolepsy. These diseases are grave and must be treated by a specialist.

However, snoring, sleep talking or screaming, sleepwalking or somnambulism, agitation or restless sleep are also common sleep disorders. But they are benign and do not usually cause health problems to sleepers. However, agitation sleep and sleepwalking can cause fall or other bodily injury to the sleeper. Snoring and screaming sleep can bother the neighbor. Snoring is more common in men than in women. Alcohol can increase the risk of snoring.

2.1.3.4 Prevention and Treatment of Sleep Disorders

For the prevention of some sleep disorders such as sleep loss and insomnia, change of lifestyle is necessary. More physical activity such as classic aerobic activity combined with mind-body exercises such as Tai Chi, Yoga, or Qigong can help you sleep better at night and may ameliorate certain types of sleep disorders such sleep loss and moderate insomnia. Choice of foods also plays an important role in the amelioration of certain sleep diseases.

To prevent sleep loss and insomnia, a dinner must be taken about three hours before going to sleep. Avoid coffee, tea, alcohol, cigarettes, dark chocolate, indigestible foods like meat with fat as well as hard spices such as chili pepper during dinner. Dinner must be rich in vegetables and sugary fruits. Taking some teaspoons of honey diluted in water before going to bed or when awakening at midnight may prevent sleep loss or accelerate sleep again. You can also replace honey with some light snacks to help with sleeping. Vitamins, antioxidants, and minerals in foods can play important roles in the prevention of many sleep disorders (94).

For hard insomnia, consulting a specialist is necessary. There are many drugs to fight insomnia such as barbiturates, benzodiazepines, antidepressants, melatonin, and so on (93). Their therapeutic effects are immediate, but their side effects are also important. Only the doctor can determine the necessary dosage and the duration of the treatment. Do not abuse these drugs. In terms of alternative medicine, acupuncture may be helpful to treat chronic insomnia, but this therapy is still not recognized by healthcare organizations (100). The results of this practice depend on the specialist. However, acupuncture does not give side effects. For hypersomnia and narcolepsy, no treatment can cure these two sleep disorders.

It should be noted that using a floor fan in the room while sleeping can cause problems for your health. Indeed, a fan may be necessary for sleep when it is hot. However, when the fan is orientated to the body directly, especially to the face or the legs, it can cause many health problems such as dryness of the mouth, throat, skin, nostrils, irritation of the eyes, and cramps (101). In addition, it can cause asthma or allergy due to the blast of air containing dusts, molds, spores, or pollen directly into your throat and bronchial tubes. Therefore, to avoid these risks to your health while sleeping with a fan, do not point the fan directly at your body, or use a fan that rotates and with a timer (101).

Sleep position can influence your health and the quality of your sleep. Most people sleep on their sides, but this position can cause shoulder and hip pain. Also, sleeping on your right side may even aggravate heartburn. You should try sleeping on your left side if you get heartburn. The best position is sleeping on your back, which only 8% of people do (102). It is the best position for reducing aches and pain, and it does not cause heartburn because your head is elevated above your chest. However, lying on your back may increase the risk of snoring. The absolute worst sleeping position is lying on your stomach. Only 7% of people do this, but it puts pressure on your entire body. You are likely to wake up with numbness and tingling, and it can increase the chance of muscle and joint pain (102).

In conclusion, one of the bases of a healthy life is sleep. It is as important as physical activity and diet. These three factors depend on each other and create harmony for maintaining health and avoiding disease. Sleep disorders cause not only damage to an individual's life, but also to society, such as the diminution of productivity in work and invention, and the occurrence of road accidents and family tragedy.

2.1.4 Break and Hobbies

Break and hobbies are generally considered less important than a healthy diet, regular exercise, and a good night's sleep. However, all physical or mental activity needs a break after a certain time of work so that the body and brain can continue to function efficaciously. Therefore, a break of one to two hours at midday and two days of weekend are granted to all workers in industrialized countries. Moreover, a summer vacation of two to four weeks is given to workers in many countries. For example, French workers have four weeks of vacation in the summer and two weeks in the winter, while Americans have only two weeks of vacation during a year (11). So, the industrial productivity of Americans is higher than that of the French, but the French are healthier than Americans and live longer than Americans. Therefore, the health of an individual also depends on the lifestyle of a society.

By definition, hobbies are seen as beneficial leisure or non-work occupations (103). The choice of hobby depends on the preference of each individual, family or society. A hobby can be an indoor or outdoor hobby. A hobby can give good, bad, or neutral effects to the physical and mental health of an individual. In general, a hobby that needs body movement, collective competition, or social activity is considered good for health. For example, playing tennis, football, walking, biking, karaoke, and dancing are good for health. Singing, playing musical instruments, choir, concerts, painting, chatting, and socializing are good for the mood, memory, and sense of relaxation. Study, lecture, and writing are good exercise for the soul and brain. They contribute to good lifestyle because they are benefic for mental health and they may prevent certain diseases such as Alzheimer's disease (3). In contrast, playing computer or card games for long periods is not good for physical and mental health; it is the same with watching television or digital video for a long time.

Normal sex relation is necessary in healthy life and gives physical and psychological pleasure for the couple. Dysfunction of sex relation is a problem in most of societies and it has a significant effect on mental and physical health. It can be said that dysfunctional sex relation may result in various family problems (3). Bad sex relation and infertility may be due to many lifestyle factors such as bad diet, lack of exercise, sleep loss, obesity, stress, cigarette smoking, alcoholism, and also other diseases of a couple (104). Some plant foods such as galangal and ginseng tubers have stimulant effects on sexual appetite. In both Chinese and Ayurvedic (Indian) traditional medicine since ancient times, galangal tubers like *Alpinia galanga* and *Alpinia officinarum* were and are still used as aphrodisiacs for both sexes (105). Wild Korean ginseng tuber and red ginseng are also used as stimulants for sexual appetite in traditional medicine (106–107). Sildenafil or Viagra (brand name) is a medication used to treat erectile dysfunction in men, but it has many side effects such as headache, flushing, dyspepsia, respiratory tract infection, nasal congestion, and cardiovascular problems especially in cardiac people (108). Acupuncture might treat some forms of infertility in men and women, but it is not recognized by Western medicine, and the results obtained depend on the acupuncturist. Consult a healthcare specialist if you have a sexual problem.

Briefly, taking breaks is necessary for all workers, and choice of hobby is important for health. Hobbies that require body movements and competition are best for everyone. For the elderly, hobbies such as ping pong, tennis, walking, dancing, singing, conversation, meeting, and writing are beneficial for maintaining health and promoting long life.

2.2 Unhealthy Lifestyle

As mentioned previously, an unhealthy lifestyle is in contrast to a healthy lifestyle. An unhealthy lifestyle may include the regular consumption of unhealthy products such as alcohol, cigarettes, drugs of abuse (cocaine, heroin, marijuana, methamphetamine), or some unhealthy foods such as tonic drink, fast foods, and snacks. Sedentary life, computer game addiction, and frequent exposure to pollution and pesticides also lend to an unhealthy lifestyle. Many unhealthy lifestyles are due to an individual's choice, with the exception of exposure to pollution and pesticides.

Unhealthy lifestyle is the source of many illnesses such as cardiovascular diseases, obesity, diabetes, cancer, and more. It is also the cause of family and society perturbations. Among the various unhealthy lifestyles, cigarette smoking and alcoholism are the most consumed and are the cause of many diseases.

2.2.1 Harmful Effects of Cigarette Smoking

The adverse effects of cigarette smoke on human health are widely recognized. Cigarette smoking is the main etiological agent in numerous diseases, in particular chronic obstructive pulmonary disease and lung cancer, and it is a known human carcinogen (109). It is the origin of about 90% of all lung cancer deaths and also of other cancers like cancers of esophagus, larynx, mouth, throat, kidney, bladder, liver, pancreas, stomach, cervix, colon, and rectum, as well as leukemia (109–111). Cigarette smoking harms nearly every organ of the body, causes many diseases, and reduces the health and the lifespan of smokers in general. Smoking also causes heart disease, stroke, hypertension, hypercholesterolemia, atherosclerosis, diabetes, rheumatoid arthritis, osteoporosis, asthma, bronchitis, infertility, and more. It impairs immune function and enhances the development of many infectious diseases (109–111). Tobacco is already the leading cause of adult death in developed countries (109). There are more than 1.1 billion tobacco smokers worldwide of which 900 million are men and 200 million are women (109). Cigarette smoking causes more than 480,000 deaths each year in the United States (110).

2.2.1.1 Composition of Tobacco Smoke

Tobacco smoke contains many chemicals that are harmful to both smokers and nonsmokers. Breathing even a little tobacco smoke can be harmful. More than 7,000 chemicals are found in tobacco smoke, and at least 250 are known to be harmful (111). Tobacco smoke contains gas and tar. Gas is formed by ozone, formaldehyde, ammonia, carbon monoxide, toluene, benzene, and more (109). Tar is constituted of many resinous particles of different sizes which are all toxic – carcinogenic, mutagenic, genotoxic, neurotoxic, immune-toxic, and so on – such as nicotine, nitrosamines, polycyclic aromatic hydrocarbons (PAH), and more (109, 111). Among the 250 known harmful chemicals in tobacco smoke, at least 69 can cause cancer such as PAH, benzene, aromatic amines, nitrosamines, acetaldehyde, cadmium, and chromium (111). However, tobacco leaves rich in selenium might decrease the immune toxicity of tobacco smoke tars (112).

2.2.1.2   Nicotine Health Effects

Nicotine, the main chemical compound in tobacco smoke, is an alkaloid of the tobacco plant, *Nicotiana tabacum*, in the Solanaceae family. Nicotine was first extracted from tobacco by German physicians Wilhelm Heinrich Posselt and Karl Ludwig Reimann (113). Nicotine in its pure form is a clear liquid with a characteristic odor. It turns brown on exposure to air. It is water-soluble and separates preferentially from organic solvents. It is an amine composed of pyridine and pyrrolidine rings. Nicotine is highly addictive and exposes people to the harmful effects of tobacco dependency (113–114). The plasma half-life of nicotine is about two hours (114). Brain imaging studies demonstrate that nicotine acutely increases activity in the prefrontal cortex and visual systems. There is release of a variety of neurotransmitters important in drug-induced reward. Nicotine also causes an increased oxidative stress and neuronal apoptosis, DNA damage, reactive oxygen species, and lipid peroxide increase (113). Predominant immediate effects as seen in animal studies and in humans consist of increase in pulse rate and blood pressure. Nicotine also causes an increase in plasma free fatty acids, hyperglycemia, and an increase in the level of catecholamines in the blood (113). In severe poisoning, there occur tremors, prostration, cyanosis, dyspnea, convulsion, progression to collapse, and coma. Even death may occur from paralysis of respiratory muscles and/or central respiratory failure with a lethal dose LD50 in adults of around 30–60 mg of nicotine. In children the LD50 is around 10 mg (113). Nicotine is one of the most addicting agents. Studies have shown that nicotine dependence is transmitted maternally and grand maternally by epigenetic mechanism. Nicotine can promote carcinogenesis by causing DNA mutations (113). Nicotine is linked to possible birth defects. Various animal studies show retarded fetal growth and lower birth weight when treated perinatally with nicotine (113–114). Prenatal nicotine also affects several neuromodulator systems, i.e., compounds that act mainly as modulators of synaptic transmission of other classical neurotransmitters (114). Nicotine replacement therapy such as dermal patches, gums, lozenges, electronic cigarettes, or nasal sprays is an effective adjunct in management of withdrawal symptoms and improves the success of cessation programs. Any substantive beneficial effect of nicotine on the human body is yet to be proven. Nicotine should be used only under supervision of trained cessation personnel, therefore its sale needs to be strictly regulated (113).

2.2.1.3   Smokeless Tobacco

Besides cigarette smoking, another type of tobacco addiction is smokeless tobacco. Smokeless tobacco is tobacco that is not burned. Since antiquity, it has been used by Native Americans and Aboriginal peoples of Australia. Consumed either orally or nasally, by chewing, sucking, or sniffing, smokeless tobacco products deliver nicotine without combustion. There are many different forms of smokeless tobacco products consumed globally, but they can be roughly divided into two categories: snuff (finely ground or cut tobacco) and chewing tobacco (whole leaf, plug or twist tobacco) (115). Although all smokeless tobacco products are addictive due to the presence of nicotine, they do not involve combustion, carry no risks associated with smoke inhalation, and are generally accepted to be less hazardous than smoking (115). However, at least 28 chemicals in smokeless tobacco have been found to cause cancer (116). The most harmful chemicals in smokeless tobacco are tobacco-specific nitrosamines, which are formed during the growing, curing, fermenting, and aging of tobacco. The level of tobacco-specific nitrosamines varies by product. Scientists have found that the nitrosamine level is directly related to the risk of cancer (116). Chewing leaf tobacco can lead to nicotine addiction and can cause cancers of the mouth, throat, esophagus, and pancreas. Chewing tobacco products may also cause gum disease, dental problem, pharyngitis, laryngitis, heart disease, stroke, and other health problems (116).

2.2.1.4 Passive Smoking

Passive smoking, also called environmental tobacco smoke, secondhand smoke, or involuntary smoking is the inhalation of cigarette smoke exhaled by a smoker or produced by a burning tobacco product in a nonsmoker (110). Cigarette smoking in public spaces such as in public transit, schools, hospitals, and cinemas is now banned since about ten years ago in many countries. Passive smoking at home can cause lung cancer, cardiovascular diseases, and atherosclerosis in nonsmoking neighbors (108, 110). In general, children exposed to environmental tobacco smoke show deterioration of lung function, more pulmonary infections, more days of restricted activity, more days in bed, more hospitalization, and more absences from school than children living in nonsmoking homes (108). Pregnant women exposed to secondhand smoke are at increased risk of having a baby with a small reduction in birth weight (110). Of course, cigarette smoking is not only harmful for the smoker, but also for his or her neighbors. For the sake of the health of yourself and your family, try to quit cigarette smoking completely.

2.2.2 Harmful Effects of Alcoholism

The harmful effects of alcohol consumption and the different types of alcohol beverages have been described in the Chapter 4 of this book. Briefly, alcohol is a psychoactive substance with dependence-producing properties. According to World Health Organization (WHO), worldwide, 3 million deaths every year result from harmful use of alcohol; this represents 5.3% of all deaths (117). The harmful use of alcohol is a causal factor in more than 200 disease and injury conditions. Heavy drinking is associated with an increase in mortality, hypertension, alcoholic cardiomyopathy, cancer, immunosuppression, and cerebrovascular events, including cerebrovascular hemorrhage (117–118). Frequent and excessive consumption of alcohol, especially strong alcohol (liqueurs and spirits), is harmful to health and can cause alcohol dependence, many dreadful ailments, road clashes, and violence (117–118).

However, some studies suggest that moderate drinking may be linked with a lower risk of heart attack and death due to cardiovascular disease and diabetes (119). Therefore, moderate consumption of certain alcohol drinks, such as wine, beer, or cider, about one cup or less a day, does not cause health problems for a majority of healthy people (119). In contrast, a recent publication found that there is 'no safe level of alcohol consumption' (120). This means that any amount of alcohol consumed is toxic to the body.

At the same quantities, some alcohol drinks are better for health than others. For example, red wine is better than white wine because red wine is prepared from red grapes which contain stronger antioxidants, like resveratrol, than white grapes (see resveratrol in Chapter 3 of this book). Resveratrol is anticancer, anti-infection, anti-diabetic, anti-aging, anti-inflammatory, immunomodulating, and a cardiovascular protector. In addition, another study found that individuals with low socioeconomic status (SES) experience disproportionately greater alcohol-attributable health harm than individuals with high SES from similar or lower amounts of alcohol consumption (121). This means that with the same quantity of alcohol consumption, rich people have fewer health problems related to alcohol than poor people because, for example, red wine of high quality is richer in antioxidants than wine of low quality.

Moreover, approximately 35–40% of the population in East Asia (China, Japan, Korea, Vietnam) have an inactive mitochondrial acetaldehyde dehydrogenase 2 (ALDH2) because of a genetic acetaldehyde dehydrogenase deficiency (122). This causes reddened face, nausea, headaches, and palpitation when consuming alcohol. Hence, alcoholism is low in these countries. People with genetic acetaldehyde dehydrogenase deficiency (ALDH2) are at much higher risk of liver cancer and esophageal cancer from alcohol consumption than individuals with fully active ALDH2 (122–123). Therefore, individuals with ALDH2 deficiency must avoid alcohol consumption.

In brief, alcoholism is harmful not only for you, but also for your family and your society. Never drive a car after drinking alcohol, even with a little portion.

2.2.3 Drug addiction and Drug Abuse

Drug addiction and drug abuse are two different bad habits of people who depend upon certain chemical compounds to satisfy their psychological and physiological needs.

2.2.3.1 *Distinction between Drug Addiction and Drug Abuse*

The definition of drug abuse is quite different from that of drug addiction (124–125).

In brief, drug addiction is the use of a drug that can cause a phenomenon of dependence to the user, such as the use of cocaine, heroin, cannabis, cigarette, alcohol, and so on. Drug abuse is a generic term for the abuse of any drug, including medicines, alcohol, and cigarettes; while drug addiction is the inability to stop using the drug due to the effect of this drug on brain. Addiction is considered to be a mental disease. The addictive drugs discussed here are opioids, cannabinoids, cocaine, and amphetamines (125).

2.2.3.2 *Harmful Effects of Drug Addiction*

Drugs causing addiction phenomena can be divided into two groups: illicit and licit drugs. Illicit or illegal drug addiction may involve cocaine, heroin, opium, cannabis, amphetamines, or lysergic acid diethylamide (LSD), among others. Legal drug addiction may involve alcohol, cigarettes, gambling, electronic games, food, and more.

2.2.3.2.1 *Cocaine Addiction*   Cocaine is a crystalline tropane alkaloid found in leaves of the coca plant. It is a mental and physical stimulant (126–127). Cocaine powder is snorted through the nose and sometimes smoked or injected. Coca leaf chewing is common among indigenous inhabitants of the Andean region (Peru, Bolivia, Colombia). Oral formulations of cocaine, such as coca tea (infusions of the leaf) and tablets, are also used in this region (127). Cocaine produces its psychoactive and addictive effects primarily by acting on the brain's limbic system, a set of interconnected regions that regulate pleasure and motivation. An initial, short-term effect gives rise to euphoria and a desire to take the drug again (128). Cocaine dependence is a significant worldwide public health problem with somatic, psychological, socio-economic, and legal implications (127). No specific effective pharmacological treatment exists for cocaine dependence. Recent advances in neurobiology have identified various neuronal mechanisms implicated in cocaine addiction and suggested several promising pharmacological approaches (127). Cocaine causes many types of intermediate-term alterations in brain cell functioning (128). Symptoms of acute cocaine toxicity includes tachydysrhythmia, stroke, severe hypertension, acute coronary syndrome, hyperthermia, seizure, acute myocardial and renal failure, cocaine-induced rhabdomyolysis, and fetal/maternal morbidity and mortality (126). Overdose of cocaine can lead to heart attack and sudden death. Long-term use of cocaine can cause fibrosis, myocarditis, and contraction band necrosis. Cocaine also can induce delirium which is often associated with aggression, hyperactivity, extreme paranoia, hyperthermia, incoherent screaming, and unusual strength (126).

2.2.3.2.2 *Heroin, Morphine and Opium Addiction*   Short-term administration of heroin or morphine produces euphoria, sedation, and a feeling of tranquility. Repeated administration rapidly produces tolerance and intense physical dependence. Overdose can cause lethal respiratory depression (125). Heroin is usually used as an illegal drug of abuse. Heroin, also known as diacetylmorphine, is a semi-synthetic compound obtained by acetylation of morphine, and is more potent than morphine (129). Heroin can be sniffed, smoked, or injected. Heroin is a strong agonist of opioid receptors. It has a short half-life of three minutes in blood after intravenous administration,

requiring drug abusers to use it several times per day to maintain the desired effect (129). Heroin is rapidly metabolized into morphine and totally absent in urine. Common side effects of heroin include respiratory depression, sleepiness, dizziness, confusion, nausea, sedation, and impaired coordination. The health risks of heroin intake are addiction, constipation, endocarditis, hepatitis, HIV, and fatal overdose. Injection of heroin can cause infection and HIV due to the transmission of virus or bacteria from contaminated syringes. In the event of overdose death, this can include signs of pulmonary edema in lung tissue sections and rhabdomyolysis, including myocardial injury (129). Morphine is an alkaloid of opium. In medicine, morphine is used mainly to treat acute and chronic severe pain. As heroin, morphine gives euphoria to the drug addict, but its effect is less rapid than that of heroin. Its side effects are similar to those of heroin. Chronic morphine abuse leads to physical and psychological dependence. Morphine withdrawal symptoms in people include sneezing, runny nose, cough, abdominal pain, diarrhea, anorexia, anxiety, and other effects (130). Morphine is rarely used by addicts because its euphoria is less intense than that of heroin.

The natural opiates include opium, morphine, and codeine (131). Opium is the latex obtained from the poppy plant namely *Papaver somniferum* belonging to the family Papaveraceae. Opium is mainly smoked with the aid of a special pipe, and sometimes prepared as a pill then swallowed. It gives to the addict a similar sensation as that of heroin and morphine, and has the same side effects. Opium addiction began since ancient times, mostly in Asia. Opiate addiction is now becoming a worldwide problem as 13–22 million people are afflicted; Asia encompasses more than half of that (131).

The opioids can be divided into subclasses based on their chemical structure as natural opium alkaloids (codeine, morphine), semisynthetic derivatives of the natural alkaloids (hydrocodone, hydromorphone, oxycodone, buprenorphine), various classes of synthetic opioids such as the anililopiperidines (fentanyl, alfentanil, sufentanil, remifentanil), diphenylpropylamine derivatives (methadone, propoxyphene, dextropropoxyphene, diphenoxylate, loperamide), and others (pentazocine, butorphanol, nalbuphine, levorphanol, tramadol), as well as the opioid antagonists (nalmefene, naloxone and naltrexone) (132).

Methadone is a chiral synthetic analgesic compound used for the treatment of heroin or opioid dependency. This therapy by substitution needs a therapeutic monitoring control of the two methadone enantiomers in biological fluids of the addict for the efficacy of methadone treatment because only one methadone enantiomer is active and varies with each individual (133). Methadone treatment can help eradicate heroin or opium addiction in drug addicts.

2.2.3.2.3 Cannabis or Marijuana and Hashish Addiction Cannabis is a flowery plant in the family Cannabaceae. The cannabis plant has two main subspecies, *Cannabis indica* and *Cannabis sativa*, and they can be differentiated by their different physical characteristics. *Indica*-dominant strains are short plants with broad, dark green leaves, while *Sativa*-dominant strains are usually taller and have thin leaves with a pale green color (134). *C. sativa* is higher in cannabinoid compounds, especially delta-9-tetrahydrocannabinol, or THC, the primary active ingredient in marijuana content, than *C. indica*. Due to its higher THC content, *C. sativa* is the preferred choice by users. It is a complex plant with about 426 chemical entities, of which more than 60 are cannabinoid compounds (134). Cannabis is also the most widely used illicit drug in the world and its use has been associated with various mental health problems, particularly in young people (134). Marijuana and hashish are both obtained from the same female *Cannabis sativa* plant. Marijuana is a dried product made from flowering tops/buds and sometimes the leaves of plant, while hashish is a resin extracted from flowering tops/buds only. The hashish effect is stronger than that of marijuana. Both marijuana and hashish have euphoric and addictive effects (134–135). Marijuana is prepared as cigarette (joint) and consumed by smoking. Hashish resin is also consumed by smoking, typically in a pipe, special vaporizer, or by chewing. Contrary to cigarette smoking, cannabis smoking has a long half-life of many days to a week, therefore cannabis smokers do not need to smoke many times a day. The effects of short-term use of cannabis are: impaired short-term memory, impaired motor coordination such as driving skills, thereby increasing the risk of road accidents, altered judgment, paranoia, and psychosis in high doses. Its effects with long-term use are addiction, altered brain development, mental health decline, poor educational outcome, cognitive impairment, diminished life satisfaction, chronic bronchitis, cough, anxiety, and chronic psychosis disorders (134–135). Marijuana use has also been associated with vascular conditions that increase the risks of myocardial infarction, stroke, and transient ischemic attacks during marijuana intoxication (135). Epidemiological studies reported a link between the use of cannabis and the development of a psychotic illness (anxiety, psychosis, memory disturbance) (146). Marijuana smoking can cause inflammation of the large airways, and lung hyperinflation (135). Cannabis is an illegal drug in a number of countries, except Canada, Uruguay, and South Africa, as well as several states in the United States.

However, cannabis can be used in therapy for certain diseases such as chronic pain, inflammation, and multiple sclerosis (135). According to the report of the Institute of Medicine, 'Marijuana and Medicine', the potential benefits of smoking marijuana include stimulating appetite, particularly in patients with the acquired immunodeficiency syndrome (AIDS) and the related wasting syndrome, as well as combatting chemotherapy-induced nausea and vomiting, severe pain, and some forms of spasticity (135). The report also indicates that there is some evidence for the benefit of using marijuana to decrease intraocular pressure in the treatment of glaucoma (134–135). Nonetheless, the report stresses the importance of focusing research efforts on the therapeutic potential of synthetic or pharmaceutically pure cannabinoids. Some physicians continue to prescribe marijuana for medicinal purposes despite limited evidence of a benefit (135). This practice raises particular concerns with regard to long-term use by vulnerable populations. For example, there is some evidence to suggest that in patients with symptoms of human immunodeficiency virus (HIV) infection or AIDS, marijuana use may actually exacerbate HIV-associated cognitive deficits (135). Therefore, the use of cannabis in the treatment of some diseases cited previously must be done with precaution because its harmful effects may be more important than its beneficial effects.

2.2.3.2.4 Amphetamine and Methamphetamine Addiction

Amphetamine and methamphetamine are synthetic compounds, psycho-stimulant drugs that cause dependence (136–138). Dependence on amphetamine and methamphetamine represent a substantial public health burden (137).

They are available in different forms such as a pure crystalline hydrochloride salt or as formulated tablets. Routes of administration are intranasal sniffing, pulmonary inhalation, injection, and oral ingestion (137–138). They give euphoria and increase energy to the user. The stimulant effects of methamphetamine and cocaine are similar, but the effects of methamphetamine may last much longer (138). Amphetamine is used as drug to treat some sleep diseases like narcolepsy, while its derivative, methamphetamine, is an illegal drug. Methamphetamine is considered a more potent derivative of amphetamine, with a longer duration of action and increased ability to cross the blood-brain barrier (136). Both compounds act on the central nervous system. They can stimulate a person to stay awake throughout the night. Their acute effects include a heightened sense of alertness, increased energy, heightened curiosity, anorexia, decreased fatigue, elevated mood, and dose-dependent effects on focus, attention, and concentration (136). In short term use, these drugs increase heart rate, blood pressure, body temperature, metabolism; cause irritability, tremor, anxiety, panic; and reduce appetite. In long-term use, they cause addiction, body weight loss, insomnia, stroke, CVD, paranoia, violent behavior, and seizure. In addition, their effects are associated with multiple morbidities, including HIV infection, hepatitis, cardiac effects, family disruptions, and prominent psychiatric consequences including psychosis (137). No pharmacotherapy has yielded convincing results for the treatment of amphetamine and methamphetamine dependence; most studies were underpowered and had low treatment completion rates (136–138).

2.2.3.2.5 Hallucinogen Addiction (LSD, Mescaline, and Psilocybin)

Hallucinogens (psychedelics) are psychoactive substances that powerfully alter perception and mood, and affect numerous cognitive processes. They are considered physiologically safe and do not produce dependence or addiction (139–140). The first generation of clinical psychedelic research began in the mid-twentieth century and focused almost exclusively on lysergic acid diethylamide (LSD), mescaline, and psilocybin (141).

Lysergic acid diethylamide (LSD) is a semi-synthetic tryptamine derived from the naturally occurring ergot alkaloid ergotamine that is present in ergot fungus (141). LSD was first synthesized in 1938 by Albert Hofmann. Its psychoactive properties, however, were not discovered until five years later (141). LSD acts primarily as a serotonergic agonist, but also shows action at dopaminergic and adrenergic receptor sites. Use of LSD in the treatment of alcoholism was one of the most widely studied therapeutic applications of psychedelics (141).

Psilocybin was first isolated in 1958 in 'magic' mushrooms named *Psilocybe* (141). It was used since antiquity for ancient ceremonies and religion rites.

Mescaline is a natural alkaloid isolated in 1896 from *Lophophora williamsii*, a small cactus native to northern Mexico and the southwestern United States, by German chemist Arthur Heffter (141). It was the first naturally occurring psychedelic alkaloid to be isolated in the laboratory.

LSD, psilocybin, and mescaline are all hallucinogens (141). When people take hallucinogens, they see, hear, or feel things that do not really exist. The acute effects of these hallucinogens are alteration of perception and feeling, hallucination, nausea, muscle twitches, and anxiety. For LSD and mescaline, increase of heart rate, body temperature, blood pressure, loss of appetite and sleep, and other troubles like sweating, dizziness, tremors, and impulsive behavior are also observed in addicts. For psilocybin, paranoia, anxiety, panic, and nausea are its main side effects. In long-term use, addiction is also observed, but this dependence is easily resolved. Besides their hallucinogenic properties, some psychedelics such as LSD have therapeutic properties such as the treatment of alcoholism and other addictions (cocaine) (139–141). Other studies examined the use of psychedelics to treat certain psychiatric disorders such as anxiety and depression, schizophrenia, and even autism (139–141).

Apart from these common addiction problems due to the use of certain natural or artificial compounds, there exist other addiction phenomena such as addiction to food, mobile phones, electronic games, gambling, playing cards, and more.

2.2.3.2.6   Food Addiction   Food addiction or eating addiction is a type of behavioral addiction that is a compulsive overeating of palatable foods. People with food addictions lose control over their eating behavior and find themselves spending excessive amounts of time involved with food and overeating (142–143). Like addictive drugs, palatable foods trigger good brain chemicals such as the neurotransmitter dopamine. As a result, people keep eating, even when they are not hungry or they know the negative consequences of overeating, such as obesity, diabetes, and CVDs (142). The evidence further suggests that certain foods, particularly processed foods with added sweeteners and fats, demonstrate the greatest addictive potential. Though both behavioral and substance-related factors are implicated in the addiction process, symptoms appear to better fit criteria for substance use disorder than behavioral addiction (143).

Food addiction differs from bulimia nervosa which is an eating disorder characterized by uncontrollable eating followed by purging such as vomiting.

2.2.3.2.7   Gambling and Electronic Game Addiction   Other addictions like gambling, electronic games, and excessive computer or television use are also harmful to health due to the lack of physical activity during a long period. These addictions can cause damage not only to different organs in the body but also to the psychic and mental activities of the gamer. For example, usage of the computer and television up to midnight may affect sleep patterns and may cause sleep disorders, obesity, and Type 2 diabetes in children and adults (3, 8). Addiction to mobile phones and computer games may lead to depression symptoms, dementia, or death (8). Playing cards for long periods is also harmful to health.

2.2.4   Harmful Effects of Medicine Abuse

By definition, the inappropriate use of any therapeutic drug is called medicine abuse. The medicine abuse described here only concerns ordinary drugs such as prescription medicines, over-the-counter (OTC) medications, and dietary supplements. In many countries, the overuse of drugs like OTC medications and supplements is a common unhealthy lifestyle (3).

2.2.4.1   Side Effects and Overuses of Medicines

The self-medication and the inappropriate prescription of drugs can be harmful to health in the short and long term. Remember that any medicine has side effects on the body. The intensity of these side effects varies depending on the drug, its dose, its duration of use, its association with other drugs or supplements, and the patient's state. Only a doctor and or pharmacist can give you necessary information about the pharmacological properties and side effects of each drug. They may also assess the benefits and risks of each drug in the treatment of a disease. Many problems concerning the risks of some drugs have been cited in the recent literature.

For example, the use of pain relievers such as nonsteroidal anti-inflammatory drugs (NSAIDs) is the origin of many other diseases reported recently. Rofecoxib (Vioxx®), a type of NSAID called a COX-2 inhibitor, caused as many as 140,000 heart attacks and strokes in the United States during the period of 1999–2004 (144). Vioxx® was removed from the market in 2004. The regrettable experience with Vioxx® raised awareness about the cardiovascular risk of NSAIDs, and led to further studies showing that the risk is not limited to Vioxx® but is associated with all NSAIDs, except aspirin (144). In 2005, then in 2015, the FDA (The Food and Drug Administration) warned that taking NSAIDs like ibuprofen and naproxen might increase risk of heart attack or stroke (144–146). Because ibuprofen (Motrin, Advil) and naproxen (Aleve) are available over the counter and are so widely used, it is important to be aware of the warnings and to take steps to limit the risk (144). Many people take NSAIDs to relieve mild to moderate pain. Examples of commonly used over-the-counter NSAIDs include ketoprofen, ibuprofen, and naproxen. Indomethacin, celecoxib, diclofenac, and others are prescription NSAIDs. The side effects of NSAIDs affecting the gastrointestinal tract and kidneys have long been known. NSAIDs may also elevate blood pressure and cause heart failure (144, 146). In brief, the warnings from the FDA concerning NSAIDs (except aspirin) include heart attack and stroke risk, not only for cardiac people, but also for people without heart disease (144–145). However, taking an NSAID for a headache, or for a few days to ease a sore shoulder is not likely to cause a heart attack or stroke. It is more prolonged use that can get risky (144). In view of the warnings, it is best for people with heart disease to avoid NSAIDs, and for everyone who is considering taking an NSAID to proceed with caution (144–145).

Recent research has found that all NSAIDs, including ibuprofen, ketoprofen, diclofenac, aspirin, and celecoxib increase the risk of miscarriage during pregnancy (147–148). So, in France, the mention: 'Prohibition for pregnant women' is now seen on the label of aspirin boxes, even at low doses (75mg).

In France, benfluorex (Mediator®), a derivative of amphetamine or fenfluramine, used in the therapy of Type 2 diabetes, hyperlipidemia and obesity since 1976, was withdrawn from circulation in 2009 because of its side effects on cardiac valves. The number of victims of Mediator® is about 2,000 deaths in France and some 10,000 patients having valvular heart disease caused by this prescription drug during its tumultuous 33 years on the market (149).

The list of drugs removed from the market due to their toxicity is long. However, an exception is reserved for thalidomide. The last one is a sedative drug used for the treatment of nausea and sickness in pregnant women in 1957–1962. It was rapidly withdrawn from the market in 1962 due to its high teratogenicity with severe birth defects in the infants of women who had been prescribed the drug as an anti-emetic (150–151). However, thalidomide was reapproved by the US

Food and Drug Administration (FDA) in 1998 due to its strong anti-inflammatory effect in the treatment of erythema nodosum leprosum (ENL), a painful inflammatory complication of leprosy (151). Thalidomide and its derivatives are now recognized as potential immunomodulatory, anti-inflammatory, and anti-angiogenic agents for the treatment of other serious diseases such as graft versus host disease and multiple myeloma (plasma cell cancer) (150–151). It is now reused for the treatment of some specific diseases cited above.

Besides the side effects of drugs, antibiotic resistance is now a problem for the treatment of many infectious diseases. Antibiotic resistance is the ability of bacteria to resist the effects of an antibiotic due to the overuse of this antibiotic previously. In many countries, especially in developing countries, antibiotics are unregulated and available over the counter without a prescription. This lack of control promotes the overuse of antibiotics. The overuse of antibiotics clearly drives the evolution of resistant bacteria. Incorrectly prescribed antibiotics also contribute to the promotion of antibiotic resistance (3, 152). Moreover, antibiotics are widely used as growth supplements in livestock. The antibiotics used in livestock are ingested by humans when they consume food, thereby, causing passive antibiotic resistance in humans. Antibiotic-resistant infections can be grave health problems that need to be resolved rapidly.

Long-term uses of antineoplastic agents or anticancer drugs (adriamycin, methotrexate, chlorambucil, cis-platin, melphalen, cyclophosphamide) and radiopharmaceuticals (radium, radioactive phosphorous, etc.) account for most of the known drug-induced cancers (153). Some immune suppressive medicines like cyclosporin, azathioprine, and analgesics like phenacetin can induce tumors (153). Some drugs suspected of being human carcinogens include anti-cancer drugs (oxorubicin, procarbazine), antifungals (griseofulvin, metronidazole), anti-epileptic drugs (phenobarbital, phenytoin), cimetidine (antiulcer), and clofibrate (anti-lipid) (153). There is evidence of an increased risk of serious infections and a dose-dependent increased risk of malignancies in patients with rheumatoid arthritis treated with anti-TNF antibody therapy (154).

In 2012, a synthetic study of 2,200 brand drugs marketed in France by Even and Debré showed that 60% of them were highly efficacious, but the remaining 40% had weak or zero efficacy (155). More precisely, 18% of the second group were weakly efficacious and the rest (22%) was totally useless. Among 2,200 brand drugs, 20% of drugs had notable side effects, sometimes grave, 5% had major risks, and 25% had diverse degrees of side effects (155). Many strong side effects were also observed among inefficacious drugs. However, this study is still not recognized by healthcare organizations in France and in Europe.

2.2.4.2 Side Effects of Over-the-Counter Medications

Over-the-counter (OTC) medicines are those that can be sold directly to people without a prescription. OTC medicines treat a variety of ailments and their symptoms, like ache and pain, coughs and colds, fever, allergy, diarrhea, constipation, acne, and others (156–157). Some OTC medicines have active ingredients with the potential for misuse at higher-than-recommended dosages. About 80% of American adults commonly take over-the-counter medications (157). This self-treatment is economic, rapid, and convenient for the user. However, the risks of this self-treatment can have many consequences. As cited above, the misuse of OTC NSAIDs like ibuprofen and naproxen can cause heart problems especially for cardiac people and the elderly, as well as miscarriage in pregnant women. OTC aspirin can provoke gastric ulcers, hemorrhage, allergy, and miscarriage for certain people. Recently, the National Agency of Drug Security of France has reported numerous cases of grave infections – even death – after intake of two OTC NSAIDS: ibuprofen or ketoprofen (158).

Even acetaminophen, the safest OTC antalgic, can cause liver disease like cirrhosis with prolonged use or high dose intake. In France, the National Agency for the Safety of Medicines and Health Products had to withdraw some medicines containing acetaminophen, aspirin, and ibuprofen, from the list of over the counter (OTC) since 15 January 2020, due to numerous accidents linked to self-medication (159). Dextromethorphan (DXM) is a cough suppressant found in many

OTC cold medicines. DXM is an opioid without effects on pain reduction and does not act on the opioid receptors. When taken in large doses, DXM causes a depressant effect and sometimes a hallucinogenic effect. Repeated use can lead to addiction similar to that of opioids (156).

People who have underlying health problems or who routinely take one or more prescription drugs would be wise to consult their doctors before taking an OTC drug. At the very least, check with the pharmacist (157). Moreover, there occur synergistic effects of OTC medications with other prescription drugs or dietary supplements. The synergistic effects can increase or decrease the effects of drugs that you use, thereby causing toxicity or inefficacy of these drugs. Indeed, be careful when using OTC medications and do not misuse or abuse them. Consult a doctor or a pharmacist before use.

2.2.4.3 Harms and Overuses of Dietary Supplements

Dietary supplements have been described in Chapter 4 of this book. Here are some main features of dietary supplements. Unlike prescription drugs and over-the counter medications, dietary supplements are not evaluated or reviewed by the US Food and Drug Administration (FDA) for safety and effectiveness (160–162). The classification of certain products used as supplements or drugs depends on the health care authority of each country. For example, dehydroepiandrosterone (DHEA) hormone is sold as supplement in the United States, but, in other countries such as France, Canada, Australia, and the United Kingdom, DHEA is a prescription drug.

Because dietary supplements are not controlled as drugs, the levels of active product in supplements can vary enormously between batch to batch and company. Moreover, they can contain harmful impurities or ingredients. A recent study comparing actual to expected concentrations of vitamin D_3 in commercially available brands revealed unacceptable deviations, with pill potency ranging from 9–146% of the stated concentration (161).

As cited in Chapter 3, prolonged use of some antioxidant vitamin and mineral supplements, such as vitamins E, D, A, niacin, selenium, iron, and iodine, can cause side effects, while the same micronutrients consumed via fresh vegetables and fruits are shown to be beneficial for health. It is now widely believed that the actions of antioxidant nutrients alone do not explain the observed health benefits of diets rich in fruits and vegetables (163). They contain not only the vitamins in question, but also other compounds such as coenzymes, cofactors, antioxidants, vitamins, and minerals that help the action of the studied vitamin. This action is due to the additive and synergistic effects of phytochemicals in fruits and vegetables that potentiate the antioxidant and anticancer activities of the studied vitamin (163). This explains why no single antioxidant or vitamin can replace the combination of natural phytochemicals in fruits and vegetables to achieve the health benefits. Moreover, the abuse of antioxidant vitamins like vitamins C, E, and carotenes can cause the formation of pro-oxidants that are harmful to health. However, in certain circumstances such as the absence of an essential vitamin or mineral in food or the need of high levels of certain essential micronutrients for the treatment of a specific disease, the supply of a specific vitamin or mineral by dietary supplements becomes necessary. For example, the supply of vitamin D and/or calcium is necessary for the treatment of certain bone diseases in the elderly. In these cases, the oversight of a doctor is necessary for this supplementation. Supplements may be obtained by chemical synthesis or natural preparation. In general, natural obtention is better than synthetic preparation. Self-medication and inappropriate use of supplements can cause health problems. The evidence suggests that antioxidants are best acquired through whole-food consumption, not from dietary supplements (163).

2.2.5 Harmful Effects of Unhealthy Foods

Unhealthy food, also called junk food or 'bad food', is a type of food that can cause harm to human health. An unhealthy diet is often high in trans-fatty acids, salt, sugar, artificial sweetener, saturated fat (lard), processed meat, margarine, soda, fume, preservative, and artificial colorants. (164). An unhealthy diet can cause health problems to consumers due to the contamination of environmental and industrial chemicals, including pesticides, insecticides, dioxins, polychlorinated biphenyls

(PCBs), pathogenic microorganisms, natural toxicants, or also due to food alterations (165). An unhealthy diet is often low in fruits, vegetables, seafoods, nuts, seeds, fibers, whole grain, milk, vitamins, minerals, antioxidants, omega-3 fatty acids, and so on. This type of diet can cause inflammatory diseases (166). An unhealthy diet may also be due to cooking mode. As cited previously, barbecuing, grilling, and frying are considered unhealthy cooking modes. Consumption of processed meats, but not red meats, is associated with higher incidence of CHD and diabetes (26–29, 167–168). The harmful effects of excessive intake of processed meat such as bacon, salami, hot dogs, ham, sausages, pâté, barbecued pork, corned beef, and beef jerky, as well as canned meat, are described in 'Chapter 6: Animal Source Foods'. Regular consumption of some processed foods, such as snack, biscuit, candy, cake, canned fruits, and margarine, is considered bad for health because these foods are made with high contents of saturated fat, trans-fat, sugar, salt and calories, with little nutritional value. Additionally, they contain many food additives and preservatives. Frequent intake of soft drinks and energy drinks may cause obesity and related health problems such as Type 2 diabetes mellitus and cardiovascular diseases. However, moderate consumption (two to three times a week) of processed meat, processed foods, and energy drinks may not be harmful to health.

2.2.6 Harmful Effects of Household Products

Many household products that can cause adverse health effects include: mothballs, air fresheners, bleach, household cleaners, antibacterial soaps, gas space heaters, insecticides for ants, flies, fleas, and ticks, herbicides for home gardens, and more (169).

2.2.6.1 Mothballs

Mothballs are sold as small white balls containing 99.9% either of naphthalene or paradichlorobenzene (PDCB), both of which become a gas with pungent odor when exposed to air. Mothballs are used to repel moths in clothing and stored carpets and to keep pests out of the house (170). The majority of exposure to naphthalene in the environment occurs through inhalation, while other pathways such as dermal contact and ingestion are rare. Naphthalene is recently classified as a possible human carcinogen (171–172). Naphthalene exposure can cause hemolytic anemia due to destruction of red blood cells with apparition of jaundice and pallor. It is also neurotoxic. Small children may eat mothballs, thinking them candy (170). Para-dichlorobenzene (PDCB) is another ingredient of mothballs used as deodorizers and fumigants. PDCB toxicity can affect liver, kidneys, skin, lungs, and the central nervous system (CNS). Chronic toxicity of PDCB often results in leukoencephalopathy, ataxia, and heterogeneous neurological manifestations (173–175). Mothballs containing either PDCB or naphthalene, can cause cancer in animals, and are potential human carcinogens (170–172). So, be careful when using mothballs as moth or pest repellents. Due to the toxicity of naphthalene and para-dichlorobenzene, avoid the use of mothballs if you have a chronic disease, or infants and children in the house. Replace mothballs by cedar chips (170).

2.2.6.2 Air Fresheners and Deodorizers

Air fresheners are products that emit a fragrance to provide an aroma to a space, or to mask an odor, with the intent of creating a pleasing indoor space. Deodorizers or air neutralizers are used to neutralize odiferous molecules by absorbing or destroying them, thus ridding the room of odor (176). Air fresheners come in numerous versions, including sprays, gels, oils, liquids, solids, automatic diffusers, and scented candles; and with instant, intermittent, or continuous release. However, air fresheners can emit and generate a range of potentially hazardous chemicals that can impair air quality and inhabitant health. Even so-called green and organic air fresheners can emit hazardous air pollutants (176). Air fresheners and deodorizers can emit over 100 different chemicals, including volatile organic compounds such as terpenes, terpenoids, eugenol, linalool, ethanol, benzene, toluene, xylene, limonene, pinene, formaldehyde, acetaldehyde, phthalates, and so on. (176–179). Air freshener and deodorizer exposures, even at low levels, have been associated with a range of adverse health effects, which include migraine headaches, asthma attacks, breathing difficulties, rhinitis, earache, mucosal symptoms, dermatitis, infant diarrhea, dizziness, neurological problems, hepatic disease, ventricular fibrillation, immune disorders, and eventual cancer risks (176–179). For instance, acetaldehyde, which can be both a primary and secondary emission from air fresheners, is associated with both acute and chronic hazards to the respiratory system, and classified as a carcinogenic hazardous air pollutant in the United States (176). Therefore, do not frequently use air fresheners and deodorizers with permanent automatic diffusers in closed spaces like the bathroom, kitchen, and car. Ventilating these spaces by opening the windows is the best choice.

2.2.6.3 Indoor Incense Smoke and Cancer

In Asian countries, incense burning is often done for religious ceremony. People usually ignite incense sticks with a flame, then these sticks continue to burn by releasing fragrant smoke (fumes). A typical composition of stick incense consists of 21% herbal and wood powder such as cinnamon, agarwood, sandalwood; 35% fragrance material (essential oils); 11% adhesive powder; and 33% bamboo stick. Incense smoke contains particulate matter, gas products, and many organic compounds (180). The gas products from burning incense include carbon monoxide (CO), carbon dioxide (CO_2), nitrogen dioxide (NO_2), sulfur dioxide (SO_2), and others. Incense burning also produces volatile organic compounds, such as benzene, toluene, and xylenes, as well as aldehydes and polycyclic aromatic hydrocarbons (PAHs) (180). These gases have harmful effects on health. When incense smokes are inhaled mostly in closed room, they can cause respiratory system dysfunction such as asthma, nasopharyngitis, and also lung cancer. Many scientific publications have highlighted the carcinogenic effects of incense smokes in experimental studies as well as in human observations (180–182). However, the results concerning lung cancer in humans are still controversial. This is due to the difference methods of making incense sticks. In short, do not burn incense sticks in closed rooms, and avoid exposing yourself to incense smoke even in the open air.

2.2.6.4 Indoor Pesticides and Herbicides

Indoors, pesticides are used to wipe out flies, mosquitoes, ants, cockroaches, pet's ticks, and so on, while herbicides are meant to kill undesirable plants or weeds in home gardens. Pesticides are also present in fruits and vegetables. Pesticides and herbicides are toxic chemicals that can cause different diseases in humans upon long exposure through contact with the skin, ingestion, or inhalation (183–187). Pulverization of pesticides is the main way they are used in the home. They can penetrate into the body by inhalation or through skin. The main harmful effect of pesticides is mutagenicity; alterations of genes or DNA damages (184). Other negative health effects that have been associated with pesticides include neurological, carcinogenic, respiratory, reproductive, gastrointestinal, endocrine, and dermatological effects (185–186). In addition, high occupational, accidental, or intentional exposure to pesticides can result in hospitalization and death (185). Aside from organic foods, pesticide residues can be found in a great variety of everyday foods and beverages, including fresh vegetables and fruits, cooked meals, water, wine, fruit juices, refreshments, and animal feeds (185). Although the levels of pesticides in foods are in conformity with official norms, the consumption of different foods with different types and levels of these chemicals can have synergistic effects on the body that render them toxic. Always keep the home clean and dry with the help of detergents. Ventilation is the best way to limit the use of pesticides indoors. The use of screens on windows prevents the intrusion of flying insects into the home. Asthmatics should reduce humidity, carpet, and wallpaper in the home to prevent mold and spore growth. If you have a garden with many plants and lawns, do not use synthetic pesticides and herbicides for the protection of your garden because you will inhale these toxic products permanently.

2.2.7 Environmental Pollution and Health

The effects of environmental pollution in health and disease are now well-established. The pollutants released into the environment come mainly from human activities such as products eliminated from industry of chemicals, mining, agriculture, energy, and transport, as well as from from household garbage and individual product use (plastic bags, bottles, etc.). The environment includes air, water, and soil. Pollutants are not only harmful to human health, but also to flora and fauna, and especially to the climate. Environmental pollution occurs when pollutants contaminate the surroundings; thereby affecting our normal lifestyles adversely. Pollutants affect people of all ages from babies and children to adults and the elderly, shortening life expectancy. About 8–9% of the total disease burden may be attributed to pollution (188). Yet it is clear that environmental and life-style factors are key determinants of human disease, accounting for perhaps 75% of most cancers (189). According to the American Cancer Society, only about 5–10% of all cancers result directly from gene defects (called mutations) inherited from a parent (190). Genetic specialists of Cancer Research UK estimate that between 3 and 10 in every 100 (3–10%) cancers diagnosed are linked to an inherited faulty gene (191). Most people who have relatives with cancer will not have inherited a defective gene. Cancer mostly occurs in older people (191). Other causes of cancer include diseases, bacteria, viruses, and more. That is why cancer occurs more often in industrialized countries than in developing and undeveloped countries.

2.2.7.1 Air Pollution

Environmental air pollution has two sources: natural activities such as volcano eruption and forest fire, and anthropogenic activities such as emanation from various industries, mining, agriculture, cars, and so on. These air pollutants may cause adverse effects on human health and the environment (192). There are four main categories of air pollutants:

- gaseous pollutants such as carbon monoxide (CO), carbon dioxide (CO2), sulfur dioxide (SO2), nitrogen oxides (NOx), ozone (O3), mercury vapor, etc.
- persistent organic pollutants like pesticides, dioxins, polychlorinated biphenyls (PCBs), polycyclic aromatic hydrocarbons (PAHs), furans, etc.
- heavy metals such as lead, mercury, cadmium, vanadium, etc.
- particulate matter such as particles in air from factories, power plants, refuse incinerators, motor vehicles, petroleum exploitation, mining, construction activity, fires, natural wind-blown dust, etc. (192).

They are often present in smokes and fumes from combustion of organic matters. Air pollution has both acute and chronic effects on human health, affecting a number of different systems and organs. It ranges from minor upper respiratory irritation to chronic respiratory and heart disease, lung cancer, acute respiratory infections in children, and chronic bronchitis in adults, aggravating pre-existing heart and lung disease, or asthmatic attacks. In addition, short- and long-term exposures have also been linked with premature mortality and reduced life expectancy (192). The increase in cases of asthma and allergies has become an important health issue worldwide. Exposure to environmental pollutants (both outdoor and indoor) may partially account for the prevalence of such diseases (193). We examine below the health effects of some products obtained from air pollution.

2.2.7.1.1 Effects of Ozone on Health

Ozone (O3) is a gas composed of three atoms of oxygen. Ozone occurs both in the earth's upper atmosphere, called stratosphere, and at ground level. In stratosphere, ozone is good for human health because it forms a protective layer that shields us from the sun's harmful ultraviolet rays (194–195). Over the first half of twentieth century, this beneficial ozone was partially destroyed by manmade chemicals such as freons, causing a 'hole' in the ozone layer. Now, this hole is diminishing due to the interdiction of freons which were previously used as refrigerant for fridges. At ground level, ozone is formed by pollution caused by human activities. As the chief component of urban smog, ozone is created by chemical reactions between oxides of nitrogen (NOx) and volatile organic compounds (VOC) in the presence of sunlight (193). Emissions from industrial facilities and electric utilities, motor vehicle exhaust, gasoline vapors, power plants, industrial boilers, and chemical plants and refineries are some of the major sources of NOx and

VOC (194–195). Ozone at ground level is a harmful air pollutant for human health and environment. Ozone is most likely to reach unhealthy levels on sunny and dry days in urban environments; therefore, many authorities limit the use of cars in town during sunny periods. Ozone is an unstable molecule that is easily broken down into oxygen O_2 by contact with water or humidity, a solid organic surface like asphalt road, or some mineral catalysts (nickel, copper, zinc). Its levels decrease at night. Breathing ozone can trigger many health problems such as chest pain, coughing, eye irritation, throat, and airway inflammation. It can also harm lung tissue and reduce lung function by worsening asthma, bronchitis, and emphysema (189, 194). People most at risk of the harmful effects of breathing ozone in the air include asthmatics, children, people with CVDs, the elderly, and outdoor workers. Ground level ozone can also have harmful effects on sensitive vegetation and ecosystems (194, 195). On high-level ozone days, staying indoors is recommended to people at risk, while limiting your outdoor activity, especially from noon to afternoon, is reserved for normal people.

2.2.7.1.2 Effects of Polycyclic Aromatic Hydrocarbons on Health   Polycyclic aromatic hydrocarbons (PAHs) are complex benzenoid compounds formed during incomplete combustion (196). The major sources of PAHs include domestic activities such as wood burning, frying, and barbecuing, as well as external origins like road traffic, fuel combustion in industry, forest fires, and more. Exposure to PAH-containing substances increases the risk of cancer in humans (196). The carcinogenicity of PAHs depends on the different chemical structure of the molecule. Fluoranthene is an important volatile PAH because it occurs at high levels in ambient air and because it has demonstrated carcinogenic property in certain test systems (196). Phenanthrene, anthracene, and pyrene also belong to PAHs and have carcinogenic property (196).

2.2.7.1.3 Effects of Polychlorinated Biphenyls on Health   Polychlorinated biphenyls (PCBs) are organic chlorine compounds that were manufactured between 1930–1977 and were predominantly used as coolants and lubricants in electrical equipment or as plasticizers in paints, plastics, and rubber products (197). PCB exposure induces various adverse health effects in animals and humans. Environmental and occupational exposures to PCBs have been associated with cancer development, adverse effects in the liver, kidney, and endocrine systems, neurodevelopmental issues, and immunological alterations. PCBs have been banned worldwide since 1977 due to their accumulation and persistence in the environment (197). No known consumer product currently manufactured in the United States contains PCBs, although some industrial processes still release them (197).

2.2.7.1.4 Effects of Dioxins on Health   Dioxins are the term used to refer to Polychlorinated Dibenzo-p-Dioxins (PCDDs) and Polychlorinated Dibenzofurans (PCDFs). Co-planar Polychlorinated Biphenyls (co-planar PCBs) possess toxicity similar to that of dioxins and are called dioxin-like compounds (198–200). In total, there are 7 PCDDs, 10 PCDFs, and 12 PCBs which are considered dioxins or dioxin-like compounds by the World Health Organization (WHO) (199).

Dioxins can be generated either naturally or by human activities (198–200). In nature, dioxins are produced through forest fires or volcanic activities. In industrial processes like chlorine bleaching of pulp paper and manufacturing of chlorinated pesticides, these compounds are produced accidentally. The incomplete combustion of municipal and domestic waste, the burning of chlorine-containing materials such as plastics, and the burning of fuels (wood, coal, or oil) produce dioxins (198–200). Heating systems in homes and emissions from cars also generate small amounts of dioxins.

Emitted in the atmosphere, dioxins and dioxin-like compounds tend to deposit on soil and water, therefore, they can contaminate the food chain (198, 199). The intake of dioxins from food has declined dramatically over the past 20 years (200). But it is human activity which has been primarily responsible for the generation of dioxins over the past two centuries. For example, in 1949, an explosion in a Monsanto chemical plant in West Virginia (USA) resulted in the exposure of workers to the dioxin-contaminated herbicide, 2,4,5-trichlorophenoxyacetic acid (199).

During the Vietnam war (1962–1973), Agent Orange, a dioxin-contaminated herbicide containing 2,4,5-trichlorophenoxyacetic acid and 2,4-dichlorophenoxyacetic acid, was used as a defoliant in Vietnam to reduce enemy ground cover (198–199). Studies of the Ranch Hand cohort have revealed that American military exposures to Agent Orange were associated with an increased risk of cancers and diabetes (199).

Adverse health effects of dioxin exposure in humans may include cancer, cardiovascular disease, diabetes, porphyria, endometriosis, early menopause, reduced testosterone and thyroid hormones, altered immunologic response, skin, tooth, and nail abnormalities, altered growth factor signaling, and altered metabolism (198–199). The International Agency for Research on Cancer under the World Health Organization has identified 2,3,7,8-tetrachlorodibenzo-p-dioxin) (TCDD) to be a polychlorinated dibenzo-p-dioxin as the most toxic of all dioxin compounds and as a carcinogen to man (198, 200). In experimental animals (rodents), high doses of dioxins during pregnancy are known to result in deformities in newborns such as cleft palate and hydronephrosis (200). Dioxins are reported to cause malfunctions in thyroid glands, atrophy of gonads, reductions in the sperm production, and suppression of the immune system in animals. Since effects on humans are not clear at present, further studies are needed of the impacts on human health (200).

2.2.7.1.5 Effects of Coal on Health
Due to its high energy generation potential, coal is used widely in power generation in different countries. The main air pollutants emitted from coal combustion include carbon monoxide, carbon dioxide, nitrogen oxides, sulfur dioxide, ozone, particulate matter and toxic minerals (mercury, lead, arsenic), volatile organic compounds, and respirable particles accumulated in air and water (201). These pollutants lead to severe environmental and health impacts including bone deformities, kidney dysfunction, asthma, cancer, CVDs, reproductive disorders, birth defect, and so on (201). Coal combustion is now banned in many countries.

2.2.7.2 Soil Pollution
'Soil pollution' refers to the presence of a chemical or substance out of place and/or present at higher than normal concentrations that has adverse effects on health (202). This occurs due to incorporation of unwanted chemicals in the soil by human activities. Industrialization, wars, mining, and intensification in agriculture (pesticides, herbicides, fertilizers) are the causes of soil pollution (202). Among them, fertilizers and pesticides used in agriculture are key causes of soil pollution, also known as land pollution. Synthetic chemical pesticides, herbicides, and fertilizers pollute soil, water, and air, harming the environment and human health (203). Excessive use of nitrate, a chemical fertilizer, leads to excess nitrogen in soil that can lead to less diversity of plant species, as well as reduced production of biomass (203). Lately, some scientists observe that glyphosate, the primary herbicide used globally for weed control, targets the 5-enolpyruvylshikimate-3-phosphate synthase enzyme in the shikimate pathway found in plants and some bacteria (204). Thus, glyphosate may affect bacterial symbionts of animals living near agricultural sites, including pollinators such as bees. The bacteria present in honeybee gut microbiota is sensitive to glyphosate. Without these bacteria, bee workers cannot grow normally, and die (204). This discovery might justify the observation that beekeepers have made about glyphosate. They call for the withdrawal of this herbicide from the market. Evidently, pesticides as well as herbicides also have benefits in agriculture. Without them, the crops of many cereals and vegetables may be damaged by parasites and insects. Recently, some natural products extracted from plants and foods have been assayed to fight some insects and parasites in plants without harmful effects on human health and environment (205). These natural products are called biopesticides (205–207).

Biopesticides are natural materials derived from animals, plants, and bacteria, as well as certain minerals, that are used for pest control (206). Biopesticides are classified into three different categories: (1) plant-incorporated protectants, (2) microbial pesticides, and (3) biochemical pesticides (207). The efficacy of biopesticides can be equal to that of conventional pesticides, particularly for crops like fruits, vegetables, nuts, and flowers (207). More research in the field of biopesticides is required to assess their effects on specific pest problems and their potential absence of side effects on human health and the environment.

In addition, mining, agriculture, and deforestation are important energy-intensive activities that impact economies and at the same time directly and indirectly cause soil, air, and land pollution (208–210). Release of industrial waste harms the soil. Food is a big contributor to landfill waste. In addition, industries generate hazardous waste from petroleum refining, mining, and plastic manufacturing. Household hazardous wastes including solvents, plastic items, motor oil, and more, are harmful to human health and the environment. More effective public health policies on hazardous waste management are urgently needed (210). Pollution is observed more in industrialized countries than in developing countries.

2.2.7.3 Water Pollution

Water pollution is any contamination of water with chemicals or other foreign substances that are detrimental to human, plant, or animal health (211). Due to the rapid growth of the world's population and the development of industries, industrial and household waste in the environment, particularly in water, is also increasing considerably. Hence, natural water is now polluted everywhere. The main pollutants infecting water include fertilizers and pesticides from agricultural runoff; chemical wastes from pharmaceutical discharges; domestic sewage and food processing waste; plastic items for individual and collective use; and lead, mercury, and other heavy metals from different industries (212). Among them, plastic items are the main concern for ecosystems worldwide (213–214).

Plastics are synthetic organic polymers. They are composed of hydrocarbons that are prepared from fossil fuel (petroleum) or other products under the action of heat (214). Plastics liberate their toxic monomers, bisphenol-A (BPA) and di-(2-ethylhexyl)-phthalate (DEHP), during decomposition into the environment or during contact with foods or human tissues. BPA and DEHP are well-known strong endocrine disruptors which can interfere with human hormone systems, and consequently, can engender a number of diseases such as infertility, sex deformation, retardation of brain development in children, and cancers of prostate, breast, thyroid (213). At present, BPA has been one of the first plastic materials to be recognized for its potential harm by the US Food and Drug Administration (FDA) (213). In response to such concerns, BPA also recently has been banned in the United States as well as in Canada and the European Union from use in infant bottles and spill-proof cups for toddlers. Do not heat or boil food in plastic containers by microwave. Replace plastic items with porcelain or glass objects. Detectable levels of bisphenol A have been found in the urine of 95% of the adult population of the United States (213).

Worldwide, nearly two billion people drink contaminated water that could be harmful to their health (211). More efforts collectively and individually are needed to resolve the problems of contaminated water that are harmful not only for humans, but also for aquatic animals and plants, which are good sources of foods for humanity. Thus, water pollution is a great problem of ecosystems that needs to be curbed rapidly.

It is now widely accepted that climate change is occurring as a result of the accumulation of greenhouse gases in the atmosphere arising from the combustion of fossil fuels from industry, cars, and heating (215). Climate change may affect health through a range of ways, like increased frequency of heat waves, increased flood and drought, changes in the distribution of vector-borne diseases, and effects on the risk of disasters and malnutrition. Adaptation to climate change requires public health strategies and improved surveillance (215). Change of individual and collective lifestyles is needed for the sake of the environment.

2.2.8 Harmful Effects of Endocrine Disruptors

Many chemicals, both natural and man-made, may mimic or interfere with the body's hormones, known as the endocrine system. Endocrine disruptors are chemicals that interfere with the hormone systems and produce adverse developmental, reproductive, neurological, and immunological effects, as well as obesity, cognitive deficiency, and other problems in mammals (216–218).

Endocrine disruptors are found in many everyday products, including some plastic bottles and containers, metal food cans, detergents, flame retardants, food, toys, cosmetics, and pesticides (216–217). Endocrine disruptors are chemicals that can interfere with the endocrine systems or alter hormone functions and produce adverse developmental, reproductive, neurological, and immune effects in both humans and animals (216–218). When absorbed in the body, an endocrine disruptor can decrease or increase normal hormone levels, mimic the body's natural hormones, or alter the natural production of hormones (216–217). Hormones frequently affected by endocrine disruptors are female sex hormones (estrogens), male sex hormones (testosterone), and thyroid hormones (thyroxin). These hormones may be overproduced or inhibited by endocrine disruptors. Consequently, exposure to endocrine disruptors may result in human health effects including lowered fertility or infertility in both sexes, sex deformation, and an increased incidence of endometriosis and some cancers such as cancers of prostate, breast, or thyroid glands and retardation of brain development in children (216–217). Research shows that endocrine disruptors may pose the greatest risk during prenatal and early postnatal development when organ and neural systems are forming (216). People may be exposed to endocrine disruptors through food and beverages consumed, pesticides applied, and cosmetics used (216). The ban of plastic bags or compounds containing endocrine disruptors (pesticides) are now the top subject claimed by many ecological organizations in the world. Therefore, consumers are advised to limit the use of plastic bags and plastic bottles, and not to throw them in the environment (road, river, ocean, field, forest, etc.), because the decomposition of plastics is harmful to human health and the environment.

3 GOOD DIET AND LIFESTYLE IN THE WORLD

In today's world, two famous well-known diets are the Mediterranean diet and the Okinawan diet. Thanks to these two diets and also to their lifestyle and climate, people in these areas generally live healthier and longer than people in other parts of the world.

3.1 MEDITERRANEAN DIET

The Mediterranean diet comprises the eating habits of people living in countries in southern Europe around the Mediterranean Sea, namely Spain, southern France, Italy, and Greece, to the Middle East and North Africa. The climate of the Mediterranean region is temperate and often sunny; hence, seafoods, fruits, vegetables, cereals, and nuts are abundant. The Mediterranean diet is known to be one of the healthiest dietary patterns in the world (219–223). The Mediterranean diet was first described by Ancel Keys in the Seven Countries Study during the 1960s as a cardioprotective diet (219, 221). The Mediterranean Diet is associated with reduced risk of coronary heart disease and protection against some cancer, Type 2 diabetes mellitus, mental health issues, cognitive decline, and more (219–223). The life expectancy for many populations in this area is ranked among the top ten in the world (see paragraph below). Although there are many different ethnicities, cultures, religions, and economies of this region, the various Mediterranean diets generally include the same key foods, namely olive oil, legumes, unrefined cereals, fruits, vegetables, nuts, and seafoods. Populations of this area consume moderately red wine and dairy products and rarely non-fish meat products (219–223). The Mediterranean diet (MD) also includes moderate consumption of fish and shellfish, white meat, eggs, and dairy products. On the contrary, consumption of red meat, processed meats, and foods rich in sugars and in fats is small in both quantity and frequency (220). The principal source of dietary lipids of the MD is olive oil. An adequate daily intake of water is necessary, and moderate consumption of red wine is recommended. Seasonality, biodiversity, and the use of traditional and local food products are also important elements in this diet. In addition, the Mediterranean diet has also qualitative cultural and lifestyle elements, such as conviviality, culinary activities, physical activity, and adequate rest (219, 220). The fruits most consumed are red grape, apple, orange, berries, prune, apricot, and olive, among others. Vegetables frequently eaten are lettuce, broccoli, tomato, carrot, endive, asparagus, and nuts. Olive oil may be the main health-promoting component of the Mediterranean diet (219–222).

The mechanisms of the Mediterranean diet's effects on health are still unclear. However, some authors have suggested that many components in foods of this diet exert the hormetic effects (223). Hormesis is a term used by toxicologists to refer to a biphasic dose response or an inverted U-shaped dose response to an environmental agent characterized by a low dose stimulation or beneficial effect and a high dose inhibitory or toxic effect (224). For example, some essential micronutrients such as selenium, fluorine, and iodine, ingested at low doses through foods, are beneficial to the body; in contrast, when they are taken at high doses, they become toxic. In the fields of biology and medicine, hormesis is defined as an adaptive response of cells and organisms to a moderate or intermittent stress (224).

3.2 Okinawan Diet

Residents of Okinawa, the southernmost islands of Japan, are well known for their long average life expectancy, high numbers of centenarians, and accompanying low risk of age-associated diseases (225). Much of the longevity advantage in Okinawa is thought to be related to a healthy lifestyle, especially the traditional diet, which is low in calories but high in nutrients, especially when it comes to phytonutrients in the forms of antioxidants and flavonoids.

The traditional diet in Okinawa is composed mainly of colorful sweet potatoes, seaweeds, green and yellow vegetables, soybean-based foods like natto, tofu, and medicinal plants (226). Marine foods, lean meats, fruits, medicinal garnishes and spices (turmeric, galangal, chili pepper), tea, and alcohol are also moderately consumed (226). The staple of the Okinawan diet is the colorful sweet potato, not rice or other grains, as well as the routine use of herbs and spices in place of salt. The traditional Okinawan diet is rich in phytonutrients and antioxidants from vegetables and fruits, but low in meat, saturated fat, sugar, salt, refined grains (rice), and full-fat dairy products (225–227). Okinawans also prefer seaweeds, especially brown seaweeds that are rich in fucoidan, a polysaccharide, and fucoxanthin, a carotenoid, both endowed with powerful antitumoral properties.

In brief, the Okinawan diet is low in calories, but rich in phytonutrients, antioxidants, omega-3 fatty acids, galangal, turmeric, and chili. Much of the longevity in Okinawa is the result of low incidence of chronic diseases such as CVDs, diabetes, obesity, cancer, stroke, and dementia (225–227). CVDs and some cancer forms are much lower in Okinawans than Japanese people in other regions of Japan as well as other people in the world (225, 227). In addition, most Okinawan centenarians practice physical activity such as housework and walking. Besides the traditional diet, three important aspects of Okinawan lifestyle are physical fitness, the social support network, and the belief of Okinawans (227). However, as the new Okinawan generation begins to imitate the lifestyle of foreigners, it is feared that the famous longevity of Okinawans may disappear soon.

3.3 Dietary Approaches to Stop Hypertension (DASH) Diet

The Dietary Approaches to Stop Hypertension (DASH) diet is, arguably, the most common physician prescribed diet to fight high blood pressure and was, in fact, originally developed by major organizations including American Heart Association, National Institutes of Health, and National Heart, Lung, and Blood Institute to do just that; hence, the acronym (228). Diagnostic testing and medications are still the mainstays of patient management. However, the importance of diet, exercise, stress reduction, and lifestyle habits cannot be ignored. The DASH dietary pattern is rich in fruits and vegetables, whole grains, low-fat dairy products, fish, poultry, beans, nuts, and seeds (228). It also contains less sodium (salt), sugar, fats, and red meat than the usual Western diet. Healthy carbohydrates in DASH include: oats, millets, brown rice, kale, broccoli, spinach, celery, collard, and low sugar fruits such as apple and orange (228). Designed with cardiovascular health in mind, the DASH diet is also lower in saturated and trans-fatty acids and cholesterol and rich in nutrients such as potassium, magnesium, calcium, protein, and fiber that are helpful for lowering blood pressure. Research on the DASH dietary pattern has shown that it not only can lower blood pressure but also improve other risk factors for CVD such as HDL cholesterol levels, triglycerides, or blood sugar. Long-term studies of the DASH dietary pattern have been associated with lower risk for hypertension and other cardiovascular diseases, diabetes, obesity and several types of cancer like colorectal cancer and stomach cancer, among other chronic age associated diseases (229).

In summary, all diets described previously have the same common base: a preference for many plant foods, seafoods, and their byproducts; an avoidance of processed meats and saturated fats; and limited consumption of red meat. The major characteristics of the Okinawan diet are low calorie intakes, preference of colorful sweet potato, tofu, turmeric, and seaweeds, and regular physical activities such as walking and doing housework. Perhaps due to these foods, their physical activities, or to their genes, Okinawans are the oldest people in the world, with the highest level of centenarians.

Although major research efforts have focused on how specific components of foodstuffs affect health, relatively little is known about a more fundamental aspect of diet – the frequency and circadian timing of meals, and potential benefits of intermittent periods with no or very low energy intakes (230). The most common eating pattern in modern societies, three meals plus snacks every day, is evolutionarily abnormal. Emerging findings from studies of animal models and human subjects suggest that intermittent energy restriction periods of as little as 16 h can improve health indicators and counteract disease processes. It will be important to develop strategies to incorporate new eating patterns into health care policy and practice, and the lifestyles of populations (230). In summary, it is better to eat less, but with 'good' foods, instead of eating a lot with 'bad' items. Indeed, diet, regular physical activity, and lifestyle play important roles in health and disease, though other factors like environmental pollution, climate, individual and national living standards, and therapeutic methods also influence the life of each person. Infectious diseases develop mainly in poor regions, while CVDs and cancer are now prevalent in industrialized countries. Cardiac crises often occur during winter or heatwaves; while long life expectancy is often found in temperate areas.

4 AGING

Aging is an extremely complex and multifactorial process characterized by gradual decline in different physiological functions that leads to degenerative diseases and death (231–233). However, the precise biological and cellular mechanisms responsible for aging remain largely elusive. Among several proposed theories of aging, the theories of mitochondria and free radicals are the most discussed (231).

Mitochondria are endomembrane systems found in most eukaryotic cells. Owing to their ability to produce adenosine triphosphate (ATP) through respiration, they became a driving force in evolution. Mitochondria are a source of chemical energy, and their functions are to perform cellular respiration and other cellular activities like signaling, cellular differentiation, cell senescence (aging process), as well as control of cell cycle and cell growth (234).

Free radicals are classified into two main species: reactive oxygen species (ROS) and reactive nitrogen species (RNS) (see Chapter 3 of this book). Reactive oxygen species (ROS) include superoxide anion (O_2^-), singlet oxygen ($^1O_2$), hydroxyl radical (HO$^\bullet$), peroxyl radical (ROO$^\bullet$), and lipid peroxyl radical (LOO$^\bullet$) (235). The human organism is equipped with very efficient antioxidative defense mechanisms that, among others, include antioxidative enzymes such as SOD, catalase, glutathione peroxidase, and glutathione reductase (233, 235). When the production of ROS is prolonged, the endogenous reserves of antioxidants become insufficient, leading to cell damage. Similarly, the production of ROS below physiological levels induces a decreased proliferative response. Both excess or decrease of ROS production can cause diseases (233, 235). Although the deleterious effects of free radicals in the aging process have been demonstrated, ROS are also important in maintaining homeostasis (233, 235).

Both theories of mitochondria and free radicals speculate that cumulative damage to mitochondria and mitochondrial DNA (mtDNA) caused by reactive oxygen species (ROS) is one of the causes of aging. Oxidative damage affects replication and transcription of mtDNA and results in a decline in mitochondrial function which in turn leads to enhanced ROS production and further damage to mtDNA (231). Indeed, excessive production of ROS and reduced antioxidant defense with age significantly contribute to aging. It seems that oxidative damage is the major cause and the most important contributor to human aging. Approaches to lowering increased ROS formation in our bodies could be implemented by avoiding exposure to exogenous free radicals, by intake of adequate amounts of antioxidants, and/or by stimulating the damage-repair systems of cells (232).

Lifestyle changes such as increased intake of vegetables and fruits, regular physical activity, and reduced calorie intake may improve health and increase longevity and contribute to the treatment of degenerative age-related diseases, like cancer, cardiovascular, and neurodegenerative diseases (232, 233). Antioxidant supplements may help to fight oxidative stress. However, synthetic antioxidant supplements can act as pro-oxidants – as oxidative stress inducers – if they are taken at high doses or in long duration. In these cases, they are also harmful to the body.

5   LIFE EXPECTANCY

5.1   FACTORS INFLUENCING LIFE EXPECTANCY

Longevity (duration of human life) and healthy aging are influenced by a lucky combination of genetic and non-genetic factors (236, 237). Non-genetic factors include the environment and lifestyle. Family studies demonstrated that about 25% of variation in human longevity is due to genetic factors (236). However, environmental improvements such as increased availability of food and clean water, better housing and living conditions, reduced exposure to infectious diseases, and access to medical care are other key factors of longevity and healthy aging (237). The difference in lifespan and healthy aging between countries with the same standard of living resides in their lifestyle, diet, environmental pollution, climate, and genetic makeup of each country. The psychological factor or mental health is another important condition for healthy aging and lifespan on an individual and collective level (238). Stress, separation, family discord, joblessness, social tension, and war are the main causes of psychological disorders that are harmful to the health of everybody. It is well known that negative emotions (depression, anger), psychosocial stress (joblessness, professional conflict), and social factors (asocial character) are related to developments of cardiovascular and mental ailments and consequently, shortening of life spans (239–240). Many studies show that individuals with the lowest level of involvement in social relationships are more likely to die than those with greater involvement (241). The best way to fight stress and to cultivate good mental health is to practice diverse physical exercises like yoga, tai chi, and collective sport (tennis, football, ping pong), and to participate in social meetings, charitable activities, and so on.

5.2   LIFE EXPECTANCY OF SOME POPULATIONS IN THE WORLD

As cited above, standard of living, lifestyle, diet, and climate are the main factors of longevity. It is not surprising that most developed countries occupy the first places in the life expectancy list, and the underdeveloped countries occupy the last places in the ranking. According to World Health Organization (WHO) data, women on average live longer than men in all major countries (242).

The countries with the lowest overall life expectancies per the WHO are Mali, Cameroon, Equatorial Guinea, Guinea Bissau, South Sudan, Côte d'Ivoire, Nigeria, Sierra Leone, Chad, Lesotho, and Central African Republic (242). They are all in sub-Saharan Africa. Their life expectancy for both sexes is between 52 to 59 years according to The United Nations Human Development Report published in 2019 (242).

The 10 first places on the list the WHO published in 2019 are Hong Kong (1st: 84.7 years for both sexes), Japan (2nd: 84.5 y.), Switzerland (3rd: 83.6 y.), Singapore (4th: 83.7 y.), Italy (5th: 83.4 y.), Spain (5th: 83.4 y.), Australia (7th: 83.3 y.), Iceland (8th: 82.9 y.), Israel (9th: 82.8 y.), and South Korea (9th: 83.8 y.) (242). As Hong Kong is not a country, therefore, Japan occupies the first place. The rankings of some industrialized countries are: France (11th: 82.5 y.), Canada (13th: 82.3 y.), Germany (24th: 81.2 y.), United Kingdom (24th: 81.2 y.), United States (35th: 78.9 y.), China (53th: 76.7 y.), and Russia (98th: 72.4 y.) (242). However, some countries with low GDP (gross domestic product) and located at similar geographies also have life expectancy nearly the same as their rich neighbors. For example, the life expectancy of the population in Greece (14th: 82.1 y.), Portugal (19th: 81.9 y.), is almost equal to their rich neighboring countries like Germany and the United Kingdom. (242). Based on the statistics cited earlier, we find that the life expectancy of a population or a country depends on many main factors, including: climate (temperate, tropical, arid, freezing), environment (mountain, forest, plains, desert, near sea or ocean), natural resources, social construction, health service, income, and pollution. For the same standard of living and environment, the life expectancy of an individual or a population is mainly linked to their diet and lifestyle, thereby, making their difference in classification.

In addition, according to Forbes (243), the world's top ten smartest countries recently classed are: Japan (1st), Switzerland (2nd), China (3rd), United States (4th), Netherland (5th), Russia (6th), Belgium (7th), United Kingdom (8th), Canada (9th), and South Korea (10th). This ranking is based on the number of Nobel Prizes won to represent historic intelligence in the past, the current average IQ (intelligence quotient) to represent intelligence of population in the present, and school test rankings to represent intelligence of the future generation (243). For the Nobel Prize, the United States occupies the first place in the world and largely overtakes other nations such as the United Kingdom (2nd place), Germany (3rd), France (4th), Sweden (5th), Japan (6th), Switzerland (6th), Russia (8th), Canada (8th), and Austria (10th) (243). For the current average IQ, Singapore occupies the first place, followed by China (2nd), Hong Kong (3rd), South Korea (4th), Taiwan (4th), Japan (6th), Finland (7th), Canada (8th), Netherlands (8th), Liechtenstein, and Switzerland (10th). School test rankings are about the same as IQ test rankings, with predominance of countries in East Asia (Singapore, South Korea, Hong Kong, Macao, Taiwan, Japan, China), as well as Russia, Kazakhstan, and Liechtenstein (243).

6 DISCUSSION

Most scientists in the world now recognize that the health and lifespan of an individual as well as a population depend on choices between good or bad habits concerning foods, drugs (cigarettes), physical activity, sleeping, mental activity, hobbies, and housekeeping. Regarding environmental pollution, the problem mainly depends on the availability of clean water and clean atmosphere. To resolve pollution, the responsibilities of industry and of government each play important roles. Changing a bad lifestyle is not easy. Addictions to tobacco, alcohol, gambling, and electronic games are not only harmful to physical and mental health, but also to their family and society. Much effort and perseverance is required to fight these addictions. Food addiction is also the cause of many ailments such as obesity, CVDs, diabetes, and more. In summary, to maintain good physical and mental health, the best way is to eat less, but with good food, practice physical exercises regularly, participate in social activities, keep house properly and preserve the environment.

Physical activity plays important roles in health and disease of all people. Physical activity contributes to prevention of cardiovascular diseases, cancer, and diabetes, and has significant health benefits for the mind. The choice of physical activity mode depends on age and accessibility to each individual.

Some diets such as the Mediterranean diet and Okinawan diet are examples of healthy lifestyle, and show that choice of foods and physical activity play important roles in maintaining health and longevity. People living in these areas have the longest lifespans in the world.

7   REFERENCES

1. Dictionary.com. (2020). Lifestyle. www.dictionary.com/browse/lifestyle.
2. Collins Dictionary. (2020). Lifestyle. www.collinsdictionary.com/dictionary/english/lifestyle.
3. Farhud D.D. (2015). Impact of Lifestyle on Health. *Iran J. Public Health*, **44**(11): 1442–1444.
4. Jensen M. (2007). Defining Lifestyle. *Environ. Sci.*, **4**(2): 63–73.
5. Vorster H.H. (2009). 1. Introduction to Human Nutrition: A Global Perspective on Food and Nutrition, pp. 1–11. In: *Introduction to Human Nutrition*. 2nd edition. Editors: M.J. Gibney, S.A. Lanham-New, A. Cassidy, H.H. Vorster. Wiley-Blackwell, Hoboken, New Jersey, 386 pages.
6. Hyman M.A., Ornish D., Roizen M. (2009). Lifestyle Medicine: Treating the Causes of Disease. *Altern. Ther. Health Med.*, **15**(6): 12–14.
7. Lourida I., Hannon E., Littlejohns T.J., Langa K.M., Hyppönen E., Kuzma E., Llewellyn D.J. (2019). Association of Lifestyle and Genetic Risk with Incidence of Dementia. *J.A.M.A. (Journal of the American Medical Association)*, **322**(5): 430–437.
8. Willett W.C., Koplan J.P., Nugent R., Dusenbury C., Puska P., Gaziano T.A. (2006). Chapter 44: Prevention of Chronic Disease by Means of Diet and Lifestyle Changes, pp. 833–850. In: *Disease Control Priorities in Developing Countries*. 2nd edition. Editors: D.T. Jamison, J.G. Breman, A.R. Measham, G. Alleyne, M. Claeson, D.B. Evans, P. Jha, A. Mills, P. Musgrove. The International Bank for Reconstruction and Development/ The World Bank, Washington, DC; Oxford University Press, New York.
9. Gadais T., Boulanger M., Trudeau F., Rivard M.C. (2018). Environments Favorable to Healthy Lifestyles: A Systematic Review of Initiatives in Canada. *J. Sport Health Sci.*, **7**(1): 7–18, January.
10. World Health Organization (WHO). (1999). Healthy Living. What Is a Healthy Lifestyle? www.kzn-health.gov.za/healthyliving.pdf.
11. Powell L.H., Shima C., Kazlauskaite R., Appelhans B.M. (2010). Lifestyle in France and the United States: An American Perspective. *J. Am. Diet Assoc.*, **110**(6): 845–847.
12. Wallace T.C., Bailey R.L., Blumberg J.B., Burton-Freeman B., Chen C-Y.O., Crowe-White K.M., Drewnowski A., Hooshmand S., Johnson E., Lewis R., Murray R., Shapses S.A., Wang D.D. (2020). Fruits, Vegetables, and Health: A Comprehensive Narrative, Umbrella Review of the Science and Recommendations for Enhanced Public Policy to Improve Intake. *Crit. Rev. Food Sci. Nutr.*, **60**(13): 2174–2211.
13. EUFIC (The European Food Information Council). (2012). Fruit and Vegetable Consumption in Europe, January 10. www.eufic.org/fr/healthy-living/article/fruit-and-vegetable-consumption-in-europe-do-europeans-get-enough.
14. Melina V., Craig W., Levin S. (2016). Position of the Academy of Nutrition and Dietetics: Vegetarian Diets. *J. Acad. Nutr. Diet.*, **116**(12): 1970–1980.
15. Minich D.M. (2019). A Review of the Science of Colorful, Plant-Based Food and Practical Strategies for Eating the Rainbow. *J. Nutr. Metab.*, **2019**, Article ID 2125070, 19 pages.
16. Comert E.D., Mogol B.A., Gokmen V. (2020). Relationship Between Color and Antioxidant Capacity of Fruits and Vegetables. *Curr. Res. Nutr. Food Sci.*, **3**: 1–10.
17. Di Gioia F., Tzortzakis N., Rouphael Y., Kyriacou M.C., Sampaio S.L., Ferreira I.C.F.R., Petropoulos S.A. (2020). Grown to Be Blue-Antioxidant Properties and Health Effects of Colored Vegetables. Part II: Leafy, Fruit, and Other Vegetables. *Antioxidants (Basel)*, **9**(2): 97, 42 pages.
18. Petropoulos S.A., Sampaio S.L., Gioia F.D., Tzortzakis N., Rouphael Y., Kyriacou M.C., Ferreira I. (2019). Grown to Be Blue-Antioxidant Properties and Health Effects of Colored Vegetables. Part I: Root Vegetables. *Antioxidants (Basel)*, **8**(12): 617, 26 pages.
19. Barrett D.M., Beaulieu J.C., Shewfelt R. (2010). Color, Flavor, Texture, and Nutritional Quality of Fresh-Cut Fruits and Vegetables: Desirable Levels, Instrumental and Sensory Measurement, and the Effects of Processing. *Crit. Rev. Food Sci. Nutr.*, **50**: 369–389.
20. Schwab W., Davidovich-Rikanati R., Lewinsohn E. (2008). Biosynthesis of Plant-Derived Flavor Compounds. *Plant J.*, **54**: 712–732.

21. Chemistry LibreTexts. (2019). 1.10: Pi Conjugation, June 5. https://chem.libretexts.org/Courses/ Purdue/Purdue%3A_Chem_26505%3A_Organic_Chemistry_I_(Lipton)/Chapter_1._Electronic_ Structure_and_Chemical_Bonding/1.10%3A_Pi_Conjugation.

22. WHO FAO (The World Health Organization and the Food and Agriculture Organization of the United Nations). (1998). Iodine. In: *Vitamin and Mineral Requirements in Human Nutrition*. 2nd edition. Report of a Joint FAO/WHO Expert Consultation, Bangkok, Thailand, September 21–30, 341 pages. https://apps.who.int/iris/bitstream/handle/10665/42716/9241546123.pdf?sequence=1.

23. Yochum L.A., Folsom A.R., Kushi L.H. (2000). Intake of Antioxidant Vitamins and Risk of Death from Stroke in Postmenopausal Women. *Am. J. Clin. Nutr.*, **72**: 476–483.

24. National Institutes of Health (NIH). Office of Dietary Supplements. (2020). Vitamin E, July 31. https:// ods.od.nih.gov/factsheets/VitaminE-HealthProfessional/.

25. Keeton J.T., Dikeman M.E. (2017). 'Red' and 'White' Meats – Terms That Lead to Confusion. *Anim. Front.*, **7**(4): 29–33.

26. McAfee A.J., McSorley E.M., Cuskelly G.J., Moss B.W., Wallace J.M.W., Bonham M.P., Fearon A.M. (2010). Red Meat Consumption: An Overview of the Risks and Benefits. *Meat Sci.*, **84**: 1–13.

27. Micha R., Wallace S.K., Mozaffarian D. (2010). Red and Processed Meat Consumption and Risk of Incident Coronary Heart Disease, Stroke, and Diabetes Mellitus. A Systematic Review and Meta-Analysis. *Circulation*, **121**: 2271–2283.

28. Micha R., Michas G., Mozaffarian D. (2012). Unprocessed Red and Processed Meats and Risk of Coronary Artery Disease and Type 2 Diabetes – An Updated Review of the Evidence. *Curr. Atheroscler. Rep.*, **14**(6): 515–524.

29. Harvard School of Public Health. (2010). Eating Processed Meats, but Not Unprocessed Red Meats, May Raise Risk of Heart Disease and Diabetes. Release: May 17. www.hsph.harvard.edu/news/ press-releases/processed-meats-unprocessed-heart-disease-diabetes/.

30. Gil A., Gil F. (2015). Fish, a Mediterranean Source of n-3 PUFA: Benefits Do Not Justify Limiting Consumption. *Br. J. Nutr.*, **113**: S58–S67.

31. Hellberg R.S., DeWitt C.A.M., Morrissey M.T. (2012). Risk-Benefit Analysis of Seafood Consumption: A Review. *Compr. Rev. Food Sci. Food Saf.*, **11**: 490–517.

32. Mozaffarian D., Rimm E.B. (2006). Fish Intake, Contaminants, and Human Health. Evaluating the Risks and the Benefits. *J.A.M.A.*, **296**(15): 1885–1899.

33. Oken E., Choi A.L., Karagas M.R., Mariën K., Rheinberger C.M., Schoeny R., Sunderland E., Korrick S. (2012). Which Fish Should I Eat? Perspectives Influencing Fish Consumption Choices. *Environ. Health Perspect.*, **120**: 790–798.

34. Bisgaard H., Stokholm J., Chawes B.L., Vissing N.H., Bjarnadóttir E., Schoos A-M.M., Wolsk H.M., Pedersen T.M., Vinding R.K., Thorsteinsdóttir S., Følsgaard N.V., Fink N.R., Thorsen J., Pedersen A.G., Waage J., Rasmussen M.A., Stark K.D., Olsen S.F., Bonnelykke K. (2016). Fish Oil – Derived Fatty Acids in Pregnancy and Wheeze and Asthma in Offspring. *N. Engl. J. Med.*, **375**: 2530–2539.

35. Marangoni F., Corsello G., Cricelli C., Ferrara N., Ghiselli A., Lucchin L., Poli A. (2015). Role of Poultry Meat in a Balanced Diet Aimed at Maintaining Health and Wellbeing: An Italian Consensus Document. *Food Nutr. Res.*, **59**, Art. 27606, 1–11.

36. Patience S. (2016). Religion and Dietary Choices, September 19. www.independentnurse.co.uk/ clinical-article/religion-and-dietary-choices/145719/.

37. Lixandru M. (2017). Chicken Eggs vs Duck Eggs: Which Is Better? December 3. www.natureword.com/ chicken-eggs-vs-duck-eggs-which-is-better/.

38. McNamara D.J. (2015). The Fifty Year Rehabilitation of the Egg. *Nutrients*, **7**(10): 8716–8722.

39. Fuller N.R., Sainsbury A., Caterson I.D., Markovic T.P. (2015). Egg Consumption and Human Cardio-Metabolic Health in People with and Without Diabetes. *Nutrients*, **7**(9): 7399–7420.

40. Réhault-Godbert S., Guyot N., Nys Y. (2019). The Golden Egg: Nutritional Value, Bioactivities, and Emerging Benefits for Human Health. *Nutrients*, **11**(3): 684, 26 pages.

41. Lopez-Jimenez F. (2020). Are Chicken Eggs Good or Bad for My Cholesterol? January 9. www.mayo-clinic.org/diseases-conditions/high-blood-cholesterol/expert-answers/cholesterol/faq-20058468.

42. Ballard O., Morrow A.L. (2013). Human Milk Composition: Nutrients and Bioactive Factors. *Pediatr. Clin. North Am.*, **60**(1): 49–74.

43. Wijesinha-Bettoni R., Burlingame B. (2013). Chapter 3. Milk and Dairy Product Composition, pp. 41–102. In: *Milk and Dietary Products in Human Nutrition*. Editors: Ellen Muehlhoff, Anthony Bennett, Deirdre McMahon. Food and Agriculture Organization of the United Nations, Rome.

44. Haug A., Høstmark A.T., Harstad O.M. (2007). Bovine Milk in Human Nutrition – A Review. *Lipids Health Dis.*, **6**(25): 1–16.

45. Pereira P.C. (2014). Milk Nutritional Composition and Its Role in Human Health. *Nutrition*, **30**: 619–627.
46. Visioli F., Strata A. (2014). Milk, Dairy Products, and Their Functional Effects in Humans: A Narrative Review of Recent Evidence. *Adv. Nutr.*, **5**: 131–143.
47. Thorning T.K., Raben A., Tholstrup T., Soedamah-Muthu S.S., Givens I., Astrup A. (2016). Milk and Dairy Products: Good or Bad for Human Health? An Assessment of the Totality of Scientific Evidence. *Food Nutr. Res.*, **60**(32527): 1–11.
48. McIntosh J. (2018). Fifteen Benefits of Drinking Water, July 16. www.medicalnewstoday.com/articles/290814.
49. World Health Organization (WHO). (2005). Nutrients in Drinking Water. http://apps.who.int/iris/bitstream/handle/10665/43403/9241593989_eng.pdf?sequence=1.
50. Pham-Huy N.L.A., He H., Pham-Huy C. (2008). Green Tea and Health. An Overview. *J. Food Agric. Environ. (JFAE)*, **6**: 6–13.
51. Chen Z-M., Lin Z. (2015). Tea and Human Health: Biomedical Functions of Tea Active Components and Current Issues. *J. Zhejiang Univ-Sci. B (Biomed. & Biotechnol.)*, **16**(2): 87–102.
52. Abe S.K., Inoue M. (2021). Green Tea and Cancer and Cardiometabolic Diseases: A Review of the Current Epidemiological Evidence. *Eur. J. Clin. Nutr.*, **75**(6): 865–876.
53. Reygaert W.C. (2017). An Update on the Health Benefits of Green Tea. *Beverages*, **3**(6): 14 pages.
54. Higdon J.V., Frei B. (2006). Coffee and Health: A Review of Recent Human Research. *Crit. Rev. Food Sci. Nutr.*, **46**(2): 1001–1023.
55. Messina G., Zannella C., Monda V., Dato A., Liccardo D., De Blasio S., Valenzano A., Moscatelli F., Messina A., Cibelli G., Monda M. (2015). The Beneficial Effects of Coffee in Human Nutrition. *Biol. Med. (Aligarh)*, **7**(4): 240–244.
56. Pourshahidi L.K., Navarini L., Petracco M., Strain J.J. (2016). A Comprehensive Overview of the Risks and Benefits of Coffee Consumption. *Compr. Rev. Food Sci. Food Saf.*, **15**: 671–684.
57. Gisslen W. (2011). Chapter 4. Basic Principles of Cooking and Food Science, pp. 63–91. In: *Professional Cooking*. Editor: Wayne Gisslen. John Wiley & Sons Inc., Copyright 2011. http://standring.weebly.com/uploads/2/3/3/5/23356120/4_-_basic_cooking__food_science.pdf.
58. Canada's Food Guide. (2019). Healthy Cooking Methods, December 11. https://food-guide.canada.ca/en/tips-for-healthy-eating/healthy-cooking-methods/.
59. Yong W., Amin L., Dongpo C. (2019). Status and Prospects of Nutritional Cooking. *Food Qual. Saf.*, **3**(3): 137–143.
60. Bylsma L.C., Alexander D.D. (2015). A Review and Meta-Analysis of Prospective Studies of Red and Processed Meat, Meat Cooking Methods, Heme Iron, Heterocyclic Amines and Prostate Cancer. *Nutr. J.*, **14**: 125, 18 pages.
61. Sobral M.M.C., Cunha S.C., Faria M.A., Ferreira I. (2018). Domestic Cooking of Muscle Foods: Impact on Composition of Nutrients and Contaminants. *Compr. Rev. Food Sci. Food Saf.*, **17**: 309–333.
62. John E.M., Stern M.C., Sinha R., Koo J. (2011). Meat Consumption, Cooking Practices, Meat Mutagens, and Risk of Prostate Cancer. *Nutr. Cancer*, **63**(4): 525–537.
63. Fabbri A.D.T., Crosby G.A. (2016). A Review of the Impact of Preparation and Cooking on the Nutritional Quality of Vegetables and Legumes. *Int. J. Gastron. Food Sci.*, **3**: 2–11.
64. Raber M., Chandra J., Upadhyaya M., Schick V., Strong L.L., Durand C., Sharma S. (2016). An Evidence-Based Conceptual Framework of Healthy Cooking. *Prev. Med. Rep.*, **4**: 23–28.
65. EUFIC (The European Food Information Council). (2015). Physical Activity and Health, July 23. www.eufic.org/en/healthy-living/article/physical-activity-and-health.
66. National Health Service (NHS) in England. (2018). Benefits of Exercise, June 11. www.nhs.uk/live-well/exercise/exercise-health-benefits/.
67. Centers for Disease Control and Prevention (CDC). (2020). Physical Activity, December 2. www.cdc.gov/physicalactivity/basics/pa-health/index.htm.
68. Miles L. (2007). Physical Activity and Health. *Nutr. Bull.*, **32**: 314–363.
69. Warburton D.E.R., Nicol C.W., Bredin S.S.D. (2006). Health Benefits of Physical Activity: The Evidence. *C.M.A.J.*, **174**(6): 801–809.
70. World Health Organization. (2020). Physical Activity, November 26. www.who.int/news-room/fact-sheets/detail/physical-activity.
71. Matthews C.E., Moore S.C., Arem H., Cook M.B., Trabert B., Hakansson N., Larsson S.C., Wolk A., Gapstur S.M., Lynch B.M., Milne R.L., Freedman N.D., Huang W-Y., de Gonzalez A.B., Kitahara C.M., Linet M.S., Shiroma E.J., Sandin S., Patel A.V., Lee I-M. (2020). Amount and Intensity of Leisure-Time Physical Activity and Lower Cancer Risk. *J. Clin. Oncol.*, **38**(7): 686–697.

72. Strath S.J., Kaminsky L.A., Ainsworth B.E., Ekelund U., Freedson P.S., Gary R.A., Richardson C.R., Smith D.T., Swartz A.M. (2013). Guide to the Assessment of Physical Activity: Clinical and Research Applications a Scientific Statement from the American Heart Association. *Circulation*, **128**: 2259–2279.

73. Harvard Health Publishing. Harvard Medical School. (2019). The 4 Most Important Types of Exercise, August 20. www.health.harvard.edu/exercise-and-fitness/the-4-most-important-types-of-exercise.

74. American Heart Association. (2018). What Type of Physical Activity is Best? March 8. www.heart.org/HEARTORG/Conditions/More/CardiacRehab/What-Type-of-Physical-Activity-Is-Best_UCM_307378_Article.jsp.

75. Health Hub. (2020). Types of Physical Activities, September 7. www.healthhub.sg/live-healthy/826/types-of-physical-activities.

76. Dairy Council of California. (2021). Types of Physical Activity. Copyright 2021. www.health-yeating.org/Healthy-Eating/Healthy-Living/Physical-Activity/Article-Viewer/Article/238/types-of-physical-activity.

77. Wang Y.T., Huang G., Duke G., Yang Y. (2017). Tai Chi, Yoga, and Qigong as Mind-Body Exercises. *Evid. Based Complement Alternat. Med.*, **2017**: Article ID 8763915, 1 page.

78. Jahnke R., Larkey L., Rogers C., Etnier J., Lin F. (2010). A Comprehensive Review of Health Benefits of Qigong and Tai Chi. *Am. J. Health Promot.*, **24**(6): e1–e25.

79. Editorial Staff of American Lung Association. (2017). Yoga, Tai Chi and Your Lungs: The Benefits of Breathing Through Exercise, September 27. www.lung.org/about-us/blog/2017/09/yoga-tai-chi-and-your-lungs.html.

80. Marks R. (2017). Qigong Exercise and Arthritis. *Medicines*, **4**(71): 1–14.

81. Sengupta P. (2012). Health Impacts of Yoga and Pranayama: A State-of-the-Art Review. *Int. J. Prev. Med.*, **3**(7): 444–458.

82. Brown R.P., Gerbarg P.L. (2009). Yoga Breathing, Meditation, and Longevity. *Ann. N.Y. Acad. Sci.*, **1172**: 54–62.

83. Bridges L., Sharma M. (2017). The Efficacy of Yoga as a Form of Treatment for Depression. *J. Evid. Based Complementary Altern. Med.*, **22**(4): 1017–1028.

84. Ross A., Thomas S. (2010). The Health Benefits of Yoga and Exercise: A Review of Comparison Studies. *J. Altern. Complement. Med.*, **16**(1): 3–12.

85. Sakamoto K., Sugimoto F., Sato Y., Fujimaki E., Tashiro Y. (1999). Dynamic Flamingo Therapy for Prevention of Femoral Neck Osteoporosis and Fractures. Part 1: Theoretical Background. *Showa Univ. J. Med. Sci.*, **11**(4): 247–254.

86. Sakamoto K., Nakamura T., Hagino H., Endo N., Mori S., Muto Y., Harada A., Nakano T., Itoi E., Yoshimura M., Norimatsu H., Yamamoto H., Ochi T. (2006). Effects of Unipedal Standing Balance Exercise on the Prevention of Falls and Hip Fracture Among Clinically Defined High-Risk Elderly Individuals: A Randomized Controlled Trial. *J. Orthopaedic Sci.*, **11**(5): 467–472.

87. U.S. Department of Health and Human Services. (2018). *Physical Activity Guidelines for Americans.* 2nd edition. Washington, DC. https://health.gov/sites/default/files/2019-09/Physical_Activity_Guidelines_2nd_edition.pdf.

88. Healthy Eating. Dairy Council of California. (2021). Physical Activity. www.healthyeating.org/nutrition-topics/general/lifestyle/physical-activity.

89. National Heart Lung and Blood Institute of National Institutes of Health (NIH), USA. (2013). Physical Activity and Your Heart, November 8. www.nhlbi.nih.gov/health-topics/physical-activity-and-your-heart.

90. Blanchard S. (Health Reporter for Mail online). (2018). Want to Live Longer? Take Up Tennis: Scientists Say the Social Sport Could Add Nearly 10 Years onto Your Life, September 5. www.dailymail.co.uk/health/article-6134379/Want-live-longer-Scientists-say-tennis-add-nearly-10-YEARS-life.html.

91. Schupp M., Hanning C.D. (2003). Physiology of Sleep. *Br. J. Anaesth., CEPD Reviews*, **3**(3): 69–74.

92. Brinkman J.E., Reddy V., Sharma S. (2020). Physiology, Sleep. In: *StatPearls [Internet].* StatPearls Publishing, Treasure Island, FL, April 29, January. www.ncbi.nlm.nih.gov/books/NBK482512/.

93. Brown R.E., Basheer R., McKenna J.T., Strecker R.E., McCarley R.W. (2012). Control of Sleep and Wakefulness. *Physiol. Rev.*, **92**: 1087–1187.

94. Partinen M., Westermarck T., Atroshi F. (2014). Chapter 7. Nutrition, Sleep and Sleep Disorders – Relations of Some Food Constituents and Sleep, pp. 191–223. In: *Pharmacology and Nutritional Intervention in the Treatment of Disease.* Editor: Faik Atroshi. IntechOpen, 426 pages. www.intechopen.com/books/pharmacology-and-nutritional-intervention-in-the-treatment-of-disease.

95. Kwok C.S., Kontopantelis E., Kuligowski G., Gray M., Muhyaldeen A., Gale C.P., Peat G.M., Cleator J., Chew-Graham C., Loke Y.K., Mamas M.A. (2018). Self-Reported Sleep Duration and Quality and Cardiovascular Disease and Mortality: A Dose-Response Meta-Analysis. *J. Am. Heart Assoc.*, **7**(e008552): 1–26.

96. Grunstein R.R. (2012). Global Perspectives on Sleep and Health Issues. *J. Natl. Inst. Public Health*, **61**(1): 35–42.

97. Crosta P., Dasgupta R. (2020). Insomnia: Everything You Need to Know, July 28. www.medicalnewstoday.com/articles/9155.php.

98. Chan M.A., Kim J., Avena-Woods C., Pisano M. (2019). Obstructive Sleep Apnea: A Review. *US Pharm.*, **44**(7): 16–19.

99. Osman A.M., Carter S.G., Carberry J.C., Eckert D.J. (2018). Obstructive Sleep Apnea: Current Perspectives. *Nat. Sci. Sleep*, **10**: 21–34.

100. Cao H., Pan X., Li H., Liu J. (2009). Acupuncture for Treatment of Insomnia: A Systematic Review of Randomized Controlled Trials. *J. Altern. Complement. Med.*, **15**(11): 1171–1186.

101. Reddick M. (Sleep Advisor Magazine). (2020). Is Sleeping with a Fan on Safe? – Can It Make You Feel Sick? June 8. www.sleepadvisor.org/sleeping-with-a-fan-on/.

102. Dodgson L. (Science Alert). (2018). There's One Sleep Position That's Better Than Others, According to Experts, April 9. www.sciencealert.com/best-sleep-position-side-back-stomach-science.

103. Larry Z.D. (2018). Towards a Definition of "Hobby": An Empirical Test of a Proposed Operational Definition of the Word Hobby. *J. Occup. Sci.*, **25**(3): 368–382.

104. Sharma R., Biedenharn K.R., Fedor J.M., Agarwal A. (2013). Lifestyle Factors and Reproductive Health: Taking Control of Your Fertility. *Reprod. Biol. Endocrinol.*, **11**: 66, 15 pages.

105. Raviraja Shetty G., Monisha S. (2015). Pharmacology of an Endangered Medicinal Plant *Alpinia Galanga* – A Review. *Res. J. Pharm. Biol. Chem. Sci. (RJPBCS)*, **6**(1): 499–511.

106. Lee Y-M., Yoon H., Park H-M., Song B.C., Yeum K-J. (2017). Implications of Red Panax Ginseng in Oxidative Stress Associated Chronic Diseases. *J. Ginseng Res.*, **41**(2): 113–119.

107. Leung K.W., Wong A.S.T. (2013). Ginseng and Male Reproductive Function. *Spermatogenesis*, **3**(3): e26391-1–e26391-6.

108. Langtry H.D., Markham A. (1999). Sildenafil. *Drugs*, **57**: 967–989.

109. Saha S.P., Bhalla D.K., Whayne Jr T.F., Gairola C.G. (2007). Cigarette Smoke and Adverse Health Effects: An Overview of Research Trends and Future Needs. *Int. J. Angiol.*, **16**(3): 77–83.

110. Centers for Disease Control and Prevention. (2020). Health Effects of Cigarette Smoking, December 10. www.cdc.gov/tobacco/data_statistics/fact_sheets/health_effects/effects_cig_smoking/index.htm.

111. National Cancer Institute of NIH. (2017). Harms of Cigarette Smoking and Health Benefits of Quitting, December 19. www.cancer.gov/about-cancer/causes-prevention/risk/tobacco/cessation-fact-sheet.

112. Pham-Huy C., Nguyen P., Marchand V., Claude J.R., Duc H.T. (2001). Selenium and Tobacco Smoke Tars: In Vitro Effects on Different Immunocompetent Cells. *Toxicology*, **164**: 111–112. Presented in International Congress of Toxicology XI, Brisbane (Australia), July 7–12.

113. Mishra A., Chaturvedi P., Datta S., Sinukumar S., Joshi P., Garg A. (2015). Harmful Effects of Nicotine. *Indian J. Med. Paediatr. Oncol.*, **36**(1): 24–31.

114. Wickström R. (2007). Effects of Nicotine During Pregnancy: Human and Experimental Evidence. *Curr. Neuropharmacol.*, **5**(3): 213–222.

115. University of Bath (United Kingdom). (2020). Smokeless Tobacco, June 8. www.tobaccotactics.org/index.php?title=Smokeless_Tobacco#cite_note-1.

116. National Cancer Institute. (2010). Smokeless Tobacco and Cancer, October 25. www.cancer.gov/about-cancer/causes-prevention/risk/tobacco/smokeless-fact-sheet.

117. World Health Organization (WHO). (2018). Alcohol, September 21. www.who.int/en/news-room/fact-sheets/detail/alcohol.

118. Iranpour A., Nakhaee N. (2019). A Review of Alcohol-Related Harms: A Recent Update. *Addict Health*, **11**(2): 129–137.

119. Kloner R.A., Rezkalla S.H. (2007). To Drink or Not to Drink? That Is the Question. *Circulation*, **116**(11): 1306–1317.

120. Burton R., Sheron N. (2018). No Level of Alcohol Consumption Improves Health. *Lancet*, **392**(10152): 987–988.

121. Probst C., Kilian C., Sanchez S., Lange S., Rehm J. (2020). The Role of Alcohol Use and Drinking Patterns in Socioeconomic Inequalities in Mortality: A Systematic Review. *Lancet*, **5**(6): e324–e332.

122. Wang W., Wang C., Xu H., Gao Y. (2020). Aldehyde Dehydrogenase, Liver Disease and Cancer. *Int. J. Biol. Sci.*, **16**(6): 921–934.

123. Brooks P.J., Enoch M.A., Goldman D., Li T.K., Yokoyama A. (2009). The Alcohol Flushing Response: An Unrecognized Risk Factor for Esophageal Cancer from Alcohol Consumption. *PLoS Med.*, **6**(3): e50, 0258–0263.

124. Kunst J. (2019). What Is the Difference Between Drug Abuse and Addiction? March 4. www.amethystrecovery.org/drug-abuse-addiction-difference/.

125. Camí J., Farré M. (2003). Drug Addiction. *N. Engl. J. Med.*, **349**: 975–986.

126. Richards J.R., Le J.K. (2020). Cocaine Toxicity. In: *StatPearls [Internet].* StatPearls Publishing, Treasure Island, FL, January. www.ncbi.nlm.nih.gov/books/NBK430976/.

127. Karila L., Gorelick D., Weinstein A., Noble F., Benyamina A., Coscas S., Blecha L., Lowenstein W., Martinot J.L., Reynaud M., Lépine J.P. (2008). New Treatments for Cocaine Dependence: A Focused Review. *Int. J. Neuropsychopharmacol.*, **11**(3): 425–438.

128. Nestler E.J. (2005). The Neurobiology of Cocaine Addiction. *Sci. Pract. Perspect.*, **3**(1): 4–10.

129. Oelhaf R.C., Azadfard M. (2020). Heroin Toxicity. In: *StatPearls [Internet].* StatPearls Publishing, Treasure Island, FL, January. www.ncbi.nlm.nih.gov/books/NBK430736/.

130. Listos J., Łupina M., Talarek S., Mazur A., Orzelska-Górka J., Kotlińska J. (2019). The Mechanisms Involved in Morphine Addiction: An Overview. *Int. J. Mol. Sci.*, **20**(4302): 1–23.

131. Nabipour S., Ayu Said M., Hussain Habil M. (2014). Burden and Nutritional Deficiencies in Opiate Addiction- Systematic Review Article. *Iran J. Public Health*, **43**(8): 1022–1032.

132. LiverTox. (2020). Opioids. In: *Clinical and Research Information on Drug-Induced Liver Injury (Internet).* National Institute of Diabetes and Digestive and Kidney Diseases, Bethesda, MD, 2012, November 24. www.ncbi.nlm.nih.gov/books/NBK547864/.

133. Pham-Huy C., Chikhi-Chorfi N., Galons H., Sadeg N., Laqueille X., Aymard N., Massicot F., Warnet J.M., Claude J.R. (1997). Enantioselective High-Performance Liquid Chromatography Determination of Methadone Enantiomers and Its Major Metabolite in Human Biological Fluids Using a New Derivatized Cyclodextrin-Bonded Phase. *J. Chromatogr. B*, **700**(1–2): 155–163.

134. Atakan Z. (2012). Cannabis, a Complex Plant: Different Compounds and Different Effects on Individuals. *Ther. Adv. Psychopharmacol.*, **2**(6): 241–254.

135. Volkow N.D., Baler R.D., Compton W.M., Weiss S.R.B. (2014). Adverse Health Effects of Marijuana Use. *N. Engl. J. Med.*, **370**(23): 2219–2227.

136. Siefried K.J., Acheson L.S., Lintzeris N., Ezard N. (2020). Pharmacological Treatment of Methamphetamine/Amphetamine Dependence: A Systematic Review. *CNS Drugs*, **34**(4): 337–365.

137. Brensilver M., Heinzerling K.G., Shoptaw S. (2013). Pharmacotherapy of Amphetamine-Type Stimulant Dependence: An Update. *Drug Alcohol Rev.*, **32**(5): 449–460.

138. Karila L., Weinstein A., Aubin H.J., Benyamina A., Reynaud M., Batki S.L. (2010). Pharmacological Approaches to Methamphetamine Dependence: A Focused Review. *Br. J. Clin. Pharmacol.*, **69**(6): 578–592.

139. Nichols D.E. (2004). Hallucinogens. *Pharmacol. Ther.*, **101**(2): 131–181.

140. Nichols D.E. (2016). Psychedelics. *Pharmacol. Rev.*, **68**(2): 264–355. Erratum in: *Pharmacol Rev*, April, **68**(2): 356.

141. Garcia-Romeu A., Kersgaard B., Addy P.H. (2016). Clinical Applications of Hallucinogens: A Review. *Exp. Clin. Psychopharmacol.*, **24**(4): 229–268.

142. Casarella J. (WebMD). (2020). Food Addiction, July 17. www.webmd.com/mental-health/eating-disorders/binge-eating-disorder/mental-health-food-addiction#1.

143. Gordon E.L., Ariel-Donges A.H., Bauman V., Merlo L.J. (2018). What Is the Evidence for "Food Addiction?" A Systematic Review. *Nutrients*, **10**(477), 30 pages.

144. Curfman G. (Harvard Health Publishing, Harvard Medical School). (2019). FDA Strengthens Warnings That NSAIDs Increase Heart Attack and Stroke Risk. Posted July 13, 2015. Updated June 27, 2019. www.health.harvard.edu/blog/fda-strengthens-warning-that-nsaids-increase-heart-attack-and-stroke-risk-201507138138.

145. US Food and Drug Administration (FDA). (2015). FDA Strengthens Warning That Non-Aspirin Nonsteroidal Anti-Inflammatory Drugs (NSAIDs) Can Cause Heart Attacks or Strokes, July 9, 2015. www.fda.gov/media/92768/download.

146. Varga Z., Sabzwari S.R.A., Vargova V. (2017). Cardiovascular Risk of Nonsteroidal Anti-Inflammatory Drugs: An Under-Recognized Public Health Issue. *Cureus*, **9**(4): e1144, 12 pages.

147. Li D.-K., Ferber J.R., Odouli R., Quesenberry C. (2018). Use of Nonsteroidal Anti-Inflammatory Drugs During Pregnancy and the Risk of Miscarriage. *Am. J. Obstet. Gynecol.*, **219**: 275.e1–8.

148. Li D.-K., Liu L., Odouli R. (2003). Exposure to Non-Steroidal Anti-Inflammatory Drugs During Pregnancy and Risk of Miscarriage: Population-Based Cohort Study. *BMJ.*, **327**(7411): 368.

149. Mullard A. (2011). Mediator Scandal Rocks French Medical Community. *Lancet*, **377**: 890–892.

150. Pham-Huy C., Galons H., Voisin J., Zhu J., Righenzi S., Warnet J.M., Claude J.R., Duc H.T. (1997). In Vitro and in Vivo Immunosuppressive Potential of Thalidomide and Its Derivative N-Hydroxythalidomide, Alone and in Combination with Cyclosporin A. *Int. J. Immunopharmacol.*, **19**(5): 289–296.

151. Liu T., Guo F., Zhu X., He X., Xie L. (2017). Thalidomide and Its Analogues: A Review of the Potential for Immunomodulation of Fibrosis Diseases and Opthalmopathy. *Exp. Ther. Med.*, **14**(6): 5251–5257.

152. Ventola C.L. (2015). The Antibiotic Resistance Crisis. Part 1: Causes and Threats. *P.T. (Pharmacy & Therapeutics)*, **40**(4): 277–283.

153. Stolley P.D., Zahm S.H. (1995). Nonhormonal Drugs and Cancer. *Environ. Health Perspect.*, **103** (Suppl. 8): 191–196.

154. Bongartz T., Sutton A.J., Sweeting M.J., Buchan I., Matteson E.L., Montori V. (2006). Anti-TNF Antibody Therapy in Rheumatoid Arthritis and the Risk of Serious Infections and Malignancies. Systematic Review and Meta-analysis of Rare Harmful Effects in Randomized Controlled Trials. *J.A.M.A. (The Journal of the American Medical Association)*, **295**(19): 2275–2285.

155. Even P., Debré B. (2012). Guide to 4000 Useful, Useless or Dangerous Drugs. (Guide des 4000 médicaments utiles, inutiles ou dangereux). Le Cherche Midi, Paris, 2012, 905 pages (French).

156. National Institute on Drug Abuse (NIDA). (2017). Over-The-Counter Medicines Drug Facts, December 17. www.drugabuse.gov/publications/drugfacts/over-counter-medicines.

157. Brody J.E. (2015). Over-the-Counter Medicines. Benefits and Dangers, November 30. https://well.blogs.nytimes.com/2015/11/30/over-the-counter-medicines-benefits-and-dangers/.

158. Agence Nationale et de Sécurité du Médicament et des Produits de Santé (National Agency of Safety of Medicines and Health Products). (2020). Anti-Inflammatoires Non Stéroïdiens (AINS) et Complications Infectieuses Graves (Nonsteroidal Anti-Inflammatory Drugs (NSAIDs) and Serious Infectious Complications), May 20. (French). https://ansm.sante.fr/S-informer/Points-d-information-Points-d-information/Anti-inflammatoires-non-steroidiens-AINS-et-complications-infectieuses-graves-Point-d-Information-actualise-le-20–05–2020.

159. Paitraud D. (Vidal) (2019). Paracétamol, ibuprofène et aspirine: fin du libre accès en pharmacie à partir du 15 janvier 2020 (Acetaminophen, Ibuprofen, and Aspirin: End of Free Pharmacy Access from January 15, 2020). (French). www.vidal.fr/actualites/24050-paracetamol-ibuprofene-et-aspirine-fin-du-libre-acces-en-pharmacie-a-partir-du-15-janvier-2020.html.

160. Federal Trade Commission. Consumer Information. (2011). Dietary Supplements, November. www.consumer.ftc.gov/articles/0261-dietary-supplements.

161. Starr R.R. (2015). Too Little, Too Late: Ineffective Regulation of Dietary Supplements in the United States. *Am. J. Public Health*, **105**(3): 478–485.

162. Schmitz S.M., Lopez H.L., Mackay D., Nguyen H., Miller P.E. (2020). Serious Adverse Events Reported with Dietary Supplement Use in the United States: A 2.5 Year Experience. *J. Diet. Suppl.*, **17**(2): 227–248.

163. Liu R.H. (2004). Potential Synergy of Phytochemicals in Cancer Prevention: Mechanism of Action. *J. Nutr.*, **134**: 3479S–3485S.

164. Canadian Health and Scientific Organization Consensus Statement. (2016). A National Model for Defining Healthy and Unhealthy Foods and Beverages, April 15. https://hypertension.ca/wp-content/uploads/2018/12/Final-Healthy-Food-Definition_EN_with-supporters_April-15–2016.pdf.

165. Thompson L.A., Darwish W.S. (2019). Environmental Chemical Contaminants in Food: Review of a Global Problem. *J. Toxicol.*, **2019**: 2345283, 14 pages.

166. Seaman D.R. (2002). The Diet-Induced Proinflammatory State: A Cause of Chronic Pain and Other Degenerative Diseases? *J. Manipulative Physiol. Ther.*, **25**(3): 168–179.

167. Bouvard V., Loomis D., Guyton K.Z., Grosse Y., Ghissassi F.E., Benbrahim-Tallaa L., Guha N., Mattock H., Straif K. (2015). Carcinogenicity of Consumption of Red and Processed Meat. *Lancet Oncol.*, **16**(16): 1599–1600.

168. Micha R., Wallace S.K., Mozaffarian D. (2010). Red and Processed Meat Consumption and Risk of Incident Coronary Heart Disease, Stroke, and Diabetes Mellitus: A Systematic Review and Meta-Analysis. *Circulation*, **121**(21): 2271–2283.

169. Campbell L. (2014). 13 Dangerous Household Items You Should Quit Using Immediately, July 30. www.housebeautiful.com/lifestyle/cleaning-tips/tips/a1492/dangerous-household-items/.

170. Harrar S. (2012). The Danger in Mothballs, June 14. www.philly.com/philly/blogs/healthy_kids/The-danger-in-mothballs.html?arc404=true.

171. Sudakin D.L., Stone D.L., Power L. (2011). Naphthalene Mothballs: Emerging and Recurring Issues and Their Relevance to Environmental Health. *Curr. Top Toxicol.*, **7**: 13–19.

172. Jia C., Batterman S. (2010). A Critical Review of Naphthalene Sources and Exposures Relevant to Indoor and Outdoor Air. *Int. J. Environ. Res. Public Health*, **7**(7): 2903–2939.

173. Dubey D., Sharma V.D., Pass S.E., Sawhney A., Stüve O. (2014). Para-Dichlorobenzene Toxicity – A Review of Potential Neurotoxic Manifestations. *Ther. Adv. Neurol. Disord.*, **7**(3): 177–187.

174. Galbo M.J. (2004). Naphthalene and Paradichlorobenzene, pp. 275–277. In: *Poisoning & Drug Overdose*. 4th edition. Editor: K.R. Olson. Lange Medical Books/McGraw-Hill, New York.

175. Kokel D., Li Y., Qin J., Xue D. (2006). The Nongenotoxic Carcinogens Naphthalene and Para-Dichlorobenzene Suppress Apoptosis in *Caenorhabditis Elegans*. *Nature Chem. Biol.*, **2**: 338–345.

176. Steinemann A. (2017). Ten Questions Concerning Air Fresheners and Indoor Built Environments. *Build. Environ.*, **111**: 279–284.

177. Steinemann A. (2017). Health and Societal Effects from Exposure to Fragranced Consumer Products. *Prev. Med. Rep.*, **5**: 45–47.

178. Steinemann A. (2018). Fragranced Consumer Products: Effects on Asthmatics. *Air Qual. Atmos. Health*, **11**: 3–9.

179. Wolkoff P., Nielsen G.D. (2017). Effects by Inhalation of Abundant Fragrances in Indoor Air – An Overview. *Environ. Int.*, **101**: 96–107.

180. Lin T-C., Krishnaswamy G., Chi D.S. (2008). Incense Smoke: Clinical, Structural and Molecular Effects on Airway Disease. *Clin. Mol. Allergy*, **6**(3), 9 pages.

181. Tung J-C., Huang W-C., Yang J-C., Chen G-Y., Fan C-C., Chien Y-C., Lin P-S., Lung S-C.C., Chang W-C. (2017). Auramine O, an Incense Smoke Ingredient, Promotes Lung Cancer Malignancy. *Environ. Toxicol.*, **32**(11): 2379–2391.

182. Friborg J.T., Yuan J-M., Wang R., Koh W-P., Lee H-P., Yu M.C. (2008). Incense Use and Respiratory Tract Carcinomas. A Prospective Cohort Study. *Cancer*, **113**: 1676–1684.

183. Jackson-Michel S. (Healthfully). (2017). The Effects of Herbicides & Pesticides on Humans, June 13. https://healthfully.com/246750-the-effects-of-herbicides-pesticides-on-humans.html.

184. Bolognesi C. (2003). Genotoxicity of Pesticides: A Review of Human Biomonitoring Studies. *Mutation Res.*, **543**: 251–272.

185. Nicolopoulou-Stamati P., Maipas S., Kotampasi C., Stamatis P., Hens L. (2016). Chemical Pesticides and Human Health: The Urgent Need for a New Concept in Agriculture. *Front. Public Health*, **4**(148): 1–8.

186 Damalas C.A., Eleftherohorinos I.G. (2011). Pesticide Exposure, Safety Issues, and Risk Assessment Indicators. *Int. J. Environ. Res. Public Health*, **8**(5): 1402–1419.

187. Kniss A.R. (2017). Long-Term Trends in the Intensity and Relative Toxicity of Herbicide Use. *Nat. Commun.*, **8**(14865): 1–7.

188. Briggs D. (2003). Environmental Pollution and the Global Burden of Disease. *Br. Med. Bull.*, **68**(1): 1–24.

189. Sharpe R.M., Irvine D.S. (2004). How Strong Is the Evidence of a Link Between Environmental Chemicals and Adverse Effects on Human Reproductive Health? *BMJ.*, **328**(7437): 447–451.

190. American Cancer Society. (2020). Family Cancer Syndromes, August 5. www.cancer.org/cancer/cancercauses/geneticsandcancer/heredity-and-cancer#.

191. Cancer Research UK. (2018). Family History and Inherited Cancer Genes, September 3. www.cancerresearchuk.org/about-cancer/causes-of-cancer/inherited-cancer-genes-and-increased-cancer-risk/family-history-and-inherited-cancer-genes.

192. Kampa M., Castanas E. (2008). Human Health Effects of Air Pollution. *Environ. Pollut.*, **151**: 362–367.

193. Kim K-H., Jahan S.A., Kabir E. (2013). A Review on Human Health Perspective of Air Pollution with Respect to Allergies and Asthma. *Environ. Int.*, **59**: 41–52.

194. Bell M.L., Zanobetti A., Dominici F. (2014). Who Is More Affected by Ozone Pollution? A Systematic Review and Meta-Analysis. *Am. J. Epidemiol.*, **180**(1): 15–28.

195. Lippmann M. (1989). Health Effects of Ozone. A Critical Review. *JAPCA (Journal of Air Pollution Control Association)*, **39**(5): 672–695.

196. Boström C-E., Gerde P., Hanberg A., Jernström B., Johansson C., Kyrklund T., Rannug A., Törnqvist M., Victorin K., Westerholm R. (2002). Cancer Risk Assessment, Indicators, and Guidelines for Polycyclic Aromatic Hydrocarbons in the Ambient Air. *Environ. Health Perspect.*, **110** (Suppl. 3): 451–489.

197. Masuda Y. (2003). Health Effect of Polychlorinated Biphenyls and Related Compounds. *J. Health Sci.*, **49**(5): 333–336.

198. Kaleka A.S., Thind S.K. (2020). Chapter 4. Dioxins and Dioxin-like Compounds (DLCs), pp. 75–97. In: *Pollutants and Protectants: Evaluation and Assessment Techniques*. Editors: Dr. Ashita Sharma, Dr. Manish Kumar. I K International Publishing House Pvt. Ltd., New Delhi, 270 pages.

199. White S.S., Birnbaum L.S. (2009). An Overview of the Effects of Dioxins and Dioxin-Like Compounds on Vertebrates, as Documented in Human and Ecological Epidemiology. *J. Environ. Sci. Health C Environ. Carcinog. Ecotoxicol. Rev.*, **27**(4): 197–211.

200. Government of Japan. (2003). Dioxins. www.env.go.jp/en/chemi/dioxins/brochure2003.pdf.

201. Munawer M.E. (2018). Human Health and Environmental Impacts of Coal Combustion and Post-Combustion Wastes. *J. Sustain. Mining*, **17**: 87–96.

202. Rodríguez-Eugenio N., McLaughlin M., Pennock D. (2018). *Soil Pollution: A Hidden Reality*. FAO, Rome, 142 pages. www.fao.org/3/i9183en/i9183en.pdf.

203. Horrigan L., Lawrence R.S., Walker P. (2002). How Sustainable Agriculture Can Address the Environmental and Human Health Harms of Industrial Agriculture. *Environ. Health Perspect.*, **110**(5): 445–456.

204. Motta E.V.S., Raymann K., Moran N.A. (2018). Glyphosate Perturbs the Gut Microbiota of Honey Bees. *Proc. Natl. Acad. Sci. (PNAS)*, **115**(41): 10305–10310.

205. Niroumand M.C., Farzae M.H., Karimpour-Razkenari E.E., Amin G., Khanavi M., Akbarzadeh T., Shams-Ardekani M.R. (2016). An Evidence-Based Review on Medicinal Plants Used as Insecticide and Insect Repellent in Traditional Iranian Medicine. *Iran Red Crescent Med. J.*, **18**(2): e22361, 8 pages.

206. Damalas C.A., Koutroubas S.D. (2018). Current Status and Recent Developments in Biopesticide Use. *Agriculture*, **8**(13), 6 pages.

207. Senthil-Nathan S. (2015). A Review of Biopesticides and Their Mode of Action Against Insect Pests, pp. 49–63. In: *Environmental Sustainability*. Editors: P. Thangavel, G. Sridevi. Springer, New Delhi. https://doi.org/10.1007/978-81-322-2056-5_3.

208. Onder M., Ceyhan E., Kahraman A. (2011). Effects of Agricultural Practices on Environment. 2011 International Conference on Biology, Environment and Chemistry, Singapore. *IPCBEE*, **24**: 28–32. IACSIT Press, Singapore. http://ipcbee.com/vol24/6-ICBEC2011-C00015.pdf.

209. Artiola J.F., Walworth J.L., Musil S.A., Crimmins M.A. (2019). Chapter 14 – Soil and Land Pollution, pp. 219–235. In: *Environmental and Pollution Science*. 3rd edition. Editors: Mark L. Brusseau, Ian L. Pepper, Charles P. Gerba. Academic Press. https://doi.org/10.1016/B978-0-12-814719-1.00014-8.

210. Fazzo L., Minichilli F., Santoro M., Ceccarini A., Della Seta M., Bianchi F., Comba P., Martuzzi M. (2017). Hazardous Waste and Health Impact: A Systematic Review of the Scientific Literature. *Environ. Health*, **16**(107), 11 pages.

211. National Institute of Environmental Health Science. (2020). Safe Water and Your Health, August 11. www.niehs.nih.gov/health/topics/agents/water-poll/index.cfm.

212. Schwarzenbach R.P., Egli T., Hofstetter T.B., von Gunten U., Wehrli B. (2010). Global Water Pollution and Human Health. *Annu. Rev. Environ. Resour.*, **35**: 109–136.

213. North E.J., Halden R.U. (2013). Plastics and Environmental Health: The Road Ahead. *Rev. Environ. Health*, **28**(1): 1–8.

214. Law K.L. (2017). Plastics in the Marine Environment. *Annu. Rev. Mar. Sci.*, **9**: 205–229.

215. Haines A., Kovats R.S., Campbell-Lendrum D., Corvalan C. (2006). Climate Change and Human Health: Impacts, Vulnerability and Public Health. *Public Health*, **120**: 585–596.

216. National Institute of Environmental Health Sciences. (2021). Endocrine Disruptors, February 9. www.niehs.nih.gov/health/topics/agents/endocrine/index.cfm.

217. Yang O., Kim H.L., Weon J.I., Seo Y.R. (2015). Endocrine-Disrupting Chemicals: Review of Toxicological Mechanisms Using Molecular Pathway Analysis. *J. Cancer Prev.*, **20**(1): 12–24.

218. La Merrill M.A., Vandenberg L.N., Smith M.T., Goodson W., Browne P., Patisaul H.B., Guyton K.Z., Kortenkamp A., Cogliano V.J., Woodruff T.J., Rieswijk L., Sone H., Korach K.S., Gore A.C., Zeise L., Zoeller R.T. (2020). Consensus on the Key Characteristics of Endocrine-Disrupting Chemicals as a Basis for Hazard Identification. *Nat. Rev. Endocrinol.*, **16**: 45–57.

219. Davis C., Bryan J., Hodgson J., Murphy K. (2015). Definition of the Mediterranean Diet: A Literature Review. *Nutrients*, **7**: 9139–9153.

220. Castro-Quezada I., Blanca Román-Viñas B., Serra-Majem L. (2014). The Mediterranean Diet and Nutritional Adequacy: A Review. *Nutrients*, **6**: 231–248.

221. Georgousopoulou E.N., George E.S., Mellor D.D., Panagiotakos D.B. (2020). Chapter 6. Mediterranean Lifestyle: Linking Social Life and Behaviors, Residential Environment, and Cardiovascular Disease Prevention, pp. 67–71. In: *The Mediterranean Diet*. 2nd edition. Editors: Victor R. Preedy, Ronald Ross Watson. Academic Press, 614 pages, ISBN 9780128186497.

222. Demarin V., Lisak M., Morovic S. (2011). Mediterranean Diet in Healthy Lifestyle and Prevention of Stroke. *Acta Clin. Croat.*, **50**(1): 67–77.

223. Martucci M., Ostan R., Biondi F., Bellavista E., Fabbri C., Bertarelli C., Salvioli S., Capri M., Franceschi C., Santoro A. (2017). Mediterranean Diet and Inflammaging Within the Hormesis Paradigm. *Nutr. Rev.*, **75**(6): 442–455.
224. Mattson M.P. (2008). Hormesis Defined. *Ageing Res. Rev.*, **7**(1): 1–7.
225. Willcox D.C., Willcox B.J., Todoriki H., Suzuki M. (2009). The Okinawan Diet: Health Implications of a Low-Calorie, Nutrient-Dense, Antioxidant-Rich Dietary Pattern Low in Glycemic Load. *J. Am. Coll. Nutr.*, **28** (Suppl.): 500S–516S.
226. Willcox D.C., Scapagnini G., Willcox B.J. (2014). Healthy Aging Diets Other Than the Mediterranean: A Focus on the Okinawan Diet. *Mech Ageing Dev.*, **136–137**: 148–162.
227. Salen P., de Lorgeril M. (2011). The Okinawan Lifestyle: A Modern View of an Ancestral Healthy Lifestyle. *World Rev. Nutr. Diet. (World Review of Nutrition and Dietetics)*, **102**: 114–123.
228. Challa H.J., Ameer M.A., Uppaluri K.R. (2020). DASH Diet to Stop Hypertension. In: *StatPearls [Internet]*. Treasure Island, FL, May 23. www.ncbi.nlm.nih.gov/books/NBK482514/.
229. Fung T.T., Hu F.B., Wu K., Chiuve S.E., Fuchs C.S., Giovannucci E. (2010). The Mediterranean and Dietary Approaches to Stop Hypertension (DASH) Diets and Colorectal Cancer. *Am. J. Clin. Nutr.*, **92**: 1429–1435.
230. Mattsona M.P., Allison D.B., Fontana L., Harvie M., Longo V.D., Malaisse W.J., Mosley M., Notterpek L., Ravussin E., Scheer F.A.J.L., Seyfried T.N., Varady K.A., Panda S. (2014). Meal Frequency and Timing in Health and Disease. *Proc. Natl. Acad. Sci. (PNAS)*, **111**(47): 16647–16653.
231. Cui H., Kong Y., Zhang H. (2012). Oxidative Stress, Mitochondrial Dysfunction, and Aging. *J. Signal. Transduct.*, **2012**, Article ID 646354, 13 pages.
232. Poljsak B., Milisav I. (2013). Chapter 14. Aging, Oxidative Stress and Antioxidants, pp. 331–353. In: *Oxidative Stress and Chronic Degenerative Diseases – A Role for Antioxidants*. Editors: B. Poljsak, I. Milisav. InTech, London.
233. Gemma C., Vila J., Bachstetter A., Bickford P.C. (2007). Chapter 15. Oxidative Stress and the Aging Brain: From Theory to Prevention. In: *Brain Aging: Models, Methods, and Mechanisms*. Editor: D.R. Riddle. CRC Press /Taylor & Francis, Boca Raton, FL.
234. Friedman J.R., Nunna J. (2014). Mitochondrial form and Function. *Nature*, **505**(7483): 335–343.
235. Pham-Huy A.L., He H., Pham-Huy C. (2008). Free Radicals and Antioxidants in Disease and Health. *Int. J. Biomed. Sci.*, **4**(2): 89–96.
236. Passarino G., De Rango F., Montesanto A. (2016). Human Longevity: Genetics or Lifestyle? It Takes Two to Tango. *Immun. Ageing*, **13**(12): 1–6.
237. Genetics Home Reference. MedlinePlus. National Library of Medicine (NLM). (2020). Is Longevity Determined by Genetics? September 18. https://ghr.nlm.nih.gov/primer/traits/longevity.
238. Diener E., Chan M.Y. (2011). Happy People Live Longer: Subjective Well-Being Contributes to Health and Longevity. *Appl. Psychol. Health Well-Being*, **3**(1): 1–43.
239. Mental Health Foundation. (2016). *Fundamental Facts About Mental Health*. Mental Health Foundation, London. www.mentalhealth.org.uk/sites/default/files/fundamental-facts-about-mental-health-2016.pdf.
240. Everson-Rose S.A., Lewis T.T. (2005). Psychosocial Factors and Cardiovascular Diseases. *Annu. Rev. Public Health*, **26**: 469–500.
241. Umberson D., Montez J.K. (2010). Social Relationships and Health: A Flashpoint for Health Policy. *J Health Soc. Behav.*, **51** (Suppl.): S54–S66.
242. Chamberlain L. (2021). Life Expectancy for Countries, May 17. www.infoplease.com/world/health-and-social-statistics/life-expectancy-countries.
243. Madden D. (2019). Ranked: The 25 Smartest Countries in The World, January 11. www.forbes.com/sites/unicefusa/2019/01/11/married-in-the-fifth-grade-in-yemen/#536792776e30.

9 Food Interactions, Sirtuins, Genes, Homeostasis, and General Discussion

1 INTRODUCTION

In this chapter, we will discuss food interactions, sirtuins, gene and its components, homeostasis, and finally, the general discussion and conclusion of the book. These are recent and topical issues in the global scientific literature.

2 FOOD INTERACTION

There are many types of food interactions, including interaction between different components of a food, interaction of food with drug, and interaction of food with physical activity.

When an interaction potentializes the effects of each component of a food much more than when they are used alone, in this case, the effect is called synergism or synergy. In other words, a synergistic effect is the situation where the combined effect of two components is much greater than the sum of the effects of each agent given alone (1). For example, a product A gives 5 calories, and a product B gives 10 calories, but when product A is combined with product B at the same time in the body, the sum of these 2 products obtained now becomes 20 calories or more, and not 15 calories. The 20 calories obtained instead of 15 calories theoretically are due to the synergistic effect between the interaction of product A with product B in the human body.

When their combined effect is equal to 15 calories, this phenomenon is named an additive effect. Additive effects occur more in the body than synergistic effects (1).

Antagonism is the opposite of synergism. It is the situation where the combined effect of two or more compounds gives less effects than the individual effects; for example, $5 + 10 < 15$. Antagonistic effects are the basis of many antidotes for poisonings or for medical treatments (1).

Potentiation results when one substance that does not normally have a toxic effect is added to another chemical, making the second chemical much more toxic; for example, $0 + 2 > 2$ (1).

Here, the discussion is limited to the synergistic effects of nutrients, phytochemicals, biological materials, drugs, and toxins in the human body.

2.1 SYNERGISTIC EFFECTS OF NUTRIENTS AND PHYTOCHEMICALS

Each food has its own unique profile of nutrients with different composition and concentration. Nutrients in foods include macronutrients and micronutrients (see Chapters 1 and 2). Each animal or plant food contains not only some main macronutrients such as proteins, carbohydrates, and lipids, but also some tens to hundreds of micronutrients like vitamins, antioxidants, coenzymes, cofactors, and minerals. Moreover, plant foods also contain many phytochemicals that can be classified as phenolics, terpenoids (carotenoids), alkaloids, nitrogen-containing compounds, and organosulfur compounds. Phenolics and terpenoids are abundant in plant foods, while alkaloids are mostly present in medicinal plants. Nutrients and phytochemicals act together and help each other for their absorption, metabolism, and elimination during digestion. There are about 8,000 phytochemicals

DOI: 10.1201/9781003220817-9

present in whole foods and over 5,000 phytochemicals that have been identified in various fruits and vegetables, but a large percentage still remain unknown and need to be identified before their health benefits are fully understood (2). These compounds differ in molecular size, polarity, and solubility, and these differences may affect the bioavailability and distribution of each phytochemical in different macromolecules, subcellular organelles, cells, organs, and tissues (2). The combination of different foods increases the absorption of each phytochemical or nutrient present in each food, thereby increasing its efficacy in health maintenance and disease prevention. Pills or tablets simply cannot mimic the balanced natural combination of phytochemicals present in fruit and vegetables (2). It is now widely believed that the actions of antioxidant nutrients alone do not explain the observed health benefits of diets rich in fruits and vegetables, because taken alone, the individual antioxidants studied in clinical trials do not appear to have consistent preventive effects (2–3). The additive and synergistic effects of phytochemicals in fruits and vegetables are responsible for their potent antioxidant activities against different chronic diseases. Meta-analyses of hundreds of studies showed that the actions of phytochemicals administered as dietary supplements alone do not explain the observed health benefits of diets rich in fruits, vegetables and whole grains; thereby showing no long-term benefits for vitamin supplements (4). The evidence suggests that antioxidants or bioactive compounds are best acquired through whole-food consumption, not from dietary supplements (3). Indeed, each biochemical or phytochemical in whole natural food is more potent and less toxic than the same compound used alone in form of dietary supplements, because in whole food, there are other compounds (coenzymes, cofactors, etc.) that help its absorption as well as its elimination. This is the case for vitamins, antioxidants, and minerals. Our understanding of the molecular mechanisms underlying such synergistic effects is still limited, but it appears that different combinations of complementary modes of actions are involved (4).

At the same time, phytochemicals or micronutrients that are extracted from foods or plants and used alone or in association with drugs or other biological compounds, are also helpful and necessary for the treatment of many diseases due to their high doses and ease of usage in their galenic form (capsule, tablet). Moreover, extraction and purification techniques allow the elimination of other toxic compounds potentially present in whole leaves, tubers, fruits, stems, or barks, and the preservation of the extracted phytochemical for a long time. In general, for disease prevention, whole food consumption is better than dietary supplements. But, for the treatment of a specific disease, a single phytochemical or micronutrient may become more potent and practical than whole food. The supplementation of some micronutrients is also necessary in the event of their absence in the diet, such as iodine, fluorine, iron, and vitamin B12.

2.2 Synergy Mechanisms of Phytochemicals in Cancer

Carcinogenesis is a complex multistep process, and oxidative damage is linked to formation of tumors through several mechanisms that play different crucial roles (2–4). Oxidative stresses induced by free radicals cause DNA damage, which, when left unrepaired, can lead to base mutation, single and double strand breaks, DNA cross-linking, and chromosomal breakage and rearrangement (2). This potentially cancer-inducing oxidative damage might be prevented or limited by dietary antioxidants found in fruit and vegetables. The mechanisms of action by which phytochemicals can modulate cancer risk include both blocking initiation and suppression of the later stages, involving promotion, progression, angiogenesis, invasion, and metastasis (4).

Blocking initiation of carcinogenesis by phytochemicals involves prevention of free radicals (reactive oxygen species) attack on DNA, altered metabolism of procarcinogens in favor of conjugation and excretion of reactive metabolites, inhibition of carcinogen uptake into cells, and enhanced DNA repair (4). Many chemo-preventive compounds possessing antioxidant or free radical scavenging potential are polyphenol molecules, which include flavonoids (tannins and condensed tannins) and non-flavonoid compounds. Flavonoids are found in tea, red grapes, apples, persimmon, cocoa, chocolate, kiwi, blackberry, apricots, peach, onion, ginkgo, nuts, beans, soybeans, tofu, and more. Some major non-flavonoid compounds include curcumin in turmeric spice, resveratrol in red grapes, red wine, peanuts, and xanthones in mangosteen, and canistel. Terpenoids are also a large group of phytochemicals which include many well-known strong antioxidants and anticancer compounds such as paclitaxel in Pacific yew, caroteinoids like carotenes, lycopene, lutein, fucoxanthin, astaxanthin, in carrot, tomato, kale, broccoli, and microalgae. These phytochemicals protect the human body against oxidative stress which is one of the causes of many cancer forms (see Chapter 5, monograph Flavonoids and Terpenoids).

Suppression mechanisms of tumor cells include growth inhibition by induction of cell cycle arrest or apoptosis. Fucoidan, a natural polysaccharide of brown seaweeds, has anti-cancer activity against various cancer types by targeting key apoptotic molecules. It can protect against toxicity associated with chemotherapeutic agents and radiation. Thus, the synergistic effect of fucoidan with current anti-cancer agents is of great interest (5). A significant number of flavonoids, alone and in combination, have been shown to induce suppression of tumor cells. Tricin, a novel flavonol in rice bran, was shown to inhibit the growth of breast tumor cells or to decrease the number of intestinal adenomas in mice (4). Many studies have reported that phytochemicals in common fruit and vegetables can have complementary and overlapping mechanisms of action, including modulation of detoxification enzymes, scavenging of free radicals, stimulation of the immune system, regulation of gene expression in cell proliferation and apoptosis, and inhibition of angiogenesis, invasion, and metastasis (2–4). More recently, evidence is emerging that specific combination of phytochemicals may be far more effective in protecting against cancer than isolated compounds. Moreover, drug-phytochemical interactions have also been observed, indicating possibilities for improved cancer therapeutic strategies (4).

Although high doses of single phytochemicals may show potent anticarcinogenic effects, the chemo-preventive properties of interactions among various dietary ingredients that potentiate the activities of any single constituent may better explain the observed preventive effect of whole foods and diets in many epidemiological studies (4). Natural remedy advocates are constantly recommending multiple supplements from various plant or herb extractions. For example, curcumin, a strong antioxidant of turmeric spice, is a potent anticarcinogen in vitro. But in humans, this property becomes weak because curcumin is poorly absorbed by the small intestine, thereby decreasing its efficacy in the prevention or treatment of cancer, inflammatory diseases, and CVDs. However, when turmeric is eaten in the same time with black pepper or galangal spice, the bioavailability of curcumin is now multiplied by 100 to 1,000 times (see Chapter 5, monograph Turmeric). Other examples of synergy between different foods are abundant. For example, resveratrol, a polyphenol present in red grape and red wine, can protect cancer and cardiovascular diseases by activating sirtuins. In contrast, resveratrol supplement alone does not give this same healthy effect as red grapes because in red grapes, there are the coenzyme NAD^+ and other phytonutrients that might help resveratrol to activate sirtuins.

2.3 SYNERGY EFFECTS OF PHYTOCHEMICALS IN CARDIOVASCULAR DISEASES

Cardiovascular disease (CVD) is the leading cause of death before cancer in developed countries. Epidemiological studies have shown that regular consumption of fruits and vegetables is linked to reduced incidence or mortality from CVD among adults. Therefore, many healthcare organizations in Europe and the United States recommended consuming five or more servings of fruit and vegetables daily for reducing the risk of both cancer and heart disease (2, 6).

The etiology of CVD is very complex, and overproduction of oxidants is one of the main pathogenic factors. Oxidative damage can cause endothelial cell injuries and deleterious vasodilator effects (6). It has been shown that antioxidant polyphenols present in diverse vegetables and fruits could improve the endothelial function of heart and vessels, and therefore play an important role in the prevention of CVD (2, 6–7). Polyphenols could also protect the cardiovascular system, not only from oxidative stress but other damage, because they possess other physiological effects, such as blood pressure reduction and inflammation decreasing action (2, 6–7). Dietary flavonoid intake was inversely associated with mortality from coronary artery disease and inversely related with incidence of myocardial infarction (2, 6). In a study in Finland, intake of apples and onions, both high in quercetin, a flavonoid polyphenol, was inversely correlated with total mortality and coronary mortality (2). In a Japanese study, total intake of flavonoids (quercetin, myricetin, kaempferol, luteolin, and ficetin) and isoflavones (daidzein and genistein) was inversely correlated with the plasma total cholesterol and low-density lipoprotein (LDL) cholesterol concentrations (2, 8). Among 30 vegetables and fruits analyzed by the Japanese study, the major source of flavonoids was onions (45.9%) and that of isoflavones was tofu (37.0%) (8). Onion contains all 5 flavonoids cited previously, and is the richest in quercetin, while parsley is the richest in myricetin among the 30 studied foods (8). These results suggest that a high consumption of both flavonoids and isoflavones often present in Japanese foods by Japanese women may contribute to their low incidence of coronary heart disease compared to women in other countries (8).

Mechanisms for the prevention of arteriosclerosis by antioxidants have been proposed. The mechanism of oxidized LDL cholesterol has been suggested as the atherogenic factor that contributes to heart disease (2). Dietary antioxidants neutralize oxidized LDL cholesterol (bad cholesterol), thereby preventing atherosclerosis, a disease of the arteries characterized by the deposition of fatty material on their inner walls. In addition, phytochemicals have been shown to have roles in the reduction of platelet aggregation, modulation of cholesterol synthesis and absorption, and reduction of blood pressure. Recently, C-reactive protein, a marker of systemic inflammation, has been reported to be a stronger predictor of cardiovascular disease than LDL cholesterol, suggesting that inflammation is a critical factor in cardiovascular disease (2, 7). Inflammation not only promotes initiation and progression of atherosclerosis but also causes acute thrombotic complications of atherosclerosis. Therefore, the anti-inflammatory activity of phytochemicals obtained from the combination of different plant foods may play an important role in the prevention of CVDs (2).

Plants rich in polyphenols are onion, red grapes, curcuma, berries, nuts, apple, parsley, beans, soybeans, persimmon, tea, jute mallow, spinach, and more.

2.4   Synergy Effects of Phytochemicals in Inflammatory Diseases

Inflammation is defined as a series of immunological, biochemical, and/or cellular alterations in response to exogenous or endogenous stimuli such as infection, injury, and irritation, caused by microbes, viruses, molds, chemicals, allergens, and more (7, 9). Both chronic and acute phase inflammatory processes act locally and systematically to activate cells associated with inflammatory process (macrophages, endothelial cells, and fibroblast) to induce inflammatory mediators like reactive oxygen (ROS), nitric oxide (NO), interleukins, prostaglandin E2, tumor necrosis factor alpha (TNF-α), cytokines, interferon gamma, and cyclooxygenase 2 (COX-2) (7, 9–11).

Inflammation includes acute inflammation and chronic inflammation. Acute inflammatory diseases are acute bronchitis, sore throat from a flu, tonsillitis, acute appendicitis, and so on. Chronic inflammatory diseases include asthma, rhinitis, allergy or hypersensitivity, muscular pain, osteoarthritis, arthritis, psoriasis, gout, inflammatory bowel diseases (Crohn's disease, ulcerative colitis), chronic rheumatoid arthritis, systemic lupus erythematosus, and more. Rheumatoid arthritis and lupus are auto-immune diseases. Chronic inflammation is another important factor that may cause or assist in the pathogenesis of many chronic diseases including CVD, cancers, and Type 2 diabetes (6).

Fruits, vegetables, and seafoods contain high levels of antioxidants that show anti-inflammatory effects, but their mechanisms of actions have not been completely identified (7, 9–11). The discovery of drugs that can be used for the treatment of inflammatory and allergic diseases is important in human health. Drug discovery from plants involves a multidisciplinary approach combining botanical, ethnobotanical, phytochemical, and biological techniques. Several natural product drugs of plant origin are in clinical use (10). Wide ranges of phytoconstituents are responsible for anti-inflammatory activity including phenolics, terpenoids, and alkaloids (10). The phenolics and triterpenoids in fruits and vegetables showed higher anti-inflammatory activity than other compounds. In food legumes, lectins and peptides had anti-inflammatory activity in most cases (9). In chronic inflammatory diseases, an imbalance between oxidant generation and defense mechanism or inadequate presence of antioxidant molecules results in the state known as oxidative stress. Growing evidence indicates that chronic and acute excess generation of oxidants under pathophysiologic conditions is pivotal in the development of chronic inflammatory diseases such as premature atherosclerosis progression, neurodegenerative disorder, cancer, CVDs, and pulmonary fibrosis (7). Numerous pieces of evidence reported curcumin (rhizome of *Curcuma longa*), EGCG (tea), and resveratrol (grapes, berry) as potential natural anti-inflammatory compounds because of their strong antioxidative properties. Curcumin has been shown to exert protective effect against neuronal degeneration by scavenging oxidants and free radicals (7). The combination of these phytochemicals between them or with other nutrients such as omega-3 in seafoods, increase their protective activity against oxidative stress considerably in comparison to the same phytochemicals used alone. Recently, some authors demonstrated the synergistic anti-inflammatory effects of curcumin, a polyphenol of turmeric spice, combined with docosahexaenoic acid (DHA) or eicosapentaenoic acid (EPA), two omega-3 fatty acids present in fish oil or seafood, by an in vitro experiment (12). They found that the combination of curcumin with DHA or EPA clearly showed the synergistic anti-inflammatory effect, as well as antioxidative stress effects of curcumin and DHA or EPA, and these effects are stronger than each compound used alone (12). Another study reported that curcumin enhanced the synthesis of DHA from its precursor, α-linolenic acid (ALA), which is mainly present in plant foods, and elevated levels of enzymes involved in the synthesis of DHA (active form of omega-3 fatty acids) in both liver and brain tissues. Furthermore, in vivo treatment with curcumin and ALA reduced anxiety-like behavior in rodents (13). Taken together, these data suggested that curcumin enhanced DHA synthesis, resulting in elevated brain DHA content, and this synergistic action could be used in the prevention of anxiety disorders in humans, in particular in vegans who do not eat fish and other animal foods (13). Moreover, asthma, muscular pain, and arthritis might be prevented or treated by combining fish oils or sea foods with curcuma tuber and galangal spice because they are all strong anti-inflammatory and antioxidant agents and have synergistic actions between them. The combination of phytochemicals of different foods might also prevent or treat obesity and Type 2 diabetes (6, 11).

However, more efforts are needed to elucidate the mechanisms of actions of herbs and plant foods, and to establish their potential utility as therapeutic agents in the treatment of many inflammatory diseases. Several mechanisms of action have been proposed to explain the anti-inflammatory actions of phytochemicals. They include: antioxidative activities; modulation of cellular activities of inflammation-related cells (mast cells, macrophages, lymphocytes, and neutrophils); modulation of proinflammatory enzyme activities such as phospholipase A2 (PLA2), cyclooxygenase (COX), and lipoxygenase (LOX) and the nitric oxide (NO) producing enzyme, nitric oxide synthase (NOS); modulation of the production of other proinflammatory molecules; and modulation of proinflammatory gene expression (10).

In brief, the synergy action between foods is demonstrated by the two famous healthy diets well known in the world: the Mediterranean diet and the Okinawan diet. People of the Mediterranean region and Okinawa isle live longer and healthier than other populations due to their diet. Thus, combining different foods to find their positive synergistic effect on health is a difficult but worthwhile task, and requires patience and knowledge.

2.5 Food-Drug Synergy and Food-Drug Interaction

When certain foods or their nutrients are combined with some drugs, two distinct consequences of this combination can occur: food-drug synergy and food-drug interaction.

In the case of food-drug synergy, a certain whole food or its nutrient can potentiate the pharmacological activity of the combined drug in comparison to the same drug taken alone without this food. Therefore, this type of food-drug synergy is beneficial for the therapy of certain diseases.

In the case of food-drug interaction, the intake of a certain food at the same time with a drug can decrease the therapeutic effect of the drug or can increase its toxic effect in the body due to the interference of the food nutrient in the metabolism of this drug.

2.5.1 Food-Drug Synergy

Food-drug synergy includes the following: the interaction of a food (or food component) and a specific drug that confers a greater health benefit than either the food (or food component) or drug alone; the additive effects of a drug in combination with a food (or food component) that confer a health benefit; and the ability of a food (or food component) to attenuate or negate a negative side effect of a drug (14). Many research about the association of food or diet with drugs have been investigated to potentiate the studied drug in the therapy of many dreadful diseases such as cancer, CVDs, and neurodegenerative diseases.

2.5.1.1 Food-Drug Synergy in Cancer Therapy

Many research papers have shown a better outcome in cancer treatment when the chemotherapeutic drugs are combined with foods or their nutrients (14–15). Flavonoids and other antioxidants of plant food when used alone could produce beneficial, detrimental, or insignificant effects in cancer patients, while if they are combined with other anticancer compounds (i.e., natural compounds or chemotherapy drugs), their effects are more likely to be beneficial or at least not harmful (15).

The treatment of colorectal tumor with 5-Fluorouracil, an anticancer drug, combined with quercetin or leuteolin (flavonoid) increased apoptosis (programmed cell death) with a significant effect for quercetin which involved the activation of the apoptotic mitochondrial pathway (15). In another study, the flavonoid silibinin strongly synergized the antiproliferative effect of doxorubicin drug in prostate carcinoma cells. This combination was associated with an increase in carcinoma cell arrest and apoptosis compared with treatment of each compound alone. Silibinin also causes synergistic cytotoxic effects when combined with chemotherapeutic drugs against breast and lung cancer cells (15). Curcumin was shown to be effective in combination treatment. The combination of curcumin with either cisplatin or oxaliplatin drug increased significantly the cytotoxic effect on ovarian cancer cells by increasing apoptosis (15). Fucoidan, a natural component of brown seaweed, has anti-cancer activity against various cancer types by targeting key apoptotic molecules. It also has beneficial effects as it can protect against toxicity associated with chemotherapeutic agents and radiation. Thus, the synergistic effect of fucoidan with current anti-cancer agents is of considerable interest (5).

Some association of green tea with drugs may be useful (synergistic effect). The combination of green tea and chemotherapy medications, specifically doxorubicin, adriamycin, sulindac, and tamoxifen, has increased the effectiveness of these medications in laboratory tests, but these results have not yet been demonstrated in clinical studies (16–17). *In vitro* and animal studies provide strong evidence that green tea polyphenols may possess the bioactivity to prevent or inhibit some forms of cancer. However, the results from epidemiological and clinical studies of the relationship between green tea and cancer prevention, especially prostate cancer and breast cancer, are mixed (16).

2.5.1.2 Food-Drug Synergy in Cardiovascular Disease Therapy

Recent evidence suggests that combining fish oil with statin therapy may beneficially alter lipid profiles more than each compound used alone (18). When statin drugs such as atorvastatin or simvastatin are taken with fish oil, a byproduct of fish flesh, their effects in the treatment of hypercholesterolemia and/or hypertriglyceridemia in patients with coronary heart disease are more effective than the effects of statins and fish oil alone (18). Indeed, this combination therapy may be an optimal therapeutic approach for correcting dyslipidemia in cardiac people (18).

The effect of fish oil supplementation in combination with nifedipine, a calcium channel blocker drug used to treat hypertension and dyslipidemia, has also been tested in humans. Interestingly, when fish oil was combined with nifedipine, total and LDL cholesterol concentrations were significantly reduced by 12.0 and 15.0%, when compared with baseline, while blood pressure decreased to a similar extent as what was noted with the nifedipine therapy alone (18). While no studies to date have examined the adverse interactions between fish oils and lipid altering drug therapies, only one trial has evaluated the interaction between fish oils and other dietary fat constituents on indicators of cardiovascular disease risk. The results demonstrated that the supplementation of EPA and DHA lead to the lowering of oleic acid concentrations in serum phospholipids. Since oleic acid has been shown to exert certain favorable effects on the cardiovascular system, the decline of oleic acid as a result of excess of omega-3 fatty acid supplementation can be regarded as a potential problem. Thus, future research should focus on defining the optimal balance of these two fatty acids (oleic acid and omega-3 fatty acid) when they are used as a combination therapy for cardiovascular disease (18).

2.5.1.3   Food-Drug Synergy in Other Disease Therapy

Green tea may also increase the effectiveness of certain antibiotics such as levofloxacin by reducing bacterial resistance to treatment (16). Green tea can prevent dental caries and some oral infections such as periodontal disease thanks to its catechin polyphenols. Results from both human and animal studies have demonstrated how green tea works against bacteria that cause cavities in teeth (16). Several human studies have shown that bacteria present in dental plaque stopped growing when people rinsed their mouths with tea 5 times for 30 seconds over a period of 15 minutes (16). Brushing the teeth with fluorine toothpaste, then rinsing the mouth with tea infusion is the best way to prevent dental caries and other oral infections.

Another in vitro study demonstrated the synergism between 13 antimicrobial drugs (penicillin, oxacillin, vancomycin, ampicillin, cephalothin, cefoxitin, chloramphenicol, gentamicin, netilmicin, tetracycline, erythromycin, cotrimoxazole, ofloxacin) and 8 plant extracts, including guava (*Psidium guajava*), clove (*Syzygium aromaticum*), lemongrass (*Cymbopogon citratus*), 'guaco' (*Mikania glomerata*), ginger (*Zingiber officinale*), garlic (*Allium sativum*), mint (*Mentha piperita*) and 'carqueja' (*Baccharis trimera*), against *Staphylococcus aureus* strains (19). This in vitro research verified the antimicrobial activities of the studied herbal extracts, and confirmed their synergism with these antibiotics. Clove, guava, and lemongrass presented the highest synergism rate with antimicrobial drugs, while ginger and garlic showed limited synergistic effect (19). Relevance of anti-inflammatory and antioxidant activities of exemestane, a synthetic steroidal inhibitor drug, and its synergisms with sulforaphane, a phytochemical in broccoli, Brussels sprouts, and cabbage, were also demonstrated by different cell line tests in vitro and in vivo in mice for disease prevention (20). The synergy of exemestane drug and sulforaphane phytochemical may prevent not only breast cancer, but also other chronic diseases that arise from inflammation, oxidative stress, and DNA-damaging electrophiles.

In summary, the study of phytochemical-drug synergy is still sparse, but its potentials in the prevention and treatment of some chronic diseases are of great interest in the future, because the synergy of diet with drugs may strengthen the efficacy of drugs alone, and may also decrease side effects.

2.5.2   Food-Drug Interaction

Consuming certain foods or their nutrients with some drugs at the same time can cause negative health effects in certain cases because of the interaction of food and drugs in the body. The food-drug interaction can decrease or increase the prescribed dose of drug in the body because certain foods can modify the metabolism of drugs or vice-versa. Therefore, the interference of certain food on the fate of drugs in the body can make drugs ineffective or conversely, more toxic. The intake of drugs with food or without food is also another condition for the efficacy of drug.

Food-drug interactions are defined as alterations of pharmacokinetics or pharmacodynamics of a drug or nutritional element or a compromise in nutritional status as a result of the addition of a drug (21). Pharmacokinetics is the study of the time course of drug absorption (A), distribution (D), metabolism (M), and excretion (E) by the body. The four phases of pharmacokinetics are abbreviated as ADME. Pharmacokinetics enables us to know the therapeutic effects of a drug. Pharmacodynamics refers to the physiologic or clinical effects of a drug in the body, or the study of the therapeutic action of a drug in the body (21). Food-drug interactions can result in two main clinical effects: either a decreased bioavailability of a drug, which predisposes to treatment failure, or an increased bioavailability, which increases the risk of adverse events and may even precipitate toxicities (21–23).

The influence of dietary substances on drug effects depends on numerous variables ranging from physicochemical properties of the drug to host factors such as enzymes and transporters in the gastrointestinal tract as well as in the entire body. The interactions may affect not only blood levels of drugs through pharmacokinetic change, but also the actual pharmacodynamic effects of drugs. Some foods attenuate or enhance drug effects and toxicity by interfering with drug actions, mechanisms, and the pharmacodynamics of the drug (22). Physiologic and physicochemical mechanisms underlying food effects on drug disposition are well characterized. However, biochemical mechanisms involving drug metabolizing enzymes and transport proteins remain underexplored. Several plant or animal foods or plant-derived beverages or dietary supplements have been shown to modulate enzymes such as intestinal cytochrome P450, especially cytochrome P450 3A4 enzymes, and/or phase II conjugation enzymes and protein transporters in the intestine, leading to altered pharmacokinetic and potentially negative pharmacodynamic outcomes (23). Some examples of food-drug interactions are as follows.

2.5.2.1   Interaction of Grapefruit Juice with Drugs

Grapefruit juice is a classic example of a selective intestinal cytochrome P450 3A4 inhibitor (21–27). Note that this interaction applies to grapefruit juice, not the whole fruit itself. Grapefruit juice is rich in furanocoumarins (bergamottin) suggesting that all major furanocoumarins contribute to the inhibitory effects of grapefruit juice (26–27). Consumption of grapefruit juice has increased the oral bioavailability of various drugs, including antihypertensive agents such as calcium channel blockers (e.g., amlodipine, felodipine, nifedipine, verapamil, etc.), statin drugs (atorvastatin, simvastatin, lovastatin), benzodiazepines (midazolam, triazolam), antihistamines (terfenadines), beta-blockers (talinolol, acebutolol), and immunosuppressants (cyclosporine, tacrolimus) (21–27). Antihypertensive drugs cited earlier (calcium channel blockers) interact with grapefruit juice by increasing their levels in the body, thereby causing side effects like orthostatic hypotension (21–27). Another well-known food-drug interaction is grapefruit juice and statin drugs (atorvastatin, simvastatin, lovastatin) which are used to treat hyperlipidemia and hypercholesterolemia. Grapefruit juice, in large quantities, can increase blood levels of statins metabolized by this pathway and cause side effects, most notably, muscle toxicity, which may manifest as myalgia, rhabdomyolysis, or myopathy (21–27). However, not all statins exhibit this interaction; only the three statins cited earlier are influenced by grapefruit juice (24). Sildenafil (Viagra), vardenafil (Levitra), and tadalafil (Cialis), used for erectile dysfunction, can also increase blood levels with concurrent use of grapefruit juice, but this interaction is unpredictable. Patients may have a slightly higher risk of adverse reactions, such as priapism, hypotension, and visual disturbances (24). Estrogen-containing oral contraceptives are also affected by grapefruit juice, but modestly (24). Clomipramine, a tricyclic antidepressant, is also affected by grapefruit juice (24). Patients taking erythromycin antibiotic and consuming grapefruit juice have an increased risk for cardiovascular symptoms, including cardiac dysrhythmias (21). Benzodiazepine tranquilizers such as diazepam, temazepam, and midazolam, taken together with grapefruit juice, can cause side effects such as drowsiness and prolonged sedation due to their higher blood levels (21, 24). Grapefruit juice doubles the oral systemic effects of budesonide, an anti-inflammatory corticoid, increasing the risk of the already prevalent glucocorticoid effects (24). Coadministration of grapefruit juice with antiarrhythmic drugs (amiodarone, quinidine, disopyramide, and propafenone), and anti-cancer agent (vinblastine) can increase their blood levels and cause diverse side effects (22, 24). Another significant grapefruit juice interaction concerns immunosuppressants: tacrolimus (FK-560) and cyclosporine, which are both used following organ transplantation (21, 24). Grapefruit juice can also increase blood levels of sertraline, an antidepressant used for therapy of anxiety and obsession, thereby causing side effects (21). Overall, grapefruit juice rich in furanocoumarins can increase the levels of many drugs due to its inhibition of the cytochrome P450 3A4, an intestinal enzyme used for the metabolism of xenobiotics like drugs; therefore, taking drugs and grapefruit juice together can increase drug side effects and may cause drug poisoning. It is recommended to avoid the use of grapefruit juice during drug therapy (21–27).

2.5.2.2 Interaction of Caffeine with Drugs

Many common drugs interfere with the metabolism of caffeine, resulting in an increase in caffeine blood levels (24). Consumption of caffeinated beverages late at night in combination with these medications may result in sleepless nights. In addition, this may enhance caffeine's diuretic effect. Ciprofloxacin (antibiotic), cimetidine (drug for peptic ulcer and acid indigestion), and oral contraceptives and prednisone (hormone) inhibit the metabolism of caffeine, resulting in increased effects of caffeine, which can cause insomnia (24). Conversely, caffeine inhibits the metabolism of theophylline drug, which shares a similar chemical structure with caffeine, and can increase the serum concentrations of theophylline. Pharmacists should warn patients taking theophylline that caffeine-containing beverages may predispose patients to adverse theophylline-related effects, such as nervousness, insomnia, and cardiac arrhythmia (24). Using bronchodilators for asthma like albuterol and theophylline with foods and drinks rich in caffeine such as coffee, cola drinks, teas, cocoa, chocolate, high-energy drinks, and some soft drinks can increase insomnia and excitability.

2.5.2.3 Interaction of Tea Infusion with Drugs

Tea is the most widely consumed beverage in the world, except water (16, 22–23). The majority of clinical studies to date evaluating the effect of repeated green tea administration on cytochrome P450 activity has not demonstrated clinically significant interactions (22–23). However, drinking tea may contribute to iron deficiency, and in infants, tea has been associated with impaired iron metabolism and microcytic anemia because tea is rich in tannins (catechins), which form with iron present in food or used as dietary supplement, a complex that has difficulty to cross the intestinal barrier (16).

2.5.2.4 Interaction of Alcohol Drinks with Drugs

Drug interactions with alcohol drinks (beer, wine, liquor, whisky) are numerous and significant (24). Some examples are benzodiazepines, antidepressants, antihistamines, anticonvulsants, antipsychotics, barbiturates, muscle relaxants, analgesics, non-steroidal anti-inflammatory drugs (NSAID), and narcotics (24). When these drugs are taken concurrently with alcohol, patients are at an increased risk of ataxia, somnolence, respiratory depression, and motor impairment, which can lead to falls, accidents, and injury (24). Excessive use of acetaminophen, an analgesic, with regular alcohol intake increases the risk of hepatotoxicity (24, 28). A disulfiram reaction (facial flushing, vomiting, tachycardia) can occur if alcohol is ingested with drugs such as metronidazole (antibiotic), sulfonylureas (antidiabetic drugs), or isoniazid (antibiotic for the treatment of tuberculosis) (24). Disulfiram reaction refers to an adverse effect caused by disulfiram, a drug used to treat chronic alcoholism. This drug causes an unpleasant reaction to alcohol. Nonsteroidal Anti-inflammatory Drugs (NSAIDs) like aspirin, ibuprofen, celecoxib, diclofenac, ketoprofen, naproxen, can cause stomach bleeding, and this effect becomes higher if they are taken with alcoholic drinks (28). Alcohol consumption can irritate the gastrointestinal mucosa and increase gastric acid secretions, which may lead to gastritis. Do not drink alcohol with narcotics such as opiates, morphine, heroin, and cocaine, because alcohol can increase the dangerous side effects of narcotics and this association can cause central nervous system depression, coma, or death (28).

2.5.2.5 Interaction of Dairy Products or Calcium-Fortified Foods with Drugs

Contrary to grapefruit juice and caffeine, dairy products rich in calcium such as milk, yogurt, or foods or beverages fortified with calcium, may decrease drug absorption because the drug binds to calcium to form a chelate calcium-drug. Therefore, some drugs become ineffective when taken at the same time with foods rich in calcium (24). For example, antibiotics such as ciprofloxacin, levofloxacin, cefuroxime, or tetracycline, may be rendered ineffective when taken at the same time as dairy products or calcium supplement (24). It is the same for bisphosphonate drugs (alendronate, risedronate, ibandronate) and antacids if they are taken together with milk or calcium-fortified beverages. In addition, methotrexate (an anticancer drug) levels are decreased with the consumption of milk-rich foods. As a general rule, the administration of dairy products and/or calcium supplements should be separated from the interacting drug by at least two to four hours for avoiding the diminution of therapeutic drug effects (24).

2.5.2.6   Interaction of Protein-Rich Foods with Drugs

Protein-rich foods can interfere with or potentiate the absorption of various medications such as antihypertensive beta-blocker drugs (propranolol, metoprolol, oxprenolol, etc.), anti-asthmatic drug (theophylline), and anti-Parkinsonian's drugs (levodopa, carbidopa) (24). Consuming a meal high in protein and taking propranolol concurrently can increase the beta-blocker's bioavailability, thereby increasing its side effects like bradycardia, hypotension, and bronchoconstriction (24). In contrast, high-protein diets can decrease concentration and efficacy of carbidopa, levodopa, and theophylline, resulting in low drug efficacy and aggravation of disease (24).

2.5.2.7   Interaction of High-Fat Meals with Drugs

Many drugs have their pharmacokinetics modified by fatty foods (24). For example, griseofulvin, an antifungal medication, has a significantly increased absorption when taken with food, especially a high-fat meal. Thus, griseofulvin is recommended to be taken with a fatty meal to benefit from this interaction.

2.5.2.8   Interaction of Fiber with Drugs

Fiber, like oatmeal and vegetables can bind drugs, resulting in decreased drug concentrations. For example, patients with diabetes who try to decrease their cholesterol levels by eating oatmeal after taking metformin, a drug used to treat Type 2 diabetes, might be worsening their diabetic control because metformin binds to fiber, decreasing its levels in blood (24). Levothyroxine, a drug used to treat hypothyroidism, is altered when taken with fiber. Digoxin and penicillin are also affected by this food-drug interaction. However, other derived penicillin drugs do not appear to be altered by the use of dietary fiber such as oatmeal, sweet potatoes, corn, bran, cereals, vegetables, and seeds (24).

2.5.2.9   Interaction of Tyramine-Containing Foods with Drugs

Tyramine is a biochemical widely found in foods and beverages such as meat, cheese, fermented foods, beans, peanuts, bananas, nuts, chocolate, and red wine. It has a significant interaction with monoamine oxidase inhibitors (MAOIs). These drugs are used to treat depression and Parkinson's disease. Linezolid, a newer oxazolidinone antibiotic, has some MAOI properties, thus showing characteristics and potential for this interaction (22, 24). Therefore, linezolid should be used cautiously in patients taking serotonin selective reuptake inhibitors (SSRIs). Lastly, isoniazid, a mainstay in the treatment of tuberculosis, also exhibits MAOI effects and should not be taken with tyramine-containing foods (24).

2.5.2.10   Interaction of Green, Leafy Vegetables with Warfarin Drug

Warfarin is an anticoagulant drug used to treat blood clots such as vein thrombosis and pulmonary thrombosis, and to prevent stroke in cardiac patients. The most notorious food-drug interaction regarding warfarin occurs with green, leafy vegetables, due to their rich vitamin K content (24). Vitamin K is used for blood coagulation and to treat or prevent hemorrhage. Warfarin and vitamin K present in vegetable foods have opposite mechanisms of action. Increasing vitamin K-rich food intake will result in reducing the efficacy of warfarin (24). Therefore, people under warfarin therapy are advised to consume leafy vegetables moderately for the good efficacy of warfarin therapy. Soy milk, char grilled foods, and sushi containing seaweed may also decrease the effect of warfarin (24). Cranberry juice, in contrast, can significantly potentiate the anticoagulant effects of warfarin (24). Dried goji berries may potentiate the anticoagulant effect of warfarin and increase the risk of bleeding.

2.5.2.11   *Interaction between Meal intake and Drug Absorption*

In many cases, the presence or the absence of a meal in the stomach can influence the oral absorption of a drug (21). Some medicines may work faster, slower, better, or worse if they are taken on a full or empty stomach. The absorption rate of a drug, its absorption magnitude, or both can be changed in relation to the stomach state. Meal intake stimulates gastric and intestinal secretions, which usually improve the dissolution of drugs and facilitate absorption (21). Meals with higher fat content stimulate the release of bile salts, which increase the intestinal uptake of highly lipophilic drugs or of substances which require bile salts for optimal absorption. In addition, a high fat content of the food also stimulates the release of cholecystokinin, which slows gastrointestinal motility and increases the contact time between the drug and the intestine and possibly also absorption (21). In certain cases, some drugs can upset the stomach, if it is empty. However, the potential physico-chemical interactions cited above, the potential binding of drug and food contents, the dose of the drug administered, and the composition of the meals make drug absorption in the presence of food unpredictable in specific cases. For that reason, the bioavailability of drugs should be tested with and without concurrent meal intake. It has been shown that certain drugs should be taken with food to maximize absorption (21). Among these drugs are: the antibiotics cefuroxime and erythromycin; lovastatin, a statin used for the treatment of hypercholesterolemia; and lithium, an alkaline salt used for psychiatric diseases. On the other hand, several drugs should not be taken with food to allow optimal absorption: the antibiotics ampicillin, ciprofloxacin, doxycycline or tetracycline; captopril (used for the treatment of hypertension); or indinavir, used for AIDS therapy (21). In general, it is important to carefully read the instructions for use before taking medicine, as well as ask your doctor or pharmacist. Avoid taking certain medicines at the same time with some foods or drinks cited earlier such as alcohol, grapefruit juice, and food or beverages containing caffeine.

2.6   Synergy of Physical Activity and Diet

The combination of regular physical activity with good diet plays important roles in the prevention of a number of dreadful chronic diseases like cardiovascular disease (CVD), cancer, bone disease, obesity, and diabetes. The combination of two forms of lifestyle including physical activity and good diet is better than each form used alone. Moderate physical activity intensifies the effects of nutrients, antioxidants, vitamins, and phytochemicals present in the diet, because physical activity stimulates their metabolism as well as their biological activity in the body. Physical activity and good diet are described in Chapter 8 of this book.

2.6.1   Synergy of Physical Activity and Diet in Cardiovascular Diseases

Research on the synergistic effect of physical activity and diet on cardiovascular diseases suggests that there may be more benefit combined than with either intervention alone. A 2014 population-based cohort study of Swedish men 45 to 79 years of age during 12 years showed that the combination of high-quality diet and physically active lifestyle was associated with a significant reduction of CVD risk compared with those who adopted none of the healthy lifestyle behaviors (29). In this study, high-quality diet is defined as a diet rich in fruits, vegetables, nuts, and seafoods, and low in saturated and trans-fats, with moderate consumption of alcohol and tobacco cessation; while good physical activity includes at least 40 minutes of walking or biking per day and 1 hour of additional physical activity per week (29). Increases in healthy diet and physical activity by any level are associated with reduced cardiovascular risk.

2.6.2   Synergy of Physical Activity and Diet in Cancer Prevention

Cancer occupies the second-most cause of death after cardiovascular diseases in developed countries. One-third of cancer deaths can be attributed to unhealthy or 'bad' diet and lack of physical activity, including overweight and obesity (30). Another one-third is caused by exposure to tobacco products. Although genetic susceptibility influences the risk of cancer, most of the variation in cancer risk across populations and among individuals is due to factors that are not inherited (30). Maintaining a healthy weight, staying physically active throughout life, and consuming a healthy diet can substantially reduce the lifetime risk of developing cancer, as well as influence overall health and survival after a cancer diagnosis (30). These same behaviors are also associated with a decreased risk of developing cardiovascular disease and diabetes (30). For example, to reduce the risk of prostate cancer, eat at least 2.5 cups of a wide variety of vegetables and fruits rich in carotenes and lycopene each day, stay physically active, and achieve a healthy weight (30). Moreover, the best nutrition- and physical activity-related advice to reduce the risk of colon cancer is to increase the intensity and duration of physical activity, limit intake of red and processed meat, consume recommended levels of calcium, ensure sufficient vitamin D status, eat more vegetables, fruits, and dairy products like yogurt and milk, avoid obesity and central weight gain, and avoid excess alcohol consumption (30). In addition, chronic constipation may cause colon cancer. The best way to avoid constipation is to combine exercise with foods rich in fibers like prune, date, and pure fruit juice. Although genetic susceptibility influences the risk of cancer, most of the variation in cancer risk across populations and among individuals is due to factors that are not inherited (30). Indeed, the synergy of physical activity with healthy foods helps fight cancer, obesity, overweight, cardiovascular diseases, and other diseases more efficiently.

2.6.3   Synergistic Effects of Physical Activity and Diet on Bone Mass Development

Bone mineral content and bone mineral density accrual is mainly determined by genotype. Approximately 70% of the variation in bone density is determined by heredity. The remaining 30% depends on the phenotype, in which physical activity and/or nutrition can induce physiological responses allowing levels of higher bone mass attainment (31). Food intake provides the necessary components for adequate metabolic functions in bone. Calcium, phosphorus, vitamin D, magnesium, proteins, and fluoride are some of the most important nutrients in bone formation and have different effects on bone mass (31). Adolescence is a period of life where major accumulation of bone mass occurs, notably during a short period of time, principally from hormonal development (31). During this period, the adequate contribution of nutrients involved in bone metabolism is critical. Milk is an ideal food for bone formation because it contains all nutrients cited previously. Moreover, these nutrients are easily absorbed through the digestive tract and transported directly by blood to bone. Many Asian people do not take bovine milk and other dairy products such as cheese and yogurt, from infancy to adulthood; therefore, their size is smaller than people who have consumed milk regularly since infancy.

Additionally, exercise has been shown to elicit osteogenic responses in bone development; indeed, it seems to potentiate, for example, the effect of calcium supplementation on bone mass (31). Gymnastics and sports are necessary for bone growth, especially for infants and adolescents. It is well known that participation in physical activity during puberty may result in greater bone mass accumulation, and also that physical activity protects against bone fractures later in life, especially, in old age (31).

Similarly, some nutritional strategies such as calcium supplementation may also benefit skeletal development, although there are controversies in this regard. The combined effect or interaction between physical exercise and calcium supplementation has been shown, and it seems to be more efficacious in bone development than just exercise or calcium alone. However, the interaction between exercise and food intake or specific diets in bone mass acquisition is not clear and further investigations are needed (31). Take note that the list of various types of synergies cited here is not exhaustive.

2.7 INTERACTIONS OF NUTRIENTS, PHYSICAL ACTIVITY WITH COVID-19 INFECTION

Coronavirus disease 2019 (Covid-19) is a severe acute respiratory infectious disease caused by a novel virus strain, SARS-CoV-2 (Severe Acute Respiratory Syndrome Coronavirus-2) (32–33). The very first case of the novel Covid-19 was originally reported in Wuhan, Hubei Province, China, in December 2019, and has quickly spread over almost every country in the world with a high mortality rate (34–35). On 30 January 2020, this dreadful respiratory infectious disease was declared by the World Health Organization to constitute a public health emergency and later, a pandemic disease (32, 35). The number of cases across the globe is increasing rapidly, and so far, no standard drug has proved to be effective for Covid-19 infection, which has a high death rate in immunocompromised patients (35). The use of personal protective equipment (masks, antibacterial gels, gloves), social distancing, quarantines, and even border closures to reduce the number of cases, have been introduced in several countries for the containment and prevention of this pandemic since its beginning (32).

The initial clinical symptoms of Covid-19 are similar to all types of viral pneumonia, with varying degrees of severity (32). Some infected subjects (children and young people) may remain asymptomatic. Among the subjects showing symptoms, 80% of patients had a mild illness, 14% of patients showed severe illness, and 5% of patients developed critical illness requiring intensive care or mechanical ventilation assistance. Elderly people and people with comorbidities such as weakened immune system, chronic pulmonary disease, diabetes, and heart disease have an increased risk of severe illness (32). The viral genome encodes a main protease (Mpro) of SARS CoV-2, which plays a crucial role in the production of viral proteins and is a key component of the viral replication. This protease is considered as a prime target for anti-Covid-19 drug development (35). The viral mutation has been linked to extreme difficulty in developing effective vaccines and drugs against coronaviruses. Anti-Covid-19 vaccines were not yet developed during the year 2020. This is why some researchers have tried to use certain natural nutrients to prevent or stop the spread of this pandemic in this period. Various studies have revealed that some micronutrients such as vitamins D, A, E, C, and minerals (zinc, copper, selenium, iron) have key roles in supporting the human immune system and reducing risk of infections (33–34). In addition, some phytochemicals such as ursolic acid and its derivatives (oleanolic acid, carvacrol), catechins, quercetin, gallic acid, gallocatechin gallate, curcumin, gingerol, and allicin were potential inhibitors against main protease of Covid-19 (35–37). Ursolic acid and its derivatives are found in various vegetables such as the leaves of rosemary, marjoram, lavender, thyme, oregano, sage, eucalyptus, loquat, hawthorn, fruits (apple fruit peel), and berries (see Chapter 5 of this book) (35). Curcumin, gingerol, and allicin are mainly present in turmeric (*Curcuma longa*), ginger (*Zingiber officinale*), and garlic (*Allium sativum*), respectively (36). Catechins, gallic acid, gallocatechin gallate, and quercetin are mainly found in green tea (37). On the other hand, the World Health Organization recommends avoiding or limiting alcohol consumption during this pandemic because alcohol diminishes the activity of the immune system and could promote the development of this infectious disease (38). In addition, a recent study observed that physical activity such as walking, jogging, cycling, yoga, stimulated the immune system and might reduce the Covid-19 infection (39–40). However, scientific studies on certain nutrients (ursolic acid, polyphenols, vitamin D, zinc, etc.) and physical activity cited earlier in the prevention of Covid-19 are still preliminary, inconsistent, and contradictory. A recent review discussed the possible roles of vitamin D in reducing the risk of Covid-19 and other acute respiratory tract infections and severity (41). However, other studies did not find the correlation when confounding variables are adjusted. Therefore, there is not enough evidence on the association between vitamin D levels and Covid-19 severity and mortality (41). According to the Superior Health Council of Belgium, vitamin D is not the anti-Covid-19 panacea (42). In the end of 2020 and the beginning of 2021, different types of vaccines protecting against Covid-19 have been developed and used for populations around the world.

Until today, no official health care organizations have recommended the consumption of certain foods mentioned previously (ursolic acid, polyphenols, vitamin D, zinc, etc.) or the practice of certain physical activities for the prevention or the treatment of Covid-19 infection, although they are immunostimulants. Therefore, the official prevention of Covid-19 infection recommended by different governments and international healthcare organizations is vaccination, the wearing of masks in public, the usage of antibacterial gels for hands, quarantine, social distancing, and the ventilation of indoor spaces. Indeed, vaccines represent the best strategy for primary prevention of Covid-19 infection (43). However, frequent consumption of some immunostimulant foods cited above and low intake of alcohol drinks as well as regular physical activity might help the anti-Covid vaccination be more efficacious.

2.8 INTERACTIONS OF PROBIOTICS AND PREBIOTICS WITH INTESTINAL MICROBIOTA OR GUT FLORA

2.8.1 Intestinal Microbiota or Gut Flora

The intestinal microbiota or gut flora has become an important aspect of human health. The intestinal tract of mammals is colonized by a large number of microorganisms that are referred as the gut microbiota (44). The human gut is a huge complex ecosystem where microbiota, nutrients, and host cells interact extensively – a process crucial for gut homeostasis and host development with a real symbiotic relationship (45). Human microbiota include bacteria, viruses, fungi, archaea, and protists. In addition to metabolic benefits, symbiotic bacteria provide the host with several functions that promote immune homeostasis, immune responses and protection against pathogen colonization. The ability of symbiotic bacteria to inhibit pathogen colonization is mediated via several mechanisms including direct killing, competition for limited nutrients, and enhancement of immune responses (44). The human gastrointestinal tract contains approximately 10^{14} (trillions) microbes with about 4,000 strains in the intestinal microbiota of a healthy individual (46–48). At birth, the human gut is sterile, but is then colonized immediately after birth (48–49). The microbial colonization of the infant gut is known to play a key role in immunological and metabolic pathways impacting short and/or long-term human health and disease (50–51). Gut microbial life is essential for assisting with the digestion of food substances to release nutrients, exerting control over pathogens, stimulating or modulating the immune system within the gut and beyond, and influencing many systems such as the liver, brain, and endocrine system (46, 51). Consequently, an imbalance of gut microbiota in early life, also called dysbiosis, may be the cause or at least may lead to the progression of various pathologies such as infectious diseases, gastrointestinal cancers, inflammatory bowel disease, asthma, atopic dermatitis, allergic diseases, obesity, diabetes, cardiovascular diseases, and neurological disorders (46, 49, 51–54). In addition, the gut microbiota facilitates the course of protein/amino acid digestion and absorption by decomposing complex subunits and changing the metabolic mechanisms of the host cell. This renders the nutrients easily absorbable by the host and has the capacity to facilitate the de novo synthesis of essential amino acids, which are implicated in amino acid homeostasis in the host (55). The gut or colon is the main host organ of microbiota in humans, but other organs like skin, mouth, nose, stomach, and vagina also contain microbiota, though in lesser amounts (49). Gut bacterial diversity is mainly affected by the diet, which may also affect its functional relationships with the host (53). During their gastrointestinal passage, the components of the diet are metabolized by intestinal bacteria. Microbial diversity of the intestine decreases in diets with higher fat content. Therefore, gut microbiota influences the biological activity of food compounds and is a target for nutritional intervention to improve health (53).

2.8.2 Probiotics

To treat or prevent some diseases due to dysbiosis (imbalance of gut microbiota), two kinds of products are used: probiotics and prebiotics. Probiotics are specific live microorganisms and prebiotics are non-digestible substrates (45). Symbiotics are defined as mixtures of probiotics and prebiotics that beneficially affect the host by impacting the microbiome within the gastrointestinal tract (47).

In 2002, the Food and Agriculture Organization (FAO) and the World Health Organization (WHO) defined a probiotic as 'live microorganisms which when administered in adequate amounts confer a health benefit on the host' (45, 47, 56–59). They are classified as non-pathogenic strains that survive gastric juices, resist bile, and colonize the gastrointestinal tract (57). Probiotics play important roles in the health of intestinal microbiota or gut flora. Probiotics include different bacteria such as *Lactobacillus rhamnosus, Lactobacillus reuteri, Lactobacillus casei, Lactobacillus paracasei, Bacillus coagulans, Bacillus clausii, Bifidobacterium infantis, Bifidobacterium longum, Bifidobacterium infantis, Streptococcus thermophilus, Escherichia coli* strain Nissle, and yeasts, including *Saccharomyces boulardii* and *Saccharomyces cerevisiae* (47). Probiotics are found in a number of fermentable foods, pills, powders, and liquid drops. Fermentable foods include dairy products and non-dairy products. Dairy products rich in probiotics are yogurt, kefir (fermented milk drink), some cheeses (mozzarella, cheddar, gouda), ice cream, and milk powder. Non-dairy foods include soy-based products (miso, natto), kimchi (Korean fermented legumes), sauerkraut (fermented cabbage), nutrition bars, and a variety of juices (59). There is a relationship between probiotics and autoimmune and inflammatory disorders. The strongest evidence in favor of probiotics lies in the prevention or treatment of five disorders: necrotizing enterocolitis, acute infectious diarrhea, acute respiratory tract infections, antibiotic-associated diarrhea, and infant colic.

Probiotic mechanisms of action include the inhibition of bacterial adhesion; enhanced mucosal barrier function; modulation of the innate and adaptive immune systems (including induction of tolerogenic dendritic cells and regulatory T cells); secretion of bioactive metabolites; and regulation of the enteric and central nervous systems (47). One of the most powerful effects of probiotics is to modulate the immune system. Probiotics strengthen both innate and adaptive immune responses through bacterial-epithelial-immune cell crosstalk. Specific probiotic and/or other gut bacteria modulated by probiotics are being found to produce multiple bioactive metabolites with anti-inflammatory properties. Probiotics are dangerous in patients with severe diseases or in those with immune deficiencies (47). In a recent publication, medical practitioners from the University of Utrecht, the Netherlands, announced that a probiotic supplement of six strains was responsible for the death of 24 patients (56). It is, however, important to note that the patients suffered from acute pancreatitis and that they were immune-compromised when treated. In another report, *L. casei* and *Lactobacillus rhamnosus* have been associated with bacteremia and endocarditis. In immunocompromised patients some lactobacilli have been associated with arthritis and meningitis (56). Therefore, consult a doctor before taking a probiotic supplement. However, foods containing probiotics cited earlier, such as yogurt, kefir, miso, kimchi, sauerkraut, are not harmful and are good for health.

2.8.3 Prebiotics

Prebiotics include oligosaccharides, resistant starch, and soluble or insoluble fibers. Prebiotics are defined as metabolic substrates that promote the growth and/or activity of beneficial microorganisms, usually in the gastrointestinal tract. Prebiotics are nondigestible by human gastrointestinal cells (47). Prebiotic substances are not hydrolyzed nor absorbed in the gastrointestinal tract but are available as substrates for probiotics, and the most commonly used ones at present are nondigestible fructo-oligosaccharides (59). Cellulose, a type of insoluble fiber, is mainly present in green vegetables, fruits, and whole grains. Although cellulose is not digested, it plays important roles in human digestion and nutrition. It stimulates the growth and/or activity of beneficial microorganisms (probiotics), usually in the gastrointestinal tract, prevents constipation, colon cancer development, hypercholesterolemia, CVDs, and Type 2 diabetes. Cellulose is used as a broom for the intestinal organs, especially for the colon, and can bind toxins and cholesterol. Its benefits include helping food move through the digestive tract more quickly, thus preventing constipation and diverticular disease (60–62).

Some plants contain significant amounts of soluble and insoluble fibers. For example, plums and prunes have a thick skin covering a juicy pulp. The skin is a source of insoluble fiber, whereas soluble fiber is in the pulp. Prunes are super fruits that may relieve constipation due to high contents of fibers and sorbitol, a laxative sugar. Grapes also contain a fair amount of soluble and insoluble fibers. Some soluble fiber products in grapes are inulin, a polysaccharide of fructose polymers, as well as other oligosaccharides like oligofructose and oligomannose. These fibers may relieve symptoms of irritable bowel syndrome, such as diarrhea, constipation, and abdominal discomfort (60–62).

Individuals with high intakes of dietary fiber appear to be at significantly lower risk for developing coronary heart diseases (stroke, hypercholesterolemia, hypertension), obesity, cancer, and certain gastrointestinal diseases. This effect is linked to its action against inflammation, oxidation, hyperlipidemia, and other physiological disorders (61). Increased intake of soluble fiber improves glycemia and insulin sensitivity in non-diabetic and diabetic individuals. Increased intake of insoluble fiber significantly enhances weight loss in obese people and can prevent a number of gastrointestinal disorders such as: constipation, gastroesophageal reflux disease, duodenal ulcer, diverticulitis, and hemorrhoids. Prebiotic fibers appear to enhance immune function (60). However, a diet high in soluble and insoluble fibers can produce significant intestinal gas (flatulence) like belching and bloating due to the fermentation of these carbohydrates in the digestive tract.

3 SIRTUINS

3.1 OVERVIEW

The first sirtuin gene, SIR2 from *Saccharomyces cerevisiae*, was originally known as MAR1 (for mating-type regulator 1). This gene controlled the ability of yeast cells to mate and was first discovered by Amar Klar et al. in yeast *Saccharomyces Cerevisiae* in the 1970s at Cold Spring Harbor Laboratory in New York (63–64). In the late 1990s a study from Leonard Guarante et al. at Massachusetts Institute of Technology (MIT), United States, demonstrated that deletion of Sir2 shortens yeast lifespan and that Sir2 overexpression extends yeast lifespan (63, 65). Sirtuin is the abbreviation of **S**ilent **I**nformation **R**egulator **T**wo (SIR2) gene first discovered in yeast previously cited (63, 66–68).

The sirtuins are a family of proteins (enzymes) that act predominantly as nicotinamide adenine dinucleotide (NAD)-dependent deacetylases, which require nicotinamide adenine dinucleotide (NAD$^+$) as an essential co-factor (63, 66–70). Acetylation and deacetylation are two important biochemical reactions to regulate the activity of proteins. All sirtuins require the coenzyme nicotinamide adenine dinucleotide (NAD$^+$) for their deacetylase or ADP-ribosyl transferase activity, linking their function tightly to cellular energy levels (66–70).

Sirtuins are present in all species from bacteria and plants to mammals (63, 66–70). In mammals, the sirtuins represent a small gene family with seven members, from sirtuin 1 to sirtuin 7. Sirtuins (Sirt1-Sirt7) constitute a class of proteins with NAD$^+$-dependent deacetylase whose activity depends on NAD$^+$ levels and thus on cellular metabolic status (66–70). Sirtuins are localized in different subcellular compartments. Sirt1 is localized in the nucleus and translocates to the cytosol under specific conditions. Sirt6 is also localized in the cytosol, rather than exclusively in nucleus. Sirt2 resides predominantly in the cytosol; Sirt3, Sirt4, and Sirt5 are mitochondrial; and Sirt7 is nuclear and nucleolar (68–70).

3.2 BIOLOGICAL ROLES OF SIRTUINS

Sirtuins are now considered to be a top-class subject in academic research as well as in various clinical applications. Their biological roles are vast and promising.

Sirtuins regulate ribosomal DNA recombination, gene silencing, DNA repair, chromosomal stability, and longevity (68–70). Sirtuins have gained considerable attention for their impact on mammalian physiology, since they may provide novel targets for treating diseases associated with aging, and perhaps for extending the human lifespan (68). Sirtuin activity is linked to gene repression, metabolic control, apoptosis and cell survival, DNA repair, inflammation, cardio-protection, neuroprotection, cancer prevention, lifespan extension, and healthy aging (70). Endogenous

Sirt1 plays a pivotal role in mediating the cell death/survival process and has been implicated in the pathogenesis of cardiovascular disease (69). Down-regulation of Sirt2 is protective against ischemic-reperfusion injury. Increased Sirt3 expression has been shown to correlate with longevity in humans. In addition, Sirt3 protects cardiomyocytes from aging and oxidative stress, and suppresses cardiac hypertrophy (69). Sirt6 has also recently been demonstrated to attenuate cardiac hypertrophy, and Sirt7 is known to regulate apoptosis and stress responses in the heart (69). Because sirtuin modulation could have beneficial effects on human diseases there is a growing interest in the discovery of small molecules modifying their activity (70). These molecules are divided into two groups called sirtuin activators and sirtuin inhibitors. Almost all the sirtuin activators of Sirt1 have been described by researchers. Resveratrol, a natural polyphenol antioxidant mainly found in red grapes, red wine, and peanuts, can activate Sirt1, and may help in the treatment or prevention of obesity, as well as in preventing tumorigenesis and aging-related decline in heart function and neuronal loss (70). However, resveratrol supplement has poor bioavailability; hence other molecules have been developed, like SRT501, SRT1720, and more, and are being studied (70). Sirtuin inhibitors such as sirtinol, AGK2 (2-cyano-3-[5-(2,5-dichlorophenyl)-2-furanyl]-N-5-quinolinyl-2-propenamide), splitomicin, cambinol, suramin, tenovin, and salermide have been identified for Sirt1, Sirt2, Sirt3, and Sirt5. Sirt1 inhibitors have been proposed in the treatment of cancer, mental retardation syndrome, immunodeficiency virus infections, and for preventing or treating parasitic diseases; whereas Sirt2 inhibitors might be useful for the treatment of cancer and neurodegenerative diseases (70).

Sirtuin activity is regulated by NAD biosynthetic pathways, and nicotinamide phospho-ribosyltransferase plays a critical role in the regulation of mammalian sirtuin activity (71). Sirt1 and Sirt5 act as deacetylases, whereas Sirt4 seems to be a mono-ADP-ribosyl transferase. Sirt2, Sirt3, and Sirt6 can display both activities (72). The activity of Sirt7 has not been clearly established, even though it has been hypothesized to act as a deacetylase (72). It is noteworthy that Sirt5 was recently described to demalonylate and desuccinylate proteins (72).

The first role of sirtuins discovered in yeast about three decades ago is the regulation of aging and the life span extension. In addition to regulating aging, sirtuin enzymes play key roles in the maintenance of organismal metabolic homeostasis and cell survival (73–74). In mammals, sirtuins are a very complicated biological response system that influences many other regulator molecules and pathways in complex manners. Responses of this system to environmental factors, as well as its role in health and disease, are currently incompletely characterized and at most partially understood (71, 75–76). These enzymes also have primarily protective functions in the development of many age-related diseases, including cardiovascular disease, neurodegeneration, and cancer. Sirtuins regulate many fundamental biological processes such as energy metabolism and mitochondrial function in response to a variety of environmental and nutritional activators or stimuli such as vitamin B3 (niacin, nicotinamide), which is a precursor of NAD, plant polyphenols (resveratrol, quercetin, piceatannol, tannins), curcumin in turmeric, and so on (75–80). These activators are found in foods, especially plant foods, and play a key role in the activity of sirtuins which declines with age and disease. In mammals, Sirt1, its activators and inhibitors, are the best studied among all sirtuins (72).

3.2.1 Roles of Sirtuins in Aging and Longevity

Sirtuins have been traditionally linked to aging and longevity. They orchestrate stress response and damage repair. Through these functions sirtuins modulate the course of aging and affect degenerative diseases (71, 73, 75–76, 81–86).

Sirtuins have been shown to regulate life span in lower organisms, including yeast, nematodes, and fruit flies (73). In mammals, it is believed that sirtuins play key roles during cell response to a variety of stresses, such as oxidative or genotoxic stress, and are crucial for cell metabolism (84). Most of these studies have described a key role for Sirt1 in regulating the metabolic response to calorie restriction, a dietary intervention that robustly extends life span across numerous species. Sirt1 does appear to promote healthy aging by protecting against several age-related pathologies (73). The strongest link between mammalian sirtuins and the antiaging effects of calorie restriction comes from Sirt3, which mediates the prevention of age-related hearing loss. Hearing loss is a gradual loss of spiral ganglion neurons and sensory hair cells in the cochlea of the inner ear, which is triggered by oxidative damage in these cells (73). Although some data put in question direct involvement of sirtuins in extending human lifespan, it was documented that proper lifestyle including physical activity and diet can influence health span via increasing the level of sirtuins (84). The search for activators of sirtuins is one of the most extensive topics of research. Some hopes are placed on natural activator compounds or nutraceuticals such as curcumin, resveratrol, vitamin B3, piceatannol, tannins, and so on (71, 73, 75–76, 81–86).

3.2.2   Roles of Sirtuins in Metabolism

All sirtuins require nicotinamide adenine dinucleotide (NAD^+) for their deacetylase or ADP-ribosyl transferase activity, linking their function tightly to cellular energy levels. Sirt1, the founding member of the sirtuin family, modulates many aspects of glucose and lipid homeostasis in almost all key metabolic tissues (72–74, 80). Sirt1 promotes gluconeogenesis, fatty acid oxidation, and cholesterol scavenging in the liver. The changes induced by Sirt1 activation are generally transcriptional in nature and are related to an increase in mitochondrial metabolism and antioxidant protection. These attractive features have validated Sirt1 as a therapeutic target in the management of metabolic disease, and prompted an intensive search to identify pharmacological Sirt1 activators (72). Other members including Sirt2, Sirt3, Sirt4, and Sirt6 are also implicated in various metabolic processes. Indeed, nearly every sirtuin has been shown to play a role in regulating metabolism and energy homeostasis, often in roles that help the cell adapt to periods of low energy input. The sirtuin system is strongly influenced by calorie restriction. In addition, sirtuins are involved in multiple metabolic pathways in lipid metabolism and adipose biology (72, 74–75, 80). A tight regulation of the equilibrium between energy intake, storage, and expenditure is required for metabolic homeostasis (74). The involvement of sirtuins in the control of energy intake in mammals remains largely unexplored. Therefore, the elucidation of the role of the various sirtuins in metabolic control is necessary for the prevention and treatment of metabolic syndrome or metabolic disorder (74, 80). Indeed, sirtuins play important roles in both calorie restriction and metabolic syndrome, although these represent opposite extremes of the same metabolic spectrum (80, 87). Metabolic syndrome is characterized by a combination of physiological parameters, including obesity, inflammation, high levels of circulating triacylglycerols (hyperlipidemia) and low-density lipoprotein (LDL) cholesterol, and low levels of high-density lipoprotein (HDL) cholesterol and high blood pressure. Metabolic syndrome or disorder is also associated with dysregulation of glucose homeostasis, which is indicative of insulin insensitivity (inability of insulin to promote normal glucose uptake by cells) (80, 87). This dysregulation can be associated with increased blood glucose levels and diabetes. Metabolic syndrome was first recognized as a risk factor for cardiovascular disease, and is associated with atherosclerosis. This syndrome also heightens risk for stroke, cancer, arthritis, CVDs and, of course, diabetes (80, 87). Lifestyle changes such as diet and physical and mental activities are the first defense in treating metabolic syndrome, followed by pharmacological intervention.

3.2.3   Roles of Sirtuins in Cardiovascular System

Sirtuins control critical cellular processes in the nucleus, cytoplasm, and mitochondria to maintain metabolic homeostasis and reduce cellular damage and inflammation for the protection of the body against a variety of age-related diseases, including cardiovascular pathologies (69, 88–89). In mammals, endogenous Sirt1 plays a pivotal role in mediating the cell death/survival process and has been implicated in the pathogenesis of cardiovascular disease (69, 88). Down-regulation of Sirt2 is protective against ischemic-reperfusion injury. Increased Sirt3 expression has been shown to correlate with longevity in humans. In addition, Sirt3 protects cardiomyocytes from aging and oxidative stress and suppresses cardiac hypertrophy (89). Sirt6 has also recently been demonstrated to attenuate cardiac hypertrophy, and Sirt7 is known to regulate apoptosis and stress responses in the heart. On the other hand, the roles of Sirt4 and Sirt5 in the heart remain largely uncharacterized (69). Among sirtuins, Sirt1 and Sirt6 are the best characterized for their protective roles against inflammation, vascular aging, atherosclerotic plaque development, and heart disease. Only Sirt6 plays a role in the protection against atherosclerotic plaque development (68).

Previous mechanistic studies have revealed that Sirt1, Sirt3, and Sirt6 demonstrate protective functions against vascular aging, while vascular function of other Sirtuins are under investigation. Thus, direct sirtuin modulation and NAD+ stimulation of Sirtuins are promising candidates for cardiovascular disease therapy in the future (83).

In brief, all sirtuins participate in the protection of the cardiovascular system; among them, Sirt1, Sirt3, and Sirt6 are its main protectors and regulators (68–69, 83, 88–89).

3.2.4 Roles of Sirtuins in Brain and Nervous System

The involvement of sirtuins in the brain during both development and adulthood has been demonstrated by different genetic and physiological analyses in animal models. The neuroprotective effect of sirtuins has been reported for both acute and chronic neurological diseases (73, 82, 90–91). Evidence from in vivo and in vitro studies have revealed that Sirt1 regulates the cellular fate of neural progenitors, axon elongation, dendritic branching, synaptic plasticity, and endocrine function (90). In addition, Sirt1 has also been implicated in protection of neurons from degeneration in models of neurological diseases, such as traumatic brain injury and Alzheimer's disease.

The protective effects of sirtuins, especially Sirt1, Sirt2, and Sirt6, against common neurological disorders, such as cerebral ischemia, axonal injury, Alzheimer's disease, Parkinson's disease, Huntington's disease, amyotrophic lateral sclerosis, and multiple sclerosis, have also been reported in a number of studies (73, 82, 87, 90–91).

Recently, studies focused on mitochondrial sirtuins and their roles in antioxidative defense. In oxidative stress and in brain aging, Sirt6 may influence DNA repair machinery and probably also telomere maintenance (82). Sirt1 and Sirt2 are also important for differentiation and migration of certain types of brain cells. In addition, Sirt2 promotes myelin formation in Schwann cells (73). Sirt1 may be a promising therapeutic target of Alzheimer's disease (90, 91).

3.2.5 Roles of Sirtuins in Renal System

Sirt1 is the main sirtuin responsible for renal protective effects. In the kidneys, Sirt1 may inhibit renal cell apoptosis, inflammation and fibrosis, and may regulate lipid metabolism, autophagy, blood pressure, and sodium balance (92–94). Therefore, its activation in the kidney may be a new therapeutic target to increase resistance to many causal factors in the development of renal diseases, including diabetic nephropathy, acute renal injury, chronic kidney disease, as well as lupus nephritis (92–94). Protective effects include the maintenance of glomerular barrier function, anti-fibrosis effects, anti-oxidative stress effects, and regulation of mitochondria function and energy metabolism (94).

Activators of the sirtuin family of proteins, including resveratrol, may be important in the development of new therapeutic strategies for treating metabolic kidney diseases, including diabetic nephropathy (92–94).

3.2.6 Roles of Sirtuins in Cancer and DNA Repair

In recent years, the roles of sirtuins in cancer biology have gained the attention of many scientists worldwide. Growing evidence demonstrates that sirtuins regulate many processes that go awry in cancer cells, such as cellular metabolism, the regulation of chromatin structure, and the maintenance of genomic stability (95). Sirtuins have involved in diverse cellular processes including DNA repair, tumor suppressor p53, energy metabolism, and tumorigenesis. Notably, genomic instability and metabolic reprogramming are two hallmarks of cancer (96). However, the ability of sirtuins to promote or suppress tumorigenesis seems to depend on the specific tumor type, cellular context, and signaling pathway affected (70, 73, 87, 95–98). Sirtuins play fundamental roles in carcinogenesis and maintenance of the malignant phenotype, mainly participating in cancer cell viability, apoptosis, metastasis, and tumorigenesis. Although sirtuin family members have a high degree of homology, they may play different roles in various kinds of cancer (98).

In tumorigenesis (cancer development), Sirt1 seems to play a contradictory role, acting as both a tumor promoter and tumor suppressor (70, 73, 87, 95–98). Sirt1 was the first sirtuin family member to be discovered and is still the most studied. Its biological role in cancer has been studied extensively, yet there are conflicting results regarding the association between the two, as Sirt1 is known to suppress or promote cancer depending on its cellular content or type (97). It is similar to survivin, a protein of the inhibitor of apoptosis family. As tumor suppressor, sirtuin1 inhibits oncogenes and oncoproteins. Sirt1 knockdown accelerated tumor xenograft formation by HCT116 cells, whereas Sirt1 overexpression inhibited tumor formation (70). High Sirt1 levels were also detected in normal colon mucosa and benign adenomas; and Sirt1 overexpression was observed in about 25% of stage I/II/III colorectal adenocarcinomas but rarely found in advanced stage IV tumors (70). On the other hand, up-regulated Sirt1 has been described in cancer cell lines as well as in tissue samples from patients with human lung cancer, prostate cancer, colon carcinoma, and chronic lymphocytic leukemia cells (70). These results raise the possibility that inhibition of Sirt1 might suppress cancer cell proliferation. However, reduced Sirt1 levels have been also reported in breast cancer and hepatic cell carcinoma compared with their normal controls, while slight increase or no change of Sirt1 levels were detected in other tumors (70).

The putative association between Sirt1 and lifespan in animal models was explained on the basis of the ability of Sirt1 to deacetylate p53 gene, thus decreasing its activity, for which it has been hypothesized that Sirt1 activity may also elevate cancer risk (70). The p53 gene plays a critical role in the body's natural defense mechanism against cancer, and the decrease of p53 gene activity can cause cancer.

Several studies support a role for Sirt2, Sirt3, and Sirt6 as tumor suppressors (73, 95). It is suggested that Sirt2 deletion may permit tumor development and that its repletion may act as a tumor suppressive therapy (70). In fact, Sirt2-deficient mice develop gender-specific tumorigenesis, with females primarily developing mammary tumors, and males developing more hepatocellular carcinoma (70).

The mitochondrial sirtuin Sirt3 regulates levels of reactive oxygen species (ROS). Loss of Sirt3 results in increased levels of ROS, which favor tumor growth (95).

Sirt6 plays a key role in DNA repair and maintenance of genomic stability in mammalian cells integrating stress signaling to prime the DNA repair machinery in response to oxidative stress (70). Sirt6 overexpression induces massive apoptosis in a variety of cancer cell lines but not in normal cells, making Sirt6 an attractive target for cancer therapy (70).

3.2.7   Roles of Sirtuins in Bone Biology

Studies have revealed that sirtuins play a critical role in normal skeletal development and homeostasis through their direct action on bone cells, and that their dysregulation might contribute to different bone diseases (99). Preclinical studies have demonstrated that mice treated with sirtuin agonists show protection against age-related, postmenopausal, and immobilization-induced osteoporosis. These findings suggest that sirtuins could be potential targets for the modulation of imbalance in bone remodeling and the treatment of osteoporosis and other bone disorders (99). Sirt1 actions in chondrocytes and bone cells are critical for normal skeletal development and homeostasis. Nonetheless, recent studies indicate that Sirt3, Sirt6, and Sirt7 also contribute to skeletal homeostasis (100). Despite these recent advances, much less is known about the roles of sirtuins in skeletal aging.

3.3   Sirtuin Activators and Inhibitors

As cited above, many natural or synthetic compounds of low molecular mass can activate or inhibit the activity of different sirtuins for therapeutic uses, and are called sirtuin modulators. The last ones include sirtuin activators and inhibitors (70). Many sirtuin modulators, used alone or in combination with other epigenetic modulators or known drugs, have been described as having beneficial effects against cancer and neurodegeneration (87). Epigenetics is the study of changes in organisms caused by modification of gene expression under the influence of the environment rather than alteration of the genetic code itself. For example, the fur of certain polar fox becomes white in winter. The activity of sirtuin enzymes in any given tissue is strongly influenced by changes in the environment, diet, and lifestyle. Some factors that have been reported to affect epigenetic expression include calorie restriction (fasting), exercise, oxidative stress, melatonin, and plant compounds like resveratrol, quercetin, proanthocyanins (75).

All sirtuin enzymes are dependent on the coenzyme NAD^+ (oxidized nicotinamide adenine dinucleotide) as a co-substrate for their activity. Sirtuin enzyme activity consumes NAD^+ and produces nicotinamide, the amide form of vitamin B3, as a byproduct. In sirtuin NAD^+ reaction, the metabolite nicotinamide acts as an inhibitor of further sirtuin activity by promoting a base-exchange reaction (75). Other metabolites issued from this reaction are also produced, but in small quantity, and their inhibitory effect is weaker than that of nicotinamide. The inhibition of nicotinamide and other metabolites affects sirtuin enzyme activity without affecting gene expression or the amount of sirtuin proteins. Therefore, supplementing different forms of vitamin B3 for the raise of NAD^+ levels, or using nicotinamide as a sirtuin inhibitor, is a strategy for the treatment of some diseases such as cancer or neurodegenerative diseases (75). It is noteworthy that NAD coenzyme can be produced in the body via direct synthesis or salvage pathway from nicotinamide ring compounds. NAD is also obtained from the diet. Nicotinamide is both a NAD^+ precursor and Sirt1 enzyme inhibitor. In the context of toxic stress, nicotinamide appears to be used preferentially to prevent depletion of NAD^+ (75). Thus, enhancing NAD^+ biosynthesis by using NAD^+ intermediates, such as nicotinamide mononucleotide (NMN), helps effectively ameliorate age-associated physiological decline. NMN has been shown to enhance NAD^+ biosynthesis, ameliorate various disease models, and slow down aging in mice (101). Without any obvious toxicity, NMN enhanced energy metabolism, promoted physical activity, improved insulin sensitivity and plasma lipid profile, ameliorated eye function, and prevented other ailments in mice (101).

3.3.1 Sirtuin Activators

Many researchers revealed that proper lifestyle, including diet and physical activity, can influence health span via increasing the levels of sirtuins (70, 75, 84).

3.3.1.1 Natural Sirtuin Activators

Some plant polyphenols obtained from food such as resveratrol, curcumin, piceatannol, kaempferol, quercetin, catechins, proanthocyanidins, fisetin, and butein can activate in vitro and in vivo sirtuins, especially Sirt1, thereby prolonging lifespan and protecting the body against degenerative diseases by the mechanisms of calorie restriction and antioxidative stress (70, 75–76, 84–87).

Resveratrol, a natural polyphenol antioxidant found mainly in red grapes, red wine, and peanuts, can activate Sirt1, and may help in the treatment or prevention of obesity, as well as in preventing tumorigenesis and aging-related decline in heart function and neuronal loss (70, 75–76). Resveratrol is responsible for the color of purple grapes, and is primarily found in their skins and seeds. Mediterranean people have longer longevity and lesser incidence of CVD than other people in the world because their diet includes resveratrol-rich red wine and red grapes as well as seafoods. However, resveratrol supplement has poor bioavailability; hence, other synthetic molecules are being developed and studied, like SRT501 and SRT1720 (70, 75–76).

Curcumin is a natural yellow polyphenol pigment extracted from turmeric tuber. Curcumin possesses multiple biological properties including antioxidant, anti-inflammatory, and anti-cancer activity, however its anti-aging effect is still being examined (84–85). Curcumin was able to extend the lifespan of organisms such as vinegar fly, nematodes, and mice, and alleviated symptoms of some diseases including age-related ones (84–85). It reduced the impact of some harmful factors such as radiation or chemicals. Curcumin possesses numerous target proteins and there are data showing that it is able to act via sirtuin activation. Several studies note that pretreatment with curcumin significantly enhances Sirt1 activation and attenuates oxidative stress (84–85). It was demonstrated that bisdemethoxycurcumin, another curcuminoid of turmeric tuber, could also antagonize oxidative stress-induced premature senescence in fibroblasts. Curcumin is a beneficial anti-pathological factor in the cardiovascular system. The neuroprotective role of curcumin is also mediated by Sirt1 induction, and observed in primary cortical neurons in vitro (84–85). On the other hand, the level of mitochondrial Sirt3 and Sirt5 increased after curcumin treatment. The effect of curcumin action strongly depends on its concentration. Curcumin belongs to hormetin, which is a compound inducing hormesis. The latter is a phenomenon dose response to an environmental agent characterized by a low dose stimulation or beneficial effect, and a high dose inhibitory or harmful effect. Sensitivity to curcumin depends on cell type and likely the phase of the cell cycle (84–85). In addition, curcumin together with physical exercise upregulates Sirt1 even more efficiently than dietary curcumin alone (84–85).

Other plant polyphenols inducing sirtuin activation include piceatannol, kaempferol, quercetin, fisetin, butein, catechins, and proanthocyanidins. They are found in tea leaves, grapes, galangal, persimmon, apple, orange, berries, cherries, nuts (walnut), beans (soybeans), olive oil, cocoa and its byproduct chocolate, ginkgo, mangosteen, pepper, chili, parsley, kale, and more. Some natural food sources rich in nicotinamide mononucleotide (NMN), a precursor of NAD+, are: edamame (immature soybeans), avocado, broccoli, cabbage, whole cucumber peel and seed, and tomato (81, 101). Vitamin B3 is also a furnisher of NAD+, an essential coenzyme of sirtuins (75).

3.3.1.2   Synthetic Sirtuin Activators

Some synthetic sirtuin activators such as SRT1720, SRT2104, SRT1460, SRT2183, STAC-5, STAC-9, and STAC-10 are considerably more potent, soluble, and bioavailable than resveratrol, and are being studied (70, 84). They have shown effectiveness in treating age-related diseases and complications associated with aging, including cancer, Type 2 diabetes, inflammation, cardiovascular disease, stroke, Alzheimer's and Parkinson's diseases, and hepatic steatosis (84).

Another compound considered anti-aging is melatonin. It is able to activate sirtuins, and its level in the human body has been observed to decline with age (84).

3.3.1.3   Physical Activity and Sirtuin Activation

Regular physical training may help improve quality of life. However, extensive physical activity induces inflammation, increases free radical production, and may impair the antioxidant defense system (84). Mildly intense exercise can act as hormetin by eliciting a mild stress, which in turn activates defense mechanisms and brings beneficial effects, including reduction of oxidative stress. Mild physical activity is a potent activator of sirtuins (84).

Sirt1 is suggested to be a master regulator of exercise-induced beneficial effects. It has been shown that long-term moderate exercise induced increase in Sirt1 level in adult rat muscle, liver, and heart (84). Similar effects were also described in humans. It has been demonstrated that in human skeletal muscle of both young and aged subjects, Sirt1 and AMPK (AMP-activated protein kinase) gene expression increase after exercise (84). Physical exercise affects the expression of sirtuin in skeletal muscle, regulating changes in mitochondrial biogenesis, oxidative metabolism, and the cellular antioxidant system. In this context, sirtuin 1 and sirtuin 3 have been the most studied (102). The reported findings suggest that an acute load of exercise activates sirtuin 1, which in turn activates biogenesis and mitochondrial oxidative capacity. Additionally, several sessions of exercise (training) activate sirtuin 1 and also sirtuin 3 that, together with the biogenesis and mitochondrial oxidative function, jointly activate ATP production and the mitochondrial antioxidant function (102).

3.3.2   Sirtuin Inhibitors

Sirtuin inhibitors can also be potentially useful as therapeutic agents because up-regulated Sirt1 has been described in cancer cell lines, raising the possibility that Sirt1 inhibition might suppress cancer cell proliferation. In addition to cancer therapy, sirtuin inhibitors have also been proposed in the treatment of Parkinson's disease, leishmaniosis, human immunodeficiency virus, metabolic syndrome, and cancer (70). Sirtuin inhibitors with a wide range of core structures have been identified for Sirt1, Sirt2, Sirt3, and Sirt5 through high-throughput and *in silico* screenings. The main sirtuin inhibitors include Splitomicin, Sirtinol, Cambinol, Salermid, Tenovin, Suramin, and HR73 (70).

Sirt1 inhibition has been proposed in the treatment of cancer, immunodeficiency virus infections, Fragile X mental retardation syndrome, and for preventing or treating parasitic diseases, whereas Sirt2 inhibitors might be useful for the treatment of cancer and neurodegenerative diseases (70).

Briefly, sirtuins are new enzymes recently discovered. Their physiological roles are vast and promising. More researches are required to determine their mechanisms and their applications in therapy. Some preliminary research revealed that their activities have been linked to metabolic abnormalities, inflammation, cancer, cardiac hypertrophy, and neurodegeneration. The uses of some natural and artificial compounds for their activation or inhibition are a hot topic for the treatment and prevention of numerous dreadful ailments.

Some natural foods such as red grapes, red wine, peanuts, tea, curcuma, galangal, and chocolate might be helpful for the stimulation of some sirtuins in humans. Maybe in the future, humans may live longer and healthier thanks to advanced research on sirtuins.

4   GENES, CHROMOSOMES, AND P53

Gene, chromosome, and p53 protein are the most important biomolecules of all living things, from bacteria and plants to animals and humans. These compounds are derived from nucleotides.

Gene was discovered in the nineteenth century by Gregor Mendel (1822–1884, Czech Republic) (103–104). He was the first scientist who laid the foundations of modern genetics with his landmark studies of heredity in the garden pea (*Pisum sativum*) (103–104). Though he did not speak of 'genes' – a term that first appeared decades later – but rather of 'elements', and even 'cell elements', it is clear why Mendel is now credited as the 'father of genetics' (103–104). Mendel formulated the laws of heredity based on his careful breeding experiments on garden pea plants (103). Later, in 1905, the term 'gene' was introduced by Wilhelm Johannsen, a Danish botanist and plant physiologist (103–104).

4.1   GENE, CHROMOSOME

A gene, the basic physical and functional unit of heredity, is made up of deoxyribonucleic acid (DNA). (103–107). A gene is a sequence of nucleotides in a particular nucleic acid (104). The nucleotide is the structural unit of a nucleic acid. It is comprised of phosphoric acid, sugar (5-carbon), and a nitrogenous base. The chains of nucleotides in a nucleic acid are linked by 3', 5' phosphodiester linkages (104). Genes control identifiable traits of an organism. Genes are segments of DNA that contain the code for a specific protein that functions in one or more types of cells in the body (106). The information stored in DNA is arranged in hereditary units, now known as genes, that control identifiable traits of an organism. In the process of transcription, the information stored in DNA is copied into ribonucleic acid (RNA), which has three distinct roles in protein synthesis (107). Some genes contain all the information necessary to synthesize a protein (enzyme). However, many genes do not code for proteins (105). In humans, genes vary in size from a few hundred DNA bases to more than 2 million DNA bases (105). Humans have about 20,000 to 25,000 genes (105–106).

Genes are contained in chromosomes in the cell nucleus and mitochondria. A chromosome is made of a very long strand of DNA and contains hundreds to thousands of genes (106). The genes on each chromosome are arranged in a particular sequence, and each gene has a particular location on the chromosome (called its locus). In addition to DNA, chromosomes contain other chemical components that influence gene function (106).

Every person has two copies of each gene, one inherited from each parent (104). In humans, somatic (non-germ) cell nuclei normally have 46 chromosomes in 23 pairs (106). Each pair consists of one chromosome from the mother and one from the father. Twenty-two of the pairs, chromosome numbers 1 to 22, the autosomes, are normally homologous (identical in size, shape, and position and number of genes). The 23rd pair, the sex chromosomes (X and Y), determines a person's sex as well as containing other functional genes. The pair of sex chromosomes determines whether a fetus becomes male or female. Males have one X and one Y chromosome. A male's X comes from his mother and the Y comes from his father. Females have two X chromosomes, one from the mother and one from the father. In certain ways, sex chromosomes function differently than non sex chromosomes. Women have two X chromosomes (which are homologous) in somatic cell nuclei; men have one X and one Y chromosome (which are heterologous) (106). The smaller Y chromosome carries the genes that determine male sex as well as a few other genes. The X chromosome contains many more genes than the Y chromosome, many of which have functions besides determining sex and have no counterpart on the Y chromosome. The X chromosome carries genes responsible for many hereditary traits (106). Because the X chromosome has many more genes than the Y chromosome, many X chromosome genes in males are not paired; in order to maintain a balance of genetic material between men and women, one of the X chromosomes in women is randomly inactivated (lyonization). A karyotype illustrates the full set of chromosomes in a person's cells (106).

4.2 DNA AND RNA

DNA (deoxyribonucleic acid) and RNA (ribonucleic acid) are chemically very similar. Both molecules belong to the nucleic acid family. The primary structures of both are linear polymers composed of monomers called nucleotides. Each nucleotide contains: a 5-carbon sugar (ribose or deoxyribose), a nitrogenous base, and at least one phosphate group (107–113). The four types of nitrogen bases are adenine (A), thymine (T), guanine (G), and cytosine (C) (108).

Cellular RNAs range in length from less than 100 to many thousands of nucleotides. Cellular DNA molecules can be as long as several hundred million nucleotides (107). The DNA molecule is a long, coiled, double helix that resembles a spiral staircase. In DNA, two strands, composed of sugar (deoxyribose) and phosphate molecules, are connected by pairs of four molecules called bases, which form the steps of the staircase (106). In the steps, adenine is paired with thymine and guanine is paired with cytosine. In DNA, hydrogen bonds between the base portions of the nucleotides hold the two chains together like rungs of a ladder. A gene consists of a sequence of bases. Sequences of three bases code for an amino acid (amino acids are the building blocks of proteins) (106).

In genomes, DNA molecules are generally very long, thin polymers with a diameter of 2 nm and a length that can extend to 10^8–10^9 nm (110). As an information store, not only must DNA be able to encode the genetic information required to specify proteins, but also it should be packaged in a compact form that allows the accessibility of that information to be regulated. In turn, the functional accessing of information may also involve structural changes in the double helix itself. These requirements for compaction, accessibility, and structural modulation imply that DNA be both flexible and able to change conformation in response to enzymatic manipulation (110).

The key difference between RNA and DNA structures is that the ribose sugar in RNA has a hydroxyl (-OH) group which is absent in DNA, and the thymine base of DNA is replaced by the uracil base in RNA (107, 111–113). The nucleotides that comprise DNA include adenine (A), guanine (G), cytosine (C), and thymine (T); whereas RNA nucleotides include A, G, C, and uracil (U). Moreover, RNA has only one long strand or chain in almost species, except in some viruses, while DNA has a double strand and looks like a twisted ladder in all species from bacteria and plants to invertebrates and humans (107, 111–113). DNA is defined as a nucleic acid that contains the genetic instructions used in the development and functioning of all known living organisms. The main role of RNA is to transfer the genetic code needed for the creation of proteins from the nucleus to the ribosome (111). This process prevents the DNA from having to leave the nucleus. This keeps the DNA and genetic code protected from damage. Without RNA, proteins could never be made. RNA molecules are not only involved in protein synthesis, but also sometimes in the transmission of genetic information (111).

In all species, there are three main types of RNA: messenger RNA (mRNA), ribosomal RNA (rRNA), and transfer RNA (tRNA) (112, 113).

Messenger RNA or mRNA accounts for just 5% of the total RNA in the cell, and is the most heterogeneous of the three types of RNA in terms of both base sequence and size (112). It carries the genetic code copied from the DNA during transcription in the form of triplets of nucleotides called codons. Each codon specifies a particular amino acid, but one amino acid can be coded by many different codons. Although there are 64 possible codons or triplet bases in the genetic code, only 20 of them represent amino acids (112).

Ribosomal RNA or rRNA is found in the ribosomes and accounts for 80% of the total RNA present in the cell (112). Different rRNAs present in the ribosomes include small rRNAs and large rRNAs, which denote their presence in the small and large subunits of the ribosome. Ribosomal RNAs (rRNAs) combine with proteins in the cytoplasm to form ribosomes or ribonucleoproteins, which act as the site of protein synthesis and have the enzymes needed for the process. These complex structures travel along the mRNA molecule during translation and facilitate the assembly of amino acids to form a polypeptide chain. They bind to transfer RNAs (tRNAs) and other molecules that are crucial for protein synthesis. In humans, small rRNAs and large rRNAs have about 1,800 and 5,000 nucleotides, respectively (112).

Transfer RNA (tRNA) is the smallest of the 3 types of RNA, with about 75–95 nucleotides, and is an essential component of translation. Its main function is the transfer of amino acids during protein synthesis (112). Additionally, some RNAs are enzymes. It was widely believed for many years that only proteins could be enzymes. RNAs are now known to adopt complex tertiary structures and act as biological catalysts. Such RNA enzymes are known as ribozymes, and they exhibit many of the features of a classical enzyme, such as an active site, a binding site for a substrate, and a binding site for a cofactor, such as a metal ion (112–113). In brief, DNA and RNA are two 'brothers': they have some common traits, but also different characters. They need to help each other for the proper functioning of their mission.

4.3   GENE MUTATION

Mutations are alterations in DNA sequences that occur during replication and result in changes in the structure of a gene (114). To prevent mistakes during replication, cells have a 'proofreading' function to help ensure that bases are paired properly. There are also chemical mechanisms to repair DNA that was not copied properly. However, because of the billions of base pairs involved, and the complexity of the protein synthesis process, mistakes may happen. Such mistakes may occur for numerous reasons (including exposure to radiation, drugs, or viruses) or for no apparent reason. Minor variations in DNA are very common and occur in most people (106).

The second form of gene mutation is inherited mutation. Inherited mutations are those that may be passed on to offspring (descendants). Mutations can be inherited only when they affect the reproductive cells (sperm or egg) (106). A number of hereditary diseases are due to single gene inheritance such as Huntington's disease, Marfan syndrome, sickle cell anemia, hemochromatosis, and so on (106). However, only about 5–10% of all cancer forms are due to inherited mutation (115–118).

The third form of gene mutation that is not due to inheritance is called acquired mutation. Acquired (or somatic) mutations occur at some time during a person's life, and are present only in certain cells – not in every cell in the body (119). Acquired mutations do not affect reproductive cells; therefore, they are not hereditary and cannot affect the descendants. They occur in somatic cells only. These changes can be caused by environmental factors such as ultraviolet radiation from the sun, pollutants, 'bad foods' and substances (cigarettes, alcohol, smoked meat, saturated and trans-fats, etc.), medicines, pesticides, and other diseases like infections by bacteria, viruses, obesity, stress, excessive movements, and so on.

In contrast, a small fraction of mutations, called natural selection, is beneficial for the evolution of species such as humankind. This kind of natural selection is very slow and caused by mutations in an interbreeding population. This slow mutation improves the health of an organism and is the mechanism of the evolution of species (106, 120). For example, the physical and intellectual forms of humankind have evolved since antiquity through the present.

In brief, based on their effects on fitness, mutations can be divided into three broad categories: the 'good' or advantageous that increase fitness, the 'bad' or deleterious that decrease it, and the 'indifferent' or neutral that are not affected by selection because their effects are too small (120).

4.4   P53 PROTEIN AND TP53 GENE

p53 is a protein with an apparent molecular mass of 53 kilodalton (kDa), hence, its name (p=protein, 53=its molecular mass) (121–131). However, based on calculations from its amino acid residues, p53 molecular mass is actually only 43.7 kDa (122). p53, also known as tumor protein 53 or tumor suppressor 53, is a protein encoded by TP53 gene (TP=tumor protein) which is located on the 17th chromosome in the nucleus of all cells (121–126). Historically, p53 was identified in 1979 by six groups of investigators, each working independently. They reported the discovery of a 53 kDa protein that was present in human and mouse cells (131). Although it was initially presumed to be an oncogene (gene engendering cancer), its character as a tumor suppressor gene was revealed in 1989 (120–121, 124).

Since its discovery in 1979, p53 has been shown to perform numerous cellular activities including regulation of the cell cycle, promotion of DNA repair, and apoptosis (programmed cell death); hence, it functions as a crucial tumor suppressor (121–131). More than 50% of human cancers are caused by a missing or damaged TP53 gene or by a loss of function mutations in TP53 gene (121–131). TP53 mutations are associated with adverse prognosis in many sporadic cancers; moreover, germline TP53 mutations are causative of the Li Fraumeni syndrome, a rare familial cancer predisposition (129).

Concerning the activity mechanism, p53 is a nuclear transcription factor with a pro-apoptotic function. Apoptosis is a natural process of programmed cell death that occurs in the body. Indeed, mutant p53 has an oncogenic potential, as more than half of the human cancers have mutated p53 (125, 128). Selective inhibition of cancer cells requires specific disruption of growth mechanisms used by these cells with limited damage to normal cells. In normal cells, the p53 protein level is low. However, when DNA is damaged by different mutagens, carcinogens, or other stress signals, this may trigger the increase of p53 protein levels, which are used to protect or repair DNA (125–129). In humans, p53 can also be damaged by different mutagens such as chemicals (pollutants, pesticides, preservatives, cigarettes, car smokes, cooking, drugs, deodorants, etc.), radiation (UV light, X rays, thermonuclear reactor, etc.), or viruses.

The TP53 gene plays an important role in the natural defense mechanism of the organism against cancer by inhibiting cell mutation and tumor propagation. Mutational inactivation is considered to be one of the most common molecular mechanisms behind the dysfunction of p53 (128). Activated TP53 gene prevents the propagation of cells with serious DNA damage – anarchic cells – thereby arresting cancer propagation. When DNA repair is complete, cells re-enter the normal cell cycle. In contrast, when cells have serious DNA damage, p53 exerts its pro-apoptotic function to eliminate cells with serious DNA damage and thereby inhibit the transfer of damaged DNA to daughter cells (128). Thus, p53 has an ability to maintain genomic integrity by suppressing anarchic cells, playing a key role in cancer prevention. However, the mechanisms by which p53 accomplishes its tumor suppressor activity are still not completely understood (130). The best described mechanism is the ability of p53 to modulate gene expression, which is necessary for its tumor suppressor activity (130). Improper function of p53 is a common cause of cancer development, cancer metastasis (propagation of cancer to other organs in the body), resistance to cancer treatment, and so on.

In 1997, two other proteins, p63 and p73, were identified beside p53 protein (124, 130). The p53 family consists of three proteins – p53, p63, and p73 – that are homologous at the amino acid level in the three primary domains of p53: transactivation domain, DNA-binding domain, and C-terminal oligomerization domain (124). p53, p63, and p73 have their own unique functions (130).

Although there have been several tens of thousands of publications on p53, scientists do not yet know how to use the immense amount of knowledge about p53 for therapeutic purposes (131). Most of the molecules found for cancer therapy, such as curcumin obtained from turmeric rhizome, for example, are still in the experimental phase and are not yet officially recognized in human therapy (125). The best way to prevent cancer is to avoid environmental factors such as chemicals, radiations, and some viruses, which could damage p53 gene activity. There are still many molecules in our body that are not yet discovered or exploited; our duty is to advance our research for their therapeutic role in many incurable diseases.

5 HOMEOSTASIS

5.1 DEFINITION

Homeostasis is derived from two Greek words: 'homeo' means 'similar' and 'stasis' signifies 'stable' (132). By definition, homeostasis is a phenomenon of equilibrum, balance, or stability of different components in a cell or organ with its environment (132–138). In other words, homeostasis is the constancy of an organism's internal environment. Homeostasis is provided by regulatory mechanisms at all levels of the organism, starting from the molecular level and up to higher systemic connections (133). Examples of homeostasis include the regulation of body temperature, and the balance between acidity and alkalinity. It is a process that maintains the stability of the organism's internal environment in response to fluctuations in external environmental conditions (134). In other words, homeostasis is a self-regulating process by which biological systems maintain stability while adjusting to changing external conditions (135). This concept explains how an organism can maintain nearly constant internal conditions that allow it to adapt and to survive in the face of a changing and often hostile external environment (135).

The concept of homeostasis was offered by the famous French scientist Claude Bernard (1813–1878) in the form of a statement that the constancy of the internal body environment is a necessary prerequisite of its independent life. The American physiologist Walter Cannon (1871–1945) at Harvard Medical School developed this idea and created a doctrine of homeostasis (133–137).

5.2 MECHANISMS

Homeostasis is regulated by a few main mechanisms: osmoregulation or balance of water and salts (electrolytes), acid-base regulation, thermoregulation, and metabolic control, such as control of sugar, fats, proteins, and hormones in the blood (132, 136). These mechanisms are performed in the body by various systems like the respiratory system, endocrine system, reproductive system, urinary system, and nervous system (132). Most physiological processes can only operate under a narrow range of conditions, which are maintained by specialized homeostatic mechanisms in the face of variations in the environment, and adjusted in response to changes in functional demands and biological priorities. However, only some of these processes are vulnerable to dysregulation and disease. For example, lipid and glucose metabolism can be derailed, leading to dyslipidemia, diabetes, and obesity, while amino acid metabolism seems resistant to homeostatic dysregulation (137). The disruption of homeostatic mechanisms can lead to disease, and effective therapy should be considered for the restoration of these homeostatic conditions (135). In other words, when these homeostatic mechanisms are in equilibrium, health is maintained; in contrast, when they are not, disease will develop. Some common diseases due to homeostatic imbalance include: diabetes, obesity, and inflammatory diseases (135–138).

The inflammatory response aims to restore homeostasis, but to achieve this goal it has to suppresses incompatible, lower-priority homeostatic processes. Therefore, inflammatory signals are antagonistic to incompatible homeostatic signals (137). Inflammatory signals are dominant over homeostatic signals because they have higher priority (137). Physiological priorities determine the hierarchy of signals. The parallels between homeostatic and inflammatory signals suggest the evolutionary origin of inflammation as a control system that complements the homeostatic control when the latter is insufficient. Chronic inflammation is an important component of numerous disease states including obesity, Type 2 diabetes, atherosclerosis, asthma, and neurodegenerative diseases (137). Water homeostasis is largely dependent on fluid intake and output and is controlled by the action of baroreceptors and osmoreceptors signaling via different pathways (138). Water homeostasis is vital for maintaining optimal health in the elderly. Due to age-related changes in thirst perception and many disabilities restricting fluid intake, dehydration is often seen in the elderly; therefore, regular fluid intake is needed for this population. However, excessive water intake is also harmful to the body and can even cause death (138).

All organisms are inseparably linked with their environment. There is no life without the environment. The environment predetermines behavior of the organism; human environments include biological, social, and spiritual spheres (133).

By extension, the balance between free radicals and antioxidants is considered a form of homeostasis. Indeed, too many free radicals or antioxidants can cause diseases, although antioxidants are considered good for health. Life requires a delicately balanced intermediate level of free radicals and antioxidants in order to maintain redox homeostasis in every cell (139) (see Chapter 3 of this book).

It is the same for the balance of omega-3 and omega-6 fatty acid levels in health maintenance. These two acids are both metabolically distinct and have opposing physiologic functions (140). An excess of omega-6 fatty acid can lead to many diseases such as inflammation (asthma, arthritis, muscular pain), and cardiovascular disease (CVD), while an excess of omega-3 fatty acid can cause hemorrhage. A proper balance helps maintain and even improve health (see Chapter 1 of this book).

In addition, the homeostasis between opposite compounds in the body is similar to the theory of yin-yang balance in traditional Chinese medicine (TCM), established for more than 2,000 years (141–142). However, in Eastern society, the yin-yang is regarded as an ideology or philosophy without definite physical meaning (141). The TCM classification of compounds as yin (feminine or negative) or yang (masculine or positive) is arbitrarily attributed and not scientifically demonstrated. In the Western world, yin-yang balance is often considered a religious belief or a principle of lifestyle (141).

In physiology, compensatory homeostasis is a self-protective process to maintain the organism's physiological function in the circle of life, and provides a window for the transition from disease to health (142). Many phenomena, including cardiac hypertrophy in heart failure, vasospasm or microvascular spasm, and ischemic hypoxia in shock, are some excellent examples of the compensation machinery in human body (142). According to Fan et al., the excessiveness and deficiency of yin-yang illustrates nicely the phenomenon of compensatory homeostasis (142).

In brief, homeostasis is defined as a self-regulating process by which a living organism can maintain internal stability while adjusting to changing external conditions (135). Homeostasis is vital for health maintenance and disease prevention.

6 DISCUSSION AND CONCLUSION

Nature has endowed the human body with several resources and mechanisms to counteract harmful effects which are either produced naturally in the body or caused by external microbes, xenobiotics, toxins, pollutants, and so on. The main natural resources used to fight the deleterious phenomena that disrupt the defense mechanisms of the body and lead to the onset of disease are foods and various natural products present in plant, animal, fungal, and mineral kingdoms. They play different roles in disease prevention. In nature, there are tens of thousands of different compounds that are still yet unexplored. In addition, plants offer an immense treasure of drugs, most of which are not yet exploited for therapeutic uses. Continuing to explore and exploit this precious treasure of natural drugs are important tasks of scientists worldwide.

More and more evidence suggest that the health benefits of fruits, vegetables, and other plant foods are attributed to synergy or interactions of bioactive compounds and other nutrients of different plant and animal foods (143). For example, turmeric is weakly absorbed when it is eaten alone, but, when it is consumed with pepper, or galangal, its bioavailability may increase considerably (144). So, according to different healthcare organizations, consumers should obtain their maximal nutrients from a balanced diet including a wide variety of plant foods (colored fruits, vegetables, nuts) with a good choice of animal foods, seafood, milk, dairy products, and some mushrooms for optimal nutrition and well-being.

The choice of healthy food and unhealthy food plays an important role in the prevention or development of many diseases. To make good choices, consumers need some knowledge concerning each food type, as well as willpower to realize these choices and patience to see the results obtained. For choosing fruits and vegetables, keep in mind that more the pronounced the color, the better the antioxidant activity. Among the same species, colored fruits and vegetables contain larger amounts of antioxidant than their less colorful counterparts. For example, black or red grapes contain more flavonoid antioxidants than white grapes; colored potatoes provide more carotenoids and flavonoids than white species. It is the same for flavored vegetables and fruits. Flavored spices like garlic, pepper, chili, turmeric, galangal, and ginger are strong antioxidants, and can protect the body against some infections and diseases.

Some inflammatory diseases such as allergic asthma, muscular pain, arthritis, and rheumatism, can be cured or ameliorated, if the patients have some scientific knowledge of these pathology. For example, asthma attacks can be prevented or diminished if the asthmatic knows that this allergic illness is caused by certain allergens like molds, pollen, and dust mites. To avoid molds and their flying spores in home, the first thing to do is to keep the home always dry by discarding water and all wet things like wallpapers, carpets, wood ceiling, ornamental plants, or flowers, because molds and spores only develop in wet space. Living in an old house or basement can cause the development of asthma more frequently than in new, dry habitations. Wet spaces and carpet are sources not only of molds, but also of dust mites, a microscopic insect. Therefore, some asthmatic people have observed that since moving out of their damp home, their asthma attacks decreased considerably or disappeared totally. Moreover, some inflammatory diseases cited previously are due to the imbalance of omega-3 and omega-6 fatty acid levels in the body (145–146). A supply of seafoods or fish oil might prevent these inflammatory diseases. Recent studies have reported that the three main bioactive metabolites (resolvin, protectin, and marsein) of omega-3 fatty acids (EPA, DHA) played beneficial effects in the treatment of allergic asthma and chronic lung inflammation (145). Therefore, the use of fish oils might treat chronic allergic asthma (145–146). However, an excess of fish oil or omega-3 intake can cause hemorrhage. Consult a specialist before taking fish oil or omega-3 supplement for the treatment of any inflammatory disease.

Homeostasis is an important mechanism of our body to maintain health. When the equilibrium of different biological compounds in our body is broken, disease will appear. Too much or too little water is harmful to the body. It is the same for free radicals or antioxidants. Although excess of free radicals is considered to be harmful to health, their lack in the body can also cause serious disease because the immune system needs them to fight microbes and anarchic cells (139). It is the same with antioxidants, despite their benefits for health. Therefore, abusive intake of antioxidants and vitamin supplements can cause disease. Both lack and excess of food, physical, and mental activity are harmful to health.

Physical activity is another important factor in health maintenance and disease prevention. Depending on age, moving the body regularly in different ways – from simple movement like walking, aerobics, dance, Tai Chi, and yoga, to intensive sports and athletics – is a necessary practice for everybody. Indeed, major systems, including the skeletal, muscular, metabolic, circulatory, digestive and endocrine systems, need body movement to develop and function properly. Therefore, physical activity can fight obesity, overweight, and insomnia, and may prevent many chronic diseases.

Physical activity is also necessary for mental activity, and can fight stress. Collective sports like tennis and football are better for mental health than individual sports like solo jogging. Take note that excess of physical activity is harmful to the body and can cause death.

Sleeping is a physiological activity necessary to the good functioning of all organs especially the brain. Sleep duration varies with age; on average, eight hours a day for adults and more for children. Insomnia may be resolved by regular exercises, yoga or Tai Chi. Coffee, tea, chocolate, and tonic drinks can cause sleep loss. That is why it is recommended to avoid consuming these caffeine-rich foods after dinner.

It should be emphasized that only 10% of cancer development is hereditary (115–118). About 30% of acquired cancer are due to 'bad foods' and unhealthy lifestyles like cigarette smoking, physical inactivity, and stress. The rest comes from other diseases like obesity, aging, infection by viruses (hepatitis, AIDS) or bacteria; industrial pollutants; dioxins; pesticides, herbicides used in agriculture; some chemicals for domestic uses like mothballs, chemical deodorants, incense smokes, insecticides; some drugs (immunosuppressant and antineoplastic agents); radioactivity; nuclear energy; UV-B of sunlight; car fumes; and so on.

Recently, the discovery of different sirtuins, a family of nicotinamide adenine dinucleotide (NAD^+)-dependent enzymes, has opened the door for important projects concerning the treatment of many dreadful ailments such as cancer, cardiovascular diseases, neurodegenerative diseases, and diabetes. Moreover, sirtuins and their natural and artificial activators and inhibitors might help extend lifespan and rejuvenate the body. More researches are needed for the applications of sirtuins in human therapy in the future.

It is noteworthy that most nutrients such as proteins, enzymes, amino acids, carbohydrates, nucleosides, antioxidants, and vitamins in animal and plant organisms are chiral compounds, and exist under single stereoisomer form only. For example, all natural amino acids are l-isomer (levo-rotatory) and all natural sugars (carbohydrates) are d-isomer (dextrorotatory). The same chiral artificial products obtained by chemical synthesis are often under racemic form – a mixture of two stereoisomers, such as d-isomer and l-isomer, S- and R-enantiomers, or cis- and trans-isomers. Our body is a great factory of chiral selectors, and could well distinguish the stereoform of a biological compound. Although they have the same chemical structure, most enantiomers of racemic products exhibit marked differences in biological activities such as pharmacology, toxicology, pharmacokinetics, and metabolism. That means our organism is smart enough to differentiate between 'good' and 'bad' isomers present, although both isomers have the same apparent chemical structure (147). That is why some chiral dietary supplements obtained by chemical synthesis do not have the same biological or therapeutic properties as their corresponding natural compounds present in foods.

Continuing to explore the immense treasure that Nature has created on this earth is necessary not only for developing new foods and medicines for human health, but also for solving hunger and famine in many parts of the world today. Natural beneficial compounds exist not only in plants and animals, but also in minerals, soil, sea, water, mushrooms, yeasts, molds, insects, and more. For their discovery, a coordination of research involving different scientists is needed. This book proposes various research topics related to food, lifestyle, health, and disease. In summary, it should be emphasized that avoiding cigarettes, alcohol, bad food, and stress, is considered as important as consuming a healthy diet rich in nutrients, antioxidants, and vitamins.

There is a proverb: 'Turn your tongue seven times before you speak', one might ask: 'Think seven times before you eat and drink'! Indeed, our health mainly depends on our choice of food, drink, and lifestyle.

7   REFERENCES

1. Canadian Centre for Occupational Health and Safety (CCOHS). (2019). Synergism. What Is Meant by the Term "Synergism"? Document, January 23. www.ccohs.ca/oshanswers/chemicals/synergism.html.

2. Liu R.H. (2003). Health Benefits of Fruit and Vegetables Are from Additive and Synergistic Combinations of Phytochemicals. *Am. J. Clin. Nutr.*, **78**(3): 517S–520S.

3. Liu R.H. (2004). Potential Synergy of Phytochemicals in Cancer Prevention: Mechanism of Action. *J. Nutr.*, **134**: 3479S–3485S.

4. de Kok T.M., van Breda S.G., Manson M.M. (2008). Mechanisms of Combined Action of Different Chemopreventive Dietary Compounds: A Review. *Eur. J. Nutr.*, **47** (Suppl. 2): 51–59.

5. Atashrazm F., Lowenthal R.M., Woods G.M., Holloway A.F., Dickinson J.L. (2015). Fucoidan and Cancer: A Multifunctional Molecule with Anti-Tumor Potential. *Mar. Drugs*, **13**: 2327–2346.

6. Zhang Y-J., Gan R-Y., Li S., Zhou Y., Li A-N., Xu D-P., Li H-B. (2015). Antioxidant Phytochemicals for the Prevention and Treatment of Chronic Diseases. *Molecules*, **20**: 21138–21156.

7. Upadhyay S., Dixit M. (2015). Role of Polyphenols and Other Phytochemicals on Molecular Signaling. *Oxid. Med. Cell Longev.*, **2015**, Art. 504253, 15 pages.

8. Arai Y., Watanabe S., Kimira M., Shimoi K., Mochizuki R., Kinae N. (2000). Dietary Intakes of Flavonols, Flavones and Isoflavones by Japanese Women and the Inverse Correlation Between Quercetin Intake and Plasma LDL Cholesterol Concentration. *J. Nutr.*, **130**: 2243–2250.

9. Zhu F., Du B., Xu B. (2018). Anti-Inflammatory Effects of Phytochemicals from Fruits, Vegetables, and Food Legumes: A Review. *Crit. Rev. Food Sci. Nutr.*, **58**(8): 1260–1270.

10. Bellik Y., Boukraa L., Alzahrani H.A., Bakhotmah B.A., Abdellah F., Hammoudi S.M., Iguer-Ouada M. (2013). Molecular Mechanism Underlying Anti-Inflammatory and Anti-Allergic Activities of Phytochemicals: An Update. *Molecules*, **18**: 322–353.

11. Carrera-Quintanar L., Roa R.I.L., Quintero-Fabian S., Sanchez-Sanchez M.A., Vizmanos B., Ortuno-Sahagun D. (2018). Phytochemicals That Influence Gut Microbiota as Prophylactics and for the Treatment of Obesity and Inflammatory Diseases. *Mediators Inflamm.*, **2018**, Art. 9734845, 18 pages.

12. Saw C.L.L., Huang Y., Kong A-N. (2010). Synergistic Anti-Inflammatory Effects of Low Doses of Curcumin in Combination with Polyunsaturated Fatty Acids: Docosahexaenoic Acid or Eicosapentaenoic Acid. *Biochem. Pharmacol.*, **79**(3): 421–430.

13. Wu A., Noble E.E., Tyagi E., Ying Z., Zhuang Y., Gomez-Pinilla F. (2015). Curcumin Boosts DHA in the Brain: Implications for the Prevention of Anxiety Disorders. *Biochem. Biophys. Acta*, **1852**: 951–961.

14. Thompson L.U., Ward W.E. (2005). Preface. In: *Food-Drug Synergy and Safety*. Editors: Lilian U. Thompson, Wendy E. Ward. CRC Press LLC, Boca Raton, FL, 488 pages.

15. Al Zaharna M., Cheung H-Y. (2014). Achieving Synergistic Effects by Combining Different Phytochemicals for the Prevention and Treatment of Cancer. *Hong Kong Pharm. J.*, **21**(1): 20–24.

16. Pham-Huy N.L.A., He H., Pham-Huy C. (2008). Green Tea and Health. An Overview. *J. Food Agric. Environ. (JFAE)*, **6**: 6–13.

17. Chen Z-M., Lin Z. (2015). Tea and Human Health: Biomedical Functions of Tea Active Components and Current Issues. *J. Zhejiang Univ. Sci. B*, **16**(2): 87–102.

18. Varady K.A., Jones P.J.H. (2005). Lipid Sources and Plant Sterols: Effect of Food and Food – Drug Synergy on Cardiovascular Disease Risk, pp. 11–25. In: *Food-Drug Synergy and Safety*. Editors: Lilian U. Thompson, Wendy E. Ward. CRC Press LLC, Boca Raton, FL, 488 pages.

19. Betoni J.E., Mantovani R.P., Barbosa L.N., Di Stasi L.C., Fernandes Junior A. (2006). Synergism Between Plant Extract and Antimicrobial Drugs Used on Staphylococcus Aureus Diseases. *Mem. Inst. Oswaldo Cruz*, **101**(4): 387–390.

20. Liu H., Talalay P. (2013). Relevance of Anti-Inflammatory and Antioxidant Activities of Exemestane and Synergism with Sulforaphane for Disease Prevention. *Proc. Natl. Acad. Sci. USA*, **110**(47): 19065–19070.

21. Genser D. (2008). Food and Drug Interaction: Consequences for the Nutrition/Health Status. *Ann Nutr Metab.*, **52** (Suppl. 1): 29–32.

22. Choi J.H., Ko C.M. (2017). Food and Drug Interactions. *J. Lifestyle Med.*, **7**(1): 1–9.

23. Won C.S., Oberlies N.H., Paine M.F. (2012). Mechanisms Underlying Food-Drug Interactions: Inhibition of Intestinal Metabolism and Transport. *Pharmacol Ther.*, **136**(2): 186–201.

24. Hulisz D., Jakab J. (2007). Food-Drug Interactions. Which Ones Really Matter? *US Pharm.*, **32**(3): 93–98.

25. Sarker S.K., Tun K.D., Eva E.O., Paul R. (2015). Grapefruit Juice: Nutritional Values and Drug Interactions. *Int. J. Integr. Med. Sci.*, **2**(10): 186–189.

26. Kiani J., Imam S.Z. (2007). Medicinal Importance of Grapefruit Juice and Its Interaction with Various Drugs. *Nutr. J.*, **6**(33), 9 pages.

27. Kahraman C., Arituluk Z.E., Cankaya I.I.T. (2020). The Clinical Importance of Herb-Drug Interactions and Toxicological Risks of Plants and Herbal Products. In: *Medical Toxicology.* Editors: Pinar Erkekoglu, Tomohisa Ogawa. IntechOpen, April 12. www.intechopen.com/books/medical-toxicology/the-clinical-importance-of-herb-drug-interactions-and-toxicological-risks-of-plants-and-herbal-produ.

28. Noureldin M., Krause J., Ng V., Tran M. (2010). Drug-Alcohol Interactions: A Review of Three Therapeutic Classes. *US Pharm.*, **35**(11): 29–40.

29. Lanier J.B., Bury D.C., Richardson S.W. (2016). Diet and Physical Activity for Cardiovascular Disease Prevention. *Am. Fam. Physician*, **93**(11): 919–924.

30. Kushi L.H., Doyle C., McCullough M., Rock C.L., Demark-Wahnefried W., Bandera E.V., Gapstur S., Patel A.V., Andrews K., Gansler T. (2012). American Cancer Society Guidelines on Nutrition and Physical Activity for Cancer Prevention. Reducing the Risk of Cancer with Healthy Food Choices and Physical Activity. *CA Cancer J. Clin.*, **62**: 30–67.

31. Vicente-Rodríguez G., Ezquerra J., Mesana M.I., Fernández-Alvira J.M., Rey-Lopez J.P., Casajus J.A., Moreno L.A. (2008). Independent and Combined Effect of Nutrition and Exercise on Bone Mass Development. *J. Bone Miner. Metab.*, **26**: 416–424.

32. Wang C., Wang Z., Wang G., Lau J.Y-N., Zhang K., Li W. (2021). COVID-19 in Early 2021: Current Status and Looking Forward. *Sig. Transduct. Target Ther.*, **6:** 114, 14 pages.

33. Akhtar S., Das J.K., Ismail T., Wahid M., Saeed W., Bhutta Z.A. (2021). Nutritional Perspectives for the Prevention and Mitigation of COVID-19. *Nutr. Rev.*, **79**(3): 289–300.

34. Calder P.C. (2020). Nutrition, Immunity and COVID-19. *B.M.J. Nutr. Prev. Health*, **3**(e000085): 74–92.

35. Kumar A., Choudhir G., Shukla S.K., Sharma M., Tyagi P., Bhushan A., Rathore M. (2020). Identification of Phytochemical Inhibitors Against Main Protease of COVID-19 Using Molecular Modeling Approaches. *J. Biomol. Struct. Dyn.*: 1–11. https://doi.org/10.1080/07391102.2020.1772112.

36. Oso B.J., Adeoye A.O., Olaoye I.F. (2020). Pharmacoinformatics and Hypothetical Studies on Allicin, Curcumin, and Gingerol as Potential Candidates Against COVID-19-Associated Proteases. *J. Biomol. Struct. Dyn.*, 12 pages. https://doi.org/10.1080/07391102.2020.1813630.

37. Ghosh R., Chakraborty A., Biswas A., Chowdhuri S. (2020). Evaluation of Green Tea Polyphenols as Novel Corona Virus (SARS CoV-2) Main Protease (Mpro) Inhibitors – An *in Silico* Docking and Molecular Dynamics Simulation Study. *J. Biomol. Struct. Dyn.*: 1–13.

38. World Health Organization. (2020). Alcohol and COVID-19: What You Need To know. www.euro.who.int/__data/assets/pdf_file/0010/437608/Alcohol-and-COVID-19-what-you-need-to-know.pdf.

39. Sallis R., Young D.R., Tartof S.Y., Sallis J.F., Sall J., Li Q., Smith G.N., Cohen D.A. (2021). Physical Inactivity Is Associated with a Higher Risk for Severe COVID-19 Outcomes: A Study in 48 440 Adult Patients. *Br. J. Sports Med.*: 1–8.

40. Shahrbanian S., Alikhani S., Ahmadi Kakavandi M., Hackney A.C. (2020). Physical Activity for Improving the Immune System of Older Adults During the COVID-19 Pandemic. *Altern. Ther. Health Med.*, **26** (Suppl. 2): 117–125.

41. Ali N. (2020). Role of Vitamin D in Preventing of COVID-19 Infection, Progression and Severity. *J. Infect. Public Health*, **13**: 1373–1380.

42. Conseil Supérieur de la Santé de Belgique. (2021). Vitamine D, Zinc et Covid-19. Rapport n° 9620. Janvier 2021 (French), 23 pages (Report 9620 – Vitamin D, Zinc and COVID-19). www.health.belgium.be/sites/default/files/uploads/fields/fpshealth_theme_file/210119_css-9620_vitd_zn_covid_vweb.pdf.

43. Scarabel L., Guardascione M., Bo M.D., Toffoli G. (2021). Pharmacological Strategies to Prevent SARS-CoV-2 Infection and Treat the Early Phases of COVID-19. *Int. J. Infect. Dis.*, **104**: 441–451.

44. Pickard J.M., Zeng M.Y., Caruso R., Núñez G. (2017). Gut Microbiota: Role in Pathogen Colonization, Immune Responses, and Inflammatory Disease. *Immunol. Rev.*, **279**(1): 70–89.

45. Butel M-J. (2014). Probiotics, Gut Microbiota and Health. *Méd. Mal. Infect.*, **44**(1): 1–8. https://doi.org/10.1016/j.medmal.2013.10.002.

46. Lin L., Zhang J. (2017). Role of Intestinal Microbiota and Metabolites on Gut Homeostasis and Human Diseases. *BMC Immunol.*, **18**(2): 25 pages.

47. Liu Y., Tran D.Q., Rhoads J.M. (2018). Probiotics in Disease Prevention and Treatment. *J. Clin. Pharmacol.*, **58** (Suppl. 10): S164–S179.

48. Sekirov I., Russell S.L., Antunes L.C., Finlay B.B. (2010). Gut Microbiota in Health and Disease. *Physiol. Rev.*, **90**(3): 859–904.

49. Daliri E.B-M., Lee B.H. (2015). New Perspectives on Probiotics in Health and Disease. *Food Sci. Hum. Well.*, **4**(2): 56–65.

50. Rodríguez J.M., Murphy K., Stanton C., Ross R.P., Kober O.I., Juge N., Avershina E., Rudi K., Narbad A., Jenmalm M.C., Marchesi J.R., Collado M.C. (2015). The Composition of the Gut Microbiota Throughout Life, with an Emphasis on Early Life. *Microb. Ecol. Health Dis.*, **26**: 26050, 17 pages.
51. Sarkar A., Yoo J.Y., Valeria Ozorio Dutra S., Morgan K.H., Groer M. (2021). The Association Between Early-Life Gut Microbiota and Long-Term Health and Diseases. *J. Clin. Med.*, **10**(3): 459, 23 pages.
52. Neis E.P.J.G., Dejong C.H.C., Rensen S.S. (2015). The Role of Microbial Amino Acid Metabolism in Host Metabolism. *Nutrients*, **7**(4): 2930–2946.
53. Carrera-Quintanar L., Roa R.I.L., Quintero-Fabian S., Sanchez-Sanchez M.A., Vizmanos B., Ortuno-Sahagun D. (2018). Phytochemicals That Influence Gut Microbiota as Prophylactics and for the Treatment of Obesity and Inflammatory Diseases. *Mediators Inflamm.*, **2018**, Art. 9734845, 18 pages.
54. Mach N., Fuster-Botella D. (2017). Endurance Exercise and Gut Microbiota: A Review. *J. Sport Health Sci.*, **6**(2): 179–197.
55. Wu L., Tang Z., Chen H., Ren Z., Ding Q., Liang K., Sun Z. (2021). Mutual Interaction Between Gut Microbiota and Protein/Amino Acid Metabolism for Host Mucosal Immunity and Health. *Anim. Nutr.*, **7**(1): 11–16.
56. Dicks L.M.T., Botes M. (2010). Probiotic Lactic Acid Bacteria in the Gastro-Intestinal Tract: Health Benefits, Safety and Mode of Action. *Benef. Microbes*, **1**(1): 11–29.
57. Bocchi S., Sagheddu V., Elli M., Lim C.Y., Morelli L. (2020). The Synergistic Interaction Between Probiotics and Food Affects Their Beneficial Features. *Adv. Nutri. Food Sci.*, **2020**(2), 12 pages.
58. Zielińska D., Kołożyn-Krajewska D. (2018). Food-Origin Lactic Acid Bacteria May Exhibit Probiotic Properties: Review. *Biomed. Res. Int.*, **2018**, Art. 5063185, 15 pages.
59. Kechagia M., Basoulis D., Konstantopoulou S., Dimitriadi D., Gyftopoulou K., Skarmoutsou N., Fakiri E.M. (2013). Health Benefits of Probiotics: A Review. *ISRN Nutr.*, **2013**: 481651, 7 pages.
60. Anderson J., Baird P., Davis R., Ferreri S., Knudtson M., Koraym A., Waters V., Williams C. (2009). Health Benefits of Dietary Fiber. *Nutr. Rev.*, **67**(4): 188–205.
61. Gerschenson L.N., Rojas A.M., Fissore E.N., Basanta M.F., De'Nobili M.D., González C.M.O., Zukowski E.F. (2021). Chapter 4. Dietary Fibre. In: *Food Bioactives and Health*. Editor: C.M. Galanakis. Springer Cham, Switzerland. https://doi.org/10.1007/978-3-030-57469-7_5.
62. Mudgil D., Barak S. (2013). Composition, Properties and Health Benefits of Indigestible Carbohydrate Polymers as Dietary Fiber: A Review. *Int. J. Biol. Macromol.*, **61**: 1–6.
63. Michan S., Sinclair D. (2007). Sirtuins in Mammals: Insights into Their Biological Function. *Biochem. J.*, **404**(1): 1–13.
64. Klar A.J., Fogel S., Macleod K. (1979). MAR1-a Regulator of the HMa and HMalpha Loci in Saccharomyces Cerevisiae. *Genetics*, **93**(1): 37–50.
65. Naiman S., Cohen H.Y. (2012). The Contentious History of Sirtuin Debates. *Rambam Maimonides Med. J.*, **3**(4): e0022, 7 pages.
66. Guarente L., Mostoslavsky R., Kazantsev A. (2018). *Introductory Review on Sirtuins in Biology, Aging and Disease*. 1st Edition. Academic Press, Elsevier, Cambridge, USA, 220 pages.
67. Horio Y., Hayashi T., Kuno A., Kunimoto R. (2011). Cellular and Molecular Effects of Sirtuins in Health and Disease. *Clin. Sci. (Lond)*, **121**(5): 191–203.
68. D'Onofrio N., Servillo L., Balestrieri M.L. (2018). SIRT1 and SIRT6 Signaling Pathways in Cardiovascular Disease Protection. *Antioxid. Redox Signal.*, **28**(8): 711–732.
69. Matsushima S., Sadoshima J. (2015). The Roles of Sirtuins in Cardiac Diseases. *Am. J. Physiol. Heart Cir. Physiol.*, **309**(9): H1375–H1389.
70. Villalba J.M., Alcain F.J. (2012). Sirtuin Activators and Inhibitors. *Biofactors*, **38**(5): 349–359.
71. Imai S. (2010). A Possibility of Nutriceuticals as an Anti-Aging Intervention: Activation of Sirtuins by Promoting Mammalian NAD Biosynthesis. *Pharmacol. Res.*, **62**(1): 42–47.
72. Canto C., Auwerx J. (2012). Targeting Sirtuin 1 to Improve Metabolism: All You Need Is NAD? *Pharmacol. Rev.*, **64**: 166–187.
73. Sebastián C., Satterstrom F.K., Haigis M.C., Mostoslavsky R. (2012). From Sirtuin Biology to Human Diseases: An Update. *J. Biol. Chem.*, **287**(51): 42444–42452.
74. Yu J., Auwerx J. (2009). The Role of Sirtuins in the Control of Metabolic Homeostasis. *Ann. N. Y. Acad. Sci.*, **1173**(01): E10–E19.
75. Kelly G. (2010). A Review of the Sirtuin System, Its Clinical Implications, and the Potential Role of Dietary Activators Like Resveratrol: Part 1. *Altern. Med. Rev.*, **15**(3): 245–263.
76. Kelly G. (2010). A Review of the Sirtuin System, Its Clinical Implications, and the Potential Role of Dietary Activators Like Resveratrol: Part 2. *Altern. Med. Rev.*, **15**(4): 313–328.

77. Moraesa D.S., Moreira D.C., Andrade J.M.O., Santos S.H.S. (2020). Sirtuins, Brain and Cognition: A Review of Resveratrol Effects. *IBRO Rep.*, **9**: 46–51.

78. Zendedel E., Butler A.E., Atkin S.L., Sahebkar A. (2018). Impact of Curcumin on Sirtuins: A Review. *J. Cell Biochem.*: 1–10.

79. Caldas A.P.S., Rocha D.M., Bressan J., Hermsdorff H.H. (2021). Dietary Fatty Acids as Nutritional Modulators of Sirtuins: A Systematic Review. *Nutr. Reviews*, **79**(2): 235–246.

80. Mayack B.K., Sippl W., Ntie-Kang F. (2020). Natural Products as Modulators of Sirtuins. *Molecules*, **25**(3287), 29 pages.

81. Imai S., Guarente L. (2014). NAD$^+$ and Sirtuins in Aging and Disease. *Trends Cell Biol.*, **24**(8): 464–471.

82. Jesko H., Wencel P., Strosznajder R.P., Strosznajder J.B. (2017). Sirtuins and Their Roles in Brain Aging and Neurodegenerative Disorders. *Neurochem. Res.*, **42**(3): 876–890.

83. Kida Y., Goligorsky M.S. (2016). Sirtuins, Cell Senescence, and Vascular Aging. *Can. J. Cardiol.*, **32**(5): 634–641.

84. Grabowska W., Sikora E., Bielak-Zmijewska A. (2017). Sirtuins, a Promising Target in Slowing Down the Ageing Process. *Biogerontology*, **18**(4): 447–476.

85. Grabowska W., Suszek M., Wnuk M., Lewinska A., Wasiak E., Sikora E., Bielak-Zmijewska A. (2016). Curcumin Elevates Sirtuin Level but Does Not Postpone in Vitro Senescence of Human Cells Building the Vasculature. *Oncotarget*, **7**(15): 19201–19213.

86. Carafa V., Rotili D., Forgione M., Cuomo F., Serretiello E., Hailu G.S., Jarho E., Lahtela-Kakkonen M., Mai A., Altucci L. (2016). Sirtuin Functions and Modulation: From Chemistry to the Clinic. *Clin. Epigenetics*, **8**(61): 21 pages.

87. Guarente L. (2006). Sirtuins as Potential Targets for Metabolic Syndrome. *Nature*, **444**: 868–874.

88. Winnik S., Auwerx J., Sinclair D.A., Matter C.M. (2015). Protective Effects of Sirtuins in Cardiovascular Diseases: From Bench to Bedside. *Eur. Heart J.*, **36**(48): 3404–3412.

89. Feng X., Wang Y., Chen W., Xu S., Li L., Geng Y., Shen A., Gao H., Zhang L., Liu S. (2020). SIRT3 Inhibits Cardiac Hypertrophy by Regulating PARP-1 Activity. *Aging (Albany NY)*, **12**(5): 4178–4192.

90. Fujita Y., Yamashita T. (2018). Sirtuins in Neuroendocrine Regulation and Neurological Diseases. *Front Neurosci.*, **12**(778): 17 pages.

91. Zhang F., Wang S., Gan L., Vosler P.S., Gao Y., Zigmond M.J., Chen J. (2011). Protective Effects and Mechanisms of Sirtuins in the Nervous System. *Prog. Neurobiol.*, **95**(3): 373–395.

92. Kitada M., Kume S., Takeda-Watanabe A., Kanasaki K., Koya D. (2012). Sirtuins and Renal Diseases: Relationship with Aging and Diabetic Nephropathy. *Clin. Sci. (Lond).*, **124**(3): 153–164.

93. Dong Y.J., Liu N., Xiao Z., Sun T., Wu S-H., Sun W-X., Xu Z-G., Yuan H. (2014). Renal Protective Effect of Sirtuin 1. *J. Diabetes Res.*, **2014**: 843786, 8 pages.

94. Wakino S., Hasegawa K., Itoh H. (2015). Sirtuin and Metabolic Kidney Disease. *Kidney Int.*, **88**(4): 691–698.

95. Chalkiadaki A., Guarente L. (2015). The Multifaceted Functions of Sirtuins in Cancer. *Nat. Rev. Cancer*, **15**: 608–624.

96. Mei Z., Zhang X., Yi J., Huang J., He J., Tao Y. (2016). Sirtuins in Metabolism, DNA Repair and Cancer. *J. Exp. Clin. Cancer Res.*, **35**(182): 14 pages.

97. Islam S., Abiko Y., Uehara O., Chiba I. (2019). Sirtuin 1 and Oral Cancer (Review). *Oncol. Lett.*, **17**: 729–738.

98. Zhao E., Hou J., Ke X., Abbas M.N., Kausar S., Zhang L., Cui H. (2019). The Roles of Sirtuin Family Proteins in Cancer Progression. *Cancers*, **11**(12): 1949, 22 pages.

99. Li Q., Cheng J.C., Jiang Q., Lee W.Y. (2021). Role of Sirtuins in Bone Biology: Potential Implications for Novel Therapeutic Strategies for Osteoporosis. *Aging Cell*, **20**(2): e13301.

100. Almeida M., Porter R.M. (2019). Sirtuins and FoxOs in Osteoporosis and Osteoarthritis. *Bone*, **121**: 284–292.

101. Houtkooper R.H., Pirinen E., Auwerx J. (2012). Sirtuins as Regulators of Metabolism and Health Span. *Nat. Rev. Mol. Cell Biol.*, **13**(4): 225–238.

102. Vargas-Ortiz K., Pérez-Vázquez V., Macías-Cervantes M.H. (2019). Exercise and Sirtuins: A Way to Mitochondrial Health in Skeletal Muscle. *Int. J. Mol. Sci.*, **20**(11): 2717.

103. Portin P., Wilkins A. (2017). The Evolving Definition of the Term "Gene". *Genetics*, **205**(4): 1353–1364.

104. Biology Online. (2021). Gene, February 27. www.biologyonline.com/dictionary/gene.

105. Genetics Home Reference. (2021). What Is a Gene, March 22. https://medlineplus.gov/genetics/understanding/basics/gene/.

106. Finegold D.N. (2019). Genes and Chromosomes, October. www.msdmanuals.com/home/fundamentals/genetics/genes-and-chromosomes.

107. Lodish H., Berk A., Matsudaira P., Kaiser C.A., Krieger M., Scott M.P., Zipursky L., Darnell J. (2003). Chapter 4: Basic Molecular Genetic Mechanisms, pp. 100–145. In: *Molecular Cell Biology*. 5th edition. W.H. Freeman & Co Ltd., 1152 pages. www.mustafaaltinisik.org.uk/s-MolecularCellBiology.pdf.
108. Rettner R. (2021). What Is DNA? March 25. www.livescience.com/37247-dna.html.
109. Alberts B., Johnson A., Lewis J., Raff M., Roberts K., Walter P. (2002). The Structure and Function of DNA. In: *Molecular Biology of the Cell*. 4th edition. Garland Science, New York. www.ncbi.nlm.nih.gov/books/NBK26821/.
110. Travers A., Muskhelishvili G. (2015). DNA Structure and Function. *FEBS J.*, **282**(12): 2279–2295.
111. Cuffari B., Mandal A. (2020). What Is RNA? February 6. www.news-medical.net/life-sciences/What-is-RNA.aspx.
112. Cheriyedath S., Greenwood M. (2021). Types of RNA: mRNA, rRNA and tRNA, May 25. www.news-medical.net/life-sciences/-Types-of-RNA-mRNA-rRNA-and-tRNA.aspx.
113. Lodish H., Berk A., Zipursky S.L., Matsudaira P., Baltimore D., Darnell J. (2000). Section 4.4. The Three Roles of RNA in Protein Synthesis. In: *Molecular Cell Biology*. 4th edition. W.H. Freeman, New York. www.ncbi.nlm.nih.gov/books/NBK21603/.
114. Lodish H., Berk A., Zipursky S.L., Matsudaira P., Baltimore D., Darnell J. (2000). Section 8.1, Mutations: Types and Causes. In: *Molecular Cell Biology*. 4th edition. W.H. Freeman, New York. www.ncbi.nlm.nih.gov/books/NBK21578/.
115. Rahner N., Steinke V. (2008). Hereditary Cancer Syndromes. *Dtsch. Arztebl. Int.*, **105**(41): 706–714.
116. Samadder N.J., Giridhar K.V., Baffy N., Riegert-Johnson D., Couch F.J. (2019). Hereditary Cancer Syndromes. A Primer on Diagnosis and Management, Part 1: Breast-Ovarian Cancer Syndromes. *Mayo Clin. Proc.*, **94**(6): 1084–1098.
117. American Cancer Society. (2020). Family Cancer Syndromes, August 5. www.cancer.org/cancer/cancercauses/geneticsandcancer/heredity-and-cancer#.
118. Cancer Research UK. (2018). Family History and Inherited Cancer Genes, September 3. www.cancerresearchuk.org/about-cancer/causes-of-cancer/inherited-cancer-genes-and-increased-cancer-risk/family-history-and-inherited-cancer-genes.
119. Genetic Home References, US National Library of Medicine, NIH. What Is a Gene Mutation and How Do Mutations Occur? March 25. https://ghr.nlm.nih.gov/primer/mutationsanddisorders/genemutation.
120. Loewe L., Hill W.G. (2010). The Population Genetics of Mutations: Good, Bad and Indifferent. *Philos. Trans. R. Soc. Lond. B Biol. Sci.*, **365**(1544): 1153–1167.
121. Brady C.A., Attardi L.D. (2010). p53 at a Glance. *J. Cell Sci.*, **123**(Pt 15): 2527–2532.
122. Mishra P.A., Chaudhari H.R., Desai J.S., Khan U.N.A. (2013). p53. An Overview. *Int. J. Pharm. Pharm. Sci.*, **5**(3): 59–65.
123. Goldstein I., Marcel V., Olivier M., Oren M., Rotter V., Hainaut P. (2011). Understanding Wild-Type and Mutant p53 Activities in Human Cancer: New Landmarks on the Way to Targeted Therapies. *Cancer Gene Ther.*, **18**(1): 2–11.
124. Freed-Pastor W.A., Prives C. (2012). Mutant p53: One Name, Many Proteins. *Genes & Dev.*, **26**: 1268–1286.
125. Talib W.H., Al-hadid S.A., Wild Ali M.B., AL-Yasari I.H., Abd Ali M.R. (2018). Role of Curcumin in Regulating p53 in Breast Cancer: An Overview of the Mechanism of Action. *Breast Cancer (Dove Med. Press)*, **10**: 207–217.
126. Campo E., Cymbalista F., Ghia P., Jäger U., Pospisilova S., Rosenquist R., Schuh A., Stilgenbauer S. (2018). TP53 Aberrations in Chronic Lymphocytic Leukemia: An Overview of the Clinical Implications of Improved Diagnostics. *Haematologica*, **103**(12): 1956–1968.
127. Kastenhuber E.R., Lowe S.W. (2017). Putting p53 in Context. *Cell*, **170**: 1062–1078.
128. Ozaki T., Nakagawara A. (2011). Role of p53 in Cell Death and Human Cancers. *Cancers (Basel)*, **3**(1): 994–1013.
129. Mantovani F., Collavin L., Del Sal G. (2019). Mutant p53 as a Guardian of the Cancer Cell. *Cell Death Differ.*, **26**: 199–212. https://doi.org/10.1038/s41418-018-0246-9.
130. Bourdon J-C. (2007). p53 Family Isoforms. *Curr. Pharm. Biotechnol.*, **8**(6): 332–336.
131. Vogelstein B., Sur S., Prives C. (2010). p53: The Most Frequently Altered Gene in Human Cancers. *Nat. Educ.*, **3**(9), 6 pages.
132. Palaparthi S. (2017). Role of Homeostasis in Human Physiology: A Review. *J. Med. Physiol. Ther.*, **1**(2): 1–5.
133. Kryzhanovsky G.N. (2004). Some Categories of General Pathology and Biology: Health, Disease, Homeostasis, Sanogenesis, Adaptation, Immunity. New Approaches and Notions. *Pathophysiology*, **11**: 135–138.

134. Torday J.S. (2015). Homeostasis as the Mechanism of Evolution. *Biology*, **4**: 573–590.
135. Billman G.E. (2020). Homeostasis: The Underappreciated and Far Too Often Ignored Central Organizing Principle of Physiology. *Front. Physiol.*, **11**(200): 1–12.
136. Modell H., Cliff W., Michael J., McFarland J., Wenderoth M.P., Wright A. (2015). A Physiologist's View of Homeostasis. *Adv. Physiol. Educ.*, **39**(4): 259–266.
137. Kotas M.E., Medzhitov R. (2015). Homeostasis, Inflammation, and Disease Susceptibility. *Cell*, **160**(5): 816–827.
138. Bak A., Tsiami A. (2016). Review on Mechanisms, Importance of Homeostasis and Fluid Imbalances in the Elderly. *Curr. Res. Nutr. Food Sci. Jour.*, **4**(Special Issue 3): 1–7.
139. Pham-Huy A.L., He H., Pham-Huy C. (2008). Free Radicals and Antioxidants in Disease and Health. *Int. J. Biomed. Sci.*, **4**(2): 89–96.
140. Simopoulos A.P. (2008). The Importance of the Omega-6/Omega-3 Fatty Acid Ratio in Cardiovascular Disease and Other Chronic Diseases. *Exp. Biol. Med. (Maywood)*, **233**(6): 674–688.
141. Ou B., Huang D., Hampsch-Woodill M., Flanagan J.A. (2003). When East Meets West: The Relationship Between Yin-Yang and Antioxidation-Oxidation. *FASEB J.*, **17**: 127–129.
142. Fan X-J., Yu H., Ren J. (2011). Homeostasis and Compensatory Homeostasis: Bridging Western Medicine and Traditional Chinese Medicine. *Curr. Cardiol. Rev.*, **7**(1): 43–46.
143. Liu R.H. (2013). Health-Promoting Components of Fruits and Vegetables in the Diet. *Adv. Nutr.*, **4**: 384S–392S.
144. Hewlings S.J., Kalman D.S. (2017). Curcumin: A Review of Its' Effects on Human Health. *Foods*, **6**(92): 1–11.
145. Miyata J., Arita M. (2015). Role of Omega-3 Fatty Acids and Their Metabolites in Asthma and Allergic Diseases. *Allergol. Int.*, **64**: 27–34.
146. Wendell S.G., Baffi C., Holguin F. (2014). Fatty Acids, Inflammation, and Asthma. *J. Allergy Clin. Immunol.*, **133**(5): 1255–1264.
147. Nguyen A.L., He H., Pham-Huy C. (2006). Chiral Drugs. An Overview. *Int. J. Biomed. Sci.*, **2**: 85–100.

Index

For Product Safety Concerns and Information please contact our EU
representative GPSR@taylorandfrancis.com
Taylor & Francis Verlag GmbH, Kaufingerstraße 24, 80331 München, Germany

www.ingramcontent.com/pod-product-compliance
Lightning Source LLC
Chambersburg PA
CBHW080122220326
41598CB00032B/4923